Safe Stretch

A comprehensive guide to stretching which takes into account the similarities and differences between people

First Edition

Rowland Benjamin D.O.

Copyright © 2015
First Edition September 2015

Published by R Benjamin
P.O. Box 245,
North Perth,
WA 6906,
Australia
E-mail: rb@informaction.org

Safe Stretch

ISBN 978-0-9943209-0-2

Preface

Stretching is an excellent way of keeping fit without the need for expensive and often inaccessible equipment. Once learned, the exercises can be practiced at home safely. They may complement or compensate for work done in sports and other areas of exercise for example weight training. They are appropriate for anyone following a sedentary lifestyle or an athletic lifestyle. Short muscles limit joint mobility and appropriate stretching helps prevent muscle and ligament injuries.

Safe Stretch is both for beginners and those who are advanced in stretching. It is an instruction book suitable for the lay person, interested in learning to stretch and who just needs a few safe stretches to do at home and doesn't want or need to know more, and it is an authoritative and reliable reference book on stretching for professionals who want to know more about the anatomy and greater detail about what happens when you stretch.

Safe Stretch contains a comprehensive list of safe and effective stretching techniques. It covers three types are stretching exercises: active stretching, passive stretching and post-isometric stretching. The book explains which muscles are stretched and which joints move during a particular stretch. It recommends which muscles should be stretched and which joints or areas should be moved for a particular need and for specific individuals and it recommends which areas should not be stretched.

Safe Stretch is clear, easy to read, user friendly and contains hundreds of photographs and line drawings showing stretches for every part of the body, as well as anatomy illustrations explaining which muscles are being stretched and which joints are being moved. The bullet points take you through the techniques step-by-step. There are lots of exercises and the book contains a good theoretical background explaining why you are doing a particular stretch. It contains a treasure trove of information for anyone interested in stretching and is a useful reference book.

Stretching works well with massage and other manual therapy techniques. The stretches can be used prescriptively for a wide range of problems encountered by the therapist. The book is useful for anyone who works with their own body or works on other people's bodies. In the first group are manual workers, musicians, dancers, yoga students, personal trainers, sports coaches, athletes and anyone engaged in sports activities. In the second group are masseurs, osteopaths, physiotherapists, chiropractors, manual therapists, yoga teachers, naturopaths, medical doctors, exercise physiologists, Pilates teachers and aerobics class instructors.

Safe Stretch is divided into an introduction, three parts and an appendix. Part A. Technique contains the individual exercises, one to a page, - each exercise divided into the starting position and the technique. Part B. Anatomy, Biomechanics and Safety contains the muscle and joint anatomy for the stretches - each section briefly reviews the starting position and then looks at the direction and range of movement, target tissues, and safety for the technique. Part C. Tables contains the icon tables for the practical things each stretch can be used for i.e. sports, jobs, hobbies etc. Although the book is comprehensive it is also concise. It focuses on specific areas of the body, and targets specific muscles and muscle groups without unnecessary repetition. Similar active, passive and post-isometric stretches are combined and fit on one page but when space isn't available they have their own page.

In part C of the book, about one hundred different daily and weekly stretching routines have been assembled to complement sports, work and other activities, and these are based on the 200 stretches in part A of the book. The stretches that make up these routines are listed as small icons in tables in part C. The stretches have been selected according to criteria such as the anatomy and which muscles and joints are used or not used sufficiently in the sport or activity. An explanation of how the stretches are selected for the different activities is provided in the appendix of the book together with a set of tables listing the movements performed during the various sports or other activities. The tables provide a logical explanation for the stretches chosen for the daily and weekly stretching routines.

All the exercises listed in this book are based on sound anatomy and biomechanics. Stretches are described for every major part of the body, starting with the head, cervical, thoracic and lumbar spine, then working down the shoulders, arms and hands, hips, knees and ankles and finishing with the feet and toes.

Safe Stretch introduces the basic science of flexibility in language that anyone can understand once the terminology of anatomy is understood and all the anatomical terms used in this book are defined in the appendix.

Why this book has been written

There are many stretching books on the market. They have beautiful drawings - the anatomy of the bones merges with an outline of the body so one can appreciate which muscles are being stretched. Mostly they are excellent books with good exercises. The disadvantage of many of these books is they assume everyone is the same and adopt a one-size-fits-all position to their stretching exercises. A potentially dangerous exercise to one person may be fine for another person.

People are different in terms of their size, shape, posture, the elasticity of their ligaments and muscles, and people are different functionally in terms of flexibility and stability. We have many shared features but we are also individuals with subtle differences and large variations exist in people. Also people change as they get older, their tissues change and become more fibrous. So a good stretching exercise for a teenager may not be good for a person in their late twenties, middle age person or older. Different types of people have different needs and require different stretching routines. For stretching to be safe, individual postural needs must be taken into account. Generally stretching should focus on stretching the most restricted joints and/or the shortest, tightest muscles.

Who is this book written for?

This book is written for all people young and old, stout and thin, inflexible and supple. There are stretches for a wide range of different people and different circumstances. Part 3 of the book divides the stretches into tables, so people can select different stretches for different reasons – for doing similar stretches in a variety of positions, or covering different parts of the body, or for targeting specific areas of the body. And there are tables of stretches for different types of people and for different activities and sports.

Icons explained

Each stretch in the book is given an icon, which make it possible to combine the stretches in different ways and create routines for different sports, jobs and popular activities.

Safe Stretch includes weekly or daily routines for desk work, heavy work, driving a car, riding a motorcycle, pregnancy, and a range of other activities and circumstances. It has stretches for people who regularly play a musical instrument including the guitar, violin, piano, cello, drums, wind instruments and singing.

Safe Stretch covers Abseiling, Aerobics, Archery, Arm wrestling, Batting as in Cricket, Bodyboarding, Boxing and Martial Arts punching, Catching a ball as in Baseball, Cricket, Rounders and Softball, Climbing, Over-arm Bowling as in Cricket, Cue sports as in Billiards and Snooker, Cycling, Solo Freeform Dancing (Pop, Disco, Techno), Partner Dancing (Waltz, Foxtrot, Quickstep, Tango), Darts, Golf, High jump, Hockey, Horse riding, Ice Skating, Juggling, Kicking a ball as in Soccer and Football, Long jump, Polo, Rowing, such as in canoeing and kayaking, Skateboarding, Skydiving, Tennis, Throwing a ball as in Baseball, Rounders, Softball and Volleyball, Walking, running and sprinting, Windsurfing, as well as stretches for specific gymnastics exercises such as Squats, Jumping jacks, Calf raises, Push-ups, Pull-ups, Dips, Sit-ups, crunches and curl-ups.

Some stretches are useful for preventing injuries and some are useful in assisting in the treatment of injuries. Safe Stretch covers the following soft-tissue problems: rotator cuff strains, lower back strains, neck and shoulder pain, tension headaches, wrist pain and plantar fasciitis with associated calcaneal spurs.

As well as providing routines for specific activities and circumstances part C of Safe Stretch groups the stretches according to Region (regional tables) and Joint Movement (movement tables). In the regional tables the stretches are listed in numerical order, starting with the head and ending with the feet. They are primarily based on anatomical region and secondarily by the direction of movement. In the movement tables the stretches are primarily based on joint movement and direction of movement, and secondarily by anatomical region. The movement tables start with the anterior occiput and end with toe flexion.

These tables can be used to design your own stretching routine. The icons are organised in such a way that you can pick from each section to get a well-rounded stretching program or combine them in different ways for different purposes. The instructions are clear and the icons are linked back to the original page which describes in detail how to stretch the muscle.

The goals of this book are to help you create a stretching program that: is safe and reduces the probability of injury; gives you optimum flexibility – mobility with stability; gives you the best results for the time spent – stretching for busy people; is personalized to your unique body type and needs.

In summary, this book was written to provide a comprehensive list of stretching techniques, to foster greater awareness of variations that exist in the human form and of hypermobility in particular and to provide a list of safe stretching techniques for these uniquely different individuals.

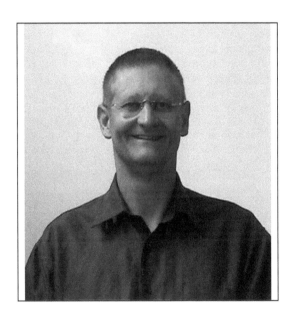

Biography

The author, Rowland Benjamin has worked as an Osteopath for thirty years and in the field of massage, yoga and stretching for nearly forty years. In the late 1970s he established yoga schools in Australia and the U.K. He worked with yoga and massage for several years before training as an Osteopath at the N.S.W. College of Natural Therapies and the Pacific College of Osteopathic medicine, Sydney, Australia. He set up his first practice as an Osteopath in July 1985 in Sydney, Australia. In 1987 he worked for a year in Liverpool, U.K. as an Osteopath and completed postgraduate studies at The British School of Osteopathy, London.

Rowland started working as a lecturer in 1987 teaching 'Natural medicine' for Liverpool City Council and 'Natural living' at Burton Manor College, Cheshire, in the U.K. Since then he has lectured in many subjects including: Alternative medicine, Natural living, Soft tissue technique,

Surface anatomy, Transverse friction, Deep tissue massage, Contemporary health issues, Life skills, Hydrotherapy and Advanced massage at various colleges in Perth, Western Australia.

During his career as an Osteopath Rowland has worked in Australia and the UK in private practice and as a locum assisting other Osteopaths. His first book Myofaction – Myofascial Manipulation was published in 2002 and has sold widely throughout the world.

The author has travelled extensively throughout Australia, New Zealand, Asia, the Middle East, Europe, Africa, North America, the Caribbean, Central America and South America. He has travelled in China and Russia and extensively in Australia, India and the United States. He has worked as an independent environmental activist and lobbyist for nearly forty years and currently runs Information for Action and its website www.informaction.org. In the 1990s he engaged in a musical career for a few year, writing and performing his song in the Australia and the UK. Since 2010 he has been engaged in the construction of a Permaculture based orchard and nature area in Bridgetown, Western Australia where he resides. Progress of work at Bridgetown Hillside Garden can be viewed at www.bhg.org.au. He continues to practice evidence based and anatomy based manual therapy using self-help systems such as stretching to empower his patients. He has practices in Perth and Bridgetown, Western Australia.

This book is the product of five years of work stretching, taking photographs of people stretching, graphic design work creating line drawings from the photographs, graphic design and other computer drawing work producing anatomy diagrams, reading books and webpages about anatomy, physiology and stretching, thinking about the mechanics behind the stretches and describing them in words that everyone can understand.

Safe Stretch has come about because of an injury to my back doing yoga in 1979 which propelled me into a career in osteopathy and the prescribing of stretching exercises to patients. The injury made me think about my body and the way I was stretching. Safe Stretch is a prequel to my next book Safe Yoga. In order to explain how to do yoga safely, I decided that I first needed to explain stretching and how to stretch safely. I needed to describe the individual stretches for building up to a safer form of yoga and provide alternatives to some of the more risky yoga postures. A book that explains a safer yoga system is surely needed.

Acknowledgments

I would like to thank Jacob Cheah, Simone Hoar, Diane Hollett, Justine Mackay, Jaala Matheson and Melanie Taylor for their help and patience as models for the book. I would also like to thank Michele Finlay for proof reading the techniques in part 1 of the book and Jason Kiely AEP, BSc (Ex & Hlth Sc), Post Grad Dip Ex Rehab, Dip Rem Massg for checking the anatomy and proof reading the introduction and part 2 of the book. I would like to thank Mike Eales for keeping my computers running and Leo Wai Kwan Lee for setting up the Safe Stretch website www.safe-stretch.info and helping with other computer problems. I would like to thank Nick Milne, Theresa Melotti and Lisette Kaleveld for their referrals and ideas. Tim Wilson is an artist and teacher of cartoon drawing and was instrumental in preparing the artwork for the front cover and introduction. Finally I would also like to thank my partner Nirada for her support.

This first edition of Safe Stretch is dedicated in memory to my friend Stuart Ashbil. Stuart posed as a model for this book and was an environmentalist, teacher of sustainability and a fine yoga teacher. He was an inspiration to children and adults, by what he said and how he lived his life, someone who really made a difference towards the conservation of the biodiversity of this planet for future generations and as an end in itself.

Contents

Part A. Technique
Chapter | Name, type of stretch & areas stretched | Technique name & position

minimus sidelying with the knee bent

Part B. Anatomy, Biomechanics and Safety
Direction, Range of Movement, Target tissues, Variations, Safety, Vulnerable areas & Key
Chapter | Name | Type of stretch & areas stretched

xviii

The mechanics of stretching

Gross anatomy

Part C. Stretching routines and combinations

Stretching programs

Introduction to Safe Stretch

Part 1. Theoretical considerations

Part 2. Practical aspects of stretching

Introduction

Part 1. Theoretical considerations

Benefits of stretching

Stretching is a powerful tool that has many benefits. When done safely, stretching can be useful for either a sedentary or active lifestyle, by improving and maintaining joint mobility, muscle flexibility and muscle tone. It can help make simple movements such as putting your shoes on easier, give you a better posture, increase your fitness, reduce muscle tension and ease muscle pain after exercise. It can also help compensate for inactivity or a sedentary lifestyle, as well as prevent injury occurring during work, sport and other types of exercise.

Stretching is useful as a warm up or for cooling down after vigorous exercise, for lengthening short muscles after activity. It is also useful for exercise involving muscle contraction or as a result of inactivity and for enabling muscles to exert force over a wider range of movement.

Stretching is an important component to staying healthy and supple. It improves muscle stamina and endurance and can lead to a better quality of life. It can be done anywhere, anytime and best of all it is free!

The benefits of stretching can be divided into physical benefits, physiological benefits and psychological benefits. Although they are broken down into the individual bullet points, many ot the bullet points listed below, are interconnected and overlapping.

Stretching can:

- enhance performance
- increase muscle flexibility
- help prevent injury
- help you relax
- develop and maintain mobility of joints
- make you feel better
- improve circulation (capillary, lymphatic and venous)
- increase strength (especially active stretching)
- warm up your body before strenuous activity
- cool down your body after strenuous activity
- reduce muscle tension
- stimulate nerves, glands, organs and other tissues
- rejuvenate muscles, tendons and ligaments
- increase muscle tone and power without increasing muscle bulk
- raise vitality
- help weight loss by burning calories
- improve posture
- increase physical fitness
- help with postural fatigue
- help improve balance and neuromuscular control
- improve concentration and self discipline
- lengthen short muscles
- improve body awareness
- help the immune system and reduce illness
- reduce joint disease
- increase fluid movement within joints which nourishes cartilage
- improve mental clarity
- stimulate the release of hormones such as endorphins which produce a feeling of wellbeing and euphoria.

Problems with stretching

Although there are great benefits from doing stretches, there are also dangers. Over-stretching or poorly localised stretching can cause too much joint mobility or hypermobility and problems such as sprains, strains and joint instability. This book provides stretches that are safe and teaches you how to avoid these sorts of problems. Stretching also has limitations and does not provide all the physical needs required by the body. For example, it does not provide aerobic fitness, coordination or skill development and has limited capacity at building muscle strength. It should therefore not be considered as a total fitness program but as complementary to other exercise systems.

Individual differences

Everyone is different. A 'one size fits all' approach to stretching is dangerous. Individual differences in muscle flexibility and joint mobility are due to a combination of genetic factors, lifestyle factors and natural ageing processes. In additon, postural forces, major injuries, repeated minor traumas, our mental and emotional state and how we use our body, cause our body to change over time, resulting in significant individual differences between people.

Safe Stretch is a stretching book which acknowledges these differences, taking them into account when recommending stretching exercises. It considers firstly if muscles need stretching, and if they do, which need strong stretching and which need light stretching. It also considers that some muscle groups may in fact need strengthening to maintain joint stability, and strengthening is a component of active and post-isometric stretching techniques.

The book explains how to stretch, providing a list of stretches that are safe or relatively safe if done correctly and which individuals in particular need to stretch these areas of the body. Some classical stretches and yoga postures (asanas) are totally unsafe, and should not be done under any circumstances! Because humans are different, some stretches will be safe for some people and not safe for others. Whenever these relatively safe stretches are included in the book, the risks and contraindications are clearly explained.

Two main factors – genetics and lifestyle influence our body and shape us in a variety of ways and they must be considered when designing the type of stretching program that best suits our needs. Ageing also affects our tissues and range of movement and must also be taken into account when designing a safe stretching program.

Genetic factors

Our genes are the blueprints of our body and they determine the shape and structural composition of our body and its function. They determine the thickness of our bones, elasticity of our ligaments, size and strength of our muscles and many other things. These in turn influence our functions, including muscle flexibility and joint mobility and stability.

Endomorph stocky type	Large bone mass, joint size, muscle bulk and ligament thickness ensure that the body offers the greatest resistance to stretching and provides maximum stability.
Ectomorph slim type	Lighter frame with smaller bone mass, joint size, muscle and ligament mass producing greater flexibility, making stretching easier but without the benefit of stability.

Body types

A huge range of variation exists in the shape of human beings. One system has classified tall thin people into ectomorphs, short stocky people into endomorphs and broad shouldered middle types of people into mesomorphs. I should point out that stocky refers to the intrinsic body shape and does not mean someone who is overweight.

The shape of the human body is important because the relative size and shape of the bones influences the range of joint movement and that determines joint stablility, muscle flexibility, and other functions.

3

Bone and joint structure either facilitates greater range of movement or reduces it. A slim person will tend to have a greater range of movement than a stocky person, and a stocky person will tend to have greater joint stability than a skinny person. While it is generally true that body shape influences range of movement and therefore flexibility, there are other genetic factors acting to increase or decrease range of movement, by either exaggerating the influence of body shape or countering it, and there are also lifestyle factors.

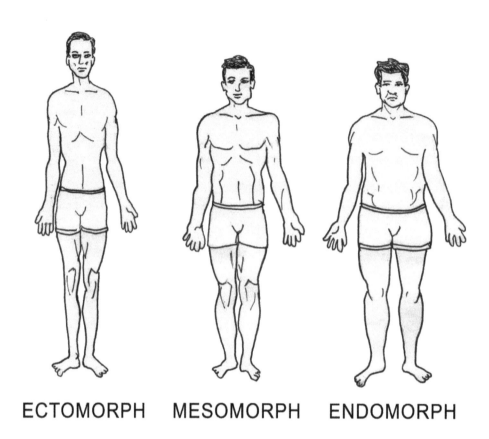

ECTOMORPH   MESOMORPH   ENDOMORPH

Body types

Gender
Gender differences influence functions such as stability and flexibility in men and women. On average, women carry more body fat than men, which gives them a more rounded appearance, but men have larger bones and muscles than women, which translates into greater muscle strength. Adult males tend to be taller than adult females and have relatively longer legs.

In general, women have greater joint mobility than men. This is most marked in girls and young women and the difference becomes less into adulthood. Hip and sacroiliac joints are more flexible throughout life in women than men.

Race
Racial differences in flexibility are not as great as gender differences. There may be greater joint mobility in Africans, Scandinavians, and some Europeans, who on average tend to be taller than Asians, who tend to be more stocky.

Ligament elasticity
The elasticity of the ligaments is a major genetic factor influencing the range of movement in joints and therefore muscle flexibility because the primary role of ligaments is to provide support to joints. Ligaments do not contract to produce movement like muscles, they are tough elastic structures that hold the body together.

Not all ligaments in the body are the same. They differ in size and composition in different joints of the body. They are made from different combinations of materials, mainly proteins, and it is the relative amounts of these materials that determines their properties such as strength and elasticity. The same ligaments can also be different in different people. The compostion of the proteins can vary, so some people have stronger ligaments and some have more elastic ligaments than others.

Elastin, a type of protein, is the main material that gives ligaments their elasticity. Different levels of elastin are found in the same ligaments in different people. In other words, different people are born with different amounts in their body. The greater the amount of elastin in the ligament the more flexible it will be. Collagen, another type of protein, is the main material that gives ligaments their strength. Thus the ratio of elastin to collagen is an important factor governing range of movement, not only in ligaments but tissues in general. The more elastin, the more elastic your tissues will be and the more collagen, the stronger your tissues will be.

Differences in range of movement exists across all human beings, which are genetically determined. There are people at one end of the human spectrum who are very flexible or congenitally hypermobile, there are people at the other end of the spectrum who are more stiff or hypomobile and in the middle are the majority of people who fall somewhere between flexible and inflexible. Range of movement roughly follows a bell curve, where the majority have average flexibility and a minority at either extremes have either low or high flexibility.

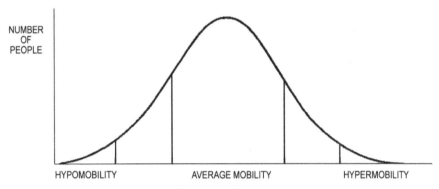

Range of joint mobility in humans

Considerations for body type
Hypermobility is greater mobility than normal, so for example, the person with hypermobility can passively bend their fingers backward 90 degrees, bend their thumbs backwards to their wrists, bend their knee or elbow joints backwards past the straight position or bring their legs behind their head. It can affect one joint, many joints or the whole body.

Up to 10 per cent of the human population may have some degree of hypermobility, with women three times more likely to have it than men. Hypermobility can be associated with certain types of diseases such as Ehlers-Danlos syndrome, Loeys-Dietz syndrome or Marfan syndrome but more commonly it is just the extreme end of a spectrum of mobility in normal healthy people.

Hypermobility may go unnoticed or be expressed through minor complications such as locking of fingers, joint clicking noises, joints that bend past neutral or normal anatomical limits (double jointed), muscle fatigue as muscles work harder to compensate for weak ligaments and flat feet (pes planus) as the ligaments in the foot collapse under the weight of the body.

If trauma, overstretching or overuse are superimposed on top of the hypermobility then it can lead to problems such as back pain from postural fatigue, nerve compression problems, tendinitis, bursitis and increased frequency of sprains such as twisted ankles, joint instability, and partial or complete dislocations. Hypermobility can also lead to chronic pain, disability and conditions such as early-onset osteoarthritis.

Hypermobility can occur during late pregnacy as the body is flooded with hormones such as relaxin, which increases ligament laxity in preparation for the birth process. Pregnancy is also accompanied by increased weight gain and a more anterior weight distribution affecting the body's centre of gravity. There may be an increased cervical and lumbar lordosis, an increased thoracic kyphosis, protraction of the scapular, an anterior pelvic tilt, an anterior head posture and hyperextension of the knees. Lower back pain and carpal tunnel syndrome are some of the unwanted side effects that can occur during pregnacy. Sometimes, symptoms occur after the pregnancy if the body fails to adapt to a return to normal hormone levels.

Although there are obvious problems associated with hypermobility, there are some benefits and hypermobility can confer advantages to certain individuals. For example, musicians may have a greater reach with their fingers on a musical instrument, and yogis and gymnasts can bend into more extreme positions.

Generalised hypermobility is determined by genes but localised hypermobility is associated with overstretching or trauma. Ligaments may be damaged by a single event such as a major injury or strong forceful stretch, or from repeated multiple minor injuries and poor stretching technique. When a ligament is stretched past its elastic limit the ligament becomes too lax to give adequate support to the joint it is meant to protect.

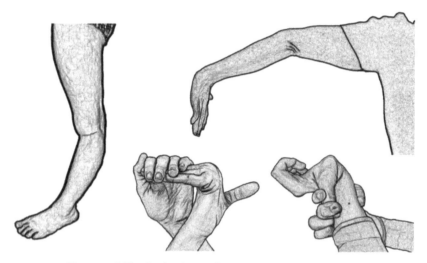

Hypermobility in the knee, fingers, elbow and thumb

Joint hypermobility occurs when the stretch or force from an injury exceeds a certain anatomical threshold. When the joint is returned to the relaxed, non-stretch position, the overstretched ligament does not return to its original length and no longer supports the joint adequately. Joints with lax ligaments are less stable and more vulnerable to further injury.

Instead of increasing the hypermobility evenly over the whole body, overstretching tends to localise it to just a few joints and to specific regions of the body and make those joints even more hypermobile. Overstretching localises the hypermobility because bones and joints differ in shape throughout the body and this affects the type and the range of movement that is possible. The structure of vertebrae in particular affects which joints move most and which move least when the spine is put through a range of movement such as a stretching exercise. Localised hypermobility also tends to occur in the spine because the rib cage tends to restrict movement in the thoracic spine and forces most of the movement to occur in the cervical and lumbar spine.

Localised and generalised hypermobility are frequently found together. The localisation becoming a complication and an exaggeraton of the generalised form of hypermobility. Localised hypermobility is less of a problem for very stiff people when they stretch because they start from a lower flexibility baseline and as they continue to stretch, their less elastic ligaments resist the over stretching.

6

Good structural integrity and an optimum ligament tightness is necessary for support, stability and good joint function. When there is ligament laxity then moderate to strong stretching is inappropriate because it will perpetuate the laxity. It takes considerable time for overstretched ligaments to return to their original level of tightness. Several months of mild stretching or even the complete abstinence of stretching may be necessary for sprained ligaments to tighten up. Sometimes quite different types of non-stretching exercises may be helpful for this. Tennis is a good way to strengthen spinal ligaments, as well as knee and ankle collateral ligaments, and wrist and elbow ligaments in the active upper limb. Standing up sailing or crewing on a small boat is another option for strengthening spinal and lower limb ligaments.

Other genetic factors

Other genetic factors influencing flexibility includes the viscosity or stickiness of the synovial fluid, the smoothness of the joint cartilage, the size, shape and elasticity of the muscles, and the thickness and elasticity of the fasciae. Posture is influenced by both genetic and lifestyle factors and as it has a such a major influence on our flexibility it will be considered separately under its own heading.

Lifestyle

Our behaviour changes us both structurally and functionally. The types of physical activity, including lack of physical activity and other lifestyle factors modify the structure of our tissues, and this in turn influences the stability, mobility, flexibility and other functions of our body.

The frequency and the intensity we use our muscles affects their strength. The frequency we stretch as well as how far we stretch our muscles affects their length and flexibility. Under-activity and poor posture are characteristics of a sedentary lifestyle, which can include hours of sitting at a desk, driving a car and watching television. If these activities, or lifestyle choices are continued over months or years, this will result in muscle atrophy, weakness and shortness, reduced elasticity in ligaments and greater viscosity of synovial fluid, all of which can lead to loss of cartilage and increased joint stiffness.

Because people differ so widely in terms of their lifestyle, they will therefore need different stretching routines. A person involved in heavy manual labour, or a very active person will need different stretching exercises compared with a moderately active or sedentary person.

The mind and mental health

Anxiety, depression and mental issues can increase muscle tension, which can change our posture and cause stiffness. Mental problems can vary from mild levels of stress to serious mental illness. The areas most commonly affected are the neck, shoulders and upper thoracic, however the abdomen, buttocks and lumbar regions can also be involved. The chin pushed or protruding forwards, a dowager's hump in the upper thoracic, rounded shoulders and kyphosis in the middle thoracic, are the classic examples of a depressive posture. They result in stiffness in the spine and shortness in the muscles in front of the chest. Elevated shoulders and chin pushed forwards are the classic examples of an anxiety posture. These result in stiffness in the neck and shoulders and shortness in the muscles above the shoulders, especially the trapezius and levator scapulae.

Stretching brings about a reduction in muscular tension and should be part of a total program to help a person deal with the effects of stress on the body. Stretching provides a sense of relaxation in the mind and in the body.

Exercise is one of the best things you can do for the health of your brain. It is good for improving mood, memory and learning. It is effective at lifting depression and works like an antidepressant by stimulating the release of chemicals in the brain called endorphins, which create feelings of happiness and euphoria. Studies show that exercise even works for people who are diagnosed as clinically depressed. If however you are clinically depressed do not suddenly withdraw your antidepressant medication and replace it with exercise.

Exercise also improves memory by increasing levels of brain chemicals which make connections between brain cells. Specifically it helps regulate the function of neurotransmitters such as dopamine. Exercises that challenge the brain are especially good for developing these connections, including ball games, certain dance routines and complex fitness movements. Also important is aerobic exercise like swimming, running and walking.

Although stretching does not fall into the category of challenging, endurance or aerobic exercise, it may have some benefits regarding mental development. Whatever the benefits, stretching should be combined with these other forms of exercises to increase muscle flexibility and joint mobility and to help prevent injury. In this respect, stretching is an important complementary exercise.

If you don't currently exercise, start by introducing stretching at home. After a week or two introduce walking, gradually building up to twenty minutes or more, or if it is practical, go swimming at the local pool. Later try experimenting by playing a game of tennis or squash with a friend or joining a dance group or gym class, depending on your age and current level of fitness.

Localised or generalised stiffness

Stiffness can affect the whole body or it can be localised to one joint, over several joints or to a small area of the body. It depends on whether the stiffness is caused genetically, by lifestyle, trauma, or because of postural or emotional reasons. Joint stiffness can occur quickly or it can happen slowly over many years. If it occurs gradually then other joints may compensate for the stiffness by becoming hypermobile and/or by becoming sprained more frequently.

Temporary stiffness may lead to permanent stiffness from osteoarthritis, ankylosis and other forms of joint degeneration. This is usually localised to just one joint such as a hip joint or an area of the body such as the lower lumbar spine, or it may involve the entire spine such as with ankylosing spondylitis. Also as joints are interconnected with muscles, stiffness in joints will lead to muscle dysfunction including shortness.

The types of stretches selected, the areas or joints selected for stretching and the intensity of stretching required to get a positive result, depend a lot on whether the stiffness is generalised and spread out across many joints, or localised to just one joint or a few small areas. Also it is important to remember that the muscles and joints of the body are interconnected and stretching one joint or one area of the body might influence other areas.

Ageing

Ageing is the process of molecular and cellular changes that occur to an individual over the course of their lifetime with various effects on their structure and function. The accumulation of molecular errors that compromise cell functions occurs because of genetic, lifestyle, environmental and other factors.

Ageing is the accumulation of damage in molecules, cells and tissues over a lifetime, reducing a persons capacity to maintain homeostasis in stress conditions, and increasing the risk for many diseases such as cancer, cardiovascular disease and premature death.

Stiffness tends to increase in all soft tissues with age. It can become more localised to certain regions. Key areas affected by ageing include the lower cervical spine, the upper and middle thoracic spine, the lower lumbar spine, and the weight bearing joints of the lower limb - the feet, knees and hips.

Joints become stiffer with age because the ligaments shorten and lose some elasticity. Muscles may be infiltrated with fat and become fibrous, tougher and less elastic. They tend to lose tone even with regular exercise. Body mass decreases as muscles atrophy and with loss of muscle mass there is reduced strength. Changes within the nervous system also contributes to reduced muscles tone and strength.

After about 60 years of age there is loss of muscle fibre number and size and an increase in the amount of connective tissue, the non-contractile part of the muscle situated between and around the muscle fibres. Ageing generally results in a decrease in both the elasticity of muscles and tensile strength of ligaments. This can result in a decrease in joint mobility and a greater chance of ligament injury due to trauma or overstretching.

Ageing results in changes in the bones, muscles and joints which results in changes to posture and gait. Ageing also results in changes in cartilage, synovial membranes, synovial fluid, the skin and hair. There is loss of cartilage in most joints but especially the hips, knees and fingers.

In young people the fasciae has wave-like undulations or crimps in their fibres that give it greater elasticity. With regular healthy loading through exercise, the crimps can be maintained into old age but the tendency is for the fasciae to become flatter, less wave-like and therefore less pliable as the fibres become more multi-directional and cross-linked together.

Bone mass, density and mineral content decreases with age, intervertebral discs become thinner, spurs form on vertebra (osteoarthritis) and the spinal column becomes progressively curved (kyphosis) and shorter. As the length of the spine decreases there is a loss of overall height, while the arms and leg appear relatively longer.

The flexed posture is arguably the most common feature of ageing. This may be due to a combination of sedentary lifestyle and degenerative changes, especially osteoporosis and other types of bone loss. A flexed throracic spine will lead to compensatory postural changes such as an forward head posture, as well as reduced movement of the ribs and diaphragm, decreased lung volume and compromised arterial, venous and lymphatic circulation.

Osteoporosis increases with age, especially in women, resulting in a greater incidence of broken bones, including compression fractures in the spine. Although stretching and exercise are important to counter bone loss, caution should be taken when stretching in women over 50 years and men over 60 years, or if osteoporosis has been diagnosed.

Age related changes are influenced by our genes and lifestyle. Genetic factors cannot be changed easily but lifestyle factors can. Lack of movement and exercise has a major influence on our bodies and on ageing. Movement is essential for health. It is necessary for maintaining structural integrity and a wide range of functions in the body. Inactivity accelerates ageing, it has a major impact on the ageing of joints and on stiffness generally. Movement is important for keeping fluids moving around joints and nourishing the cartilage. Without movement, the cartilage lining our joints gets thinner and this eventually leads to degeneration. The effects of inactivity on muscles is atrophy, fibrous changes and fatty infiltration. These are almost the same as the changes described above for ageing and in many respects degeneration and ageing go together and are the same.

Few people go through life without injuring themselves and as we grow older we accumulate more damage to our tissues. Injuries to a muscle or joints lead to the development of fibrous tissue from scarring or adhesions. These should be a temporary tissues, a bridge between the damaged tissue and the fully formed new tissue but injuries commonly get left untreated, or are not treated effectively or the damaged tissues are allowed to rest too long, and so retain this temporary fibrous scar tissue in between their normal or healthy tissue. As fibrous tissue is less elastic and less strong than the original tissue that it is trying to replace, the result is stiffness and weakness.

Age related stiffness or hypomobility causing hypermobility

Although the stiffness occuring in the tissues of the body with increasing age is usually a generalised type of stiffness or hypomobility affecting the whole body, there is the potential for hypermobility to develop in localised areas of the spine when stretching with too much force. Ageing is inevitable and everyone will get stiffer with passing years. Regular stretching counters increasing stiffness and helps maintain healthy muscles and joints throughout a persons lifetime but overstretching can cause problems. Stretching will keep you flexible but it must be done safely.

How you stretch depends on whether you are new to stretching or have been stretching for many years and are relatively supple. It also depends on whether you have joint disease or have had an artificial joint replacement.

Posture

Posture is concerned with the carriage of the body as a whole, the head, spine and the position of the arms and legs. Good posture depends on optimal muscle tone, power and flexibility and on having appropriate balance between the agonists and antagonist muscles at the front and back of the body, and between the muscles on the left and right sides. Good posture also depends on appropriate ligament support around the joints.

Prolonged sitting or standing, particularly in the presence of a slouched forward posture, eventually results in changes to muscle tone, power and elasticity. The posteriorly positioned muscles have to work harder against the continuous action of gravity pulling the body forwards and downwards. Overworked muscles eventually fatigue and start to undergo structural changes. They become more fibrous, less elastic and less efficient in contracting. Pectoralis major and minor and anterior scalene tend to shorten while erector spinae, trapezius and rhomboid major and minor tend to lengthen and become more fibrous. Levator scapulae in particular is found to become more fibrous, partly due to effects of gravity, but also due to habitual over-contraction associated with patterns of overuse and stress.

Gravity and posture

Gravity has a profound effect on the human body over a lifetime, including the soft tissues which determine our posture, height and the placement of our organs. Gravity causes our discs to lose fluid throughout the day and this results in a height loss of up to two centimetres between awakening in the morning and going to sleep at night. Most of the fluid returns to the disc overnight, but it never returns 100 per cent and over a lifetime a person can permanently lose between three and five centimetres in height from the spine. After the age of twenty, the spine loses about one centimetre in height every fifteen years due to compressive force of gravity. This means our body becomes stockier and our arms and legs look relatively longer as we get older.

One consequence of a lifetime of gravity compressing our soft tissues is a reduction in our range of movement. Flexibility is lost in the spine as the discs become thinner and it is lost throughout the body generally, as ligaments and fasciae become more distended over time. This is compounded by the loss of elasticity in our muscles and ligaments, loss of mineralisation and other changes in our bones, as well as loss of cartilage lining our joints. These are the result of ageing processes that are partly governed by our lifestyle, but mainly governed by our genes which control cellular repair and replacement.

In addition to the effects on our spine gravity stretches the skin causing wrinkles and other outward effects of ageing, connective tissue supporting organs causing them to prolapse or move from their rightful place in the body, ligaments and fasciae changing the shape of our body, and veins distending them and causing varicose veins which results in sluggish circulation and swelling in the feet.

Genes and posture

The genes we inherit from our parents play a major role in determining shape of our posture as we develop. The chance interplay between the dominant and recessive genes of our mother and father are expressed as the many variations of human posture. Genes produce structural and functional characterists that confer benefit or detriment to posture. The size and shape of our bones, joints and muscles and the laxity of our ligaments and other factors, influence how we develop and are pre-programmed by our genes. If we are lucky we will have the structural foundations for a good posture and if we are unlucky we will have to work harder to maintain a good posture.

A scoliosis is a lateral curvature of the spine. The curve may be located in the cervical, thoracic, thoracolumbar, lumbar or sacroiliac spine. When a scoliosis develops the spine bends sideways and rotates along its vertical axis – in the same direction to the sidebending in the cervical spine but usually in the opposite direction to the sidebending in the thoracic and lumbar spine. Most rotation occurs at the apex of the curve. A scoliosis may have single, double or multiple curves. The curves may be in either direction but the left lumbar and right thoracic curves are the most common.

A lordosis is a normal inward (concave) curvature of the lumbar or cervical spine. A hyperlordosis is an increased or excessive lordosis, commonly referred to as a sway back. A kyphosis is a normal outward (convex) curvature of the thoracic spine. A hyperkyphosis is an increased or excessive kyphosis and is commonly referred to as a hunchback.

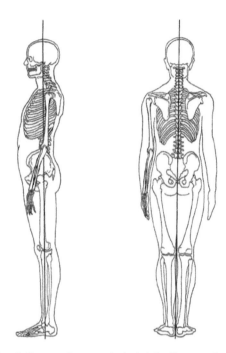

Plumb line and normal skeletal alignment
Viewed from the side (left) and viewed from behind (right)

The genes we inherit at birth, like the hand of cards we are dealt in a card game, are mostly fixed. How we live our life is analogous to how we play our cards. With appropriate exercise and good use of our body throughout life, we can mitigate the expressions of our genes. As we get older, our posture tends to become more exaggerated. So a person with a mild spinal curvature as a young adult will tend to develop a more severe curvature as they get older. How hard we work to counter the effect of gravity shaping our genetically inherited posture will determine the outcome as we get older.

Exaggerations or deviations of the body's shape from the norm create unique challenges for the body. Genetic variation leads to a range of different postures in humans. A kyphosis or lordosis may be increased or decreased or reversed, and a scolisis may be left or right, single or multiple. A scoliosis will interact with a kyposis and lordosis, creating the potential for many different postures.

Different postures interact with gravity in different ways to produce a range of different effects on muscles. Pathologies like osteoarthritis also appear after the age of forty, resulting in localised loss of joint movement and this interacts with posture to produce muscle changes. Greater muscle activity produces muscle hypertrophy (increase in size), shortening, and increase in strength. Reduced muscle activity produces atrophy (decrease in size), lengthening and weakness.

The optimum spine is well balanced over the intervertebral disc to facilitate the movement of nutrients throughout the disc. An extreme increase or decrease of lordosis, kyphosis or scoliosis will impair nourishment to the disc by placing greater pressure on the one side of the annulus fibrosus, reducing fluid and nutrient flow.

Ligaments play a major role in maintaining posture. The size of the ligament, the types of collagen and the alignment of the collagen within the ligament, and the presence or absence of elastin within the ligament are some of the genetic factors that affect joint stability and flexibility.

Large strong tight ligaments result in greater stability, and surrounding muscles need to work less to maintain posture - but there is the potential for greater stiffness. In contrast small weak lax ligaments result in greater mobility, and surrounding muscles need to work harder to maintain posture. Both extremes have advantages and disadvantages. Joints with tight ligaments are stable but stiffer and prone to injury. Joints with lax ligaments are sprained more easily, associated intervertebral and fibrocartilagenous discs are injured more frequently and muscles tend to get bigger, tighter and more fibrous because they have to work harder to provide the stability which the ligaments do not provide.

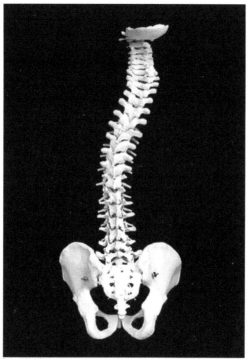

Scoliosis - posterior view of spine and pelvis

Specific examples of ligament laxities caused by genes include: knee hyperextension (genu recurvatum), atlanto-occipital and metacarpophalangeal joint hyperextension, flat feet (pes planus) plus thumb, wrist, glenohumeral and spinal joint hypermobility. Other structural variations with a strong genetic basis are knock knees (genu valgum), bow legs (genu varum), high arch (pes cavus), and bunions (hallux valgus).

These structural deviations may cause problems locally or result in compensatory postural problems elsewhere in the body or they may not result in any problems. A reduced medial longitudinal arch characteristic of pes planus may be rigid and present in both the weight bearing and the non-weight bearing foot, or it may be flexible and only present in the weight bearing foot. It may be made worse by lifestyle factors, especially the wearing of shoes. Knee hyperextension may be associated with fixed plantarflexion and restricted ankle dorsiflexion. It may result in posterior joint capsule stress and lengthening, and over time lead to cartilage loss and degeneration. An anterior pelvic tilt due to lax hip ligaments may be associated with an increased lumbar or lumbosacral lordosis, an increased thoracic kyphosis, sacroiliac changes and a forward head posture - classical characteristics of poor posture. Postural extremes may cause abnormal compressive forces on joints, resulting in cortical thickening in bones, abnormal wear on cartilage, shortening and overstretching of ligaments and muscles, as well as other changes.

Curvatures of the spine

A good posture is one with a straight spine or a very mild S-shaped curve (scoliosis) when viewed from the back, and mild to moderate anterior-posterior curves, when viewing the spine from the side, in other words a modest thoracic kyphosis and lumbar and cervical lordosis. A poor posture is one with an extreme scoliosis and exaggerated anterior-posterior curves, or a reversal of the normal curves, in other words spinal curvatures showing a marked deviation from the norm - an increased lordosis, kyphosis or scoliosis, or a reduced kyphosis or lordosis (flat back), or a reversed lordosis or kyphosis (back to front curvature).

Gravity is constantly pushing the body downwards and to counter gravity our postural muscles have to contract to hold us upright. A good posture with neutral spinal alignment and optimal curvature responds more efficiently to gravity, and with the least amount of effort, compared to a poor posture where the body is further from its centre of gravity. When we have a good posture, the muscles only need to contract lightly and intermittently, allowing longer muscle rest periods. With a poor posture the body is a long way forwards, backwards or to one side of an imagined plumb line going through the middle of the body; and the long levers that are created by these extremes of spinal curvature effectively increases the weight of the body, placing greater stress on the joints and higher work load on the muscles, which have to contract more strongly and continuously. Muscles supporting a poor posture have less rest time therefore have a higher probability of failing sooner than the same muscles supporting a good posture.

Mild curves require the least amount of energy to maintain them because they are better lined up with gravity, whereas extreme curves require a higher level of energy to maintain them because they are further away from the centre of gravity, and as more energy is expended holding poor postures upright, this can eventually result in pain, lowered vitality and tiredness.

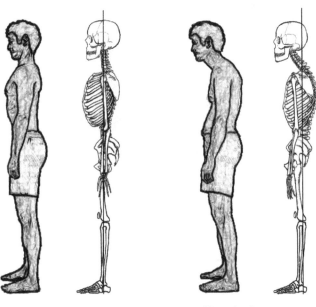

Normal posture   **Slouched posture**

There are several different variations of thoracic kyphosis. It can be a generalised over large areas of the thoracic spine or it can be localised in a 'Gibbus deformity' in the middle of the thoracic spine or a dowager hump at the top. Also the kyphosis can be combined with a scoliosis, adding sidebending and rotation to the flexion curvature. There may also be areas of extension, usually at or around T4 and in the lower thoracic or thoracolumbar area.

The forward head posture is a complex combination of anterior occiput, lower cervical lordosis and scoliosis. There may also be areas of flexion involved. It results in compression of the posterior facet joints and posterior disc, shortening of the posterior ligaments and joint capsule, closing and narrowing of the intervertebral foramina. There may be a reduction in blood supply and fibrous development in the posterior cervical muscles as a result of constantly having to contract isometrically to counter the pull of gravity on the head. Over time there may be degenerative changes in the lower cervical spine, especially between C5 and C6, nerve root irritation, and changes in the temporomandibular and shoulder joints.

In the optimal posture, an imaginary plumb line bisects the body into two symmetrical halves. When viewed from the front, the head is straight with no tilting or rotation, and the eyes, clavicle, shoulders, and hips are level and parallel to the ground. Viewed from behind, the plumb line falls down the spine and the mid-line of the body, and the medial borders of the scapulae are parallel. The inferior angles of the scapulae, lateral contour of the ribs, waist angles, iliac crests, gluteal folds, hips, knees and malleoli are equidistant from the plumb line.

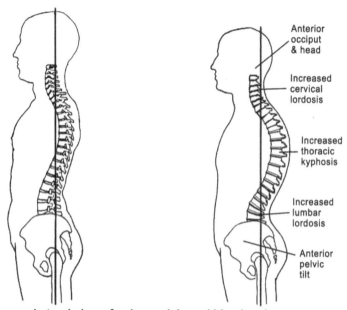

Lateral view of spine, pelvis and hip showing
optimal posture (left) and exaggerated posture (right)

Viewed from behind, the spine is rarely perfectly straight and many people have some lateral curvature of the spine, in other words a mild scoliosis. A scoliosis is usually well established by early adolescence and may simply be a reflection of how strong the dominant side of our body is. In contrast to an ambidextrous person, a person with strong left handedness or strong right handedness will have greater muscle development on one side of their body and this right-left muscle imbalance is likely to have a major influence on the formation of a scoliosis. The stronger spinal and shoulder muscles of the dominant side will pull the spine to that side, and other areas in the body will automatically compensate.

Some people have a primary scoliosis and one or two compensatory secondary curves, while other people have multiple scoliotic curves. Greater complexity occurs when a scoliosis is combined with a kyphosis or lordosis or reverse curve. A postural problem rarely occurs in only one plane. It affects the whole body including the upper and lower limbs.

There are several types of scoliosis or lateral spinal curvatures. An adolescent idiopathic scoliosis as the name suggests, develops in adolescence and may be caused by a hormonal imbalance, a problem with the vestibular system and it may be genetic. This type of scoliosis has extreme fixed structural curves. It involves asymmetric growth in the vertebral bodies, discs, ligaments and muscles down one side of the body. Fortunately it is relatively rare and falls outside the scope of this book.

In contrast to the adolescent idiopathic scoliosis, the functional scoliosis is not structural and therefore can be reversed to a much greater extent if treated early and the cause of the problem removed. Common causes of a functional scoliosis include an anatomical short leg, muscle imbalance and postural overuse favouring one side of the body.

14

If a short leg is causing the scoliosis then a heel lift in the shoe of the short leg may be required if the leg difference is greater than about 1 cm or if the scoliosis does not compensate well for the shortness, especially as people get older. Another common problem which can cause a scoliosis is a twisting in the pelvis known as a sacral torsion. This will need to be fixed before addressing the scoliosis. Also a muscle that becomes strained or irritated can go into spasm, causing a scoliosis. Although this may be extremely painful it is usually of short duration and once the acute symptoms have gone the scoliosis will usually self correct.

Other less common causes of scoliosis include abnormalities in vertebrae at birth (congenital scoliosis), disorders of the central nervous system such as cerebral palsy (neuromuscular scoliosis), infections and fractures of the spine.

Lifestyle factors influencing posture

In addition to being genetically determined, a good or bad posture is also partly the result of lifestyle and behaviour factors, including a person's psychoemotional state. Posture may be affected by a temporary loss of concentration and intention to stay straight, perhaps due to tiredness, or by a lack of discipline and will power or by deeply ingrained physical and mental habits established over a long period of time. A depressed mental state may result in muscle fatigue, anxiety may result in muscle tension, and both of these can affect posture.

Sitting causes many problems for the posture and is the single most important cause of bad posture after genetics. Common problems are slouching and not balancing the spine and upper body over the sit bones (ischial tuberosities), crossing the legs and taking the weight of body over one sit bone and forcing the spine into a compensatory sidebending scoliosis, protruding the chin and moving the head into an forward (anterior translation) position, sitting too long so that the hamstrings, hip flexors and other muscles remain in a shortened state. Office workers who sit for long hours on the job are most susceptible to structural changes in muscle and degenerative changes in joints and intervertebral discs.

Postural challenges at work may have adverse effects on structure and function. Each profession has unique postural problems and injuries. Shop assistants, bricklayers and surgeons adopt static standing postures. Computer operators, secretaries and office workers adopt sitting postures. Musicians, dentists and machine operators adopt asymmetrical postures. Athletes, football players and runners adopt strong dynamic postures. The mechanical stresses for each of these is different and requires different stretching exercises.

Shoe-wearing influences the shape of our feet, our posture and the way we walk. Chimps have a floppy middle section in their feet to allow them to grip a branch but humans evolved a rigid midfoot to enable bipedal walking. When shoes were adopted many centuries ago, they took over the role of the foot in providing rigidity and in some people the foot became flat and floppy.

There is a lot of diversity among individuals in the shape and range of joint movement of the foot. This is especially true for the midfoot, which is stiff in some people and has a large range of movement in others. Shoes can cause some people to develop flat feet, whereas others continue to maintain a relatively normal arch. Flatness is not ideal for efficient walking and running because of the reduced elastic recoil when the foot comes to the toe-off phase, which can lead to postural compensations such as external rotation in the hips and increase flexion in the sacroiliac joints and increased lumbosacral extension and changes higher in the spine.

Effects of good or bad posture

In addition to its mechanical effect on muscles and joints, posture affects a wide range of other body functions including the circulation of blood and lymph, respiration and nerve function. A good posture optimises breathing and the circulation of bodily fluids, and it facilitates optimal organ function and movement. An increased thoracic kyphosis affects the rib cage and the diaphragm, reducing rib movement and limiting respiration. This can lead to reduced oxygenation throughout the body. It can also compromise internal organ performance by increasing pressure throughout the abdomen.

Loss of range of movement caused by bad posture is particularly noticeable in the shoulder joints, rib cage and thoracic, lumbar and cervical spine. There is an interconnection between posture and muscle. Poor posture results in fibrous and short muscles, and unless these fibrous and short muscles are stretched, they affect posture.

When there is good posture, there is a neutral spine with an optimum curvature and optimum alignment of the body segments. There is a vertical ilium with a sacrum tilted forward midway between flexion (nutation) and extension (counter-nutation), lumbar (L1 - L5) bent backwards in a natural lumbar lordosis, thoracic (T1 - T12) bent forwards in a natural kyphosis and cervical (C1 - C7) bent backwards as a cervical lordosis. When the pelvis is in neutral, the anterior superior iliac spines and pubic symphysis fall in the same vertical line. From the sagittal view, the plumb line should bisect the ear, odontoid process of C2, the cervical vertebral bodies, the centre of the glenohumeral joint, the lumbar vertebral bodies, the centre of the acetabulum, just posterior to the patella and through the tarsals of the feet. Although a scoliosis is common in many people, in the ideal posture a plumb line should run vertically down the midline of the body dividing it symmetrically into right and left halves with equal weight on left and right feet.

Solutions

We can work towards a better posture with postural awareness, and with stretching and strengthening exercises but our genes ultimately limit what is physically possible. Only the good fortune of a healthy genetic inheritance can provide us with an ideal posture. And then it is up to us to keep it that way. If through problems at birth or because of our genes we inherit a poor posture, we may be able to improve it, but it will require hard work. It may be a big challenge for us just to keep it from deteriorating under the influences of gravity and lifestyle. But it is up to us. What we make of our posture depends on the environment we grow up in and how we use our body, including safe stretching.

In general, muscles that are abnormally shortened and fibrous need stretching, and muscles that are abnormally lengthened and weak need strengthening. Low level stretching may also be used to relieve pain occurring as a result of postural fatigue in the latter group of muscles.

Stretching also acts to counter extreme postural deviations that take the body far away from its centre of gravity - increased thoracic kyphosis, anterior occiput or scoliosis. Of course, for stretching to have any long term effect it must be combined with lifestyles change.

The universal posture

The standard postural model so far described and the one found in most anatomy books has the anterior-posterior curvature of the spine as a lumbar lordosis, thoracic kyphosis and cervical lordosis. A more accurate representation of the human posture is the universal human posture. The universal posture has greater complexity than the standard postural model and is closer to the reality found in practice.

The universal posture includes an anterior occiput, flexed upper cervical spine, extended lower cervical spine, flexed upper thoracic spine, extended group of vertebrae centred around T4, flexed middle thoracic spine, extended thoracolumbar spine, flexed lumbar spine and extended lumbosacral spine.

There are many variations of human structure and not everyone fits the universal posture model. But if your body does fit the universal model then it can be useful for adopting the right stretching techniques. If your body is completely different from the universal model then a unique stretching program is required. It is also important to deduce which areas of your body are hypomobile and which are hypermobile. Common hypermobile areas are described below.

In contrast to the anterior-posterior curvatures of the spine, the lateral curvatures show greater variability and much more complex patterns. Here are some of the many different possible scoliotic curves.

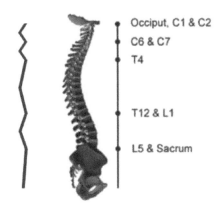

The universal posture

- The lumbar spine is divided equally between one third straight, one third sidebent left and one third sidebent right.

- The lower thoracic or thoracolumbar spine tends to compensate for the lumbar curve by sidebending in the opposite direction.

- Because most people are predominantly right handed and their right shoulder muscles depress the right shoulder, the thoracic spine is predominantly sidebent right. The right sidebending can occur in the upper thoracic, lower thoracic or throughout the whole thoracic spine.

- The middle thoracic is divided equally into right and left sidebending depending on whether the scoliosis is a single 'S' curve or multiple curves.

- The cervical spine is predominantly sidebent left in compensation for the thoracic spine sidebending right but may be sidebent in any direction.

- The shape the thoracic spine adopts depends on:

    o If the scoliosis is a single 'S' shape curve or a more complex series of curves.
    o How it interacts with the anterior-posterior curves and the position of the sacrum.

- The lateral curvature of the whole spine is influenced by:

    o Whether the spine is in neutral position or an increased or reversed cervical or lumbar lordosis or thoracic kyphosis.
    o Any leg length discrepancy will have a crucial influence on the shape of the spine.

Flexibility, mobility and stability

Flexibility and mobility are not the same. Mobility is the same as movement, and is the primary function of joints which should move freely and through a full range of movement. Flexibility is the same as extensibility, an important attribute of skeletal muscles, and is the ability of a muscle or group of muscles to lengthen through a range of motion.
Mobility is influenced by a range of factors including:

1. Muscle flexibility - a joint won't move well if the muscles around it don't fully elongate.
2. Muscle contractibility - a joint won't move well if the muscles around it don't fully contract.
3. Ligament (and/or capsule) integrity - a tight ligament will limit joint movement, whereas a lax ligament will permit too much movement thereby affecting stability

4. Tendon integrity - when a tendon is irritated this may result in tendonitis and pain
5. Synovial membrane integrity - when irritated or thickened (synovitis) this may result in rheumatoid arthritis
6. Cartilage thickness - the loss of which may result in osteoarthritis.
7. History - especially with regard to joint trauma, infection and use.
8. Other factors - genetic and lifestyle.

A joint can have average mobility, increased mobility or decreased mobility. Loss of mobility (hypomobility) may be due to damage to any structure within or around a joint whereas too much mobility (hypermobility) is usually due to damage to a ligament resulting in laxity - an injury or repeated overstretching or genetic factors.

A muscle can have average flexibility, increased flexibility or decreased flexibility. Loss of flexibility may be due to a muscle being held in a shortened position too long or having increased tension and or some type of structural change like fibrosis, scarring or adhesions. Muscle flexibility is only part of what constitutes overall body movement.

Stability is concerned with the proper alignment of joints so that the bones are taking most of the stress, not the overlying connective tissues. If you lack adequate stability then you will compensate by using more muscle effort and put greater strain on tendons and ligaments.

Ligaments are vital structures maintaining joint stability and they are the final line of joint protection when joints are moved to the limits of their range. A joint is most healthy when ligament tension is normal - not too stiff and not too lax.

If a joint moves beyond the viscoelastic limit of its ligaments, affecting their overall structural integrity, then they will no longer function as effectively in supporting the joint. A single forceful injury, many milder assaults or repeated overstretching of the joint may result in ligament laxity, localised hypermobility and joint dysfunction. Good muscle tone will help maintain posture for a while but problems may develop if muscle tone is lost.

Mobility and flexibility testing

Mobility and flexibility are tested using active and passive movements. Active testing involves voluntary contraction of the muscle or muscles overlying the joint or joints to produce the movements i.e. you do the moving. Passive testing can also be done yourself on most of the joints in the upper and lower limbs by using an arm or both arms to move the limb while you relax. But in the spine it needs to be done by another person, usually a therapist, who moves the spine through a full a range of movement while you relax. Active motion tests muscle flexibility, mobility and nerve function. In contrast, passive motion is limited to only testing mobility (but will be positive for muscle spasticity from an upper motor neuron syndrome).

Not all loss of motion can be helped with stretching. The effectiveness of a stretch is determined by the mobility of the joint. You will not be able to stretch a muscle to its full capacity if it passes over a joint with a mobility restriction. Stretching increases muscle flexibility but it does not always increase a joint's range of motion.

The effectiveness of stretching also depends on the cause of the loss of motion, the type of tissue involved and the severity of the problem. Stretching will help when there is a tissue extensibility dysfunction such as a short, tense or fibrous muscle. Passive stretching may help when there is a joint mobility dysfunction - or it may not. It will not fix a joint dysfunction if the problem is too great. Sometime capsular adhesions, tight ligaments or mechanically locked up joints require targeted joint articulation or mobilisation techniques, which can be self-directed but are usually done by a manual therapist.

Joint mobilisation

The best way to mobilise a stiff joint and increase its range of movement is to position the joint where the tissues around the joint have the least possible tension and then use passive joint-play movements to free up the joint. For example if there is restricted dorsiflexion in an

18

ankle joint, stretching the calf muscles will not fix the problem. The ankle joint will first need to be mobilised.

Here is a basic description of a technique to mobilise an ankle: With your foot planted on the ground, flex your knee to relax the gastrocnemius muscle and to introduce some ankle dorsiflexion. Now imagine looking down on a clock face with your toes pointing to the twelve o'clock position. Move your knee diagonally forwards and to the left to the ten o'clock position. Move your knee in small circles and later in progressively larger circles increasing dorsiflexion and sideways movement as you do so. Then take your knee to the eleven o'clock position and repeat the circles. Then go diagonally forwards and to the right to the one and two o'clock positions, and finally to the twelve o'clock position, increasing dorsiflexion with each position. This is one example of a passive joint mobilisation technique, in this case assisted by the weight of the body. All the passive stretches described in this book may indirectly help mobilise restricted joints but they are primarily directed at increasing flexibility in muscles and joint mobilisation is outside the scope of this book.

When stretching to increase joint mobility, it is important to aim for getting an optimum level of mobility - enough so the ligaments are stretched within safe limits and the joint is freed up but not so much that the ligaments are over-stretched and damaged.

Mild versus strong stretching
When stretching muscles you should aim for an optimum level of muscle flexibility. If a muscle is very short because its tissues have changed structurally it will need stronger stretching than a muscle that is moderately short because it is tense due to a resetting by the nervous system. Milder maintenance stretching will work for tense muscles, temporarily increasing their length and decreasing their tone, and this level of stretching will need to be continued because the muscle will usually return to its original tense shortened state over time.

Stronger developmental stretching is needed for chronically short muscles, a hamstring for example. Developmental stretching has a more permanent effect on the length of muscles because it results in micro-tearing of the fibres which then, over time, realign in a more lengthened position. In contrast to maintenance stretching, developmental stretching is better at increasing flexibility and the result is longer lasting. As well as lengthening short muscles, developmental stretching augments improvements in range, quality and control of body movement, which gets translated into improved performance and joint health.

With strong stretching there is always the danger of taking the muscle or ligament beyond its optimum level of flexibility and losing stability, so great care should be taken. Stretch areas that you know are tight and have a history of tightening up - joints that are stiff and muscles that are short.

Active versus passive stretching
Active stretching is safer than passive stretching because the range of joint motion is limited by the tension of the muscle moving the joint (agonist) and how far it can contract, and by the tension of the muscle being stretched (antagonist) and how much it is able to relax. Although reciprocal inhibition of the antagonists facilitates the relaxation and hence stretching of the antagonist muscles, the nervous system will not allow a healthy joint to be overstretched.

Approaching the problem of joint dysfunction will depend on both location and mobility: whether the joint is within the spine or the limbs, and whether the joint is hypomobile or hypermobile. If a joint in one of the upper or lower limbs is hypomobile, localised passive stretching combined with mobilisation techniques can be use. Active and post-isometric stretches may also help improve the range of movement of a joint provided they are localised to the restricted joint. If a joint in the spine is hypomobile, it is extremely difficult to free it up yourself because it is difficult to localise your forces on the most restricted joint. A manual therapist is usually required to free up the spine. The use of a high velocity thrust or movement with impulse, which results in the classical popping or cavitating of a joint has merit for the breakup of some joint fixations but in general when it is used alone it is insufficient to mobilise a joint. To be effective the high velocity technique should be combined with an articulation technique.

Only when the joint is sufficiently freed up by the therapist should passive stretching be introduced. And it is important that the force of the stretch be localised on the most restricted joint. Active stretching is less effective at improving the mobility of restricted joints in the spine because the movement will tend to be spread over the whole spine or it will occur in adjacent joints which have good mobility, thus avoiding the restricted part.

Factors affecting muscle strength	
Age	Maximum strength occurs between the ages of 25 and 30 years and decreases thereafter
Size	The larger a muscle's cross sectional area the more force it can apply
Gender	Strength is the same until pubescence and thereafter females have on average 2/3 the strength of males

If a joint in one of the upper or lower limbs is hypermobile, build strength and tone in all the muscles passing over the joint, and use active stretching, being careful not to take the joint beyond safe structural limits. If a joint in the spine is hypermobile, do not do any stretches that will perpetuate the hypermobility, and especially avoid passive stretching techniques; engage a manual therapist to free up adjacent hypomobile areas, rest the hypermobile joint but remain active with regular walking and swimming; build strength and tone in overlying muscles with isometric and isokinetic strengthening exercises; and maintain good posture.

Passive stretching is useful for stretching tight ligaments and muscles when there is no danger of creating hypermobility in adjacent joints or exacerbating already existing hypermobility. Passive stretching techniques can increase the laxity in already lax ligaments because the nature of certain body positions creates relatively long levers, thereby taking the joint through a greater, and potentially more damaging range than active stretching.

Passive stretching should be pursued:

- when there is extreme muscle shortness and inflexibility
- when there is joint hypomobility provided there is no joint hypermobility near the joint being moved.

Active stretching should be pursued:

- When there is mild hypermobility but not when the hypermobility is extreme
- When there is muscle weakness and the muscle needs strengthening with regular contraction
- When there is muscle inflexibility but no joint hypomobility.

When a joint is hypomobile it should be mobilised as a priority over stretching the overlying muscles. Muscle shortness is not desirable but the muscle cannot be stretched effectively until the joint hypomobility is fixed. Prolonged muscle shortness can lead to joint hypomobility but muscle shortness is more likely to be a consequence of the joint hypomobility rather than the cause. Allowing the muscle to remain short indefinitely is not good but the joint restriction is the primary problem.

Joint hypomobility is best treated using passive stretching. With passive techniques the overlying muscles are relaxed and gravity and/or leverage from another limb can be used to move the joint. After a few days of working on the joint problem, begin stretching the overlying muscle as well because the joint problem and the muscle shortness are entwined and both need fixing.

If full range of joint movement cannot be achieved using self-directed techniques such as passive stretching then consult a manual therapist, who will use appropriate articulation techniques to the joint. If through previous injury or abnormal wear of the cartilage a joint undergoes degenerative changes and these have progressed to osteoarthritis then movement will be severely curtailed. There will be a sudden, abrupt and solid end-feel to the movement of the joint. Mobility will be extremely restricted and it will cease earlier in its range than expected, in one or several directions or there will be no movement at all.

If there is osteoarthritis in a joint, then mobilisation will not work. If the restriction is not responding to passive stretching and other self-directed techniques then it is important to get a diagnosis.

Osteoarthritis is a progressive disease, the degenerative changes to the joint are permanent and irreversible; the earlier it is diagnosed the sooner a strategy can be put in place to prevent other joints from becoming arthritic or hypermobile and the sooner a pain management program can be put in place for the arthritis. Suspected osteoarthritic changes should be confirmed or ruled out by X-ray.
Without joint movement, effective muscle stretching may be difficult or impossible.

Effective stretching of a muscle will depend on:

1. The level of joint degeneration – mild, moderate or advanced osteoarthritis.
2. Whether the muscle passes over one, two or more joints; because if the muscle passes over another joint and it is healthy, then you can use the other joint to stretch the muscle.
3. How other joints compensate for the degeneration because you do not want to create hypermobility in the compensating joints by overstretching their overlying ligaments.

Osteoarthritis limits the amount of joint movement available for stretching, so alterative techniques need to be used. To lengthen a short muscle, which passes over an arthritic joint you need to combine stretching (depending on available joint movement) with self-mobilisation techniques:

1. Fixed transverse pressure on the muscle with your fingertips or thumb (inhibition)
2. Sliding over the width of a muscle using your fingertips or thumb (kneading)
3. Holding down the tendon or the end of a muscle with your fingertips or thumb (pinning).

Hypermobility and hypomobility
The body is healthy and functions optimally when it has good overall mobility; it is less healthy when it has areas of stiffness (hypomobility) or areas of increased mobility (hypermobility). Some people are flexible throughout most of body, while others are flexible in one area or joint but not in others. Sometimes hypermobility and hypomobility occur together in different areas of the body and sometimes they occur alone. Whether they exist alone or together depends on genetic factors influencing mobility and how long the hypomobility or hypermobility has existed.

Any joint can be hypermobile or hypomobile but problems with extreme mobility are more common in the spine. Single isolated areas of hypermobility or hypomobility can exist but more often there is an area of hypermobility associated with an area of hypomobility. There may be many areas of alternating hypomobility and hypermobility running down the spine. They may be unrelated but more often they are linked together.

Extremes mobility are more common in the spine because the spine consists of a long chain of vertebrae with a large number of joints. The facet joints are all plane joints with a similar shape but they differ in their orientation. Another factor affecting the hypermobility-hypomobility polarisation is the part of the spine that is connected to a relatively inflexible rib cage. Any region of the spine can become hypomobile or hypermobile but there are reoccurring patterns of hypo-hypermobility and some generalisation can be made about flexibility in the different regions of the spine.

Hypermobility is more common in the thoracolumbar region and in the upper cervical spine. It sometimes occurs in the middle and lower lumbar, sacroiliac, middle cervical spine and in an area of the thoracic centred around T4. Hypomobility most commonly occurs in the upper, middle and lower thoracic spine and sometimes occurs in the middle lumbar spine. In the upper and lower limbs hypermobility more frequently occurs in the hip, knee, shoulder, elbow, wrist, thumb, finger joints.

Types of Flexibility

There are two main types of flexibility:

- Active flexibility
- Passive flexibility

Active flexibility or movement is the ability to adopt and maintain a position solely using the voluntary contraction of a muscle, and under voluntary conscious control. It occurs when an agonist muscle or group of muscles stretches its antagonist muscle or muscles, without any assistance from body weight (gravity), another body part or limb, an external prop, or another person. An agonist, also known as a prime mover, is a muscle that produces the primary contraction and motion at a joint and an antagonist is a muscle with the opposite function.

Passive flexibility or movement is the ability to adopt and maintain a position using assistance from body weight (gravity), another body part or limb, an external prop or another person. It is described as involuntary movement. The muscle or group of muscles being stretched must be relaxed.

Passive flexibility is always greater than active flexibility for the same joint. Also passive flexibility results in greater muscle lengthening than active flexibility. This is because during active stretching, muscle contraction creates tension which limits the range of movement. During passive stretching all the muscles around the joint are relax and more movement is possible.

Factors affecting muscle flexibility	
Age	Flexibility decreases with age
Body type	Thinner people are more flexible than stocky people
Gender	Females are more flexible then males
Temperature	Flexibility increases up to 37 degrees centigrade
Movement	Inactivity reduces flexibility
Injuries	The severity and the number of injuries reduce flexibility. Also flexibility depends on how recent the injury occurred.
Disease	Muscle, nerve and joint disease may reduce flexibility

Although passive stretching produces greater range of movement, active stretching can be very useful because it builds strength, is a better measure of functional flexibility and is generally safer than passive stretching. In general, active stretching mainly increases active flexibility and passive stretching mainly increases passive flexibility.

Stability and flexibility

Good posture is also about creating the right balance between muscle tone and muscle flexibility. In general, increased muscle tone creates greater stability, while increased muscle flexibility creates greater range of movement. In some respects these are conflicting requirements, meaning the greater there is of one, the less there is of the other. There is an optimum level of stability and flexibility.

Low flexibility, particular during ballistic type movement such as throwing or kicking a ball, means less muscle extensibility and this translates into a greater rate of muscle injury. Evidence clearly shows a correlation between short hamstrings and hamstring tears. This is generally true for all short muscles. Short muscles have less maneuverability and during sports or periods of peak demand are prone to greater injury. In contrast to muscle shortness, high flexibility results in a greater number of joint dislocation and ligament sprains. The best way to find the right balance between stability and flexibility is with an exercise program that stretches the right muscles and strengthens the right muscles.

Muscles contribute towards mobility and stability. Mobility is produced through bony levers acting through rotation around a joint. Stability is produced through the longitudinal pull of a muscle down the shaft of a bone, by the tension of ligaments and the congruence of joint surfaces. When a joint has maximum congruence, which is usually in full extension, it has the highest level of stability and is said to be in the close-packed position. When a joint has minimum congruence, which is usually in partial flexion, it is almost totally dependent on muscle contraction for stability and is said to be in the loose-packed position.

Other factors limiting range of movement

Internal influences:

- The type of joint
- The bony structure
- Internal resistance within a joint
- Muscle mass (excessive muscle bulk)
- The elasticity of muscle tissue (ageing, scarring, fibrous changes)
- The elasticity of tendons and ligaments (ageing, scarring, fibrous changes)
- The elasticity of skin
- The tone of the muscle
- The level of fatty tissue
- Insufficient or abnormal chemical composition of synovial fluid
- Insufficient or unhealthy cartilage

External influences:

- Fitness levels with respect to muscle flexibility and joint mobility
- The external temperature (flexibility increase with temperature)
- The time of day (the body has greatest flexible between about 2pm and 4pm in the afternoon)
- Restrictive clothing
- The level of hydration

Types of stretches

Not all stretches are the same. They differ in the way they are executed, their effects on the body and their levels of safety. There are two main kinds of stretches - dynamic stretches and static stretches. Dynamic stretching uses controlled muscle contraction to generate continuous swinging or to-and-fro movements to take a joint through its stiffness barrier. Dynamic stretching is often just a slowed down movement, mimicking the same kinds action used in a particular sport, and it is commonly used as a warm up exercise for the sport. The amplitude and speed of the movement is gradually increased until the joint reaches the limits of its range of movement. Leg swings and arm circles are examples of dynamic stretches.

When dynamic stretching incorporates the momentum of a body part and a bounce at the end of the range to move through stiffness, this is known as ballistic movement or ballistic stretching. Dynamic and ballistic stretches both involve muscle contraction and relatively fast movement to push through the stretch reflex, the body's automatic protection mechanism to overstretching, whereas ballistic stretching with its use of momentum and the bouncing action is less controlled.

In contrast to dynamic stretches, static stretches use slow progressive ratchet-like movement, often combined with breathing with the body part held in a fixed position during the inhalation and moves into the stretch on the exhalation. Although dynamic stretching is commonly used in aerobic classes, gymnastics and by sports training professionals there are dangers associated with this type of stretching, especially the ballistic stretching. Dynamic stretching pushes the body part through the stretch reflex and can cause micro-trauma to muscles, ligaments, tendons and intervertebral discs, and sometimes there can be serious damage to the tissues if the movement is done forcefully. This book places a great deal of emphasis on safety, and as a result only static stretches are covered. Many of the static stretches described in this book can however be done as dynamic stretches.

There are three main kinds of static stretches:

- Active stretches
- Passive stretches
- Post-isometric stretches

Active stretches are done when the person doing the stretch uses their own muscle contraction to overcome the resistance offered by a muscle or muscles on the opposite side of the limb or the opposite side of the spine. Passive stretches are done when the person doing the stretch uses one limb to stretch another limb or body part, or when one person holding the limb or body part moves it while the other person relaxes. Post-isometric stretches are done by first contracting the muscle that you intend to stretch - but not allowing any movement, and then after it has been allowed to relax for a couple of seconds introducing movement which produces the stretch. Post-isometric stretches are also known as proprioceptive neuromuscular facilitation or PNF stretches.

During all types of static stretching, a muscle or group of muscles is stretched by slowly moving the limb or body part into a position and then holding the position for a short period of time. When a movement is slow and the muscle being stretched is relaxed there is resistance offered by the elasticity of the muscle or ligament but there is less reaction from the muscle being stretched. Within every muscle, running parallel with each muscle fibre is a muscle spindle, a sensory receptor which gives the brain information about muscle length to prevent damage. When triggered the muscle spindle will cause the muscle to contract and any further stretching will be strongly resisted by the muscle. This is the stretch reflex. When any movement or stretch is done too quickly we can activate the stretch reflex, which causes the muscle being stretched to contract and shorten, rather than stretch and lengthen. We need to bypass or reduce the full effect of the muscle spindle by combining breathing with slow controlled movement.

Muscle injury may occur when a strong stretch reflex is activated during stretching. High levels of tension are generated within the muscle as the fibres contract and are stretched at the same time. One goal of stretching is to lengthen muscle fibres and stretching is optimal when the muscle is relaxed. The faster a muscle is stretched the higher the stretch reflex. More muscle cells are made to contract as greater numbers of muscle spindles trigger a stretch reflex. It is advantageous therefore to stretch as slowly as is practical.

Although one of the main goals of stretching is to increase and then maintain an optimum level of flexibility within a reasonable time frame, it is important not to rush the stretch because initiating the stretch reflex will be counterproductive.

There are three main advantages of active stretching:

- It stretches muscles on one side of the body/limb
- It strengthens muscles on the other side of the body/limb, thereby increasing muscle tone, which is important for maintaining good posture
- It decreases muscle tension in both the stretched and strengthened muscles

The disadvantage of active stretching is it does not take the joint through as great a range of movement as passive stretching. Of the three main types of stretching techniques, active stretching is the most useful for developing muscle strength.

Medical conditions requiring caution

If this is your first attempt at stretching or if you have not stretched for a while, then go lightly. There are huge benefits from simply taking your joints through a normal range of movement. Just moving to the end of a comfortable range and without stretching. Many of the stretches in this book can be done as simple movements and this is recommended for people recovering from illness or who are eldery.

Joint degeneration, hypomobility and hypermobility

Joint degeneration is synonymous with ageing and hypomobility. It is an important cause of hypomobility, which may lead to a gradual overall stiffness or a combination of hypomobility and hypermobility. When a joint or several joints are hypomobile, forceful stretching may result in hypermobility, as the body attempts to maintain a similar degree of overall flexibility. Stretching should avoid causing or exaggerating joint hypermobility. If stretching exaggerates movement in hypermobile areas of your spine, then you need reduce the intensity of the stretching and focus on stretching the areas of restriction.

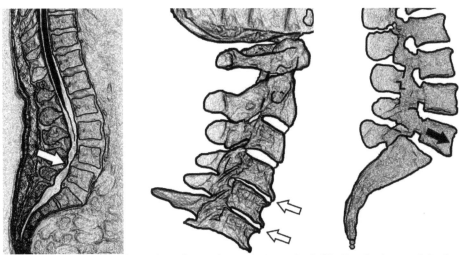

Pathologies affecting the spine: Central canal stenosis (left), Cervical spondylosis or osteoarthritis (middle) and Spondylolisthesis or a pars defect (right)

Osteoarthritis

Osteoarthritis is a form of joint disease or degeneration involving inflammation of one or more joints. It can occur as a result of trauma to a joint, including minor trauma such as lifting a load that is too heavy, infection in a joint, secondary compensations from another joint, genetic factors and natural ageing processes. It is most commonly found in the weight bearing joints such as the hips and knees, and in the lower lumbar and lower cervical spine. With osteoarthritis the protective cartilage that cushions the ends of bones wears down, causing swelling, pain and the development of osteophytes, or bone spurs, all of which result in the localised reduction in the range of movement of the joints affected.

Stretching is an important way of helping to prevent osteoarthritis. It produces periodic loading and unloading of the cartilage which stimulates the water content and health of the cartilage, and it stimulates the movement of synovial fluid within the joint thus nourishing the cartilage, and it may also help with maintaining the synovial fluid chemical composition.

With osteoarthritis there is localised structural damage and permanent loss of movement. Over time the body normally tries to compensate for this loss of movement by increasing movement in adjacent joints. Stretching can be useful for easing muscle and joint pain associated with osteoarthritis but it is important not to force movement when there is osteoarthritis because it may exaggerate the compensatory mobility and lead to hypermobility in the adjacent joints. The same is true for pre-existing congenital problems or other joint diseases such as rheumatoid arthritis and psoriatic arthritis.

Central canal stenosis

Central canal stenosis is a narrowing of the space within the spinal column as a result of degenerative changes in the intervertebral discs or bony vertebral changes from osteoarthritis or other arthritides, impacting on the canal containing the spinal cord. Bilateral symptoms such as burning in the feet are common. Flexion helps remove or reduces the symptoms in some case of central canal stenosis. Flexion may be combined with sidebending or rotation. Central canal stenosis may also be caused by spinal tumours and normal ageing processes.

Spondylolisthesis (Pars defect)

A spondylolisthesis is a break in a vertebra, causing the body the vertebra to slide forwards in varying degrees of severity. The break is usually at L5 vertebra but may be at L4 or rarely at any level in the spine. Abdominal strengthening exercises may be beneficial for a pars defect at L4 or L5 if there is an increased lumbosacral angle or lordosis and weak abdominal muscles. This may be combined with lumbar sidebending stretches for creating a better balance in muscle tone between the front of the body and the back. Keep the lumbar in neutral or slight flexion when doing the sidebending stretching and avoid lumbar extension, especially at the lumbosacral junction.

Over activity and under activity

A large percentage of muscle and joint problems arise from under-activity, and in stark contrast, another large percentage of muscle and joint problems arise from over-activity or faulty activity. Sometimes both under-activity and over-activity occur together. It is not uncommon for a person with a predominantly sedentary job and lifestyle to engage in bursts of high impact activities such as jogging, jumping weight training and high intensity sports. Alternating between long periods of under-use and short periods of overuse where joints are subject to intense loading and unloading can result in microtrauma to joints and soft tissues.

Under-activity includes prolonged sitting and a sedentary lifestyle in general, bed rest as a result of illness or injury, immobilisation and prolonged external strapping. Over-activity and faulty activity includes repetitive activities, faulty exercise, over-exercise, contact sports, extreme martial arts, dangerous sports and the wrong kind of movements in general.

Under-activity can cause contracture and shortness of muscles, fasciae, ligament and joint capsules, adhesions between the synovial folds, atrophy of cartilage and local osteoporosis. It can also result in ligament and muscle weakness. Joints subjected to continuous loading can also have adverse effects to the surrounding tissues including weakness and microfailure in tendons and ligaments, degenerative changes in cartilage, and fibrous changes in muscles.

Stiffness and inactivity are cyclic and feed off each other. A sedentary lifestyle and a lack of movement causes muscle stiffness. Stiffness leads to disuse, which leads to weakness, more stiffness and inactivity, and so on in a descending spiral. This inactivity spiral eventually melds with genetic factors potentially leading to permanent degenerative changes in muscles and joints. Stretching helps counter the effects of a sedentary lifestyle and slows joint degeneration and ageing. A good long-term goal is to maintain your range of motion as long as possible.

Immobilisation affects muscles in a variety of ways depending on the muscle, the duration and whether it is immobilised in a shortened or lengthened state. A muscle immobilised in a shortened state will show a reduction in the contractile component and an increase in the non-contractile component plus a general loss of overall muscle size and a decrease in functionality, especially with respect to being able to generate tension. The muscle will adapt to its shortened state with resistance to passive and active lengthening and loss of joint range of movement.

Ligamentous creep, a long-lasting elongation of vital stabilising ligaments can begin after only 30 minutes in a fixed position, so it is good to change your postures frequently, by taking short walks and short exercise breaks throughout the day to help prevent this creep, as well as longer walks and longer exercise periods to promote general fitness. Use resistance and combinations of isometric and isotonic concentric and eccentric exercises in different directions to improve the strength in muscles and ligaments.

Mobility in terms of active and passive range of movement varies between individuals and depends on:

a) Body shape – small, tall, stocky and thin (genetic).
b) Ligament laxity – hypomobility, average or hypermobility (genetic).
c) Age
d) Wear and tear of joints.
e) Posture - tends to be exaggerated with time (developmental).
f) Diseases such as osteoarthritis, ankylosing spondylitis, rheumatoid arthritis, past fractures.
g) Unique variation in structure
h) Surgery
i) History of activity or lack of it during work and recreation

Gravity, psychoemotional factors, patterns of misuse and overuse, tissue changes due to ageing or disease often combine to produce changes in the structure of the tissues. Also maladaptation as we evolved to bipedalism from quadrupedalism is often cited as a factor in influencing our structures. These can lay down the conditions for faulty use patterns to develop within the body. Mild daily activities might not result in obvious signs or symptoms of structural weaknesses, only when the body is stressed or taken to the limits of exercise will it develop problems such as pain. An activity such as a competitive sport might be the trigger to accelerate structural breakdown.

Part 2. Practical aspects of stretching

How to use this book

If you are not familiar with a stretch or it is your first time doing a stretch then first read the entire description and use the photographs to complement your understanding of the technique. Do not rely on the photographs alone. When you have an overall appreciation of the stretch then follow the bullet points consecutively. Use the anatomical diagrams to get a better knowledge of which muscles you are stretching and the direction of the stretch.

If you are familiar with a stretch but this is your first time using this book I recommend reading through the bullet points and making sure you have not overlooked something or developed any bad habits. If there is a more advanced version of the stretch, do the basic version first to established good technique. Do not jump to the advanced version first. Sometimes working through the basic version of the stretch will give you fresh insights. Read the description and use the supporting photographs.

Although you may have less flexibility or greater flexibility than the person in the photograph, the purpose of the photograph is to show you the basic elements of the stretch. Do not just copy the person in the photograph. Focus on your own body and stretch according to your unique needs. If for example the person in the photograph is doing a forward bend and their hamstring flexibility enables them to bring their head to their knees, this may be fine for them but may not be appropriate for you. Each technique informs you which muscle or muscles should be targeted. Work within you own limitations and do not try and mimic exactly the movements of another person. Similarly with stretching classes, do not compare yourself with the person next to you. They may have a genetic advantage or they may have been stretching since they were very young.

If you are stretching at home make sure there are no distractions that will interfere with your concentration. Turn off the television and your mobile phone. If you have children make sure they have someone supervising them or they are engaged in an activity in another part of the house so that they will not disturb you. Similarly if you have pets make sure they remain in the garden or another part of the house while you stretch. You will not be able to concentrate on stretching if you have a child or dog climbing all over you. Make sure you empty your bladder and bowel before stretching. Wear clothing that permits easy movement such as a track suit top and pants, tights, leotard or bathing costume.

Is stretching safe?

Stretching is generally one of the safest forms or exercise, especially when compared with sports which have a high level of body contact. But with any exercise there are no absolute guarantees of safety, there are only probabilities. The purpose of this book is to encourage stretching but to also highlight when a stretch has potential problems. A stretch may be contraindicated when an injury or joint disease is present or for someone who is congenitally hypermobile, or for someone over 50 years, or a variety of other reasons.

Safe Stretch contains many stretching exercises. Some are safer than others, but no stretch is completely risk free. When you are applying physical stresses to the body, you are challenging the body's tissues. You are helping the tissues to become stronger but you are also placing a greater demand on the body. If a muscle, tendon or ligament has been weakened by inactivity, injured by overactivity or repetitive activities, or fatigued by gravity then it may be more vulnerable to injury. Injuries do occur during stretching; most of the dangers associated with stretching occur when the joints are taken to extreme ranges of motion. Precautions need to be taken to prevent this.

A stretch may be safe when done correctly but unsafe when done incorrectly. *Safe Stretch* clearly describes how the individual stretches should be done and highlights if there are potential problems with certain exercises. For example in the post-isometric techniques 1.7g and 1.7h, the bullet point says, 'Do not pull on the head'. This is a safe technique if you don't pull on the head, but people continue to strain muscles and sprain ligaments in their neck because they have not been warned of the dangers.

Props used in stretching

The floor
The use of a high density foam mat on the floor will make stretching more comfortable. Get one that does not slip and is firm. If you do not have access to a mat, lying on a carpet may be more comfortable than doing the stretches on a wooden floor.

A chair
A chair is useful for supporting the body or maintaining balance when doing a stretch standing, as a platform for the buttock bones and to keep the spine straight when doing a stretch seated. It is also used to increase internal and external rotation in the hips.

The best way to maintain an upright sitting position when seated is by tilting the top of your pelvis forward and holding it in this position while balancing the weight of your upper body over your sit bones (ischial tuberosites). Alternatively, use a chair with a lumbar back support to keep the pelvis and spine vertical.

A wall
A wall is useful for support, keeping the spine or body straight and vertical, as a reference point and as an unyielding object.

Rolled towel
Have a rolled up towel available for lying over to extend the thoracic spine during some of the stretching exercises. Also have a strap, belt or small towel available, which may be grasped at one end and used for pulling into a stretch, particularly if you are not very flexible.

Daily considerations when stretching

Warming up in the morning
Warming up is the process of raising your core body temperature – perhaps by as much as one or two degrees Celsius. On awakening in the morning, warm up with a hot shower or some activity before you start stretching. A good warming up activity might be simple rotation movements of the joints but within their normal range of movement or cleaning around the house for five or ten minutes. Go for a short walk or run. Give yourself time to wake up. Perhaps have a hot drink without milk for easier digestion. Don't push your body too hard first thing in the morning. If the outside temperature is especially cold or you are very stiff then you should pay even greater attention to warming up before you stretch.

Evening stretching
Soft tissue flexibility increases with temperature and use. In the evening the body is warmer, stretching will be easier and you can push your body a bit harder. Think of the morning stretch as a wake up stretch and think of the evening stretch as a developmental stretch where you can increase flexibility. But don't overstretch if you have already achieved an adequate level of flexibility.

Stretches for different situations
a) The warm up stretch
This is best for relieving tension or postural fatigue or as a warm up before sport or first thing in the morning. The warm up stretch is done with light force and maybe done once or twice on each side.

b) The maintenance stretch
This is useful for the maintenance of flexibility. Use a moderate force. A muscle or group of muscles should be stretched at least twice a day.

c) The developmental stretch

To increase the length of a muscle, a developmental stretch may be used. Greater force can be applied. The stretch can be done up to five times.

Food

Do not eat before stretching. Stretching can be done with food in the stomach but it is better done on an empty stomach. Ideally allow an hour after a snack or three hours after a large meal before stretching. How long you wait before you start stretching depends on what you have eaten, how much you have eaten and how long ago you have eaten. It also depends on how long and hard you wish to stretch. An intense session of stretching is not recommended after a meal. However a mild 5 minute stretch can be done almost any time of day.

There are two main problems with combining stretching and digesting food. Firstly during digestion, blood is directed to the gut by the nervous system to digest food and there is therefore less blood available for the muscle. Stretching involves muscle contraction and the competition between the muscle and the gut for blood can lead to poor digestion and cause problems in the muscle such as cramping. Secondly there is the problem of the mass of food in the stomach causing mechanical pressure and strain to the abdominal wall and other organs, especially in stretches involving forward bending.

Eating is less of a problem for stretching than it is for weight training or aerobic exercises such as running, which involves strong muscle contraction but muscle problems are possible if stretching is done on a full stomach.

Stretching routine

Develop a regular routine of safe stretching. It can be 10, 20 or 30 minutes or one hour and it can be once or twice daily. It can be every day or every other day. Never drop your stretching routine below ten minutes twice a week.

If you don't want to or can't adopt a regular routine because you are too busy, or have an unstructured life, or you just can't follow a routine, then stretch when you can. A short stretch can be done almost any time of day. Stretching can range from a couple of minutes 'quick stretch' to a one hour workout. If you are in a hurry, or if you just want to quickly ease tension, or if you have to wait for something, or if you have time to kill then a couple of minutes of stretching is fine. But if you are an athlete or have a particular goal to reach then up to an hour of stretching may be needed.

How much you stretch in one session may vary and will depend on how tight your muscles are and how much time you have available.

If you are already flexible either because you are genetically very flexible or because you have achieved it through hard work, it may be necessary to keep stretching to maintain flexibility and for warming up before exercise - but do not overstretch.

The order of stretching muscles

Stretching is safest if the stretches are done in the right order. Commonly, a stretching exercise stretches more than one muscle. The stretch targets a primary muscle but also stretches several secondary muscles or synergists. Sometime the secondary muscles will be so tight the person feels the secondary muscles being stretched before they feel the primary muscles. If the stretch isn't stretching the right muscles then there may be problems. The secondary muscles may be vulnerable to injury.

The secondary muscles should not be allowed to become the main barrier to the movement. If this is the case, then it is important to stretch the secondary muscles first. For example if a stretch for the hamstrings pulls on the lower back muscles before the hamstrings, then it is important to stretch the lower back muscles with a sidebending stretch to loosen them up before stretching the hamstrings. Stretch the lower back muscles with sidebending before attempting flexion at the hip to help prevent ligament sprains in the lumbar and sacroiliac joints.

Here are some rules about the best order to do stretching, with 1 being the most important and 8 the least:

1. Stretch the lower back muscles with sidebending before stretching other muscles such as the hamstrings and adductors.
2. Stretch the lower back muscles with sidebending before attempting flexion or extension at the hip.
3. Stretch the shoulder muscles such as trapezius and levator scapula before stretching the cervical muscles.
4. Warm up before stretching the cervical spine particularly first thing in the morning.
5. Stretch the pectoralis major before attempting shoulder abduction stretches such as the hanging stretches.
6. Stretch your hip abductor muscles after stretching your back and before stretching other lower limb muscles.
7. Stretch your gluteus maximus before stretching your iliopsoas or hamstrings.
8. Stretch your calves before stretching your hamstrings.

Pain during stretching

Stretching some muscles may be painful. Stretching the hamstrings is nearly always painful because the sciatic nerve passes along its length in the posterior part of the thigh. Stretching the calf muscles is painful if the muscles are very tight but the pain diminishes as the muscles get longer with regular stretching. The most painful stretch of all is the combined hamstring and calf stretch of the 'lower dog' stretch. Again this is because the sciatic nerve is under maximal stretch. Other muscles may be painful when stretched but this is a 'good pain' and should not be considered pathological.

Other tissues affected by stretching

Stretching exercises stretch and compress muscles, ligaments, cartilage, nerves, blood vessels, glands and organs. Compression and stretching moves fluids around and within the tissues, thereby facilitating cellular exchange.

Stretching can increase strength and endurance. This is particularly true for active stretching where muscles are used to stretch their antagonists, and to a lesser extent post-isometric stretching, where isometric contraction is used prior to stretching and to a much lesser extent during passive stretching where one limb or body part is used to stretch another limb or body part.

Muscle pain after exercise

Use light stretches for muscle soreness after a heavy exercise workout. Focus on stretching the muscles that have been contracted most during the exercise, which are usually the same muscles that are sore.

Injury

When muscles become tight and short, this increases the chances of injury. Common injuries include tennis elbow, rotator cuff tendon tears, wrist tendonitis and muscle strains, particularly in the hamstrings, quadriceps and calf muscles.

There are many causes of sports injuries including poor technique, overuse, direct impact, overloading of muscles and joints and structural abnormalities such as short muscles. Research has clearly demonstrated a strong correlation between chronically short muscles and injury. Stretching is a useful way of lenthening these short muscles and for correcting muscle imbalances. For example short hamstrings may lead to a hamstring strain and lower back injury, and short pectoralis major muscles may lead to a rotator cuff injury. Inflexibility is not good and regular stretching clearly helps reduce the probablility of some injuries.

But research also indicates that static stretching immediately before high demanding sports events does not reduce sports injuries and in fact may increase them. The reasoning is that static stretching interferes with the stretch reflex, desensitising the muscle spindle, thereby weakening muscle and decreasing the amount of force it can produce. It is also argued that for a period of time after stretching, the muscle doesn't have much strength because the actin-myosin filaments of the muscle fibres are pulled so far apart they cannot form enough cross-bridges to produce a strong contraction. This may especially be a problem for power sports such as jumping, sprinting and skating.

Researchers also argue that static stretching has a pain-relieving effect, masking pain that may serve as a warning to stop the activity before injury occurs. Others also claim stretching after a vigorous sports activity doesn't reduce soreness in muscles the next day. They reason that delayed onset muscle soreness is caused by micro-tearing in the muscle and that only rest and time will repair the damage. It is known that strong muscle contraction and strong stretching can both cause micro-tearing. It is therefore likely that strong stretching immediately after vigorous exercise would make muscle soreness worse. But it is my opinion that a light stretch may have some benefit.

Evidence suggests that initially after stretching a muscle is weaker, and a consensus is gradually emerging that static stretching should not be used prior to a competitive event. Clearly, stretching has benefits when done by athletes well before events. But there is no consensus about how soon before an event the static stretching should cease. It may depend on the type of sport and the intensity of the stretching. Power sports are likely to be the most vulnerable because they require the most explosive muscle contractions. It may take minutes for a muscle to recover after a light stretch and it may take days for a muscle to recover and adapt after a strong developmental type stretch.

The mechanism for the theory that static stretching causes weakness is based on the sliding filament theory of muscle contraction. According to this theory the actin-myosin filaments are pulled so far apart during passive stretching that they are unable to form enough cross-bonds for a strong contraction. While this may be true over the shorter term, over longer periods of time a stretched muscle will adapt to its new length, forming new cross-bonds and the longer muscle is likely to be as strong as or stronger than before.

Static stretching has an important role in producing and maintaining flexibility and preventing injury. But it needs to be done at the right time. If top performance for a major sporting event is required then static stretching should clearly be done well before the sporting event. The goal of stretching should be optimum flexibility, combined with strengthening for stability. Correct warming up before high level sport should involve activities that use controlled movement over a full range, including dynamic stretching. These will improve coordination, muscle response, reduce post-exercise pain levels and reduce injuries.

The barrier concept

A barrier is an obstruction that restricts free movement in a joint in the body and can be a normal or abnormal barrier. Types of normal barrier include the anatomical barrier, which is the total range of movement that can be produced in a joint; the elastic barrier, which is the range that passive movement can produce; the physiological barrier, which is the range that active movement can produce. An abnormal barrier is a pathological barrier that may occur within the limits of motion at any joint. An abnormal barrier occurs when there is restricted movement due to structural changes in muscle, fasciae, ligament, joint capsule and skin, as well as localised oedema, osteophytes or due to the effects of pain.

The anatomical barrier is an absolute non-negotiable barrier such as a bone or ligament that serves as the final limit to motion in a joint, beyond which tissue damage occurs. The physiological barrier is a soft tissue tension that limits the voluntary motion of a joint. Further motion to the elastic barrier can be done passively but the physiological barrier is the limit of active motion.

Active motion is movement of a joint by the muscles around that joint to the physiological barrier and is limited to the range that can be produced voluntarily. Passive motion is movement induced in a joint using another body part, usually an upper limb, gravity or another person, while the muscles around the joint being moved are relaxed.

Passive movement is always greater than active movement. Active stretching can increase movement up to the physiological barrier and passive stretching can increase movement up to the elastic barrier. In general, during active stretching, muscle and joint protection mechanisms will not let the joint go beyond its barrier, whereas during passive stretching weaker protection mechanisms and a greater potential for the use of excessive force means that the joint can be forced beyond its barrier.

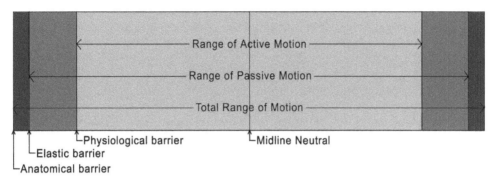

Range of movement at a joint

The stretching process and the outcome will depend on whether we are stretching to a normal barrier or through an abnormal barrier to a normal barrier. Most of the time stretching involves lengthening a short muscle to enable the joint it moves, to move to its normal barrier, either to move actively to its physiological barrier or to be moved passively to its elastic barrier.

If the muscle is healthy it may be short because it is tense or has been in a prolonged shortened state. Mild stretching is usually required to return this muscle to its natural length so that the normal barrier of the joint it controls is positioned an optimal point along its range, and is neither hypomobile nor hypermobile.

If restricted movement is due to muscle (or fascial) shortness from muscle scarring after previous trauma or fibrosis after years of postural fatigue then these structural changes will have to be fixed, either with myofascial manipulation (massage) or with stretching, and the stretching technique will need to be modified to take into account the unique structural changes in the muscle.

If restricted movement is due ligament scarring after previous trauma or damage to other articular tissues or there is an underlying systemic problem affecting the joint then these structural changes will have to be fixed with manual therapy before addressing the adaptive muscle shortness with stretching. Joint restrictions caused by structural changes in joints will benefit from stretching but there is no guarantee that stretching alone will fix these types of problem.

If there is an abnormal barrier with pathology we need to approach stretching more cautiously than if the tissues are healthy. Over-enthusiastic stretching too soon after trauma may prolong recovery and make the tissue damage worse. In acute situations an appropriate rest period is required, ranging from hours to days, depending on the severity of the problem. It is advisable to start with light stretching after the acute phase has peaked and progress towards stronger stretching and other forms of rehabilitation exercise as the condition improves. Over-enthusiastic stretching can even cause damage when the problem is chronic. Once again, an incremental approach to stretching is advised, starting slowly and increasing the stretching as the problem gets better.

The quality, range and end feel at the very end of the available range of movement can all provide useful information to the person stretching provided it can be perceived and they know how to interpret it. Body awareness is a skill that can reveal a great deal about the nature of the muscle or joint, especially if various pathologies exist.

Healthy joint movement (and muscle extensibility) is smooth, free, natural and silent, there is optimal range. If a muscle limits movement then the end feel is firm but slightly bouncy whereas if the joint capsule limits movement and there is normal tissue approximation, the end feel is firm but soft.

Short tense (hypertonic) muscles have good quality of movement but there is an increase in resistance offered by the muscle before the expected end of the range. As the barrier releases during a stretch, the person stretching may feel a softening of the tissue and an increase in motion. With extremely short hypertonic muscles, the end feel will be a tight and there may be a tugging sensation but the barrier will move with repeated stretching.

Fibrous or scarred muscles have undergone structural changes and there will be greater resistance to stretching than with hypertonic muscle. Fibrous muscle or scarring is less elastic and there is a firm hard end feel to the muscle. With muscle spasm, contracture or spasticity movement is abrupt, rubbery and may be painful. There may be extreme loss of range of movement due to high levels of muscle tightness and stiffness. There may be a muscle reflex reaction if the muscle is stretched too briskly.

Hypermobile joints with ligament laxity will feel loose and move further than expected. There may be a rapidly increasing harder end feel to the joint. The joint will tend to more easily cavitate or make an audible popping sound as the joint surfaces separate at the end of the range of movement.

Loss of cartilage will result in bone moving on bone or osteoarthritis. There will be reduced range of movement, especially in some directions, poor quality movement involving crepitus, a crackling, grating feeling or sound in the joint. The end feel is solid and may be painful. Swelling or oedema usually results in reduced range of movement due to the internal pressure of fluid within the joint. There is a soft, diffuse and boggy end feel to the joint.

Pain from muscle or joint pathology may affect the quality, range or end feel of a joint. Pain can create a joint barrier and it may elicit movement away from the source of the pain. Psychological factors can create a joint barrier which restricts movement.

Biomechanical factors

Force and speed
Force combined with speed multiplies the effect on the stretch reflex. Ballistic and fast dynamic stretches activate the stretch reflex the most and for this reason, they are potentially the most dangerous of all the stretching techniques. The dynamic yoga asana salute to the sun and many aerobic movements fall into this category.

Levers
The longer the lever action of a bone and the more power that is exerted by the person stretching the greater the force generated. There are many long lever stretches including: technique 2.1, 2.4, 2.6b, 2.8, 2.9, 3.0a, 3.1a, 4.0e, f and g 4.9, 5.1, 5.2, 5.7, 5.8, 6.0, 6.1, 6.2. 6.3, 6.4, 6.5, 6.6, 6.7, 6.9 and 7.1. Long lever stretches are not dangerous if done correctly but they are potentially dangerous because the lever amplifies the forces. Most problems arise when a long lever combines with: a powerful muscle, high speed, large amplitude and gravity, which tends to overwhelm the weaker muscles and ligaments.

Gravity
The influence of gravity on a stretch is significant and is frequently underestimated. Gravity has influence on our joints, ligaments, muscles, intervertebral discs and the position of our organs. In addition it affects our circulation and other body fluids. Gravity's downward pull increases the force on some stretches and requires certain muscles to contract to counter its effect on others. The influence of gravity on a stretch depends on the starting position, the direction of movement, and the relation of the body parts to each other as well as to gravity itself.

Optimal stretching

Working against gravity, using short levers and muscles of equal or similar strength to work against each other is generally the safest option when stretching.

When a powerful muscle or muscle group is used to stretch a weaker muscle or muscle group and leverage magnifies the force, there is potential for injury. For example the more powerful hamstring muscles can overwhelm the weaker spinal muscles and ligaments to force the joints in the spine to yield. In people with areas of hypermobility, the hypermobile joints may be subject to overstretching.

Slow movement is the safest way of stretching but practical time considerations means that there is an optimal speed of stretching. Slow active stretching is generally the safest form of stretching because active stretches do not activate the stretch reflex in the same way as passive stretches. In active stretching, there is less danger of joint sprains because the muscles being stretched (antagonists) are usually of similar strength to the muscles being contracted (agonists), and there is less danger of muscle strains because in active stretching, reciprocal inhibition relaxes the muscle being stretched. In active stretching there is more coordination between the agonists and antagonists and joint movement is within its anatomical limits.

In addition to the safety benefits, the active stretching technique also has the advantage of increasing muscle strength because a muscle is contracted against the resistance offered by the muscle and other tissues being stretched.

Speed and duration measured as breaths

Stretching is safest and most effective when done slowly and the best way to measure the time period of the stretch is to synchronise the stretch with the breathing cycle. A slow full inhalation followed by a slow full exhalation takes on average about 15 seconds. Stretch on the exhalation and hold the position on the inhalation. The exhalation stretch phase should take about 10 seconds and the inhalation hold phase should take about five seconds.

In static stretching, movement should progress forwards in one direction - like a ratchet, and it should not go backwards except when you have finished the stretch. It should not swing backwards and forwards - this is dynamic stretching.

Between three and five cycles of breathing and stretching is recommended for each muscle or group of muscles. It is appropriate to stretch one side of the body or limb then stretch the other side of the body, and then repeat the stretch on each side of the body or limb a second time. A second pass through the stretching results in a better outcome than a single one, but after the second pass there is progressively less return for the time and energy put into the stretching. In total one stretch done twice on each side of the body should take about two minutes.

Breathing

Breathe by inhaling slowly through the nose, emphasising the expansion of the abdomen rather than the chest, holding the breath a moment, then exhaling slowly through the nose or mouth. Inhaling through the nose filters, warms and humidifies the air for optimal oxygen transfer in the lungs. Do not force the breathing. The abdomen and diaphragm should remain relaxed and the breathing should be natural.

Breathing is one of the inherent movements of the body. During inhalation the curves of the spine straighten, the limbs externally rotate, and the diaphragm stretches and compresses the heart and internal organs, moving blood around the body and food through the gut. During exhalation the curves of the spine increase, the limbs internally rotate and the elastic recoil of the diaphragm and other muscles of respiration assist with venous and lymphatic return and movement of food through the gut. These rhythmic respiratory pumping actions also helps increase blood flow and remove waste products from the muscles in the body, including the ones you are stretching.

Anger and stretching

Stretching is good for anxiety, depression and reducing muscle tension after stress. But it is not good to stretch if you are angry or unable to maintain mental equilibrium. Safe stretching means being able to focus on the muscle or muscles being stretched. If you have recently been in an argument or extremely stressful situation, regain your composure before starting stretching. Walking, swimming, focusing on a task or doing something positive for ten to twenty minutes is a good way to wind down. Be mindful of your body during stretching, learn to control your ego and try to relax.

The focus during the stretch

During the stretch, focus on the muscle or muscles being stretched, the inhalation and then the exhalation of your breathing, the relative positions of the joints and the overall posture of your body. Awareness of the muscle being stretched is necessary to direct the stretching process efficiently and to prevent injury. Awareness of the breathing is necessary to relax the muscle being stretched and relax the body generally, as a timekeeper for the stretch and to keep your mind focused on the process of stretching. Awareness of the position of the joints and bones is necessary so that the body parts are coordinated, work efficiently and move safely. Awareness of the posture is necessary so the body is stable, steady and well balanced in relation to gravity.

Stretch both sides of the body or both limbs equally. If you have been taught which joints or areas of the body are tight then stretch them more. If you can discern whether one side is tighter than the other, then stretch the tighter side. If you start by stretching the tighter side first and end by stretching the tighter side then you will always stretch the tighter side one more time than the less tight side.

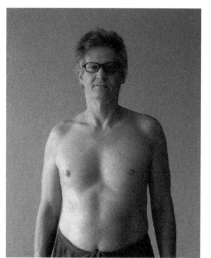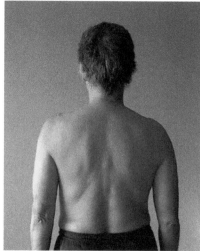

Scoliosis sidebent right with a depressed right shoulder - viewed from the front (left) and viewed from behind (right)

It is easy to see the effects of a scoliosis if we look in the mirror. One shoulder is usually higher than the other. But to appreciate the more subtle nuances of our spine is more difficult. The high shoulder is on the side of the convexity of the primary scoliosis or the highest convexity in the thoracic under the shoulder.

Localised stretches versus complex stretches

Some stretches focus on one joint and stretch a single muscle or small group of muscles, for example the triceps stretch 5.4. In contrast, other stretches are more complex, involve a large number of joints and stretch a combination of muscles, for example the multi shoulder stretch 4.8 for triceps, teres major, teres minor and infraspinatus). In general, there is greater efficiency and the stretching is safer, when you focus on stretching a single muscle or muscle group, and localise the stretch to one joint or a few joints. By limiting the number of actions involved in one stretch, you are better able focus on doing the stretch.

Active, passive and post-isometric systems

Passive stretching works because the muscle being stretched is relaxed during the stretch. Active stretching works because reciprocal inhibition of the antagonist muscle automatically relaxes the muscle during the stretch. Post-isometric stretching works because for a few seconds after the muscle is contracted there is a refractory period where the muscle automatically relaxes.

Post-isometric stretches

Post-isometric stretching is also best done when synchronised with the breathing cycle but the cycle for post-isometric stretching takes a little bit longer than the cycle for active or passive stretching. The isometric muscle contraction is done during the inhalation cycle and the movement is done during the exhalation cycle. But in between the isometric contraction and the movement, there is an additional period of a few seconds to allow the contracting muscle to relax. After a muscle contracts, it needs time to reset itself to do it again and it is during this period that the stretch is achieved.

The optimum length of time for the isometric muscle contraction and the optimum force of the contraction vary between different muscles. A small muscle such as one of the suboccipital muscles, or one or a small group of spinal muscles, generally require a short period of isometric contraction, say two to three seconds and a light force of about 200 grams. Large muscles such as the biceps brachii or rectus femoris, generally require a longer period of isometric contraction, say five to eight seconds and a heavier force of say 1000 grams.

Good localisation requires correct force and joint positioning. Poor positioning and too little force will result in insufficient firing of muscle fibres. Too much force will result in other muscles being recruited and less targeting of the right muscles. For example an isometric spinal sidebending stretch that is too strong or poorly localised may recruit the lateral abdominal muscles, quadratus lumborum, and latissimus dorsi and have negligible effect on lower thoracic erector spinae muscles, when in fact they were the target.

For safe and effective stretching, joints should be positioned correctly. Overstretching is most problematic during passive stretching because one limb or body part is used as a lever to stretch a muscle or group of muscles distant to the limb or body part. Sometimes the forces generated can overwhelm supporting ligaments and over-stretch the muscle or muscles. The start point for the stretch should be well within the ligamentous limit or elastic barrier of the joint. If the individual has generalised congenital ligamentous laxity or localised laxity due to injury or overstretching, then joints will need to be protected and stretching kept within safe limits, well away from the elastic barrier.

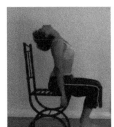 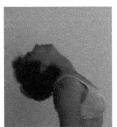 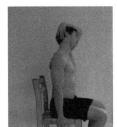 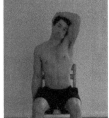

Cervical extension hypermobility   **Cervical sidebending stretches**

If an individual has hypermobility, safe stretching may mean avoiding some stretches, modifying some stretches or exercising greater caution when executing particular stretches. For example in the post-isometric sidebending stretches for the cervical spine 1.7g and 1.7h it is important not to pull on the head when relocalising to the new stretch barrier. The correct method should involve just taking up the slack or tension gained by the isometric muscle contraction.

When someone has generalised hypermobility the effects are usually easy to see in the cervical spine because cervical extension, sidebending and rotation will be greatly increased. At the end of extension the head typically drops backwards beyond the usual 90 degrees and the neck adopts 'swan-like' characteristics, and during sidebending there is kinking in the hypermobile part of the neck. Avoid overstretching hypermobile joints such as these. In the cervical spine this means for example, only partially sidebending the head and neck, and then getting most of the stretch by actively depressing the opposite shoulder.

What is the best way to begin stretching?

If you have never stretched before, start slowly and build up. There may be muscle soreness after the first couple of days, called delayed onset muscle soreness caused by microscopic tearing of the muscle fibres and some inflammation. If this occurs, then stretch the sore muscles again but more lightly. Stretching the sore muscles will hurt but it is useful for its mechanical effect and for stimulating circulation to the muscles. With increasing fitness, the condition will improve and there will be less muscle soreness. Light stretching may help with the pain but the real problem is lack of fitness and overworking muscles that are unable to cope with the type of exercise or sport. It is important to differentiate the pain from overdoing exercise with the pain caused by injury. Stretching is contraindicated in the first 24 hours after injury. Professional advice and a measured stretching program may be necessary if the injury is serious.

Injuries

If you have previously injured a muscle, ligament or tendon, any stretching of the injured area should be approached with caution or avoided. You don't have to give up stretching altogether. Just avoid the injured area and stretch the rest of the body. Get a good diagnosis of the problem and then get it fixed.

Some stretches may be contraindicated for certain problems. For example, overhead arm stretches commonly aggravate rotator cuff strains or subacromial bursitis, and lumbar backward bends may aggravate ligament sprains, and spondylolisthesis in the lower back.

Overstretching

Natural limits to movement must be respected if you are to stretch safely. The most important of these is the elastic tension of ligaments. Other factors include the elastic tension from muscles and their voluntary and involuntary contraction; the approximation of body parts; synovial fluid and internal pressure holding joint surfaces together and the effects of gravity.

Joint are more stable and better protected against injury when they are in a close-packed position. The close-packed position is useful when you need to hold a joint in a fixed position during stretching. Sometime close packing is applied to joints associated with the muscles that need stretching and sometimes it used for joints that need to remain stable for supporting the rest of the body during the stretching exercises.

The close-packed position varies in different areas of the body but it is usually at one end of a joints range of movement. It involves maximal congruence of bony surfaces, as well as maximal capsular and ligamentous tension and stability. The close-packed position in the: shoulder is abduction and internal rotation; hip is extension and medial rotation; ankle is dorsiflexion; spine is flexion; and in the elbow, wrist and knee it is when the joint is in extension. In contrast, the least-packed position in the: shoulder is partial abduction; ankle is neutral; spine is neutral; and in the elbow, wrist, hip and knee it is when the joint is in partial flexion. The sacroiliac joint is close-packed in neutral when standing and least-packed in flexion when sitting.

Some muscles and joints are more vulnerable to overstretching than others, for example the shoulder joints, sacroiliac joints and the joints of the suboccipital, cervical and thoracolumbar spine. Some joints are more vulnerable to overstretching and injury in certain directions, for example the shoulder in abduction, and the thoracolumbar and atlanto-occipital joints in extension. Some joints are more vulnerable to overstretching when there is a combination of movements and influencing factors, for example the sacroiliac joints are more vulnerable when lumbar flexion and sacral counter-nutation (extension) are combined with rotation and sidebending and the person is sitting.

Passive stretches are more likely to over-stretch than active stretches, and passive stretches that use strong muscle contraction, a lot of body weight (gravity) and long levers to stretch relatively weak muscles are usually the most problematic. The list is extensive and includes some of the stretches in this book for example the hanging passive stretch, the flexed cat standing and the scapula retractor stretch and a large number of yoga asanas including Dhanurasana (bow) Urdhva Dhanurasana (crab/wheel), Ustrasana (camel) Bhujangasana (cobra), Sarvangasana (shoulder stand) Halasana (plough), Uttanasana (standing forward bend) and most of the sitting forward bends.

Joint disease and surgery involving joint fusion or replacement with an artifical joint increase localised stiffness. Over zealous stretching can be a problem when there are extreme levels of joint stiffness. Before attempting stretching, know which areas of your spine are hypermobile and need to be protected, and which areas are restricted and need to be stretched. Movement of the spine during a stretch should be even and distributed over the whole spine. A good exercise program should differentiate between stretching and overstretching or straining.

When you stretch a muscle it is not just the actual muscle fibre that is being lengthened but also the fasciae, the connective tissues that surround the muscle, as well as the fasciae that connects the muscle to the bone. The connective tissues make up about one third of the muscle and when we stretch a muscle a large proportion of the stretch occurs in the connective tissues. With too much stretching, connective tissues loses its elasticity or its ability to return to its original resting length. When this occurs, the connective tissues loses its role supporting the muscle and its associated nerves and blood vessels.

Rest

Once a week, take a day off from stretching and do something else or rest completely. It is a good idea to give the muscles a rest from the same routine. One day of rest will not result in previous levels of stiffness returning. Quite the contrary, rest allows your muscles to relax and rejuvenate, and then stretching is usually easier the next day.

Stretching relaxes and lengthens short tight muscles but too much stretching causes muscle fatigue and micro-tearing. Over time there is progressively less benefit from ongoing stretching and it becomes counterproductive. Instead of relaxing and lengthening, the muscles become tighter. Although there are benefits to resting muscles after stretching, too much resting may also be counterproductive.

One day of rest every week is recommended but calculating the ratio of rest to exercise depends on several factors, including the person's level of fitness and the combination of stretching with other types of exercise and sports. The most important factor influencing the rest period is the intensity of prior stretching. The stronger the stretch, the greater the level of micro-tearing; the more micro-tearing the longer the rest period will have to be. Micro-tearing will cause the muscle fibres to grow back in a slightly longer state. Micro-tearing is a normal part of the process of developmental stretching and also occurs during vigorous exercises involving strong muscle contraction, hence should not be considered problematic. It is important to realise that the muscle may be sore and it will need to be given time to recover. Light stretching or complete rest may be necessary until the pain in the muscle has gone.

What should you stretch?

When stretching it is important to know what you are stretching and why. Stretching does two simultaneous things: it elongates muscles, including their associated fasciae and it elongates the ligaments that surround the joint. It has been stressed repeatedly throughout this introduction that you should always stretch the area or areas in the body that are most restricted. But when stretching it is important to know which tissue or tissues are restricted - ligament, muscle or fasciae. As it is very difficult to examine oneself, especially the spine, this will usually require an external assessment by in manual therapist. Once an accurate assessment has been made stretch or treat the joint stiffness (hypomobility) first and then stretch the overlying short muscles and fasciae.

The tighter the muscles the more often it should be stretched, and within limits of safety, the harder it should be stretched. Muscles that are less tight may also benefit from being stretched, for example to relieve tension. You should be careful when stretching muscles associated with hypermobile joints not to overstretch the ligaments protecting that joint. By stretching a variety of different muscle groups, you will improve overall flexibility but targeted stretching is better for increasing flexibility where it is needed most. By focusing on the areas of greatest joint stiffness and muscle shortness with a well-balanced exercise programme, you are creating an even level of flexibility throughout the body.

The range of joint movement is determined by the anatomy of the body, and you should not expect to be more mobile than anatomical limits will allow. But it is important to reduce joint stiffness where it is greatest. Each joint and each area of the body has an optimum level of mobility. Flexibility can be measured in 'absolute' terms where a minimum range of movement exists for each joint and where one person's body is compared with all the other people in the world; or it can be measured in 'relative' terms, where one joint is compared just with all the other joints within their body.

Exaggerations in posture, short tight muscles, muscle weakness, vulnerable areas of the body may predispose people to developing structure problems. Greater emphasis should be placed on stretching to correct bad posture, or lengthen short muscles and strengthen weak muscles overlying vulnerable joints.

If muscles are very tight you may need to stretch them more often than once a day. Very tight hamstrings for example should be stretched every two hours until they are at a safe length and level of flexibility. Tight hamstrings contribute to repeated lower back strains and sprains by restricting pelvic movement and forcing greater lumbar and sacroiliac movement.

Stocky hypomobile people who begin stretching for the first time will generally find stretching hard because of the thickness and shape of their bones and joints, as well as the tightness of their muscles and ligaments. They will have higher levels of joint stability, which will mean a lower probability of developing localised hypermobility and injury from overstretching.

Skinny hypermobile people who begin stretching for the first time will generally find stretching easy because of the fineness of their bones and joints, and the elasticity of their muscles and ligaments. They will have higher levels of joint instability, which will mean more chance of developing localised hypermobility and a higher probability of injury from overstretching.

Joints which have been fused by surgery or become fused by degeneration have no mobilty and have the potential to cause hypermobility in adjacent joints, hence caution should be taken when stretching these areas. Longitudinal stretches are good because they create less sidebending angulation, hence there is less chance of overstretching a hypermobile joint or causing hypermobility. Use stretches 2.3, 2.4a, 2.4b, 3.7, 3.8, and 3.9. Active stretches are good, especially when done against gravity because there is less probability of overstretching and they strengthen the antagonist muscles. Use 1.3a, 2.7a, 3.0c, 3.1b, 4.0d and 7.5a.

Know your body

Before attempting any stretch, it is useful to work out which areas of your spine are the most restricted and need to be stretched. There are common vulnerable areas, which are described using the universal posture model of common postural patterns, but this model is just a generalisation as not everyone fits into its framework. Get to know your body, find out which areas of your spine are hypomobile and which are hypermobile, and get some feedback about the shape and flexibility of your spine, either by asking a qualified manual therapist to do an assessment or by doing it yourself.

Determine if you have a stocky or slender build or somewhere in between. Observe your own body and how the different areas in you body move. Work out how flexible you are. Are you generally flexible or inflexible? Are you flexible in some areas but not in others? Determine if your flexibility or inflexibility is caused genetically, by your lifestyle or by a combination of both. Develop sensitivity and feedback skills so that you may find safe joint limits when you are stretching.

Tune into your body and learn what it needs. For example, if you are tighter on one side of your body than the other, stretch the tighter side more. Also consider your job, sport and daily activities: what do these activities require and what type of positions are you in most of the time? Now adopt those stretches into your daily program which address any imbalances they create, spending more time stretching the tighter areas, the muscles and other tissues shortened and the postures that are shaped by those actions and postions.

In part 3 of this book are daily and weekly stretching routines for many sports, jobs and activities. These stretching routines come with tables which supports which stretching techniques I have selected. The stretches are based on which muscle are contracted, the areas stretched and the range of movement. If a routine for your activity is not listed in part C you can work out your own using the table idea.

Posture

As explained in the early part of the introduction under theoretical considerations, a healthy posture depends on good ligament and muscle structural integrity in areas of the body: good ligament strength and muscle tone and power to support the body and hold the joints together; with good ligament viscoelasticity and muscle flexibility to enable full range of movement but not hypermobility. A good posture is a neutral posture, where there is a healthy balance between the agonist and antagonist muscles and between all the tissues located on opposite sides of a joint or on opposite sides of the spine. In addition to the muscles, the ligaments and fasciae need to be balanced throughout the whole body.

Poor sitting or standing posture usually involves slouching forwards over long periods, leading to fatigue and eventually structural changes in the muscles attached to the back of the rib cage, thoracic spine and shoulders. These posterior positioned muscle have to work harder against the continuous pull of gravity.

The suboccipital and upper posterior cervical muscles, anterior scalene, pectoralis major, pectoralis minor, iliopsoas, the hamstrings and the calf muscle tend to shorten; while erector spinea, trapezius, levator scapulae, rhomboid major and rhomboid minor tend to lengthen and become more fibrous. Stretching should mainly be directed at lengthening the short muscles but can be used to relieve tension in muscles that may already be in a lengthened position.

Unless stretches are specifically designed to move the spine, then they should be done with a straight spine and with the head in line with the spine. Avoid the anterior head posture. Poking the chin out is a common bad habit that may result in suboccipital strain, pain and headache.

Stretching solutions

To get the best from stretching you need to stretch short muscles and stiff joints, which will be where there is maximal resistance against movement. In the limbs, loss of muscle flexibility and range of movement is quite easy to see, feel and measure in absolute terms and you can compare the right and left limb and decide in relative terms if there is restriction. But in the spine this is more difficult.

The areas of greatest sidebending restriction in the spine will usually be at the apex of the primary and secondary scoliotic curves. Restricted extension will usually occur where there is increased flexion such as an increased kyphosis or a reversed lordosis, and restricted flexion will usually occur where there is an increased lordosis or a reversed kyphosis.

To be able to localise the stretch in the right areas of your spine you need knowledge about its shape and mobility, as well as awareness about how it feels. The simplest way to learn about your spine is by engaging a competent therapist to either take photographs of your back or look at your back and draw a diagram on paper or on a computer screen and then print it out for you. Static plain film anteroposterior and lateral spinal X-rays taken standing and erect are useful. But by far the best way to get to know the shape of the spine and its mobility or lack of mobility is to take dynamic plain film X-rays of the spine in positions of full flexion, extension and right and left sidebending. In addition, useful information about areas of hypermobility may be gleamed if the spine is stressed and these positions are slightly exaggerated. Of course a skilled therapist should also be able to discern areas of hypermobility by means of palpation.

Armed with the knowledge about the state of your spine it is then necessary to develop an appreciation about how it feels. Use the diagrams, photographs or X-rays to create a mental image of your spine. Develop an awareness of your spine and superimpose this over your intellectual knowledge thereby renforcing one with the other. Feel where your spine is stiff, where it is free and where it moves too easily. When you have learned to distinguish these then you will be better equipt to localise the stretches on the most restricted part of the spine. In general your spine will have the least movement at the apices of it curvatures and this is where you need to apply your forces during the stretch. By getting to know your spine experientially you can develop a better stretching practice.

Extremes of mobility, either hypomobility or hypermobility may be localised or generalised. Extremes of posture include: an increased or decreased thoracic kyphosis, cervical or lumbar lordosis; cervical, thoracic or lumbar scoliosis; scapula protraction and scapula retraction.

The following are a list of stretches that may be used for each posture:

For an increased thoracic kyphosis:

- thoracic and lumbar extension stretches 2.5
- all the rolled towel stretches 3.6 to 3.9.

For a decreased thoracic kyphosis:

- thoracic and lumbar flexion stretches
- longitudinal sidebending stretches.

For an increased cervical lordosis:

- cervical flexion, sidebending or chin tuck stretches 1.3, 1.4 and 1.7.

For a decreased cervical lordosis:

- cervical extension stretches.

For an increased lumbar lordosis:

- lumbar or thoracolumbar flexion, sacral extension stretches 2.9 and 3.0
- pelvic tilt abdominal strengthening 7.6.

For a decreased lumbar lordosis:

- lumbar or thoracolumbar extension or sacral flexion stretches.

For a cervical scoliosis:

- cervical sidebending stretches 1.7.

For a thoracic scoliosis:

- thoracic sidebending stretches 2.0b, 2.1b and 2.2
- Hanging longitudinal stretch 2.4a.

For a lumbar scoliosis:

- thoracolumbar and lumbar sidebending 2.0a and 2.1
- Hanging longitudinal stretch 2.4a.

42

For scapula protraction:

- scapula retraction stretch 4.0c
- any stretches from 4.0 or 4.1.

For scapula retraction:

- scapula protraction stretches 4.9 and 5.0.

To find the best stretches for the different regions of the body go to part C of this book and use the movement tables - stretches based primarily on joint movement and direction and secondarily according to anatomical region.

Stretching compared with other exercise systems

A wholistic exercise programme includes five key elements:

1. Aerobic fitness which enables the lungs, heart and blood vessels to work at optimum efficiency.
2. Strength development where muscle power and tone are developed.
3. Stretching where muscles and joints are made flexible for agility and to prevent injury.
4. Stamina development to enable the body to cope with a constant workload without fatigue.
5. Neuromuscular coordination or skills for the development of the nervous system for the control of muscles.

Sport	Stamina	Suppleness	Strength
Badminton	**	***	**
Canoeing	***	**	***
Climbing	***	*	**
Cricket	*	**	*
Cycling	****	**	***
Disco Dancing	***	****	*
Partner Dancing	*	***	*
Digging	***	**	****
Football	***	***	***
Golf	*	**	*
Gymnastics	**	****	***
Hill Walking	***	*	***
Housework	*	**	*
Jogging	****	**	**
Judo	**	****	**
Lawn Mowing	**	*	***
Rowing	****	**	****
Sailing	*	**	**
Squash	***	***	**
Swimming	****	****	****
Tennis	**	***	*
Walking	**	*	*
Weightlifting	*	*	****
Yoga	*	****	*

Stretching doesn't take a lot of time, especially when compared with other exercise systems. Ten minutes stretching each day is enough to get a positive outcome.

Stretching is important for flexibility, movement, gait and joint and muscle health. But stretching doesn't cover all fitness needs very well. Stretching doesn't cover aerobic fitness, coordination, skills, stamina and strengthening needs well. These fitness needs must be provided by another exercise system. For a well balanced exercise program, stretching should be combined with an aerobic activity such as swimming or running; mind-body coordination skills such as tennis or other ball games; strengthening using weights machines, free-weights or gym-floor-workouts; and stamina building such as digging the garden, chopping wood, cleaning and most jobs involving manual labour.

Stretching complements other exercise systems and most sports well because mostly they don't increase flexibility and in many cases may decrease it. In the list on the previous page, only swimming, judo, yoga and some types of gymnastics increase suppleness.

How is stretching different from Yoga?

Localisation is important for optimum flexibility - moving the most restricted joints and stretching the tightest muscles. A problem with yoga is it tries to stretch everything and doesn't focus enough on stretching the stiff areas which are different in every individual and different in each part of the body. When yoga was created there wasn't a modern understanding of anatomical principles. Yoga asanas are part of a much larger ancient system which developed in an environment when there was little or no knowledge of anatomy or biomechanics. There are many positive benefits from practicing yoga but there are also dangers and these will be explored at a later time in another book.

Stretching in sport and exercise

Stretching should be part of a total exercise routine and integrated into every sport but it is frequently neglected. It is usually only done as part of a five minutes warm up at the beginning of training. The warm up is an important protection against injury and five minutes is insufficient. Sometimes stretching takes the form of a series of ballistic movements, quick bouncing movements which do not give the muscle sufficient time to stretch. Also stretching may be neglected at the end of training because the the person is in too much of a hurry. Stretching should be done before and after training.

Good flexibility should be the foundation for aerobic and strength training, and all sports and activities that place demand on the body because flexibility is a safeguard or buffer giving joints a greater range and protecting muscles, tendons and ligaments against injury.

Static stretching should not be used by competitive athletes immediately before high intensity sports when a high demand on the body is required. Static stretching may lead to a drop in performance and may not work well in reducing injury. For 30 minutes to an hour before peak demand only use dynamic stretching and warming up type activities. Power sports like speedskating, running and swimming in particular should avoid static stretching prior to competition because it may cause a temporary decrease in muscle strength.

Stretching classes

Although stretching can be self-taught and based on books such as *Safe Stretch*, the ideal way is to start stretching with a few one-to-one lessons from a qualified teacher. Although there are generalisations that can be made about stretching, everyone is different and each stretching routine that is prescribed and followed should be based on individual needs.

The rate of improvement in flexibility depends on the type of body that one starts with. Someone starting stretching with high levels of inflexibility will find it harder to stretch initially and may take longer to stretch than a more flexible person. In contrast, someone starting stretching from pre-existing high levels of flexibility may run into trouble because they may become hypermobile in some areas and remain stiff in other areas. People who are highly flexible may get faster results initially but if they push themselves too hard and become hypermobile this may cause problems years later. Quick results may lead this group of people to push themselves even harder. So don't get overly competitive or obsessive about getting very flexible. Stability is important and optimum flexibility should be the goal - not too much or too little. If you become overflexible if is hard to reverse. Genetically flexible people need to be cautious when stretching or when doing yoga or gymnastics, if they wish to progress safely. Overflexibility is arguably more problematic than inflexibly.

The effect of stretching on muscle strength

Stretching prior to exercise has been shown to decrease power or performance in muscles. This weakening effect depends on the type of stretching and the duration. Static stretching resulted in the lowest muscle performance followed by isometric and dynamic stretching. The weakening effect of static stretching occurs only after lengthy period of stretching. Prolonged stretching for two to three minutes reduces muscle strength but short periods of stretching for one minute or less, as prescribed by this book, have no significant effect on muscle strength. The weakness is of short duration and the muscle returns to its full strength after a few hours.

One reason for this short term weakening effect of static stretching is because there is less overlapping of the myosin and actin filaments, thus fewer cross-bridges can form between the actin and myosin for a strong contraction to occur. Another reason for the reduced muscle strength is changes may be occuring to the viscoelasticity of the muscle.

Stretching the spine

Movement in the cervical spine is relatively free in all direction. In the thoracic spine movement is mainly limited by the rib cage. The ribs protect the thoracic spine from overstretching, especially in sidebending and rotation. Rotation is limited in the lumbar by the shape and sagittal alignment of the facet joints. Whereas the cervical spine is vulnerable to overstretching in all directions, the thoracic and lumbar spine is most vulnerable to overstretching when moving into extension and flexion.

Relatively strong forces can be generated by limb muscles due to limb bones acting as levers. It is important when stretching to protect the spine against these strong forces. Those areas in the spine most vulnerable to overstretching will move first and move through a greater range of movement compared with areas of greater stiffness. Flexible parts of the spine can become even more flexible if the strong forces coming from the limbs are able to overload the spine.

Overuse patterns

Some people are unable to relax. Most often this is in the muscles of the upper body - the shoulders, neck and jaw, but it can be anywhere in the body. Stretching and exercise is an important component in helping people relax because exercise counters the effects of tension. But if the symptoms keep coming back, even with exercise, you may need to learn *Somafeedback,* a technique designed to teach people to relax, and look at other causes.

Somafeedback assesses a person's ability to relax a single muscle or a group of muscles, and corrects the muscle problems that are identified. It uses verbal and tactile techniques to encourage maximum relaxation, and to correct the tension. It works on two levels: firstly by bringing the tension problem to the conscious awareness of the person and secondly by removing the overuse behaviour that causes the tension.

Occupational overuse syndrome is different from common overuse tension. Overuse syndrome also known as repetitive strain injury or RSI, usually occurs in the fingers, hands, wrists and elbows and is caused by repetitive movements and bad posture. Better workplace design, ergonomics and sitting behaviour can help. Sometimes rest is required for a short period of time before introducing exercise.

Therapist controlled passive stretching

There are many benefits and some dangers when stretching is done passively or post-isometrically, by a therapist or physical education teacher. A stretch reflex may be activated if the therapist stretches the muscle too quickly and with too much force. Passive stretching as a form of manual therapy is outside the scope of this book. Anyone interested in manual therapy passive and post-isometric stretching should consult my previous book: Myofaction Myofascial Manipulation. www.informaction.org/myofaction

How long does stretching work?

Regular stretching increases muscle length and joint range of movement. Strengthening exercises and some active stretching exercises increase muscle tone and this helps maintain good posture and stability. Stretching with greater frequency produces longer lasting flexibility, and strengthening with greater frequency and resistance produces longer lasting stability. Both strengthening and stretching are necessary for good postural balance.

How long the body maintains good flexibility and posture after stretching depends on lifestyle genetic factors, and how much you stretch. A mild and very short stretching program will help for a few hours, a moderate stretching program over a few days will help for a few days and an intensive stretching program over several months will have longer lasting benefit. But no stretching program will have lasting benefit in the face of overwhelming lifestyle and genetic factors working against the body.

Localisation

Localisation is necessary to stretch the right muscle or muscles and to avoid stretching the wrong muscles and overstretching hypermobile joints. To achieve good localisation the person stretching needs to focus on the target muscle while being aware of the other muscles and joints, as well as the orientation of their body in space and relative to gravity.

Mostly during stretching we do not want to have to focus our attention on maintaining balance and expending unnecessary energy on not falling over; the goal is to stretch short muscles. The best way to achieve this, is to position the body in the most stable position. This may involve keeping the body's centre of gravity near the mid-point between both feet, or holding onto a chair or table for support. So, unless developing good balance is one of the goals of the stretching exercise, adopt the most stable position.

To stretch safely focus the mind on the muscle or muscles being stretched, and the joint or joints associated with those muscles. In spite of popular mythology about multitasking the mind really can only focus effectively on one thing at a time. By making a stretch complicated we dilute the focus and the effectiveness of the stretch, making ourselves vulnerable to injury or faulty movements.

Our brains can't multitask. When we attempt to do many things at once our brain frantically jumps around, switching constantly between the tasks and not doing any of them efficiently. That is one of the problems of hatha yoga asanas. We think we are doing a lot but the end result is we don't do any of the tasks efficiently. We just jump back and forth focusing on each part of the stretch or yoga asana for a few milliseconds at a time and don't stretch anything well. Multitasking could be viewed more positively as whole body awareness!

Neuroplasticity and stretching

Learning a skill

When we are learning a skill, we are developing new nerve connections between the body, the brain and spinal cord. Stretching is not as complex as gymnastics, yoga, tennis and many other sports but it is a skill and each time a stretch is done it stimulates new nerve connections.

Use patterns affecting the brain

Problems can develop when stretches are done incorrectly on a regular basis because the receptors in the muscles and joints provides the brain with information. Over time, strong nerve connections become firmly established. Faulty mechanics results in feedback loops which can be difficult to break. If faulty skills are not corrected early and the joints maintain the same pattern of movement over months or years, the new nerve connections become stronger, becoming progressively more difficult to change the bad habit. It is like the body gets stuck in an unwanted pattern of movement and eventually the mind locks it into memory.

Previously scientists thought that the brain was a relatively static organ. But we now know that over the course of a lifetime the brain can be changed in any direction, for better or worse. Brain plasticity or neuroplasticity refers to changes in neural pathways and synapses due to changes in behavior, environment, thinking, as well as physical and emotional trauma. With willpower, better skills can be learnt, including stretching.

Feedback

When learning a new skill like stretching, it is important to have good feedback and to act on it appropriately. We experience feedback within our own bodies from the sensory receptors in our skin, joints and muscles. Unfortunately sometimes the information from our body can be misinterpreted by our brain; this is especially true with respect to the spine. Feedback from our spine regarding our scoliosis is particulary unreliable. Most people think their spine is straight when in fact it is not. Most people have a mild scoliosis and many of these people have a scoliosis combined with a forward or backward curve. They may have a reversed lumbar lordosis or an exaggerated thoracic kyphosis or an anterior occiput making judgement particularly difficult.

Most people would not be able to tell you how their spine is organised. They do not know where their spine is sidebent and in which direction, left or right. The feedback system works to an extent but it doesn't work well. It works to protect the body when it is about to fall over or when there is pain but it doesn't help you understand your posture.

Causes of poor spinal feedback

Habituation, sensory adaptation and motor fatigue are three factors influencing how we feel our body. We think we are straight when in fact we are not.

- Habituation is the decrease of a response to a repeated stimulus - a learned adaptation.
- Sensory adaptation is an inability to detect a stimulus as efficiently as when first presented.
- Motor fatigue is the ability to detect a stimulus but inability to respond to it efficiently.

Over a lifetime we tend to decrease or cease to respond to the stimuli coming from the receptors in our spine. The process of developing an increasingly crooked spine increases with age but is so slow that we don't notice it. We stop responding to the stimulus because it is not relevant to our survival. Perhaps another reason is because we do not stretch enough and have become out of touch with our body.

Habituation is a form of neuroplasticity where the brain changes as skills are learned. When new skills are learned, the brain moves to a relatively fixed state and once there, it takes greater effort to move it to a new fixed state.

In the execution of repeated poor actions with poor feedback, incorrect coding takes place. A memory of the action is imprinted in the nervous system so that it does not have to be consciously learned each time, but is acted out subconsciously.

If good feedback is obtained in the initial stages of learning a skill, then proper coding results. The student may be able to then integrate this feedback into their practice; knowing this feedback to be based on sound and correct training from their teacher.

Complexity of skill and coding

The more complex a skill the more difficult it is to develop the correct coding. That is why most of the techniques in this book are simple and focused on only stretching one muscle or one group of muscles. This approach should be used when begining any new skill; break it down to individual components and build up the complexity over time.

Private tuition compared with group classes

Stretching is best learned from a qualified teacher on a one-to-one basis for the first few weeks. Beginners tend to have problems accurately localising the stretch to the correct region of the spine and keeping good spinal alignment when stretching major upper and lower limb muscles. Private tuition is more costly than group classes but in the initial stages of learning a skill like stretching it is important to get good feedback. A private teacher is better able to identify your strengths and weaknesses, correct your posture, guide your movements and help you avoid adopting bad habits. As all of the focus is on you, private lessons are more intensive and may be tiring but there is greater progress. When the techniques have been sufficiently mastered then they can be practiced at home alone.

Group exercise classes can lead to competitiveness and exhibitionism. The follow-the-teacher approach of exercise classes can be problematic because the student may not clearly see what the teacher is doing or may fail to translate the action of the teacher into the correct movement. Unless the student is physically guided into positon by the teacher they may develop a false awareness of how the stretch feels and end up doing the stretch wrongly.

Group fitness classes do have their place but they should be kept to a size that can be managed by the teacher or teachers. Also teachers must adopt a hands-on approach to give each student in the class appropriate feedback to ensure faulty-use patterns are avoided.

Activities and lifestyle affect structure

Our physical activities influence our body in many ways. Healthy activities like stretching, walking and swimming change it in positive ways and unhealthy activities like prolonged sitting or repetitive work change it in negative ways. Activities change the structure of our tissues, which influences the function of our body, including the stability and mobility of our joints and the flexibility and strength of our muscles. A sedentary lifestyle leads to atrophy, weakness and shortness in muscles and other body tissues as well as stiffness in joints. Activity done safely is a positive thing for the body but over-activity or repetitive activity can, like under-activity, leads to muscle shortness. So, stretching is good after activity or inactivity.

Factors affecting structure and flexibility

Many things can cause changes in the structure of muscles and other tissues including: psychoemotional factors, gravity acting on posture and patterns of overuse or misuse. Fibrous development is the most common change. This results in reduced elasticity in muscles and ligaments and reduced range of movement in joints.

Lengthening - temporary or long term?

Stretching modifies the shape, stability and flexibility of our body by lengthening our ligaments and muscles. This is a temporary modification because our soft tissues will return to their original shortened state if the stretch is not repeated regularly.

Ligament laxity

The primary role of ligaments is in providing support and stability to joints. Ligaments should have good structural integrity and an optimum level of tightness for this function. If ligaments are lax because of genetic reasons or damaged by overstretching or injury, then stretching is contraindicated. Stretching lax ligaments is inappropriate because it may increase the laxity. Initially, a complete abstinence of stretching may be needed to allow overstretched ligaments to return to an optimum level of tightness, combined with strengthening and other exercises to stress the joint productively. This may be followed by several months of mild stretching as the situation requires.

Overstretching hypomobility and hypermobility

If you push a stretch too hard the ligaments overlying hypermobile areas of the spine will usually yield before those in the hypomobile areas, so you must stop before you get to the point of overstretch. You must be particularly careful when using leverage-assisted passive techniques, which are usually more dangerous than active technique.

Ligament laxity from one or several events

Ligament laxity can come from a single event such as trauma or several repeated events of overstretching. The result will be similar with both events - ligaments stretched beyond their elastic limit will cause joint hypermobility and in extreme cases may cause instability.

Part A. Technique

1.1 The Lion - active stretches for the face, tongue, jaw, shoulders, cervical and thoracic spine

1.1a Lion stretch kneeling

Starting Position

- Kneel on a mat with your knees apart and your arms in front of you.
- Straighten your arms at the elbows and pull down your shoulders.
- Place the front of your wrists on your knees with your palms downwards.
- Spread and pull back your fingers and rest them on the floor.
- Push your chin forward and bend your neck and thoracic spine backward.
- Open your eyes wide and look upwards.
- Open your mouth wide, stick out your tongue and point it downwards.

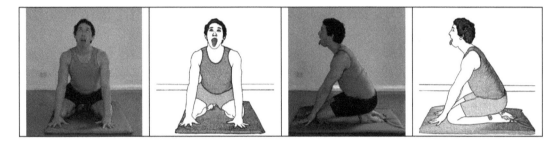

Technique

- Take a deep breath in.
- Slowly exhale and combine the following movements:

  - Partially extend your head and cervical spine
  - Fully extend your upper and middle thoracic spine
  - Depress your shoulders
  - Extend your forearms at the elbows
  - Extend and abduct your fingers
  - Open your eyes wide and look upwards
  - Open your mouth wide, depress your mandible, and stick out your tongue and point it downwards.

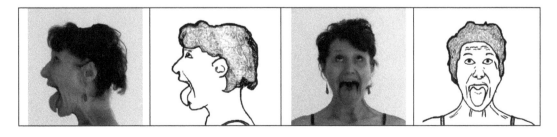

- Repeat the stretch several times, moving with each exhalation.

1.1b Lion stretch seated

Starting Position

- Sit on a stool or chair with your knees apart and your arms in front of you.
- Straighten your arms at the elbows and pull down your shoulders.
- Place the front of your wrists on your knees with your palms downwards.
- Pull back your fingers and spread them wide.
- Push your chin forward and bend your neck and thoracic spine backward.
- Open your eyes wide and look upwards.
- Open your mouth wide, stick out your tongue and point it downwards.

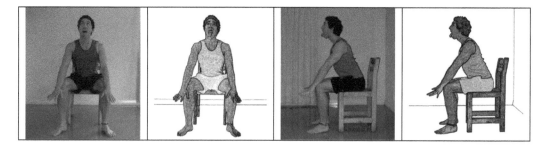

Technique

- Take a deep breath in.
- Slowly exhale and combine the following movements:

  - Partially extend your head and cervical spine
  - Fully extend your upper and middle thoracic spine
  - Depress your shoulders
  - Extend your forearms at the elbows
  - Extend and abduct your fingers
  - Open your eyes wide and look upwards
  - Open your mouth wide, depress your mandible, and stick out your tongue and point it downwards.

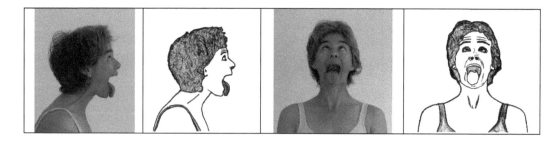

- Repeat the stretch several times, moving with each exhalation.

1.1c Lion stretch standing

Starting Position

- Stand with your knees and feet apart and your arms in front of your body.
- Straighten your arms at the elbows and pull down your shoulders.
- Place the front of your wrists on your knees with your palms downwards.
- Pull back your fingers and spread them wide.
- Push your chin forward and bend your neck and thoracic spine backward.
- Open your eyes wide and look upwards.
- Open your mouth wide, stick out your tongue and point it downwards.

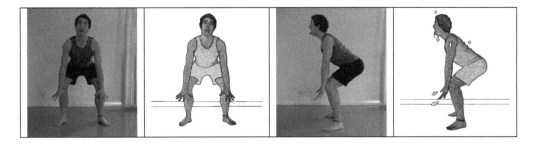

Technique

- Take a deep breath in.
- Slowly exhale and combine the following movements:

  - Partially extend your head and cervical spine
  - Fully extend your upper and middle thoracic spine
  - Depress your shoulders
  - Extend your forearms at the elbows
  - Extend and abduct your fingers
  - Open your eyes wide and look upwards
  - Open your mouth wide, depress your mandible, and stick out your tongue and point it downwards.

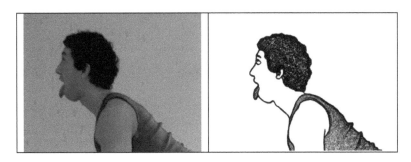

- Repeat the stretch several times, moving with each exhalation.

1.2 The Shrug - active, post-isometric and passive stretch for the face, jaw, shoulders, arms and hands

1.2 Shrug

Starting position

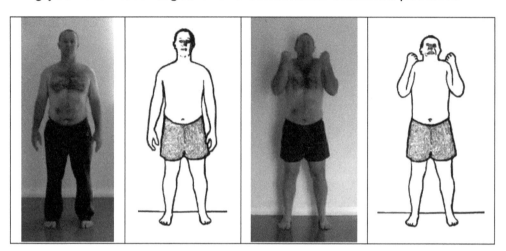

- Stand with your feet apart and arms at your sides.
- Make a fist with both hands and fully bend your forearms at the elbows.
- Lift both shoulders as high as possible but keep your elbows at your side.
- Bring your back teeth together in a comfortable clenched position.

Technique

- Take in a deep breath and hold it in.
- Close your eyes and tense your muscles in the following order:

  - Tighten your clenched fists.
  - Flex your elbows.
  - Shrug your shoulders.
  - Clench your jaw.
  - Squeeze your eyelids and eyes together.

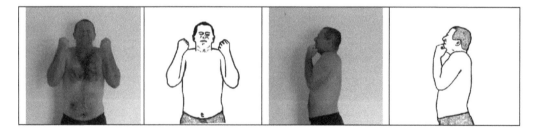

- When all the muscles are contracting together, increase the intensity of the muscle contraction to a safe maximum level for a few seconds.
- Exhale and immediately relax all the muscles.
- The shoulders and arms should be allowed to drop to the side of the body in a natural way using only gravity.

1.3 Chin tuck - active stretches for the suboccipital, cervical and upper thoracic spine

1.3a Chin tuck prone

Starting position

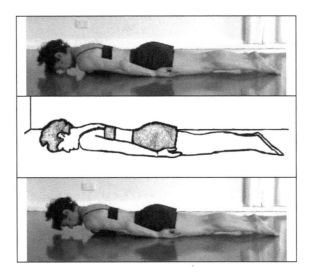

- Lay face down on a mat, on the floor or on a table.
- Both arms should rest at the side of the body with your shoulders relaxed.
- Position your head so that you rest on the point of your nose.

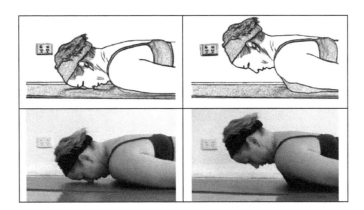

Technique

- Take a deep breath in.
- Slowly exhale as you lift your head off the floor.

- Careful execution of this technique is necessary for it to be effective.

  - As you lift your head keep it parallel with the floor and tuck in your chin.
  - Do not tilt your head and neck backwards.
  - Your shoulders, ribs and thoracic spine are the foundation that anchors your muscles and enables them to lift your head and neck off the floor.
  - Do not lift your chest or lumbar spine off the floor.
  - Your shoulders, ribs and mid to lower thoracic spine should not move.

1.3b Chin tuck standing or seated

Starting position

- Stand with your back to a wall, or away from a wall, or sit on a stool with your back straight, or sit on a chair with your back against the chair back.
- Your feet are apart.
- If you do it standing with your back against a wall, your buttocks, shoulder blades and middle thoracic spine are in contact with the wall but your heels are a few centimetres away from the wall.
- If you do it seated make sure both feet are firmly planted on the floor
- Both arms should rest at the side of the body with your shoulders relaxed.

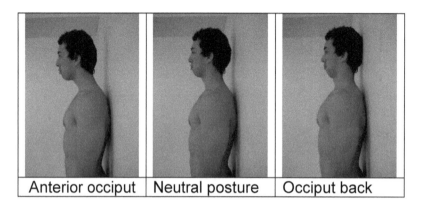

| Anterior occiput | Neutral posture | Occiput back |

Technique

- Point your chin forward but keep your head vertical.
- This is the characteristic poor posture where the occiput has moved anterior on the atlas and the upper cervical spine is in extension.
- Take your chin backward while maintaining your head in a vertical plane.
- Stop when you feel a sudden increase in tension in the back of your neck, or when the back of your head makes contact with the wall.

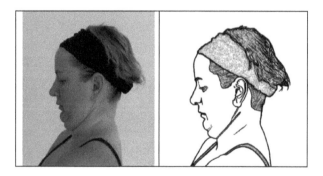

- Take a deep breath in.
- Exhale and move the back of your head backwards and upwards.
- Tuck your chin in as you lift your head.
- If you are using a wall, move the back of your head up the wall.
- Do not flex or extend your head - keep your head vertical.

1.3c Chin tuck supine

Starting position

- Lay on your back on the floor.
- Both arms should rest at the side of the body with your palms upwards and shoulders relaxed.
- Position your head so that you rest on the back of your head.
- Do not allow you head to drop backwards.
- If cannot prevent your head dropping backwards then place it on a small pillow.

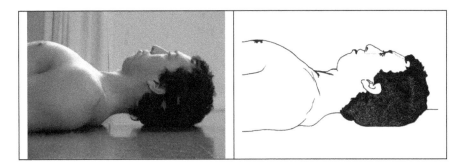

Technique

- Take a deep breath.
- Exhale and move the back of your head away from your body and along the floor.

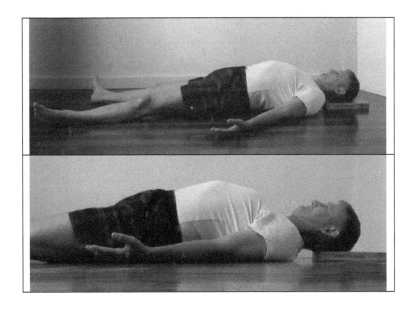

- Try to flatten out the arch in your neck.
- Tuck in the chin but do not let your head come off the floor.
- The muscles that move your head and neck are anchored onto your shoulders, spine and ribs.

1.4 Neck flexion stretches - active, passive and post-isometric flexion stretches for the suboccipital, posterior cervical and upper thoracic spine

1.4a Head & neck active flexion stretch seated

Starting position

- Sit in a chair with your feet apart and firmly planted on the floor.
- Both arms hang at the side of your body and your shoulders are relaxed.
- Maintain an upright sitting position by consciously holding your pelvis in a vertical position or use a chair with a back support.

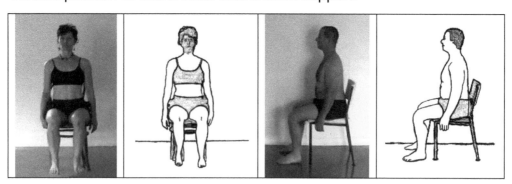

Technique

- Look straight ahead and take a deep breath in.
- Slowly exhale while looking downwards.
- Following the direction of your eyes your head and neck will flex.
- Feel the stretch in the back of the neck as your forehead moves forwards and downwards

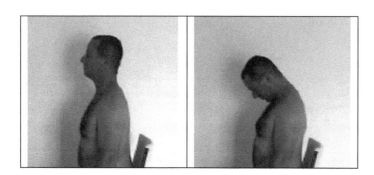

- Contract the muscles in the front of your neck with a light force to increase the stretch.
- This can be done as a passive stretch if you relax and allow the weight of your head to stretch the tissues.
- Actively depress your shoulders to localise the stretch to the upper trapezius, levator scapulae and rhomboid muscles.

1.4b Head & neck post-isometric flexion stretch supine

Starting position

- Lay on your back on a mat on the floor with your hips and knees flexed, feet apart and feet firmly planted on the floor.
- Interlace your fingers and place your hands behind your head to support and protect the suboccipital spine and control movement of your head.
- Position your hand so that your little finger covers the bottom of your occiput, middle finger covers your atlas (C1), index finger covers your axis (C2) and thumb cover C3 and vertebrae below.

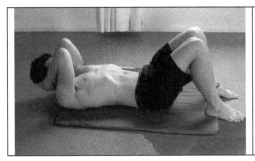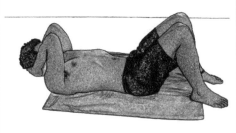

Technique

- Look straight ahead and take a deep breath and hold it in.
- Slowly exhale and look down the front of your body towards your naval.
- During the exhalation your head will move in the direction of your eye movement and you should use your hands to follow the flexion movement.
- Inhale and look up but resist any upward movement of your head.
- Exhale and once again look downwards towards your naval.
- Repeat the manoeuvre several times, each time using your hands to follow the eye movement with greater levels of head and neck flexion.
- Do not pull on your head and neck and do not push on your head and compress your neck.

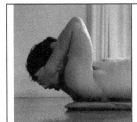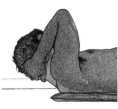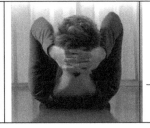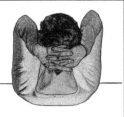

- The force generated in the neck muscles by the eye movement is light to moderate but enough to move the head.
- A passive stretch can be applied at the end of the post isometric stretch.

1.4c Head & neck localised post-isometric flexion, sidebending and rotation stretch supine

Starting position

- Lay on your back on a mat on the floor.
- Lift your head until your upper thoracic spine starts to move off the floor.
- Flex your left arm and forearm, reach behind your head and wrap your left hand around the joints at the top of your spine and the base of your skull.
- The fingers of your left hand point towards your right ear.
- Turn your head to the left and towards your left arm and forearm.

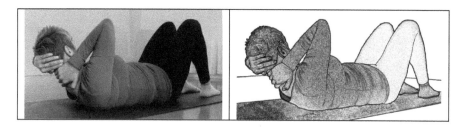

- Flex your right arm and forearm, reach behind your head and wrap your right hand around the back of your neck to fix the lower cervical spine.
- Sidebend your neck to the left by dropping your left elbow and tilting your left wrist but protect the joints at the base of the skull with your left hand.
- Localise the stretch to the desired vertebral level with your right forefinger
- Stop when you feel the initial stages of muscle resistance in each plane of movement - flexion, left rotation and left sidebending.

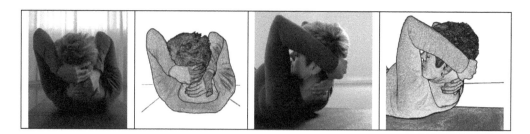

Technique

- Take in a deep breath and hold it in.
- Look upwards and to the right for about five seconds.
- Exhale and then look downwards and to the left and sidebend and rotate your cervical spine to the left with your left hand.
- Localise the stretch to the desired vertebral level with a light pressure on the right side of your spine with the forefinger of your right hand.
- Use your left hand to protect the suboccipital joints against overstretching.
- Do not pull on the head - localise the stretch to your cervical spine.
- Stop moving when you feel the initial stages of muscle resistance
- Work through each plane - flexion, left rotation and left sidebending.
- Repeat the post-isometric stretch several times
- Repeat the stretch on the other side.

1.5 Neck extension stretch - active and passive extension stretch for the cervical, upper thoracic and suboccipital spine

1.5 Head & neck extension stretch seated

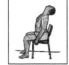

Starting position

- Sit in a chair with your feet apart and firmly planted on the floor.
- Both arms hang at the side of your body and your shoulders are relaxed.
- Maintain an erect sitting position by consciously holding your pelvis in a vertical position or use a chair with a back support.

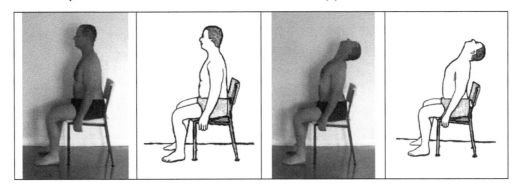

Technique

- Look straight ahead and take a deep breath in.
- Slowly exhale while looking upwards, and as you do so extend your head and neck.
- Lead with your eyes, and your head will move backwards following your eye movement until it reaches full extension.
- If you have symptoms, such as pain, dizziness or tingling in either of your arms or hands, return your head to the vertical position.

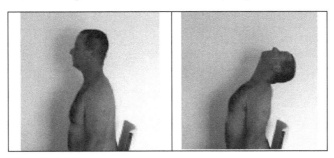

- If there are no symptoms continue with the active stretch.
- With each exhalation look upwards and backwards, and move your head further backwards into extension.
- Feel the stretch in front of your neck.
- If you cease muscle contraction and just let go of the head this becomes a passive stretch.
- Relax and allow the weight of your head to stretch the tissues.
- With the head behind its centre of gravity its weight stretches the muscles, ligaments and fascia of the anterior cervical spine and upper ribs.

1.6 Neck rotation stretch - active rotation stretch for the suboccipital, cervical and upper thoracic spine

1.6 Head & neck active rotation stretch seated

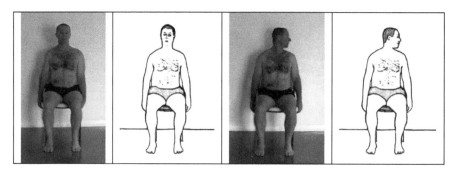

Starting position

- Sit in a chair with your feet apart and firmly planted on the floor.
- Both arms hang loosely at your side and your shoulders are relaxed.
- Sit up straight and maintain an upright sitting position by evenly positioning the weight of your body over your sit bones, the ischial tuberosites.
- Use muscle contraction, or use a chair with a back support to stay upright.
- Turn your head to the left until it is in a comfortable fully rotated position.

Technique

- Look to the left and 45 degrees upwards and then take in a deep breath.
- Exhale and actively rotate your head further left and upwards by contracting your neck rotator muscles with a light to moderate force.
- Look to the left and 45 degrees downwards and take in another breath.
- Exhale and look more to the left and downwards, as you actively rotate your head further left and downwards.
- Look horizontally directly to the left.
- Take in another deep breath.
- Exhale and look more to the left as you actively rotate your head further left.

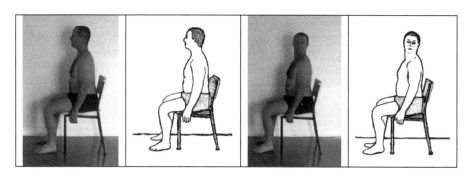

- Repeat active rotation stretch several times combining eye movement with muscle contraction each time.
- Repeat the stretch on the right side.

1.7 Neck sidebending stretches - active, passive and isometric for the suboccipital, cervical, upper thoracic and shoulders

<u>1.7a Head & neck active sidebending stretch seated with both arms free for anterior and lateral neck muscles</u>

Starting position

- Sit in a chair with your feet apart and planted on the floor.
- Your arms hang at the side of your body with your shoulders relaxed.
- With the arms and shoulders free there is less pull on trapezius.
- Sideshift your upper body to the right so that more of your weight is on your right buttock.
- Fix your eyes forwards and sidebend your head to the left.
- Keep your pelvis in a vertical position or use a chair with a back support.

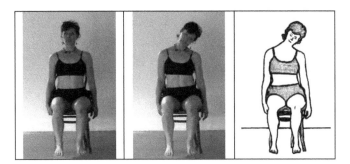

Technique

- Take a deep breath in.
- Exhale and sidebend your head further to the left by contracting the muscles down the left side of your neck with a light to moderate force.
- Feel the stretch down the right side of your neck.

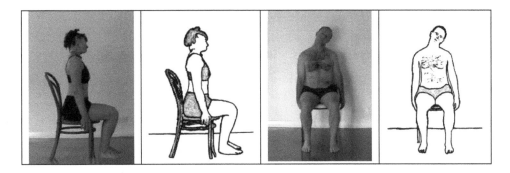

- Do not rotate your head – looking straight ahead helps.
- Do not flex or extend the head and neck – keep it in neutral.
- Return your head to the vertical position.
- Move your head backwards and simultaneously tuck your chin in.
- Exhale and sidebend your head to the left – but without tilting it.
- Head and neck sidebending combined with posterior translation localises the stretch to the front and side of your neck and the anterior scalene.
- Repeat the stretches on the left side of your neck.

1.7b Head, neck & shoulder active sidebending stretch seated with one shoulder fixed for the upper trapezius & lateral neck

Starting position

- Sit in a chair with your feet apart and firmly planted on the floor.
- Sideshift your upper body to the right so that more of your weight is on your right buttock.
- Reach down to the floor with your right hand and grasp the side of the chair near the front leg. This fixes the shoulder in a descended position.
- Sideshift your upper body back to the left a bit - stop before you feel a stretch in your right shoulder muscles.
- Maintain an upright sitting position by consciously holding your pelvis in a vertical position or use a chair with a back support.
- Fix your eyes forwards and then sidebend your head to the left.

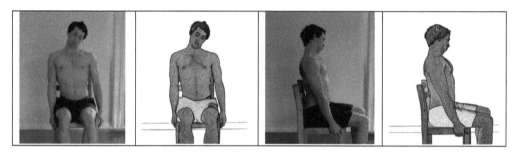

Technique

- Take a deep breath in.
- Exhale and sidebend your head to the left by contracting the muscles down the left side of your neck with a light to moderate force.
- Feel the stretch down the right side of your neck and shoulder.
- Do not allow your head to rotate – looking straight ahead helps.
- With each exhalation take the head further into sidebending.
- Keep your head and neck in neutral to stretch the fibres of upper trapezius which attach on the acromion process.
- Return your head to the vertical position.
- Move your head backwards and simultaneously tuck your chin in.
- Exhale and sidebend your head to the left – but without tilting it.
- Head and neck sidebending combined with posterior translation stretches the front and side of your neck and the clavicular fibres of trapezius.
- Repeat the stretches on the left side of your neck.

  - To localise the stretch to the suboccipital muscles and occipital fibres of trapezius tuck your chin in and flex your head a bit.
  - To increase the stretch of anterior scalene translate your head backwards but allow your chin to poke out a bit to relax trapezius.
  - To increase the stretch of sternocleidomastoid translate your head backwards and keep your chin in.

- Repeat the stretch on the left side of your neck and shoulder.

1.7c Head, neck & shoulder active sidebending stretch seated with one shoulder fixed for posterolateral fibres of trapezius & the neck

Starting position

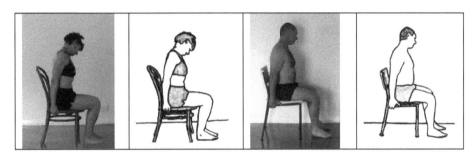

- Sit in a chair with your feet apart and firmly planted on the floor.
- Sideshift your upper body to the right so that more of your weight is on your right buttock.
- Reach down to the floor with your right hand and grasp the side of the chair near the back leg. This fixes the shoulder in a descended position.
- Sideshift your upper body back to the left a bit - stop before you feel a stretch in your right shoulder muscles.
- Maintain an upright sitting position by consciously holding your pelvis in a vertical position or use a chair with a back support.
- Fix your eyes forwards and then sidebend your head to the left.

Technique

- Take a deep breath in.
- Exhale and sidebend your head to the left by contracting the muscles down the left side of your neck with a light to moderate force.
- Feel the stretch down the right side of your neck and shoulder.
- Do not allow your head to rotate – looking straight ahead helps.
- With each exhalation take the head further into sidebending.
- Keep your head and neck in neutral to stretch the fibres of upper trapezius which attach on the acromion process.
- Return your head to the vertical position.
- Move your head forwards and simultaneously tuck your chin in.
- Exhale and sidebend your head to the left.
- Head and neck sidebending combined with head and neck flexion stretches the back and side of your neck and the fibres of trapezius attaching on the spine of the scapula.
- Repeat the stretches on the left side of your neck.

  o To localise the stretch to the occipital fibres of trapezius tuck your chin in and flex your head a bit more.

- Repeat the stretch on the left side of your neck and shoulder.

1.7d Head, neck & shoulder active sidebending stretch standing with one shoulder fixed for upper trapezius & muscle of the neck

Starting position

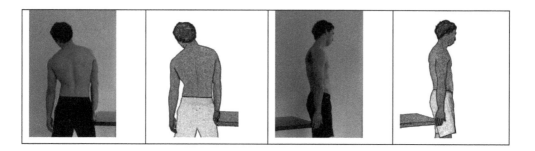

- Stand with your arms at your sides and your shoulders relaxed.
- Reach down to the floor with your right hand and grasp the side of a table.
- Select a table that is an appropriate height to allow you to stand straight without having to bend your knees yet enables you to fix your shoulder in a descended position so you can stretch your trapezius and neck muscles.
- Keep the right side of your hip in contact with the side of the table.
- Drop your left shoulder and sidebend your thoracic spine to the left to increases the stretch in your upper and middle trapezius muscles.
- Maintain an upright standing posture in the frontal plane.
- Fix your eyes forwards and then sidebend your head to the left.

Technique

- Take a deep breath in.
- Exhale and sidebend your head to the left by contracting the muscles down the left side of your neck with a light to moderate force.
- Feel the stretch in the tissues down the right side of your neck.
- Do not rotate your head – looking straight ahead helps minimise rotation.
- With each exhalation take the head further sideways.

To localise the stretch to the:

- o Occipital fibres of trapezius - tuck your chin in and flex your head.
- o Clavicular fibres of trapezius - move your head backwards without tilting it and hold on the table in front of your body.
- o Scapular fibres of trapezius and posterior neck muscles - hold the table behind your body and flex your head and neck a bit.
- o Fibres of the upper trapezius attaching on the acromion process - keep your head and neck in neutral.
- o Anterior scalene - translate your head backwards but allow your chin to poke out a bit.
- o Levator scapulae - fully rotate your head in the same direction as sidebending

- Repeat the stretch on the left side of your neck.

1.7e Head & neck active sidebending rotation stretch seated with both arms free for anterior and lateral neck muscles

Starting position

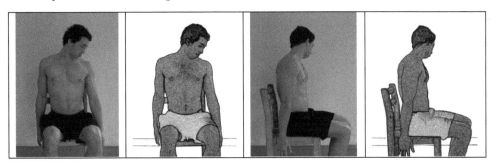

- Sit in a chair with your feet apart and firmly planted on the floor.
- Your arms hang at the side of your body with your shoulders relaxed.
- Sideshift your upper body to the right so that more of your weight is on your right buttock.
- Sidebend your head to the left until you start to feel a pull down the right side of your neck.
- Rotate your head 10 degrees to the left.

Technique

- Take a deep breath in.
- Exhale and sidebend your head to the left by contracting the muscles down the left side of your neck with a light to moderate force.
- Feel the stretch in the tissues down the back and right side of your neck.
- Rotate your head 20 degrees to the left.

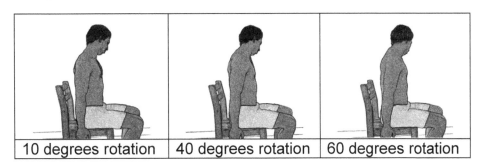

| 10 degrees rotation | 40 degrees rotation | 60 degrees rotation |

- Repeat the sidebending stretch with an exhalation.
- Rotate your head 40 degrees, 60 degrees and 80 degrees to the left and repeat the sidebending stretch with an exhalation at each position.
- With minimal levels of rotation of the head and neck sidebending mainly stretches rectus capitis lateralis, rectus capitis anterior, longus capitis, longus colli, semispinalis capitis and semispinalis cervicis.
- With greater levels of rotation there are greater levels of stretching of rectus capitis posterior major and obliquus capitis inferior, splenius cervicis, splenius capitis, iliocostalis cervicis and to a lesser extent longissimus cervicis, spinalis cervicis and the scalene.
- Repeat the stretch on the muscle of the left side of your neck.

1.7f Head, neck & shoulder active sidebending and rotation stretch seated with one shoulder fixed for levator scapulae and neck muscles

Starting position

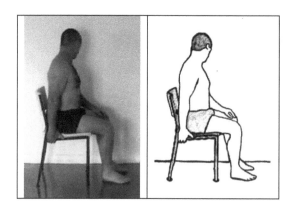

- Sit in a chair with your feet apart and firmly planted on the floor.
- Grasp the side of the chair near to its back leg with one hand.
- The other arm should hang at your side with the shoulders relaxed.
- Lean the body away from the grasping hand to take up some of the slack in the muscles in the right shoulder and arm.
- Sidebend your head to the left and fully rotate your head to the left.
- Maintain an erect sitting position.

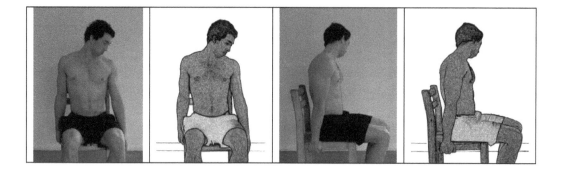

Technique

- Take a deep breath in.
- Exhale and increase sidebending of the cervical spine to the left while maintaining full rotation of your head and neck to the left.
- Contract the muscles down the front and left side of your neck with a light to moderate force.

- Feel the stretch down the side of the cervical spine and into the scapula.
- Repeat the stretch on the levator scapulae on the left side.

1.7g Head, neck & shoulder post-isometric sidebending and rotation technique seated with one shoulder fixed

Starting position

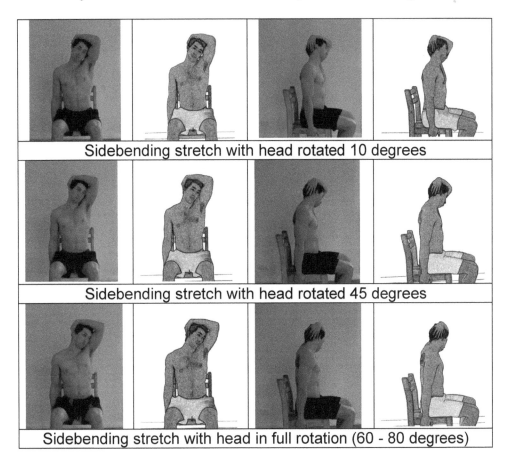

- Sit in a chair with your feet apart and firmly planted on the floor.
- Sideshift your body to the right so your weight is over your right buttock.
- Reach to the floor with your right hand and grasp the side of the chair.
- Sideshift your upper body back to the left and stop before you feel a stretch in your right shoulder muscles.
- Maintain an upright sitting position or use a chair with a back support.
- Raise your left arm, reach over your head with you left hand and grasp your head and neck at the suboccipital level.
- Sidebend your head to the left and rotate your head 10 degrees to the left.

Sidebending stretch with head rotated 10 degrees

Sidebending stretch with head rotated 45 degrees

Sidebending stretch with head in full rotation (60 - 80 degrees)

Technique

- Take a deep breath in.
- Attempt to push your head to the right but resist the movement with your left hand using an equal and opposite counterforce.
- After about five seconds cease the contraction, exhale and sidebend your head to a new stretch position - do not pull on the head.
- Rotate your head 45 degrees and then fully to the left and repeat the post-isometric sidebending technique at each position.
- Repeat the technique on the muscle down the left side of your neck.

1.7h Trapezius and levator scapulae post-isometric stretch seated with one shoulder fixed

Starting position

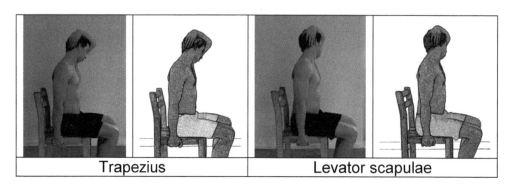

- Sit in a chair with your feet apart and firmly planted on the floor.
- Reach down to the floor with your right hand and grasp the side of the chair near to its back corner.
- Sidebend your head to the left
- Raise your left arm, reach over your head with you left hand and grasp your head and neck at the suboccipital level.

Technique

- Take a deep breath in.
- Attempt to sidebend your head to the right but resist the movement with your left hand using an equal and opposite counterforce.
- After about five seconds cease the contraction, exhale and sidebend your head to the new stretch position - do not pull on the head.
- Do not rotate the head.
- Repeat the post-isometric technique for trapezius several times.

To localise muscle lengthening on individual muscle fibres of trapezius:

- ○ Occipital fibres - tuck your chin in and flex your head
- ○ Clavicular fibres - move your head backwards without tilting it
- ○ Scapular fibres and posterior neck muscles - flex your head and neck
- ○ On the acromion process - keep your head and neck in neutral.

Trapezius	Levator scapulae

- Rotate your head to the left as far as possible but maintain sidebending.
- Take in a deep breath and hold it in.
- Attempt to sidebend your head to the right but resist the movement with your left hand using an equal and opposite counterforce.
- After about five seconds cease the contraction, exhale and sidebend your head to a new stretch position.
- Do not pull on the head.
- Maintain full rotation.
- Repeat the post-isometric technique for levator scapulae several times.
- Repeat the technique for trapezius and levator scapulae on the left side.

1.7i Levator scapulae active, passive or post-isometric stretch sidelying

Starting position

- Lay on your left side on the floor.
- Rest on your left shoulder with your left arm is straight out in front of you or bent at the elbow and tucked under your rib cage.
- Position your body so your shoulders and ribs are perpendicular to the floor.
- Reach down your right side with your right hand and place your palm flat on your right hip.
- Allow your head to drop to the floor into a left sidebent position.
- Rotate your head as far as possible to the left so the left side of your forehead rests on the floor.

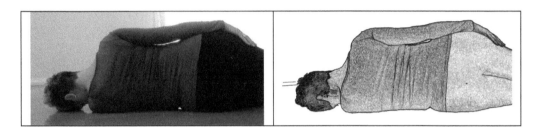

Technique

- Take a deep breath in.
- Exhale and reach further down your side, towards your feet with your right hand while increasing head and neck sidebending and rotation to the left.
- Repeat the active stretch for levator scapulae several times.

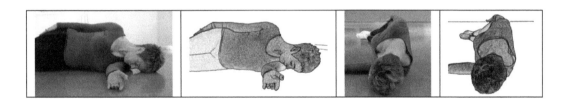

- Take another deep breath and hold it in.
- Attempt to lift your head off the floor by sidebending and rotating your head to the right.
- Use the weight of your head as a counterforce but stop before there is any movement.
- After about five seconds cease the isometric contraction, exhale and rotate and sidebend your head to the left and to a new stretch position.

- Repeat the post-isometric technique several times.
- Repeat the stretch on the other side.
- Rotation stretches levator scapulae but sidebending stretches trapezius.

1.8 Sternocleidomastoid stretch - an active stretch for the sternocleidomastoid and the cervical spine

<u>1.8 Head & neck extension, sidebending and reverse rotation stretch kneeling, seated or standing for sternocleidomastoid</u>

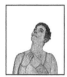

Starting position

- Kneel on the floor, sit in a chair with your feet apart or stand up straight.
- Bend your elbows and place the fingertips of your left hand over the lower part of your right sternocleidomastoid muscle just above the clavicle.
- Place the fingertips of your right hand over your left fingertips for support.
- Bend your head backwards and cervical spine and then sidebend your head left.
- Do not allow your head to rotate to the left - keep it straight or rotated right.

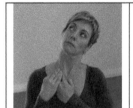 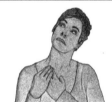 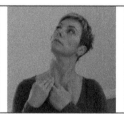 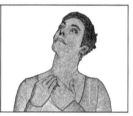

Technique

- Take a deep breath in.
- As you slowly exhale bend your head and neck further backwards and further into sidebending.
- Apply light fingertip pressure on the muscle to increase the stretch.
- Keep your fingertips to the outside and lower half of the muscle.
- Do not press on your throat.
- If you have symptoms such as pain, dizziness or tingling in either arm or hand, return your head to the vertical position and discontinue the stretch.

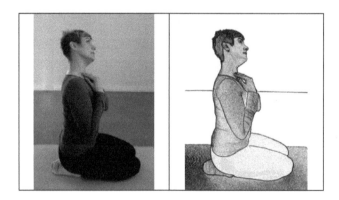

- With each exhalation move your head further backwards and further into sidebending.
- Feel the stretch in sternocleidomastoid in the front and side of your neck.
- Repeat the stretch for the left sternocleidomastoid.

1.9 Atlanto-occipital post-isometric stretch

1.9 Atlanto-occipital post-isometric technique seated

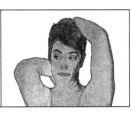

Starting position

- Sit in a chair with your feet apart and firmly planted on the floor.
- Maintain an upright sitting position by consciously holding your pelvis in a vertical position or use a chair with a back support.
- Place the fingers of your right hand behind your neck so that your little finger covers the bottom of your occiput, ring finger covers your atlas (C1), middle finger covers your axis (C2) and index finger and thumb cover C3 and vertebrae below. Your right elbow points forward.

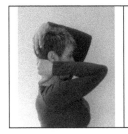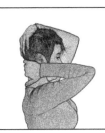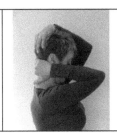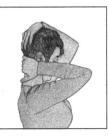

- The spinous process of your axis is the most prominent bump.
- Raise your left arm and grasp the back and right side of your head with the palm of your left hand. Your left elbow points forward and to the left.
- Flex your head and tuck in your chin - this is posterior translation.
- Stop if you feel your atlas push backwards against your fingers.
- Sidebend your head a few degrees to the left while maintaining flexion.
- Rotate your head to the right while maintaining flexion and sidebending.
- Stop rotation if the right side of your atlas presses against your fingers.

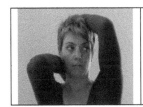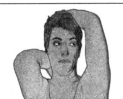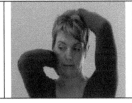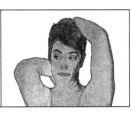

Technique

- Take a deep breath in.
- Look upwards and feel your head attempt to move backwards - but resist the movement with your left hand.
- After five seconds exhale, look downwards and allow your head to move to the new flexion barrier.
- Stop if you feel your atlas push backwards against your fingers.
- This is a subtle tucking in of your chin - do not pull on your head.
- After three eye-induced isometric contractions, relocalise sidebending left and rotation right.
- Repeat the technique on the opposite side.

2.0 Chair supported thoracic, lumbar and hip active sidebends

2.0a Lumbar and hip sidebending stretch standing

Starting position

- Stand with the left side of your body near to the back of the chair.
- Grasp the back of the chair with your left hand.
- Raise your right arm sideways until it is nearly vertical.

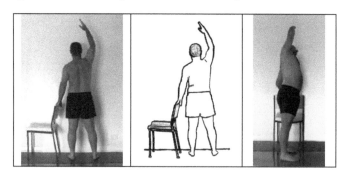

- Use the back of the chair as a pivot, and for support and control.
- Both legs remain extended - do not bend your knees.
- Your body is in the frontal plane - do not rotate your pelvis or spine.
- Your centre of gravity falls evenly across both feet – for ideal balance.
- Sideshift your pelvis and hips to the right and away from the chair.
- Flex your left elbow to lower your body and sidebend your spine left.
- Stop when you feel the initial stages of a stretch down your right side.

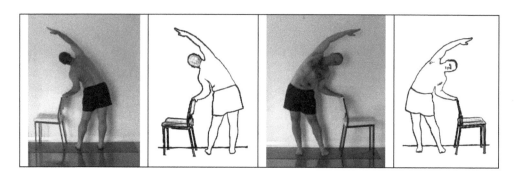

Technique

- Take a deep breath in.
- Exhale and reach 45 degrees up and to the left with your right arm.
- Keep your right elbow extended and reach strongly with your fingertips.
- Feel you are lengthening the spine rather than compressing it.
- Hold the stretch for about five seconds or the length of a full exhalation.
- Breathe in again.
- Flex your left elbow to sidebend your body further to the left.
- Stop when you feel the resistance again down the side of your body.
- Hold this position and repeat the stretch on the right side of your body.
- Repeat the stretch for the left side of the lumbar spine.

2.0b Middle and lower thoracic and thoracolumbar sidebending stretch standing

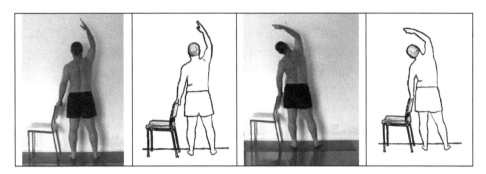

Starting position

- Stand with the left side of your body near to the back of a chair.
- Grasp the back of the chair with your left hand.
- Abduct your right arm until it is nearly vertical.
- Flex your forearm 90 degrees so your elbow points up and to the right.

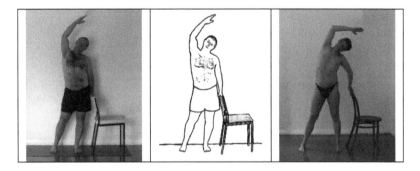

- Use the back of the chair as a pivot and for support and control.
- Both legs remain straight - do not bend your knees.
- Your body is in the frontal plane - do not rotate your pelvis or spine.
- For ideal balance, your centre of gravity should fall between both feet.
- Sideshift your pelvis and hips to the left and towards the chair.
- Flex your left elbow to lower your body and sidebend your spine left.
- Stop when you feel the initial stages of a stretch down your right side.

Technique

- Take a deep breath in.
- Exhale and sidebend your middle thoracic spine and rib cage left by:

  - Maintaining the sideshifting of your pelvis to the left
  - Sideshifting your upper thoracic spine and ribs to the right
  - Pointing the tip of your right elbow 45 degrees up and to the right

- Hold the stretch for about five seconds or the length of a full exhalation.
- Flex your left elbow to sidebend your body further to the left.
- Hold this position and repeat the stretch on the right side of your body.
- Repeat the stretch for the left side of the thoracic spine.

2.1 Wall supported thoracic, lumbar and hip passive and post-isometric sidebending stretches

2.1a Wall supported passive lumbar & hip sidebend stretch

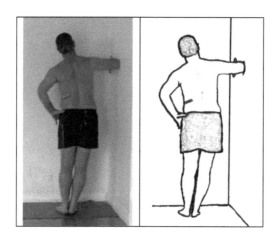

Starting Position

- Stand about 40 cm from the wall with your feet together and the right side of your body opposite a wall.
- Bend your right elbow 90 degrees and lift your shoulder up to 90 degrees.
- Place your right forearm and the palm of your right hand against the wall.
- Your right arm and forearm should be horizontal and level with your shoulder.
- Place your left hand against the side of your pelvis or hip.

Technique

- Take a deep breath in
- Exhale and move the right side of your pelvis nearer to the wall.
- Sidebend at the hip and lower lumbar spine
- Keep your knees straight.
- Do not allow your pelvis or spine to flex, extend or rotate.

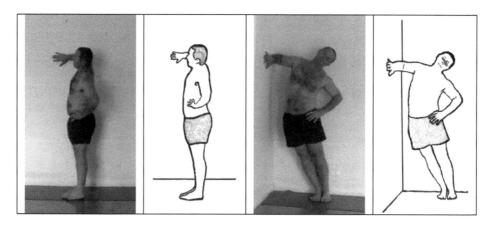

- Repeat the sidebending stretch to the left with each exhalation.
- Repeat the stretch on the other side.

2.1b Wall supported passive thoracic sidebend stretch

Starting Position

- Stand straight with your feet together and the right side of your body facing a wall and about 70 cm from the wall.
- Abduct your right arm 90 degrees.
- Place the palm of your right hand against the wall.
- Your arm should be parallel with the floor and level with your shoulder.
- Place your left hand against the side of your rib cage.

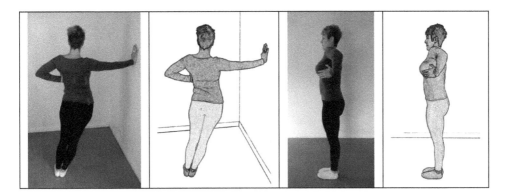

Technique

- Take a deep breath in.
- Exhale and move the right side of your rib cage nearer to the wall.
- Press against the side of your ribs to emphasis thoracic sidebending.

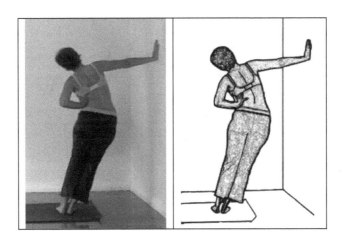

- Keep your knees extended and do not allow your spine to flex, extend or rotate.
- Repeat the sidebending stretch to the left with each exhalation.
- Repeat the sidebending stretch on the right side.

2.1c Wall supported post-isometric hip & spine sidebend stretch

Starting Position

- Stand straight with feet together and your right side facing a wall.
- Abduct your right arm 90 degrees and place your palm against the wall.
- Your right arm should be straight, horizontal and level with your shoulder.

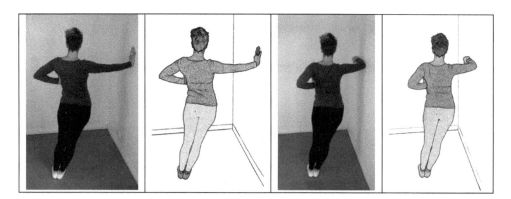

- Alternatively, flex your right elbow 90 degrees, abduct your shoulder 90 degrees and place your forearm and palm against the wall.
- Your right arm should be perpendicular with your forearm and both your arm and forearm should be horizontal and level with your shoulder.
- Place the palm of your left hand on the left side of your rib cage or pelvis.

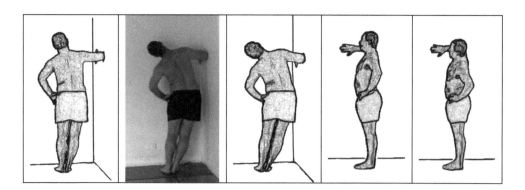

Technique

- Take a deep breath and hold it in.
- If you have rib cage contact then contract the muscles down the right side of your spine and attempt to return to the straight standing position.
- If you have pelvic contact then contract the muscles on the right side of your hip and attempt to return to the straight standing position.
- Resist this contraction with an equal and opposite counterforce from your left hand pushing against the left side of your ribs or pelvis.
- After about five seconds cease the contraction, relax your spine or hip, exhale and move your spine or hip closer to the wall.
- Keep your knees and spine straight and do not allow your spine to rotate.
- Repeat the sidebending stretch to the left with each exhalation.
- Repeat the sidebending stretch on the other side.

2.2 Thoracic and rib active sidebending stretches

2.2a Thoracic and rib sidebending stretch seated

Starting position

- Sit in a chair with your feet apart and planted on the floor.
- Bend your left elbow and place the palm of your left hand against the left side of your rib cage with your fingers pointing forwards and down the ribs.
- Sideshift your upper body to the right so that more of your weight is on your right buttock.
- Fix your eyes forwards and sidebend your head to the left.

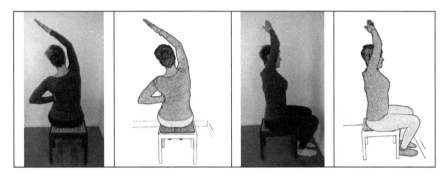

- Keep your pelvis in a vertical position or use a chair with a back support.
- Your body should remain in the frontal plane - do not rotate your spine.
- Raise your right arm until it is vertical and then reach over your head and to the left.
- Stop when you feel the initial stages of a stretch down your right side.

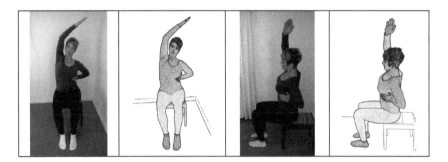

Technique

- Take a deep breath in.
- Exhale and combine the following actions:

  - Reach 45 degrees up and to the left with your right arm
  - Sidebend your head to the left
  - Press against your ribs with your left hand.

- Hold the stretch for about five seconds or the length of a full exhalation.
- Breathe in again and then repeat the sidebending stretch to the left.
- Repeat the stretch for the other side of the thoracic spine and ribs.

2.2b Thoracic and rib sidebending stretch kneeling

Starting Position

- Kneel on a mat with your knees apart and your arms in front of your body.
- Flex your left elbow and place the palm of your left hand against the left side of your rib cage with your fingers pointing forwards and down the ribs.
- Sideshift your upper body to the right so that more of your weight is on your right buttock and over your right foot.
- Fix your eyes forwards and sidebend your head to the left.

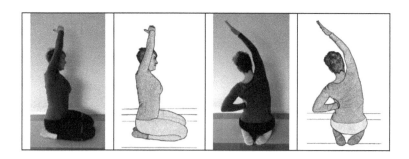

- Keep your pelvis in a vertical position.
- Your body should remain in the frontal plane - do not rotate your spine.
- Raise your right arm until it is vertical and then reach over your head and to the left.
- Stop when you feel the initial stages of a stretch down your right side.

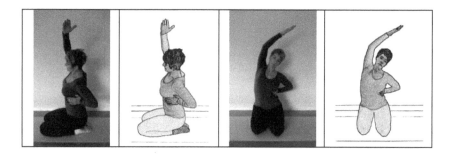

Technique

- Take a deep breath in.
- Exhale and combine the following actions:

  - Reach 45 degrees up and to the left with your right arm
  - Sidebend your head to the left
  - Press against your ribs with your left hand.

- Hold the stretch for about five seconds or the length of a full exhalation.
- Breathe in again and then repeat the sidebending stretch to the left.
- Repeat the stretch on the other side of your thoracic spine and ribs.

2.3 Kneeling lateral stretch - active stretch for the shoulder, trunk and hip

2.3 Kneeling lateral stretch

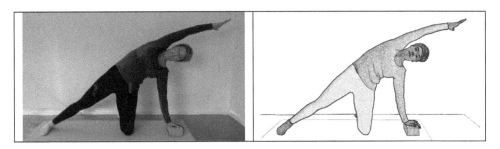

Starting position

- Kneel on a mat with a block or a small stool at your left side.
- Move your right foot to your right and straighten your leg.
- Place your left hand, palm down on the block – make sure it is far enough from your hip that your arm and forearm are vertical.
- Keep your left elbow extended – but flex your elbow if you use a stool.
- Adjust your pelvis so that it is in a vertical plane.
- Your left hip should be above your left knee and your thigh vertical.

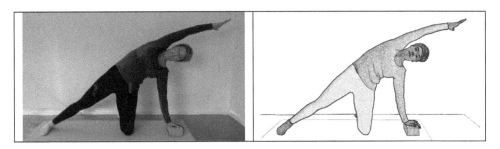

- Take your right arm over your head and reach upwards about 45 degrees but keep your arm in line with your body.
- Stop when you feel the initial stages of a stretch down your right side.
- Keep your whole body in the frontal plane - do not allow it to rotate.

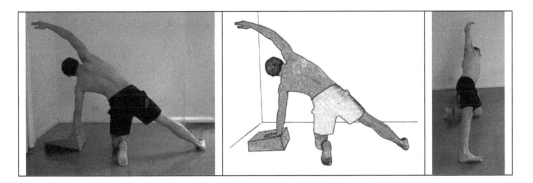

Technique

- Take a deep breath in.
- Exhale and reach about 45 degrees upwards and left with your right arm.
- Keep your right elbow extended and reach strongly with your fingertips.
- Hold the stretch for about five seconds or the length of a full exhalation.
- Feel the stretch down the whole right side of your body.
- Flex your left elbow to increase sidebending but do not allow rotation.
- Repeat the stretch several times, moving with an exhalation.
- Repeat the stretch on the opposite side of the body.

2.4 Hanging stretches - passive and post-isometric stretches for latissimus dorsi, the thoracolumbar fascia, quadratus lumborum and the lateral fibres of erector spinea

2.4a Hanging stretch erect

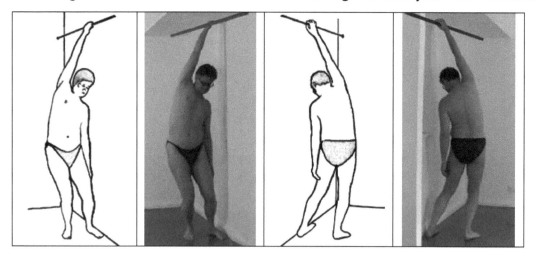

Starting position

- Stand straight and below a strong wooden horizontal pole or metal bar.
- The pole should not be so high that you have to strain or stand on tip toes to reach it and not so low that you have to squat deeply.
- The pole should be firmly attached to a wall at both ends and strong enough to support your body weight.
- Raise your right arm and grasp the pole with your right hand.
- Your right elbow should be flexed five or 10 degrees and your arm relaxed.

- Bend both hips and knees and lower your body towards the floor until your right arm is straight and you feel the initial stages of tension taken up by your ligaments and muscles down the right side of your body.

Technique

- Take a deep breath in.
- Exhale, flex your right knee and allow your right hip and pelvis to drop towards the floor.
- Allow the muscles on the right side of your body to completely relax and use the weight of your body to stretch the right shoulder, spine and hip.
- Introduce forward or backward pelvic translation, forward or backward pelvic tilt or right sideshifting of your pelvis to target specific muscles.
- Take a deep breath in and then pull down on the bar with your right arm.
- Resist any upward movement of your body with a firm stance.
- After five seconds exhale, cease the isometric muscle contraction, and then relax and allow your right hip and pelvis to drop towards the floor.
- Repeat the stretch down the left side.

2.4b Hanging stretch flexed unilateral

Starting position

- Stand up straight in front of a strong wooden vertical pole or metal bar.
- The pole should be firmly attached to something top and bottom and strong enough to support your body weight.
- Flex your body at the hips and grasp the pole with your right hand.
- Keep your arm straight and in line with your body.
- Your knees may be extended or slightly flexed.

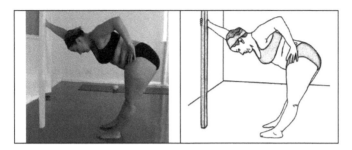

Technique

- Take a deep breath in.
- Exhale and let your right hip and pelvis drop backwards.

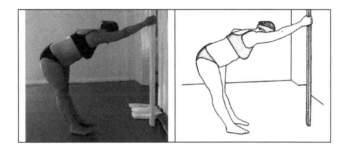

- Allow the muscles on the right side of your body to completely relax and use the weight of your pelvis to stretch the right shoulder and spine.
- Tilt your pelvis forwards or backwards or sideshift it to the right to target specific muscles.

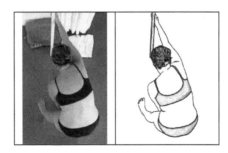

- Take a deep breath in and then pull down on the bar with your right arm.
- Resist any upward movement of your body with a firm stance.
- After five seconds exhale, cease the isometric muscle contraction, and then relax and allow your right hip and pelvis to drop backwards.
- Repeat the stretch down the left side.

2.4c Hanging stretch flexed bilateral

Starting position

- Stand straight in front of a strong wooden vertical pole or metal bar.
- The pole should be firmly attached to something top and bottom and strong enough to support your body weight.
- Flex your body at the hips and grasp the pole with both hands.
- Keep your arms straight and in line with your body.
- Your knees may be extended or slightly flexed.

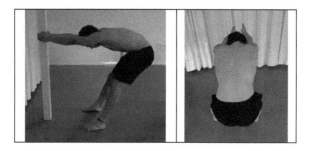

Technique

- Take a deep breath in.
- Exhale and let your right hip and pelvis drop backwards.

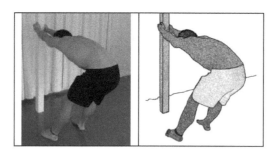

- Allow the muscles down both sides of your back to completely relax and use the weight of your body to stretch the shoulders and spine.
- Tilt your pelvis forwards or backwards or sideshift left or right or cross your arms and internally rotate your shoulders to target specific muscles.

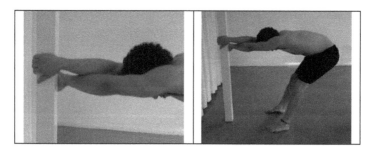

- Take a deep breath in and then pull down on the bar with both arms.
- Resist any movement of your body with a firm stance.
- After five seconds exhale, cease the isometric muscle contraction, and then relax and allow your hips and pelvis to drop backwards.
- Repeat the stretch down the left side.

2.4d Hanging passive stretch unilateral sidebending

Starting position

- Stand with your feet together with the left side of your body near to a post.
- Raise your arms until your hands are directly above your head.
- Sidebend your body at the hips and grasp the post with both hands.
- Move your pelvis to the right and away from the post.
- Keep your body in a frontal plane (no flexion, extension or rotation) by adjusting your shoulders and pelvis and keep your knees straight.

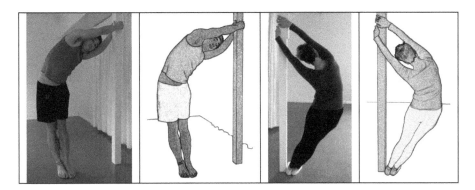

Technique

- Take a deep breath in.
- Exhale and perform one of the following actions:

  - Sideshift your pelvis to the right and further away from the post to sidebend the lumbar spine and hips to the left.
  - Move your rib cage to the right and further away from the post to sidebend the thoracic and thoracolumbar spine to the left.

- Feel the stretch in your right thigh, hip, pelvis, ribs, lumbar and thoracic.
- When the feet are near the post this increases the stretch on the hip.
- When the feet are away from the post this increases the stretch on the thoracic spine.

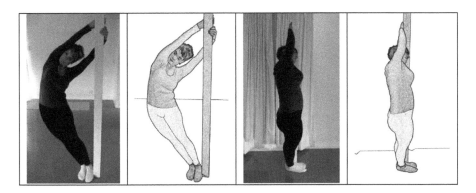

- Repeat the technique for the left side.

2.5 Upper Dog - active extension stretches for the shoulders, thoracic and lumbar spine

2.5a Upper Dog extension stretch kneeling

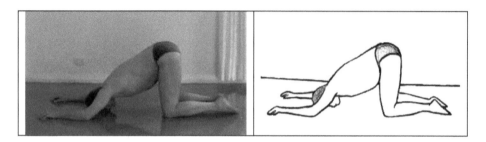

Starting position

- Kneel on the floor, preferably on a carpet or mat.
- Place your elbows, forearms and hands flat on the floor so they are parallel and shoulder distance apart.
- Place your forehead on the floor and keep your palms down.
- Your hips should be over your knees so that your thighs are vertical.
- Place your knees and feet slightly apart for better balance.

Technique

- Straighten your right elbow but keep your left elbow flexed on the floor.
- Take a deep breath in.
- Exhale and move your right shoulder, thoracic and ribs towards the floor.
- Continue to bring your right side towards the floor with each exhalation.
- Focus on the area in your thoracic spine that is most restricted.
- Sidebend left by sideshifting your upper thoracic spine to the right.
- Bend your right elbow and straighten your left and repeat on the left side.

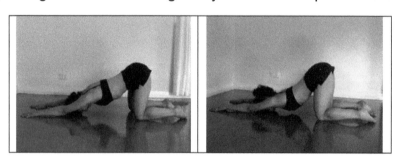

- Straighten both of your elbows.
- Take another deep breath in.
- Exhale and bring both shoulders and both sides of upper thoracic spine and rib cage towards the floor.
- Continue to bring your chest further towards the floor with each exhalation.
- Determine where your thoracic is most restricted and focus on this area.
- Introduce sidebending by sideshifting your upper thoracic spine to one side and then repeat the extension and sidebending on the opposite side.

2.5b Upper Dog extension stretch standing

Starting position

- Stand straight facing a vertical wall with your feet slightly apart.
- Place the palms of both hands on the wall, shoulder distance apart and about 30 cm above your head.
- Take a step back with one foot.
- Bend your knees and straighten your elbows.
- Place your forehead on or near the wall.
- Allow your thoracic spine to bend backwards.
- If necessary, adjust the position of your feet.

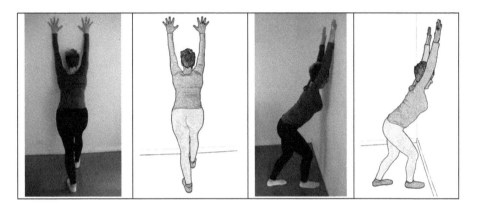

Technique

- Take a deep breath in.
- Exhale and bring your shoulders, thoracic spine and ribs towards the wall.
- Continue to bring your chest further towards the floor with each exhalation.

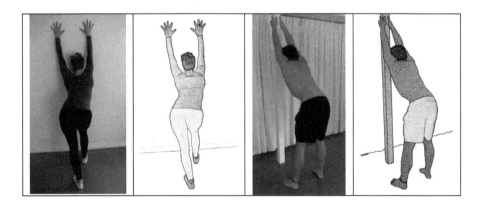

- Focus on extend your thoracic spine where it is most restricted.
- Maintain extended elbows.
- Take another deep breath in.
- Exhale and while maintaining backward bending introduce sidebending to the left by sideshifting your upper thoracic spine and shoulders to the right.
- Repeat the sidebending movement in extension for several exhalations then repeat the stretch on the other side.

2.5c Latissimus dorsi stretch kneeling

Starting position

- Kneel on the floor, on a carpet or mat facing a stool, chair or low table.
- Bring your elbows, forearms and palms together.
- This will externally rotate your arms and separate your shoulder blades.
- Lean forwards and place your elbows on the top of the stool.
- Move your knees and feet slightly apart for better balance.

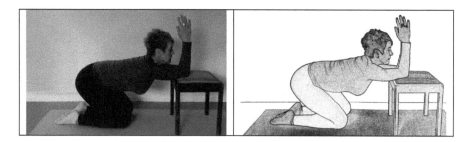

Technique

- Take a deep breath in.
- Exhale and move your pelvis backwards and towards the floor.
- Drop your chest towards the floor and elongate your spine.

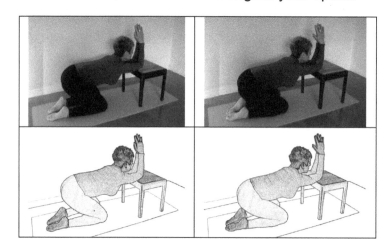

- Take another deep breath and hold it in.
- Press down on the stool with your arms and elbows.
- Resist any upward movement of your body with a firm stance.
- After five seconds exhale, cease the isometric contraction, and relax and allow your pelvis to drop backwards and towards the floor.
- Repeat the stretch bringing your buttocks further towards your feet with each exhalation.
- This is a useful technique for lengthening the spine after a spinal rotation stretch.

2.6 The Cobra - active and passive extension stretches for the shoulders, cervical, thoracic, lumbar spine and hips

2.6a Half Cobra

Starting position

- Lay on your front in the prone position on the floor with your feet apart and your toes pointing backwards.
- Flex your elbows 90 degrees and place them at the side of your body directly under your shoulders so that your arms are vertical.

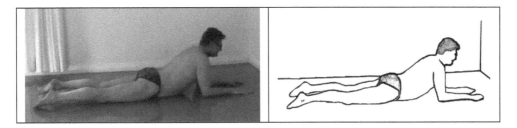

- Place your palms downwards, flat on the floor.
- Keep your spine straight so the tension on each side of your spine is even.
- Adjust your body so that the tissues are at their most relaxed state.

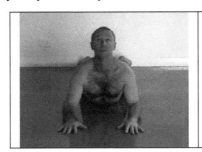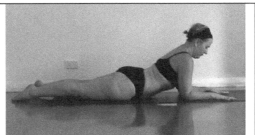

Technique

- Take a deep breath in and contract specific shoulder, spinal and hip muscles to produce targeted joint movements:

  - Move your shoulders forwards and away from your spine (protraction)
  - Move your cervical spine up and back (posterior translation) – contract your thoracic muscles
  - Push your pubic bone and hips downwards and into the floor – contract your buttocks – use a mild force

- Hold the contraction for about five seconds and then exhale and relax your shoulder, thoracic, lumbar and hip muscles completely.
- Allow your body to sink into the floor.
- Combine the movements or do them individually.
- Vary the level of contraction from mild to moderate.
- Focus on letting go in the areas of restriction.

2.6b Full Cobra

Starting position

- Lay on your front in the prone position on the floor with your feet apart and your toes pointing backwards.
- Flex your elbows and place them at the side of your body directly under your shoulders and with your palms down flat on the floor in the half cobra.

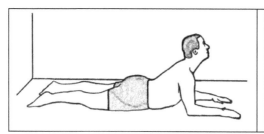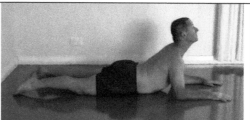

- Slide your palms a few centimetres forward along the floor to a position in line with and directly in front of your shoulders.
- Straighten your elbows until you are in a mild backward bending position.

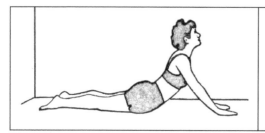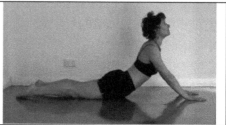

Technique

- Take a deep breath in and contract specific shoulder and spinal and hip muscles to produce targeted joint movements:

  - Move your shoulders forwards and away from your spine
  - Move your cervical spine up and back. Tuck in your chin. Don't hyperextend your head. Contract your thoracic muscles.
  - Push your pubic bone and hips downwards and into the floor. Contract your buttocks - use a mild force.

- Hold the contraction for about five seconds and then exhale and relax your shoulder, thoracic, lumbar and hip muscles completely.
- Allow your body to drop into the floor.
- These movements can be done individually or combined.
- Vary the level of contraction, from mild to moderate.
- Increase the intensity of the backward bending by bringing your hands closer to your body. Focus on extending areas of restriction.
- With greater levels of back extension there is the danger of increasing pre-existing hypermobility in joints in localised areas of the spine.
- Extend but don't hyperextend your head.

2.6c Sidebending Cobra

Starting position

- Lay on your front in the prone position on the floor with your feet apart and your toes pointing backwards.
- Flex your elbows and place them at the side of your body directly under your shoulders and with your palms down flat on the floor in the half cobra.

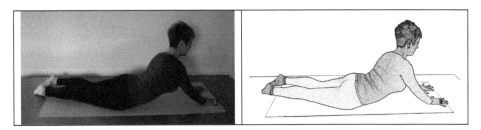

- Sidebend your thoracic, lumbar and hip to one side.
- Adopt a generalised sidebending or localise the sidebending to the thoracic, lumbar or hip joint.

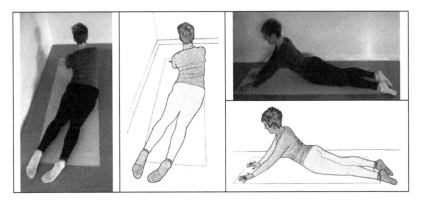

Technique

- Take a deep breath in and contract specific shoulder and spinal and hip muscles to produce targeted joint movements:

  - Move your shoulders forwards and away from your spine
  - Move your cervical spine up and back. Tuck in your chin. Don't hyperextend your head. Contract your thoracic muscles.
  - Push your pubic bone and hips downwards and into the floor. Contract your buttocks - use a mild force.

- Hold the contraction for about five seconds and then exhale and relax your shoulder, thoracic, lumbar and hip muscles completely.
- Allow your body to drop into the floor.
- These movements can be done individually or combined.
- Vary the level of contraction, from mild to moderate.
- Move your hands a few centimetres forward along the floor and then straighten your elbows and adopt the full cobra
- Attempt the full cobra with either a generalised or a localise sidebending.

2.6d Rotation Cobra

Starting position

- Lay on your front in the prone position on the floor with your feet apart and your toes pointing backwards.
- Flex your elbows and place them at the side of your body directly under your shoulders and with your palms down flat on the floor in the half cobra.

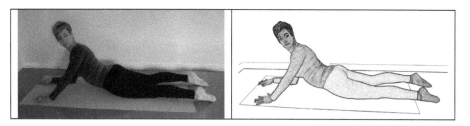

- Straighten your left elbow and allow your shoulder, spine and rib cage to rotate to the left in the backward bending position.

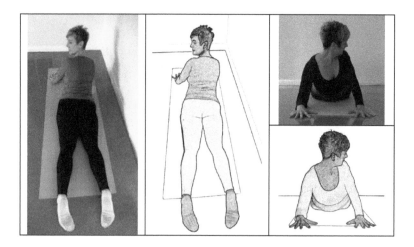

Technique

- Take a deep breath in and contract specific neck, shoulder and spinal muscles to produce targeted joint rotation:

  - Rotate your head and neck to the left
  - Move your left scapula upward, forwards and away from your spine (protraction) and rotate spine and rib cage to the left.

- Increase the rotation with each inhalation and maintain it during exhalation.
- These movements can be done individually or combined.
- Vary the level of contraction, from mild to moderate.
- Combine rotation with sidebending in half cobra and full cobra.

2.7 The Locust - active stretches for the shoulders, thoracic, lumbar spine and hips

2.7a Diagonal locust

Starting position

- Lay on your front on the floor with your feet slightly apart and your toes pointing backwards.
- Move both arms out sideways until they are in contact with the side of your head and your hands are above your head.
- Place your hands so your palms point down into the floor.
- Keep your head straight, face down and resting on your nose or chin.

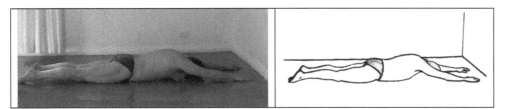

Technique

- Take a deep breath in and lift your right arm and left leg off the floor.
- Allow movement of your scapula but stop before your spine rotates or your pelvis or rib cage lifts off the floor.

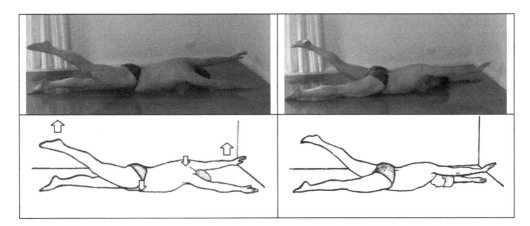

- Hold the position for five to 10 seconds.
- Only lift only one arm and one leg off the floor.
- Exhale while bringing your arm and leg back to the floor.
- Allow your limbs to relax for a few seconds.
- Repeat using the left arm and right leg.
- The diagonal action of the arm and leg helps maintain balance.
- This active stretch can be done as a single arm raise or a single leg raise.
- This stretch can be done standing with the weight of the body on one foot.
- This is useful in rehabilitation after injury or surgery or for older people.

2.7b Full Locust arms at side

Starting position

- Lay on your front in the prone position on the floor with your arms at your side, palms upwards, feet apart and your toes pointing backwards.

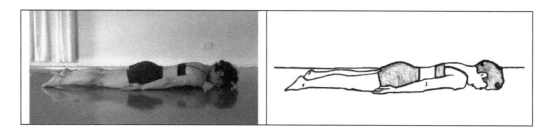

- Keep your head straight, face down and resting on your nose or chin.

Technique

- Take a deep breath in and lift your arms and legs off the floor.
- Contract your buttocks and squeeze your shoulder blades together.
- Extend your thoracic and lumbar spine but not your cervical spine.

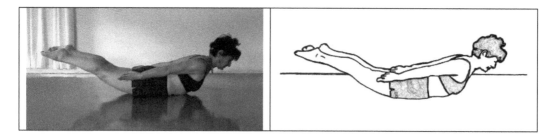

- Hold the position for five to 10 seconds.
- Your pelvis, abdomen and lower ribs remain in contact with the floor.
- Exhale and bring your arms and legs back to the floor.
- Relax your limbs for a few seconds and then repeat the active stretch.

2.7c Full Locust arms abducted

Starting position

- Lay on your front in the prone position on the floor with your arms at your side, feet apart and your toes pointing backwards.
- Move both arms out to the side until they are in contact with the side of your head and your hands are above your head.
- Alternatively bend both arms 90 degrees and bend your elbows 90 degrees.
- Place your hands
- In both cases, have the palms of your hands facing down to the floor.
- Keep your head straight, face down and resting on your nose or chin.

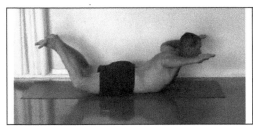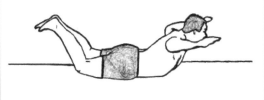

Technique

- Take in a deep breath and lift your arms and legs off the floor.
- Contract your buttocks and squeeze your shoulder blades together.
- Allow your thoracic and lumbar spines to extend but not your cervical spine.

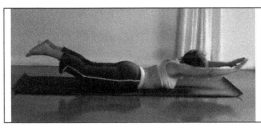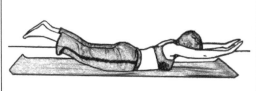

- Hold the position for five to 10 seconds.
- Your pelvis, abdomen and lower ribs remain in contact with the floor.
- Exhale while bringing your arms and legs back to the floor.
- Relax your limbs for a few seconds and then repeat the active stretch.

2.8 The Extended Cat - an active extension stretch for the shoulders, hips, and cervical, thoracic and lumbar spine

2.8 Extended Cat

Starting position

- Kneel on the floor, preferably on a carpet or on a mat.
- Place your hands palms down on the floor and shoulder distance apart.
- Your thighs are vertical and your knees are directly under your hips.
- Adjust your arms until they are straight and vertical.
- Keep your knees and feet slightly apart for better balance.
- Your spine should be in a neutral position, neither flexed nor extended.

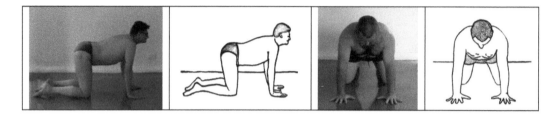

Technique

- Fully exhale.
- Slowly start to inhale while simultaneously extending your spine
- Start by bending your head and neck up and backwards.
- Move progressively down your spine extending your thoracic, lumbar and sacrum, and finally flexing your pelvis on your hips.
- By the end of the inhalation your entire spine should be fully extended.

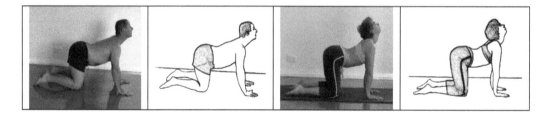

- Fully exhale again.
- Repeat the extension movement several times with each inhalation.
- Focus your attention on the areas of your spine that show the greatest resistance to extension.
- These are usually the middle and very upper thoracic spine but as everyone is unique there are exceptions to this generalisation.
- Although most stretches are done on the exhalation, the extended cat is best done on the inhalation because inhalation synchronises with the natural movement of the ribs.

2.9 The Flexed Cat - active flexion stretches for the shoulders, hips, and cervical, thoracic and lumbar spine

2.9a Flexed Cat kneeling

Starting position

- Kneel on the floor, preferably on a carpet or on a mat.
- Place your hands palms down on the floor and shoulder distance apart.
- Your thighs are vertical and your knees are directly under your hips.
- Your arms are straight and vertical.
- Keep your knees and feet slightly apart for better balance.
- Your spine should be in a neutral position, neither flexed nor extended.

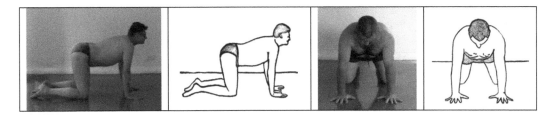

Technique

- Take a deep breath in.
- Exhale, while simultaneously flexing your spine.
- Progressively work down your spine flexing your head, cervical, thoracic and lumbar spine and sacrum.
- Your hips are fixed and so the final movement involves posteriorly tilting your pelvis thereby extending your pelvis on your hips.
- Tuck in your chin and tail bone.
- By the end of the exhalation your entire spine should be fully flexed.
- Make sure you tuck in your chin and tuck in your coccyx.

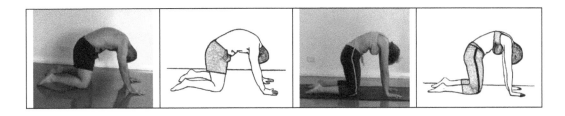

- Fully inhale again.
- Repeat the flexion movement several times with each exhalation.
- Focus your attention on the areas of your spine that show the greatest resistance to flexion.
- These are usually the thoracolumbar and lumbosacral spine but it could be anywhere in the spine.

2.9b Flexed Cat standing

Starting position

- Stand with your feet apart and your arms in front of your body.
- Flex your knees and hips about 20 degrees each.
- Cross your arms and place your right hand on your left thigh and your left hand on your right thigh just above each knee.
- Flex your head, neck, thoracic and lumbar spine.

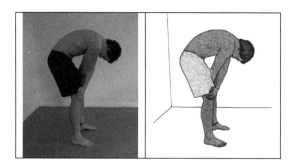

Technique

- Take a deep breath in.
- Exhale and simultaneously increase the flexion of your spine.
- Start by bending your head and neck downwards and forwards.
- Move progressively down your spine, flexing your spine through your thoracic, lumbar and sacrum to your hips.
- Try and separate your scapula (protraction) and stretch the muscles between them.
- By the end of the exhalation your entire spine should be flexed and your shoulders apart.

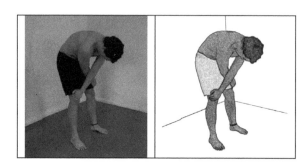

- Fully inhale again.
- Repeat the flexion movement several times with each exhalation.
- Focus your attention on the areas of your spine that show the greatest resistance to flexion.
- Do not overstretch your spine.

3.0 Knees to chest - active, passive and post-isometric flexion stretches for the lower thoracic, lumbar and hips

3.0a Passive knees to chest stretch supine

Starting position

- Lie on the floor, preferably on a carpet or mat.
- If you have an increased thoracic kyphosis or you are very stiff, place a pillow under your head to prevent your head dropping backwards and straining the muscles or ligaments in your neck.
- Flex your hips and knees.

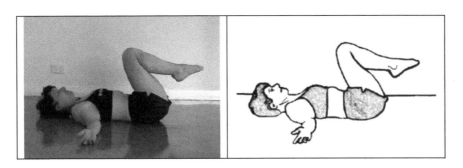

- Grasp around your knees with both hands.
- Bring your knees towards your chest but stop when you feel the initial stages of a stretch in your lower back.
- Tuck your chin in.

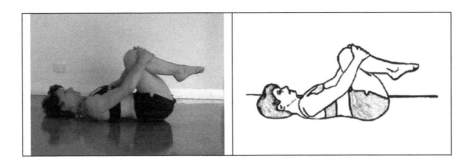

Technique

- Take a deep breath in.
- Exhale as you pull your knees towards your chest and slightly upwards towards your head.
- Feel the stretch in your lower back and buttocks.
- Take another deep breath in then exhale and repeat the stretch.

3.0b Post-isometric knees to chest stretch supine

Starting position

- Lie on the floor, preferably on a carpet or mat.
- If you have an increased thoracic kyphosis, place your head on a pillow.
- Bring your knees to your chest.
- Grasp around your knees with both hands.
- Bring your knees towards your chest.

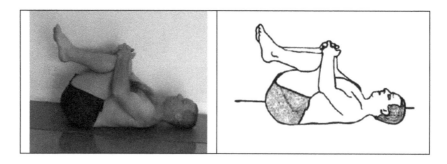

Technique

- Take a deep breath in.
- Attempt to take your knees away from your chest but resist the movement with both hands using an equal and opposite counterforce.

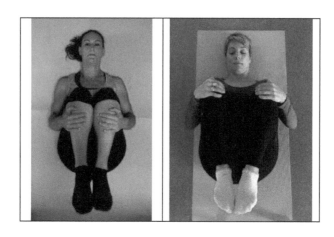

- After about five seconds cease the contraction, exhale and bring your knees further towards the floor and to the new tension barrier.
- Repeat the technique several times bringing pull your knees further towards your chest with each exhalation.

3.0c Active knees to chest stretch supine

Starting position

- Lie on the floor, preferably on a carpet or mat.
- If you have an increased thoracic kyphosis, place a pillow under your head to prevent straining the muscles or ligament in your neck.
- Fully flex your hips until your knees are as close to the chest as possible and hold this position.

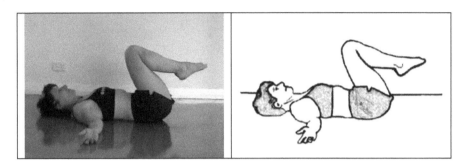

Technique

- Take a deep breath in.
- Exhale and combine the following movements:

  - Increase hip flexion by bringing your knees further towards the floor
  - Lift your coccyx up and off the floor
  - Push the back of your pelvis into the floor
  - Flatten your lumbar spine.

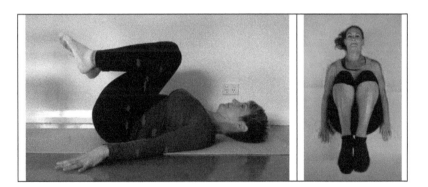

- Hold the contraction and flexed posture for three to five seconds.
- Feel the stretch in your lower back and a tightening in you abdomen.
- Inhale, relax and bring your hips and back to the starting position.
- Repeat the active stretch several times during an exhalation.

3.0d Active knees to chest stretch with rotation supine

Starting position

- Lie on the floor, preferably on a carpet or mat.
- If you have an increased thoracic kyphosis support your head with a pillow
- Bring your knees to your chest.
- Abducted your arms 90 degrees and rest them on the floor.
- Take your knees to the left by rotating your pelvis and spine.

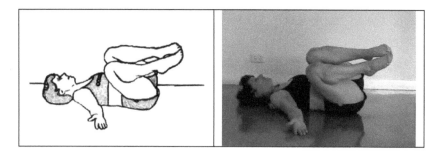

Technique

- Take a deep breath in.
- Exhale, and while maintaining hip flexion (knees to your chest) increase hip rotation by taking your knees to the left.
- You should be able to rotate your hips about 45 degrees while still maintaining balance.
- Feel the stretch in the right hip and right side of the spine.
- Repeat the stretch with each exhalation by taking your knees to the right.
- Repeat the stretch on the other side.

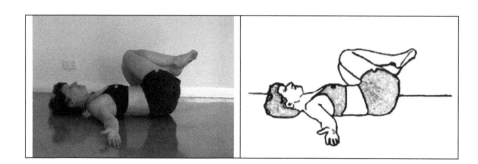

- If you are unable to maintain your balance, flex your elbow 90 degrees, grasp a table leg with your hand and use it for support.

3.0e Unilateral stretch for the lumbar and gluteus maximus

Starting position

- Lie on your back on a carpet or mat.
- Place a pillow under your head if you have a stiff flexed thoracic spine.
- Flex your right hip and knee.
- Grasp around your right knee and leg with both hands.
- Pull your right knee towards your chest.

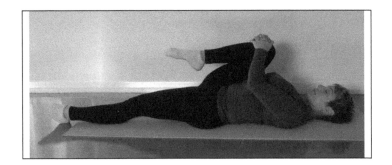

Technique

- Take a deep breath in.
- Exhale and during the exhalation pull your right knee further towards your chest and the floor.

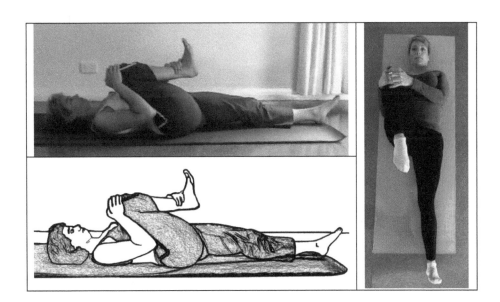

- Keep the back of your left thigh and leg in contact with the floor.
- Your left hip and left knee should be kept in full extension.
- Repeat the technique several times and with each exhalation bring your knee further towards your chest and the floor.

3.1 Spinal twist sitting - active and passive rotation stretches for the shoulders and the cervical, thoracic and lumbar spine

3.1a Passive spinal twist seated

Starting position

- Sit on a chair with your body at right angles to the back of the chair so the left side of your pelvis and thigh are in contact with the back of the chair.
- The seat should be horizontal so that you can keep a straight spine and it should be at a suitable height off the ground so that the soles of your feet are flat on the floor - alternatively place your feet on two blocks or books.

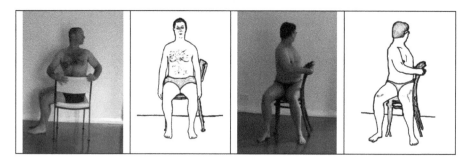

- Rotate your head, neck, shoulders and spine to the left so that you face the back of the chair.
- Grasp the back of the chair with both hands.

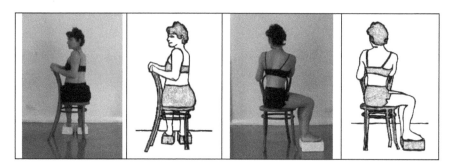

Technique

- Take a deep breath in.
- Exhale and rotate further left, towards the back of the chair by pulling on the back of the chair with your right hand and pushing with your left hand.
- Maintain rotation as you inhale and increase rotation with each exhalation.
- Passive rotation of the spine is produced using upper limb muscle contraction and leverage through the shoulder to the spine.
- Repeat the stretch by passively rotating the spine to the right.

3.1b Active spinal twist seated

Starting position

- Sit on a chair with your body at right angles to the back of the chair so the right side of your pelvis and thigh are in contact with the back of the chair.
- The seat should be horizontal so that you can keep a straight spine and it should be at a suitable height off the ground, so that the soles of your feet are flat on the floor - alternatively place your feet on two blocks or books.
- Rotate your head, neck, shoulders and spine to the left so that your upper body faces the front of the chair.

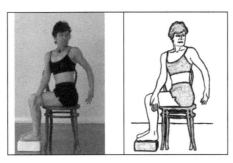

- Place your right wrist against the outside of your left thigh and fully straighten your right forearm at the elbow.
- Your wrist acts as a pivot and your thigh a fulcrum and your body moves around this fixed point of contact via the long lever of your extended arm.
- Allow your left shoulder to drop and your left arm to hang freely.

Technique

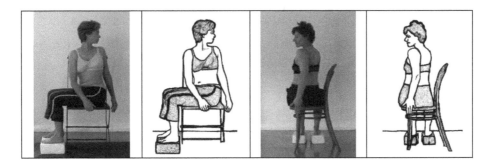

- Take a deep breath in.
- Exhale and rotate your spine and upper body further left, towards the front of the chair using your abdominal, spinal and scapular retractor muscles.
- In addition to rotating your thoracic spine and shoulders, also turn your head and neck – open your eyes and look in the direction of rotation.
- Do not grasp and pull on your body or the chair or with your hands - your right wrist simply rests on your left thigh and your body moves around this fixed point of contact, while your left arm hangs freely by your side.
- Your wrist is a pivot, your thigh is the fulcrum, and your arm is a long lever.
- Maintain rotation as you inhale and increase rotation with each exhalation.
- Repeat the stretch by actively rotating your spine to the right.

3.1c Spinal twist sitting on the floor

Starting position

- Sit on the floor with your legs straight and out in front of you.
- Flex your left hip and knee and place your left foot on the outside of your right leg, so the outside of your left ankle is resting against the outside of your right knee and the sole of your left foot is planted on the floor.
- Place the palm of your left hand on the floor about 20 cm from your pelvis.
- Rotate your spine to the left and grasp the outside of your left knee with your right hand - or if you are very flexible, place your right elbow on the outside of your left knee and your forearm down the outside of your leg.
- Fully extend your left forearm at the elbow and lift the left side of your body upwards until your spine is vertical - maybe also use your fingertips to lift.
- Rotate your head, neck, shoulders and spine fully to the left.

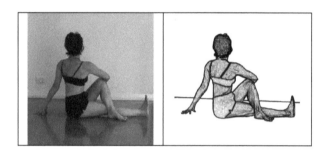

Technique

- Take a deep breath in.
- Exhale and rotate further to the left by pulling on the side of your knee with your right hand or forearm – this is the passive stretch using shoulder muscle contraction and leverage.
- Take in another deep breath while maintaining the rotation.
- Exhale and rotate further to the left by contracting the muscles in your spine – this is the active stretch.
- Increase rotation with each exhalation using the passive or the active variation or a combination of both.
- Repeat the stretch by rotating the spine to the right.

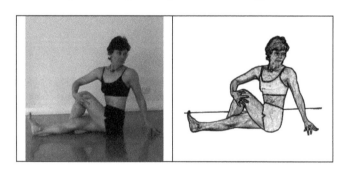

Do not do this stretch if you cannot keep an erect spine when sitting on the floor.

3.2 Spinal twist standing - active and passive rotation stretches for the shoulders and the cervical, thoracic and lumbar spine and hips

3.2a Passive spinal twist standing wall supported

Starting position

- Stand with your feet apart, about 20 cm from a wall or wire fence and with the left side of your body facing the wall.
- Flex your forearms about 90 degrees and flex your arms 45 degrees.
- Rotate your head, neck, shoulders and spine to the left so that your upper body faces the wall – but keep your pelvis at right angles to the wall.
- Place your palms flat against the wall about shoulder height.
- Alternatively place your hands against a wire fence about shoulder height with your fingers intermeshed with the wire.

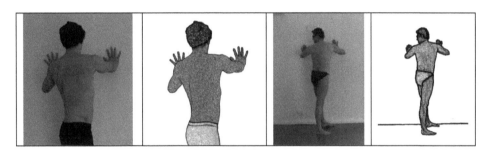

Technique

- Take a deep breath in.
- Exhale as you rotate further left by pulling on the wall with your hands.
- Maintain the rotation as your inhale and increase the rotation with each exhalation using muscle contraction and leverage from the upper limb.

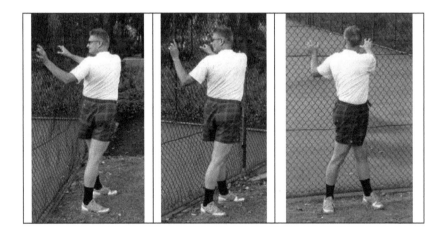

- Keep your pelvis perpendicular to the wall and your spine straight.
- Repeat the stretch by rotating the spine to the right.
- As an alternative to the wall, grasp a wire tennis fence.
- Stand side-on to the fence or wall, or if you are more flexible then start with your back to the fence or wall.

3.2b Active spinal twist standing

Starting position

- Stand with your feet apart and your arms at your sides.
- Rotate your head, neck, shoulders and spine to the left but keep your pelvis and lower limbs in a fixed position.

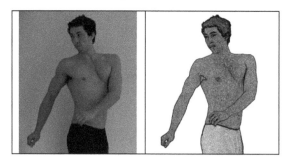

- Relax your shoulders so they are in a natural descended position.
- Your arms hang freely but follow the rotation of your body to the left.

Technique

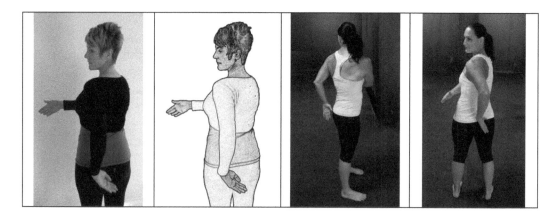

- Take a deep breath in.
- Exhale and rotate further to the left by contracting your abdominal, spinal rotators and scapular retractor muscles.
- Allow your arms to follow the rotation of your body to the left.
- Also turn your head by focusing your eyes in the direction of the rotation.
- Maintain rotation as you inhale and increase rotation with each exhalation.
- Repeat the stretch by actively rotating your spine to the right.

3.3 Spinal twist standing flexed at the hips - active rotation stretch for the shoulders and the thoracic and lumbar spine

3.3 Active spinal twist standing flexed at the hips

Starting position

- Stand with your feet 30 to 50 cm apart about 1 m from a chair or table.
- Flex your body about 90 degrees at the hips and place the palms of both hands on the back of the chair.
- Take your pelvis backwards and away from the chair and drop your shoulders and upper thoracic spine towards the floor.

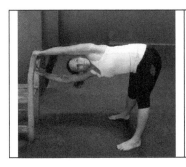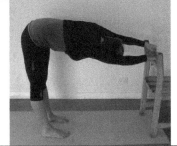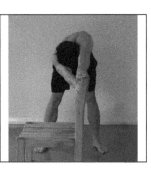

- Keep your spine, knees and arms straight.
- Rotate your spine to the left so that your upper body faces sideways.
- As an alternative to using a chair or table you can grasp a wire fence and use it to assist rotation.

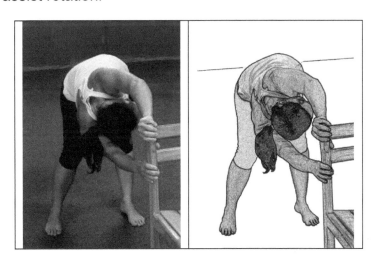

Technique

- Take a deep breath in.
- Exhale as you rotate to the left by contracting your abdominal, spinal rotators and scapular retractor muscles.
- Maintain rotation as you inhale and increase rotation with each exhalation.
- Repeat the stretch by actively rotating your spine to the right.

3.4 Spinal twist kneeling - active rotation stretch for the shoulders and the thoracic and lumbar spine

3.4 Active spinal twist kneeling

Starting position

- Kneel on the floor with your knees and feet apart, and with your thighs vertical so that your knees are directly under your hips.
- Place your hands palms down on the floor, shoulder distance apart.
- Move your left hand a few centimetres forward and flex your left forearm at the elbow.
- Lift your right hand off the floor and slide it along the floor and under your chest to the left.
- This will rotate your head, neck, shoulders and spine to the left.
- The back of your right hand, forearm and arm should rest on the floor.
- Your left elbow should be flexed about 90 degrees.

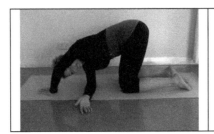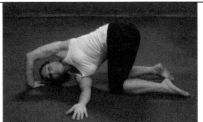

Technique

- Take a deep breath in.
- Exhale and rotate your thoracic spine to the left by reaching along the floor with your right hand while moving your left shoulder backwards.
- This movement involves contraction of your abdominal, spinal rotators and your scapular retractor muscles on the left, and your scapular protractor muscles on the right.

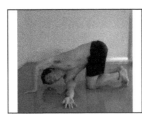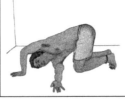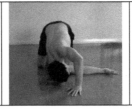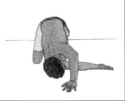

- Combine this with rotation of your head and cervical spine to the left by looking under your arm and upwards.
- Maintain rotation as you inhale and increase rotation with each exhalation.
- Repeat the stretch by actively rotating your spine to the right.

3.5 Spinal twist prone - active and passive rotation stretches for the shoulders and the cervical, thoracic and lumbar spine

3.5 Active and passive spinal twist prone

Starting position

- Lie on your front in the prone position on the floor with your feet apart and your toes pointing backwards.
- Abduct your arms 90 degrees and place your palms flat on the floor, level with your shoulders.
- Flex your left forearm at the elbow and bring your left hand closer to the side.
- Raise your head, left elbow and shoulder off the floor and your spine will rotate to the left.
- Make sure your pelvis remains on the floor.

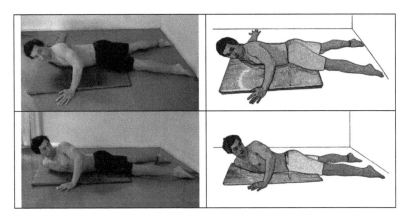

Technique

- Take a deep breath in.
- Exhale and rotate to the left by pushing with your left arm and lifting your left shoulder off the floor - this is the passive stretch.

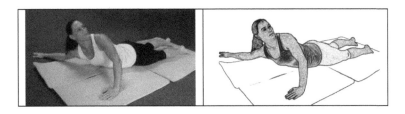

- Take in another deep breath and hold it in.
- Exhale and rotate further to the left by contracting your spinal rotators and scapular retractor muscles - this is the active stretch.
- In addition to rotating your thoracic spine and shoulders, also turn your head, focusing your eyes in the direction of the rotation.
- Maintain rotation as you inhale and increase rotation with each exhalation.
- Repeat the stretch by passively and actively rotating your spine to the right.

3.6 Rolled towel - active, post-isometric and passive stretch for pectoralis major, the ribs, thoracic and cervical spine

3.6 Pectoralis stretch supine over a rolled towel

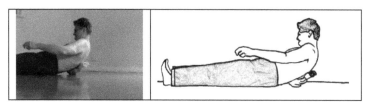

Starting position

- Sit on the floor, preferably on a carpet or mat.
- Place a tightly rolled up towel behind your back.

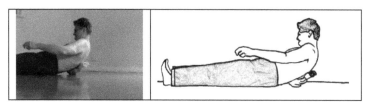

- Lie over the rolled up towel with your feet apart and your palms upwards.
- The towel should be about 4 cm in diameter and placed perpendicular to your spine at the apex of your primary forward curve or kyphosis or across any area of increased flexion in your thoracic spine.

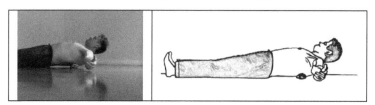

- Abduct your arms 90 degrees so that your body is in a cross position.
- Tuck your chin in as your body relaxes over the towel.

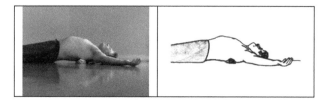

Technique

- Take in a deep breath and hold it in.
- Tense the muscles in your arms and legs by rotating them, reaching with them or pushing them into the floor.
- Exhale, relax your whole body and allow your body to sink into the floor.

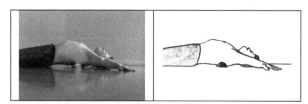

- Turn your palms down into the floor.
- Take in another deep breath and tense your muscles again.
- Exhale and relax your whole body.
- Abduct your arms further and feel an increased chest stretch.

3.7 Rolled towel - active, passive and post-isometric stretch for the shoulders, ribs, thoracic and cervical spine

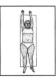

Starting position

- Sit on the floor and place a tightly rolled up towel behind and across your thoracic spine at the level of its apex - where the curve is most flexed.
- Lie over the towel with your legs and arm apart, palms upwards and your chin tucked in.
- Fully abduct your arms so they rest against the side of your head.
- You should feel an increase in pressure of your body on the towel.

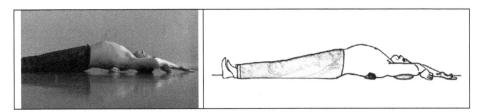

Technique

- Take in a deep breath, hold it in and with both arms and legs straight stretch one arm, both arms or combinations of arms and legs:

  o Reach along the floor, upwards and away from your head with one arm and stretch from your shoulder through to your fingertips – this stretch focuses on one upper limb
  o Reach along the floor, upwards with one arm and reach along the floor downwards with the same side leg, and stretch the whole side of your body from your fingertips to your toes or heel – this stretch focuses on the upper limb and lower limb on one side of the body
  o Reach along the floor, upwards with both arms and reach along the floor, downwards with both legs to stretch both sides of your body – this stretch focuses on the upper and lower limb on both sides
  o Reach along the floor, upwards and away from your head with one arm and reach along the floor downwards and towards your feet with the other arm – this diagonal stretch focuses on both upper limbs and the upper thoracic spine
  o Reach upwards (elevating) the arm and leg on one side of the body and reach downwards (depressing) the arm and leg on the other side – diagonal stretch focuses on upper and lower limbs, thoracic and lumbar

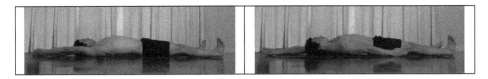

- Exhale, relax and allow your arm, shoulder and ribs to sink into the floor.
- The stretches can be done mildly, moderately or strongly.

3.8 Rolled towel - active, passive and post-isometric stretches for the shoulders, arms, forearms, wrist, hands and fingers

3.8a Bilateral anterior forearm and hand stretch supine

Starting position

- All of the stretches in 3.8 can be done sitting or standing.
- Lie on the floor with the apex of your thoracic curve over a rolled up towel, legs apart, arms straight above your head and your chin tucked in.
- Interlace the fingers of both your hands.
- Rotate your forearms so that your palms face up, away from your head.
- Extend your elbows until both arms are completely straight.
- The ulna side of your hands should be in contact with the floor or near to it.

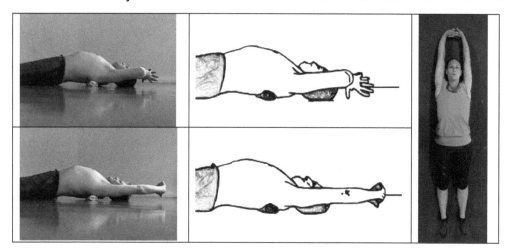

Technique

- Take in a deep breath, hold it in and perform the following movements:

  - Push your hands along the floor and away from your head
  - Maintain full elbow extension by contracting your triceps - bring your forearms together
  - Push on the ends of all the metacarpal bones with your fingers
  - Pull back on your fingers with your other hand

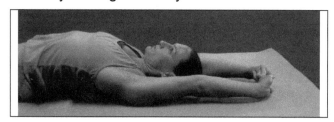

- Feel the stretch in your shoulders, arms, forearms and palms.
- Maintain hand contact with the floor or as near to the floor as possible.
- After about five seconds cease the contraction, exhale, relax your arms, and allow your whole body to sink into the floor.
- Repeat the stretch several times.

3.8b Unilateral anterior forearm and hand stretch supine

Starting position

- Lie on the floor with the apex of your thoracic spine over a rolled up towel, your legs apart, arms straight above your head and your chin tucked in.
- Interlace the fingers of both your hands.
- Rotate your forearms so that your palms face up, away from your head.
- Extend your right elbow until your arm is completely straight.
- Flex your left elbow about 20 degrees.
- Stretch the right hand and anterior forearm muscles with your left hand.
- Press against the end of your metatarsal bones with your fingertips.
- Pull back on your fingers and hand and extend your wrist.
- Try and keep your hands in contact with the floor.

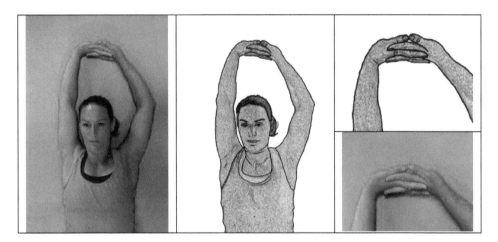

Technique

- Take in a deep breath, exhale and perform the following movements:

  - Push your right wrist along the floor and away from your head
  - Maintain right elbow extension by contracting your triceps
  - Push on the end of the row of metacarpal bones with your fingers
  - Pull back on your fingers with the fingers of your other hand.
  - Localise the stretch on individual fingers or stretch the whole hand.

- Feel the stretch in the anterior wrist and forearm and palm of the hand.
- Maintain hand contact with the floor or as near to the floor as possible.
- Repeat the stretch several times for the right upper limb, stretching on the exhalation.
- Repeat the stretch for the muscles of the left upper limb.

3.8c Unilateral anterior finger and hand stretch supine

Starting position

- Lie on the floor with the apex of your thoracic spine over a rolled up towel, your legs apart, arms straight above your head and your chin tucked in.
- Lightly hold the fingers of your right hand with your left hand.
- Rotate your right forearm so that your right palm faces away from you.
- Extend your right elbow until your arm is completely straight.
- Flex your left elbow about 20 degrees.
- Grasp the index finger of your right hand with your left hand.
- Pull back on your finger.
- Try and keep the side of your hands in contact with the floor.

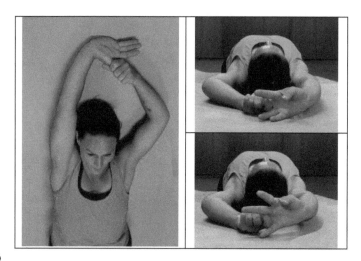

Technique

- Take in a deep breath, then exhale and perform the following movements:

    - Pull your finger back - feel the stretch from the finger, through the hand and to the wrist
    - Push your right arm along the floor and away from your head
    - Maintain right elbow extension by contracting your triceps
    - Twist your finger in one direction and then in the other direction
    - Firmly hold onto your finger and twist your hand in one direction and then in the other direction.

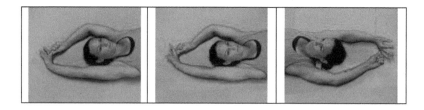

- Feel the stretch down the back of your finger, metacarpal and wrist.
- Stretch each finger and then the thumb of your right hand.
- Stretch the thumb and fingers of your left hand.

3.8d Unilateral posterior forearm and hand stretch supine

Starting position

- Lie on the floor with the apex of your thoracic spine over a rolled up towel, your legs apart, arms straight above your head and your chin tucked in.
- Interlace the fingers of both hands.
- The palms of your hands should face down towards your head and the radial side of your hands is in contact with the floor or near the floor.
- Extend your right elbow until your arm is completely straight.
- Flex your left forearm at the elbow about 20 degrees and gently pull on the back of your right hand with the fingers of your left hand.

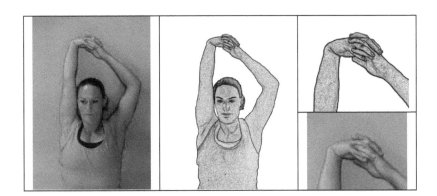

Technique

- Take in a deep breath, then exhale and perform the following movements:

  - Push your right arm along the floor and away from your head
  - Maintain right elbow extension in your right arm
  - Pull on the end of the row of metacarpal bones on the back of your right hand with all the fingers of your left hand
  - Pull on the end of individual metacarpal bones with one finger to stretch the wrist at individual carpometacarpal joints

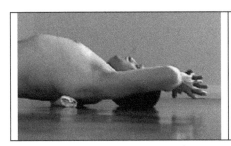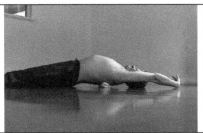

- Localise the stretch on individual fingers or stretch the whole hand.
- Feel the stretch in the posterior wrist, forearm and hand.
- Maintain hand contact with the floor or as near to the floor as possible.
- Repeat the stretch for the right side several times.
- Repeat the stretch for the muscles on the left side.

3.8e Unilateral posterior finger and hand stretch supine

Starting position

- Lie on the floor with the apex of your thoracic spine over a rolled up towel, your legs apart, arms straight above your head and your chin tucked in.
- The palms of your hands face down towards your head and the radial side of your hands are in contact with the floor or near the floor.
- Grasp the index finger of your right hand with your left hand.
- Flex your left elbow about 20 degrees.
- Extend your right elbow until your arm is completely straight.
- Pull down on your finger and flex your finger and wrist.
- Try and keep the side of your hands in contact with the floor.

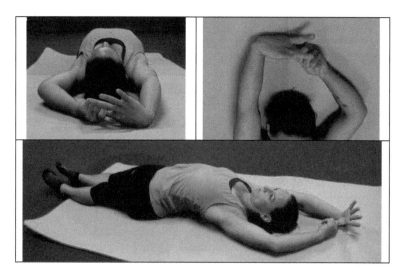

Technique

- Take in a deep breath, then exhale and perform the following movements:

  - Pull your finger down towards your head - feel the stretch from the finger, down the back of the hand and to the wrist
  - Push your right arm along the floor and away from your head
  - Maintain right elbow extension by contracting your triceps
  - Twist your finger in one direction and then the other direction

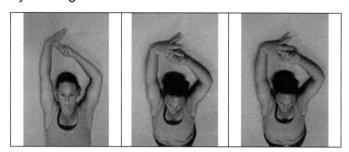

- Feel the stretch down the back of your finger, metacarpal and wrist.
- Stretch each finger and then the thumb of your right hand.
- Repeat the stretch for the thumb and fingers of your left hand.

3.9 Rolled towel - active and passive stretches for shoulder, spine, ribs and hip down one side of the body

3.9a Supine hip and spine stretch over a rolled towel

Starting position

- Lie on the floor with the apex of your thoracic spine over a rolled up towel, your left arm by your side and your right arm fully abducted so that it is in contact with the side of your head.
- Flex your left hip and knee and place your left foot on the outside of your right leg about level with your knee.
- Adduct your right hip as far as possible and then hold it in the adducted position with your left foot to lengthen the hip abductor muscles.
- Adjust your head so there is no strain on your neck by tucking in your chin.
- Slide your left hand down the side of your left thigh towards your foot so that your spine is sidebent to the left.

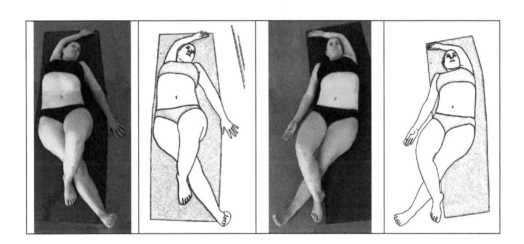

Technique

- Take in a deep breath, hold it in
- Exhale and reach your right hand over the top of your head in a 45 degree direction upwards and to the left.
- Ensure your right hand remains in contact with the floor.
- Feel the stretch down the whole right side of your body – right shoulder, ribs, thoracic, lumbar and hip.
- Move your right hip further into adduction and hold it there with your left foot.
- Repeat the stretch down the right side of the body several times, each time with an exhalation.
- Repeat the stretch on the other side.

3.9b Supine lumbar & thoracic spine stretch over a rolled towel

Starting position

- Lie on the floor with the apex of your thoracic spine over a rolled up towel, your left arm by your side and your right arm fully abducted so that your arm is in contact with the side of your head.
- Adjust your head so there is no strain on your neck by tucking in your chin.
- Slide your left hand down the side of your left thigh towards your foot so that your spine is sidebent to the left.
- The apex of any sidebending curve (scoliosis) should also be near to the point the towel crosses the spine.

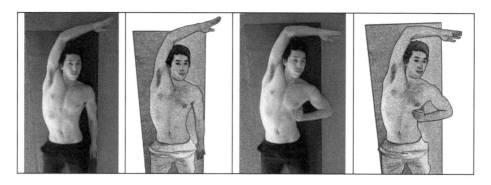

Technique

Sidebending stretch for the ribs, lower thoracic and upper lumbar spine

- Take in a deep breath and then exhale and combine the following actions:

  - Reach over the top of your head in a 45 degree direction upwards and to the left with your right hand
  - Reach down the side of your left thigh and towards your left foot with your left hand.

- Ensure your spine remains in contact with the towel and your body remains parallel with the floor – do not allow rotation of your spine.

Sidebending stretch for the ribs and middle and lower thoracic spine

- Flex your left elbow about 110 degrees and place the palm of your left hand against the side of your ribs.
- Flex your right elbow until it is in about 90 degrees flexion.
- Take in a deep breath and then exhale and combine the following actions:

  - Push your right elbow in a 45 degree direction away from your head upwards and to your right
  - Push against the left side of your ribs with your left hand

- Repeat the stretches several times on the right and on the left side.

118

4.0 Pectoralis stretches - active, passive and post-isometric stretches for pectoralis major and other anterior shoulder muscles

4.0a Easy pectoralis stretch sitting on the floor

Starting position

- Sit on the floor with your legs out in front of you and your feet apart.
- Your knees can be extended or flexed.
- Place your hands palms down, flat on the floor behind you and with your fingers pointing away from you.

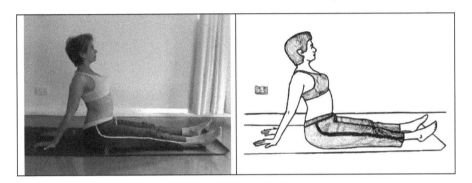

- Fully straighten your elbows until your arms are completely straight.
- Move the top of your pelvis forward and maintain an upright sitting position by contracting your hip flexor muscles.

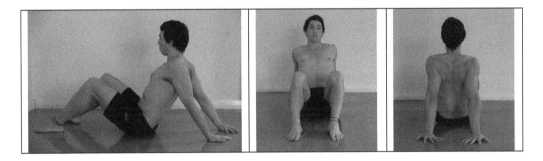

Technique

- Take in a deep breath in.
- Exhale and combine the following movements:

    o Rotate your arms, elbows and forearms outwards
    o Pull your shoulders backwards
    o Gently squeeze your shoulder blades together

- Feel the stretch in front of your shoulders and over your ribs.
- Repeat the stretch with each exhalation.

4.0b Easy pectoralis stretch standing

Starting position

- Stand with your feet apart.
- Raise your arms 20 to 30 degrees to the side and then take them 20 to 30 degrees backwards.
- Rotate your arms outwards as far as possible.
- Your palms should now point forwards, upwards and to the side.
- Spread your fingers apart.

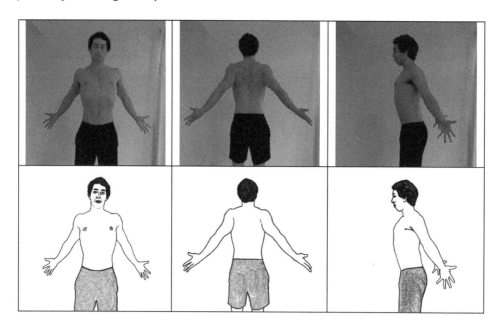

- Move your shoulders backwards.
- Stand up straight.

Technique

- Take in a deep breath in.
- Exhale and combine the following movements:

    - Move your arms backwards
    - Rotate your arms outwards – point your thumbs backwards
    - Pull your shoulders backwards
    - Gently squeeze your shoulder blades together

- Feel the stretch in front of your shoulders and over your ribs in the pectoralis muscles.
- Repeat the stretch with each exhalation

4.0c Pectoralis stretch seated in a chair

Starting position

- Sit in a chair with your feet apart and firmly planted on the floor or a block.
- Raise your arms until they are level with the shoulders or a little bit higher.
- Bend your elbows until your arms and forearms are at right angles.
- Rotate your arms outwards and backwards, rotate your forearms outwards and then take your elbows backwards as far as possible.
- Your elbows and hands move horizontally backward and parallel with the floor and your thumbs point backwards.
- Sit upright by keeping your centre of gravity over your buttock bones, contracting hip and trunk muscles or using a chair or pillow for support.

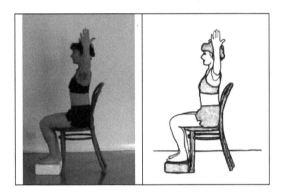

Technique

- Take in a deep breath.
- Exhale and move your elbows horizontally backwards.
- Do not allow your elbows to drop below the height of your shoulders.

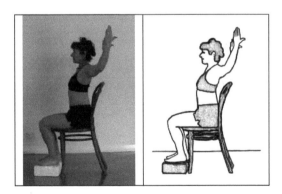

- Take in another deep breath in.
- Exhale and move your hand backwards leading with your thumbs.
- Perform these two actions either as individual alternating movements or together as one movement.
- Feel the stretch in front of your shoulders and over your ribs.

4.0d Pectoralis stretch prone

Starting position

- Lie on a carpet or mat on the floor face down.
- Bring your arms out to the side until they are in line with your shoulders.
- Bend your elbows until your arms and forearms are at right angles.
- Your arms will be rotated outwards.
- Rotate your forearms outwards so your thumbs point up towards the ceiling.

Technique

- Take in a deep breath.
- Exhale and lift your arms, elbows and forearms off the floor.
- The emphasis should be on lifting your elbows as high as possible.
- Your forearms should stay horizontal and parallel with the floor and your elbows should stay in line with your shoulders.

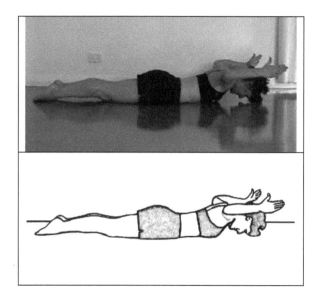

- Take in another deep breath in.
- Exhale and lift your arms, elbows and forearms off the floor but this time the emphasis should be on lifting your hands off the floor.
- Lead with your thumbs pointing them upwards towards the ceiling.
- Perform these as individual alternating movements or in combination.
- Feel the stretch in front of your shoulders and over your ribs.

4.0e Unilateral passive and post-isometric pectoralis stretch standing and wall supported

Starting position

- Stand with your feet apart and the right side of your body near a wall and your right foot is about 6 cm from the wall.
- Raise your right arm and place the palm of your hand on the wall to the right of your head and just above shoulder height.
- Place the front of your right shoulder against the wall but not your right hip.
- Move your right forearm until your elbow is straight.
- Bend your knees a little and adjust your feet for optimum balance.

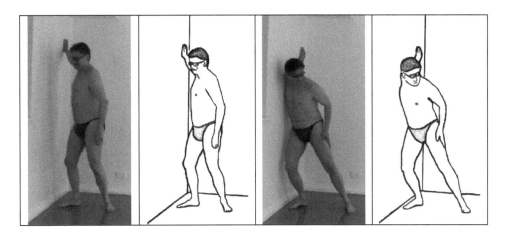

Technique

- Take a deep breath in.
- Exhale and perform the following movements:

  - Move your left shoulder away from the wall by rotating your upper thoracic spine to the left and retracting your left scapula.
  - Move your right hip forwards and parallel with the wall.
  - Move your left hip backwards and rotate your pelvis to the left, pivoting around your right hip.

- Ensure your right shoulder remains in contact with the wall and your right hip remains away from the wall.
- Feel a stretch in front of your right shoulder and ribs.
- Take another deep breath and hold it in.
- Push the whole of right arm against the wall for about five seconds.
- Resist any movement of your body with a firm stance.
- Cease the contraction, relax, exhale and perform the movements above.
- Repeat the passive or post-isometric stretch several times.
- Repeat the stretch on the left side.

4.0f Bilateral passive and post-isometric pectoralis stretch standing and doorway supported

Starting position

- Stand with your feet apart facing an open doorway or two vertical posts.
- Move your right foot through the doorway and place it on the floor so that the back of your heel lines up with the doorway.
- Lift up your arms until your hands are level with or just above your shoulders.
- Place your wrist or forearms against the side edges of the doorway.
- Bend your hips and knees and lunge forwards through the door.
- Adjust your feet for optimum balance.

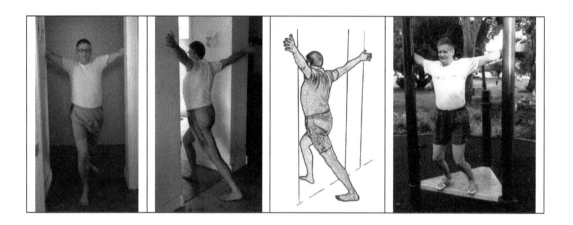

Technique

- Take a deep breath in.
- Exhale, bend your right hip and knee and move through the doorway.
- Pull your shoulders backwards and bring your shoulder blades towards your spine.
- Feel the stretch in front of both shoulders and both sides of your rib cage.
- Keep your elbows extended and your spine straight and vertical.
- Repeat the stretch with an exhalation several times.
- Take another deep inhalation and hold it in.
- Push your forearms against the edges of the doorway for about five seconds.
- Resist any movement of your body with a firm stance.
- Cease the isometric muscle contraction, completely relax all the muscles across the front of your rib cage and then exhale and move further through the doorway.
- Repeat the passive or post-isometric stretch several times.

4.0g Bilateral pectoralis stretch standing walls supported

Starting position

- Stand with your feet apart facing the corner of a room.
- Place your right foot in front of and to the right of your left foot.
- Raise your arms up to the side until your hands are level with or just above your shoulders and place the palms of your hands on each of the walls.
- Straighten your elbows so your arms are straight.
- Bend your right hip and knee and lunge towards the corner of the room.

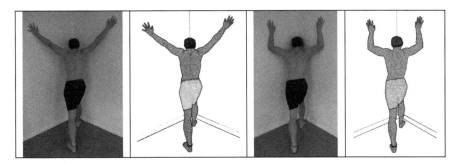

Technique

- Take a deep breath in.
- Exhale, bend your right hip and knee and move your body towards the corner of the room.
- Pull your shoulders backwards and bring your shoulder blades towards your spine.
- Keep both arms and spine straight.
- Feel the stretch in front of both shoulders.
- Bend your elbows 90 degrees and place your palms, forearms and elbows on the walls so your forearms are vertical and your arms are horizontal.
- Lunging towards the corner of the room with elbows flexed increases shoulder external rotation.
- Take another deep breath in.
- Exhale, bend your right hip and knee again and move your body towards the corner of the room.
- Pull your shoulders backwards and bring your shoulder blades towards your spine.
- Feel the stretch in front of both shoulders.
- Repeat the stretch with an exhalation several times.
- Take another deep inhalation and hold it in.
- Push your hands and forearms against the wall for about five seconds.
- Resist any backward movement of your body with a firm stance.
- Cease the isometric muscle contraction, completely relax all the muscles across the front of your rib cage and then exhale and move further into the corner of the room.
- Repeat the passive or post-isometric stretch several times.

4.0h Bilateral active pectoralis and latissimus dorsi stretch standing with pole or towel

Starting position

- Stand with your feet apart and grasp either end of a pole or towel with your hands.
- Raise your arms so the pole is above your head.
- Straighten your elbows so your arms are fully straight.

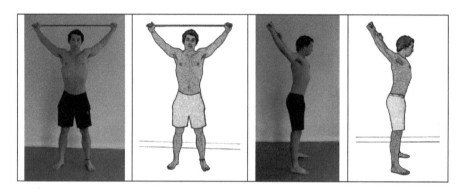

Technique

- Take a deep breath in.
- Exhale and move the pole and both hands and arms backwards.
- Pull your shoulders backwards and pull your scapula towards your spine.
- Keep both arms extended and keep your spine straight.
- Feel the stretch in front of both shoulders.
- Repeat the stretch with an exhalation several times.
- The pole or towel can be used in a variety of ways and positions.

  - Your hands can be brought closer together
  - One or both elbows can be flexed
  - One hand can be moved further backwards than the other.

- Attempt a variety of pole positions but do the movements slowly and with an exhalation.

4.1 Subscapularis stretch - passive and post-isometric stretch for subscapularis and other anterior shoulder muscles

4.1 Unilateral passive and post-isometric subscapularis stretch

Starting position

- Stand with your feet apart and the right side of your body next to a post.
- Flex your right forearm, externally rotate your right arm and place the palm of your right hand on the post.
- Your right elbow is flexed about 90 degrees and tucked close up against the right side of your body.
- Rotate your pelvis to the left until you feel the initial stages of a stretch in front of your right shoulder.
- You may need to reposition your feet so that your centre of gravity falls between them and your spine is straight.
- Relax your shoulders.

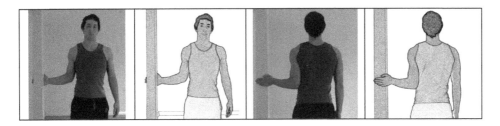

Technique

- Take a deep breath in.
- Exhale and rotate your upper thoracic spine to the left, taking your right shoulder forwards and your left shoulder backwards.
- Feel a stretch in front of your right shoulder.
- With your palm against the post and your elbow against the side of your body, turning your body to the left will externally rotate your right shoulder.
- Ensure your right elbow remains in contact with the side of your body so that it functions as a pivot during movement.
- If you are not getting sufficient stretch it may be necessary to reposition your pelvis or feet - when all the spinal rotation has been taken up, take the right hip or foot forwards.
- Take another deep breath and hold it in.
- Push the palm of your right hand against the post in a forwards and inwards direction for about five seconds.
- Resist any movement of your body with a firm stance.
- Cease the contraction, relax, exhale and perform the movements described above.
- Repeat the passive or post-isometric stretch several times.
- Repeat the stretch on the left side.

4.2 The shoulder drop - passive and post-isometric stretch for the scapula depressor muscles

4.2 The shoulder drop

Starting position

- Stand with your back to a low table or chair.
- Flex your hips and knees.
- Place your palms on the chair with your fingers over the edge.
- Walk your heels away from the chair until your legs are straight.
- Straighten your arms.
- Relax your shoulders and lower your pelvis and spine towards the floor.
- Allow your shoulders to rise but stop when you start to feel the stretch.

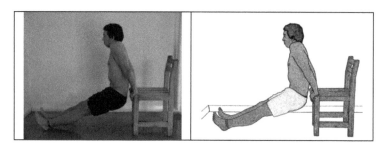

Technique

- Take a deep breath in.
- Exhale and allow your body to drop towards the floor.
- Feel the stretch down your back and deep in front of your chest.
- Keep your spine, legs and arms straight.
- Tuck your chin in and try and lengthen through your cervical spine.

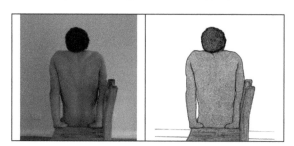

- Take in another deep breath and hold it in.
- Attempt to lift your body upward by pushing down on the chair for about five seconds but stop before there is any movement.
- Cease the isometric contraction, relax, exhale and allow your body to drop towards the floor.
- Feel the stretch down your back and deep in front of your rib cage.
- You should be able to raise your shoulders as high as your ears.
- Repeat the passive or post-isometric stretch several times.

4.3 Downward shoulder - active stretch for muscles responsible for scapular elevation

4.3 Downward shoulder stretch

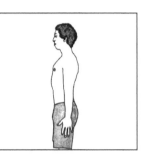

Starting position

- Stand with your feet slightly apart and arms at your sides.
- Tuck in your chin and take your head back.
- Keep your head vertical and in line with your body.

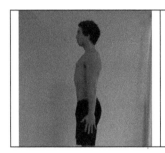

- Maintain your head over your body's centre of gravity.
- Move your shoulders downwards but keep your arms by your side.

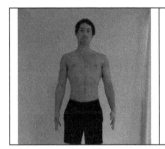
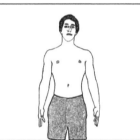

Technique

- Take a deep breath in.
- Exhale, while moving your shoulders, arms, forearms and hands downwards towards the floor.
- Keep your elbows, wrists and fingers straight - your whole body should be vertical and in a straight line.

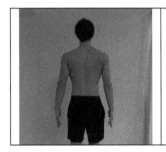
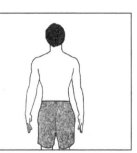

- Tuck in your chin as you reach your arms towards the floor.
- Feel the stretch over your shoulders and down the back of your cervical spine.

4.4 Shoulder abductor front stretch - a passive and post-isometric stretch for the muscles responsible for shoulder abduction and scapula retraction

4.4 Shoulder abductor front stretch

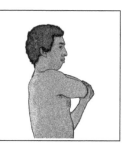

Starting position

- Stand straight with your feet apart, and your arms and shoulders relaxed.
- Flex your right elbow and then take your right hand across the front of your body, as far as you can comfortably go to the left.
- Flex your left elbow and grasp your right arm above your elbow.
- Depending the angle you wish to apply the stretch you can either cradle your right forearm in your left forearm with your wrist resting in the crease of your elbow or you can rest your wrist on the top of your shoulder.
- Pull your arm across the front of your body until you feel the initial stage of resistance from the shoulder muscles and ligaments and then stop.

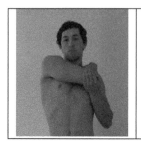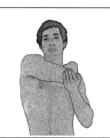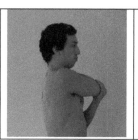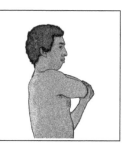

Technique

- Take a deep breath in.
- Exhale and pull your right arm across the front of your body to the left.
- Feel the stretch down the back of your right arm, behind your right shoulder and across and down the right side of your back.

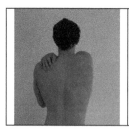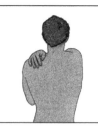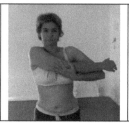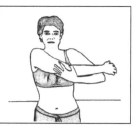

- Take another deep breath and hold it in.
- Push your right elbow and arm forwards and to the right for five seconds.
- Resist any movement of your arm with a firm grip on your right elbow with your left hand and a firm stance - no movement of your spine or pelvis.
- Cease the isometric muscle contraction, relax, exhale and then pull your right arm further across the front of your body and to the left.
- Repeat the passive or post-isometric stretch several times, increasing the stretch with each exhalation.
- Repeat the stretch for the left shoulder.

4.5 Shoulder abductor behind stretch - passive and post-isometric stretch for the shoulder abductors

4.5 Shoulder abductor behind stretch

Starting position

- Stand up straight with your feet slightly apart and your arms at your sides.
- Flex your right elbow and place your right hand behind your back.
- Reach as far as you can across your back and to the left of your spine.
- Flex your left elbow and place your left hand behind your back.
- Reach as far as you can across your back and to the right of your spine, and grasp your forearm as near to your elbow as you can.
- Pull your right arm and forearm further across your back with your left hand until you feel the initial stage of resistance from your shoulders.

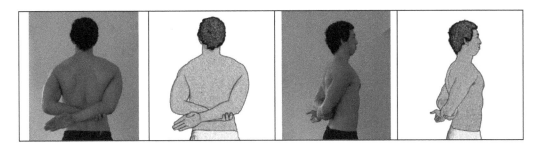

Technique

- Take a deep breath in.
- Exhale and pull your right arm and forearm further across your back.
- Feel the stretch across the top of you right shoulder and down the side of your right arm.

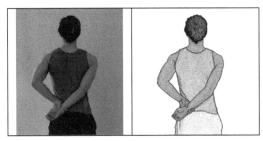

- Take another deep breath and hold it in.
- Attempt to move your right arm and elbow to your right and away from your body for about five seconds but resist the movement with a firm hold on your forearm with your left hand.
- Cease the isometric muscle contraction, completely relax your shoulder muscles, then exhale and pull your right hand and forearm further to the left and across your back with your left hand.
- Repeat the stretch several times with each exhalation.
- Relax your shoulders, stand straight and do not move your spine or pelvis.
- Repeat the stretch for the left shoulder abductors.

4.6 Palms together above head - active stretch for shoulder muscles and strengthening technique for muscles of the spine, thighs and legs

4.6a Palms together above head with forearms supinated

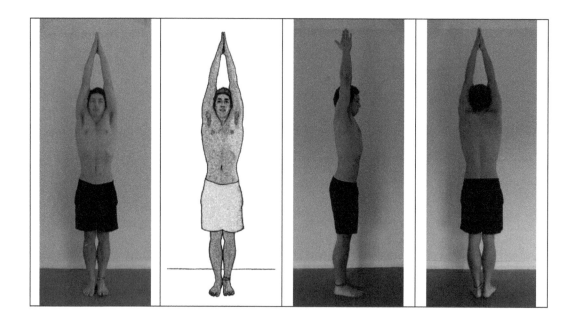

Starting position

- Stand with your feet together and arms at your sides.
- Abduct your arms until your hands are above your head.
- Bring your palms together.
- Your arms are externally rotated and your forearms supinated.
- Your elbows are straight and your head in line with your body.

Technique

- Take a deep breath in.
- Exhale and take your hands further away from your head.
- Reach towards the ceiling and feel the stretch in your thoracic spine, ribs, shoulders, arms, forearms and hands and through to your fingertips.
- Keep your elbows straight.
- Repeat the stretch several times, each time with an exhalation.

4.6b Palms together above head with forearms pronated

Starting position

- Stand with your feet apart and arms at your sides.
- Abduct your arms until your hands are above your head.
- Internally rotate your arms so your palms face outwards.
- Cross your forearms and wrists and bring your palms together.
- Your arms are internally rotated and your forearms pronated.

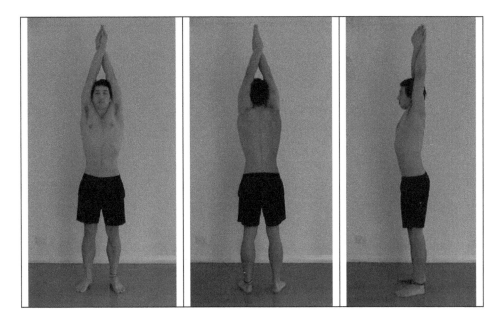

Technique

- Take a deep breath in.
- Exhale and take your hands further away from your head.
- Reach towards the ceiling and feel the stretch in your thoracic spine, ribs, shoulders, arms, forearms and hands and through to your fingertips.
- Keep your elbows straight.
- Repeat the stretch several times, each time with an exhalation.

4.7 Palms together behind back - an active stretch for pectoralis minor and a passive stretch for the flexor carpi ulnaris and other anterior forearm muscles, and wrist and finger flexor muscles and fascia of the hand

4.7 Palms together behind back

Starting position

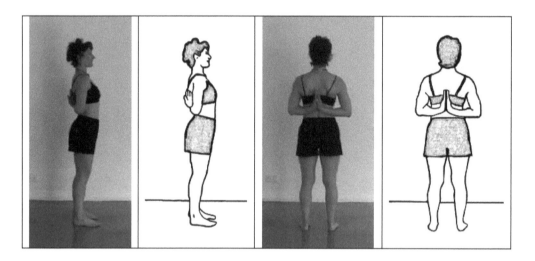

- Stand with your feet apart.
- Flex your elbows, then abduct your arms and internally rotate them.
- Your hands should now rest on your iliac crests and lateral lumbar spine.
- Slide your hands behind your back and bring your palms together.
- If this is difficult, then start with the index and forefinger of each hand touching and gradually work your way into a full contact of both palms.
- The little fingers of both hands rest against your back.

Technique

- Take a deep breath in.
- Exhale, and as you do so, contract the muscles between your spine, scapula and arms and take your elbows as far backwards as possible.
- Repeat the movement several times with an exhalation.
- Take another deep breath in.
- Exhale and as you do so, contract muscles which take your hands away from your back.
- Move your hands backwards if possible.
- Repeat the movement several times, always with an exhalation.
- Maintain full contact with both palms, including fingers and thumbs.
- Perform these two stretches together or as alternating movements.
- Feel the stretch in front of and down the sides of your ribs and in your palms and anterior forearms.
- If you are unable to bring both palms together, then try and do the arm movements individually.

4.8 Multiple shoulder muscle stretch - active and passive stretch for many shoulder muscles

4.8 Multiple shoulder muscle stretch

Starting position

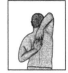

- Standing with your feet slightly apart and arms at your sides.
- Bend your left elbow to the fully flexed position.
- Lift your left arm until it is fully abducted.
- Your left arm and forearm should now be near your left ear and your left hand should rest against your upper thoracic spine.
- Internally rotate your right arm and place your right hand behind your back.
- Clasp the fingers of both hands together behind your back.
- If you are unable to clasp your hands together, grasp two points of a towel.
- Keep your head and spine straight, while relaxing your shoulders.

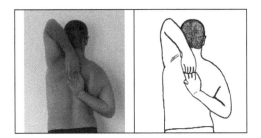

Technique

- Take a deep breath in.
- Exhale and move the point of your right elbow backwards, then to the right and then to the left, while maintaining the grip with your fingers.
- Repeat this action with an exhalation two or three times, each time readjusting your grip so your hands are closer together.

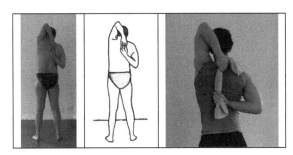

- Introduce small circles and then progressively wider these circles with your right elbow.
- Repeat the backwards, right, left, circle movements with your left elbow.
- Feel the stretch in your scapular muscles and shoulder joints.
- Make sure that all the movement is with your arms, forearms, shoulders and scapular - do not move your head, spine or pelvis.
- Relax your right shoulder.
- Keep your left elbow back - don't let your forearm push your head forward.
- Repeat the stretch on the opposite side.

4.9 Scapula retractor stretches - active, passive and post-isometric stretches for the shoulder, spine and scapula retractor muscles

4.9a Scapula retractor stretch standing

Starting position

- Stand straight with your feet apart facing a doorframe or strong pole.
- Raise your right arm and grasp the vertical pole with your right hand.
- Hold the pole at shoulder height so that your arm is horizontal.
- Bend your hips and knees and allow your body to drop towards the floor.
- Lean backwards and rotate your upper thoracic spine to the right so that your right arm moves horizontally to the left and in front of your body.
- Stop when you feel the initial stretch down the side of your right shoulder.
- Your right arm should remain straight.

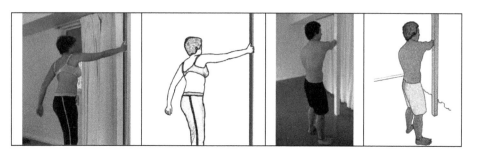

Technique

- Take a deep breath in and then exhale and combine the following actions:

  o Allow your right shoulder, upper spine and rib cage to drop backwards, using your body weight to stretch the muscles
  o Lean your body to the right - a sideshifting movement of the shoulders
  o Move your left shoulder forwards by rotating your spine to the right.

- Feel the stretch in the muscles of your right shoulder, ribs and upper and middle thoracic spine.
- Take another deep breath and hold it in.
- Pull on the pole with your right arm, attempting to move your arm and scapula backwards for about five seconds.
- Resist any movement with a firm stance - no movement of your body.
- Cease the isometric muscle contraction, relax, exhale and let your right shoulder and ribs drop backwards while taking your left shoulder forwards.
- Let go of your shoulder muscles and use the weight of your body.
- Allow your spine to rotate towards the side you are stretching.
- Feel the stretch in your right shoulder, rib cage and upper thoracic spine.
- Repeat the passive or post-isometric stretch several times, increasing the stretch with each exhalation.
- Repeat the stretch for the left shoulder.

4.9b Scapula retractor stretch squatting unilateral

Starting position

- Squat in front of a strong vertical wooden or metal pole.
- Grasp the pole with your right hand at a height that is level with or slightly above your shoulders.
- Lean backward until your right arm is straight.
- If you are unable to squat easily then grasp the pole first and then bend your hips and knees and move into the squatting position.

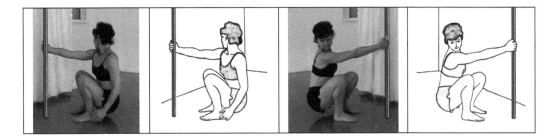

Technique

- Take a deep breath in.
- Exhale and as you lean backward with your right shoulder and right side of your spine, take your left shoulder forwards.
- Allow your spine to rotate towards the side you are stretching.

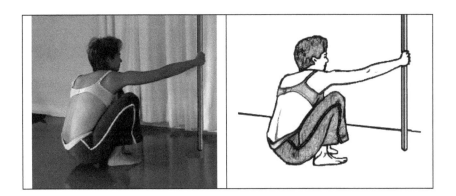

- Use the weight of your body to stretch your muscles.
- Let go of your shoulders and allow your spine to rotate to the right but keep the rest of your body in a fixed position.
- Feel the stretch in muscles across your right shoulder and rib cage as well as the right side of your upper and middle thoracic spine.
- Repeat the passive stretch several times, increasing the stretch with each exhalation.
- Repeat the stretch on the left side.

4.9c Scapula retractor stretch squatting bilateral

Starting position

- Squat in front of a strong vertical, wooden or metal pole.
- Grasp the pole with your hands at a height that is slightly above your shoulders.
- Lean backwards until your arms are straight.
- If you are unable to squat easily, then grasp the pole first and then bend your hips and knees and move into the squatting position.

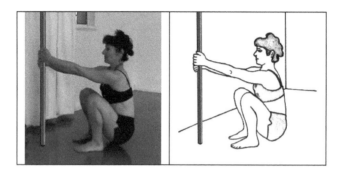

Technique

- Take a deep breath in.
- Exhale and allow your upper body to drop backward.
- Maintain a firm hold on the pole but relax your shoulder muscles.
- Feel the stretch in muscles across the back of your upper thoracic spine, ribs and shoulders.
- Repeat the passive stretch several times, increasing the stretch with each exhalation.
- Use the weight of your body to stretch your shoulder, ribs and spine.

4.9d Scapula wrap stretch standing

Starting position

- Stand up straight.
- Lift your right arm, reach forward and then take your right hand to the left and around the left side of your rib cage.
- Grasp your ribs and lateral border of your left scapula with your right hand.
- Repeat the process with your left arm, grasping your ribs and the lateral border of your right scapula with your left hand.
- Make sure your arms and forearm fit comfortably together and wrap around your rib cage.

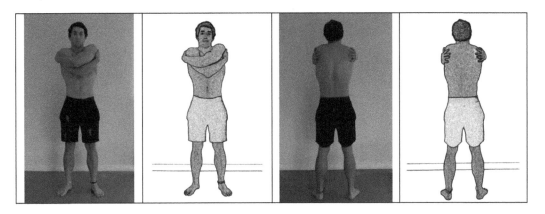

Technique

- Hold your ribs firmly with both hands.
- Take a deep breath in and hold it in.
- Contract your shoulder retractor muscles and attempt to pull both scapulae backwards and towards your spine for about five seconds.
- Tense your shoulder muscles and squeeze your body hard like you are giving yourself a bear hug.
- Resist any movement with a firm stance and firm hold on your ribs.
- After five seconds cease the isometric muscle contraction, relax, exhale and then lift your hands and arms off your rib cage, and reposition them further around your rib cage.
- Feel the stretch in muscles between your scapula and thoracic spine.
- Repeat the post-isometric stretch several times, increasing the stretch with each exhalation.

4.9e Scapula active retractor stretch standing

Starting position

- Stand up straight.
- Flex your hips and knees
- Place the palm of your left hand on top of your left thigh and flex your left elbow about 20 degrees.
- Use your left arm to help keep a fixed posture and to steady your body during the stretch.

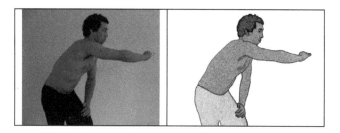

- Raise your right arm and reach forward, down and away with your hand.
- Your spine is straight and angled slightly forward on your hips.
- Your right arm should be straight and angled down towards the floor.
- The angle of your right arm relative to your spine will determine which muscles are stretched but should average at about 90 degrees.

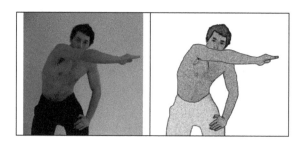

Technique

- Take a deep breath in.
- Exhale and reach forward and away with your right hand and arm and at the same time rotate your thoracic spine to the right.
- Feel the stretch in the muscles at the back of your right shoulder, rib cage and upper and middle thoracic spine.
- Keep a firm stance – do not move the rest of your body.
- Repeat the active stretch several times, each time with an exhalation.
- Repeat the stretch for the left shoulder.

5.0 Shoulder external rotator stretches - passive, post-isometric and active stretches for muscles responsible for shoulder external rotation and scapular retraction

5.0a Shoulder external rotator stretch

Starting position

- Stand with your feet slightly apart and arms at your sides.
- Flex your right elbow 90 degrees and abduct your arm 45 degrees.
- Internally rotate your right arm and place the back of your right hand against the right side of your lower back.
- Your right wrist rests on the crest of the right side of your pelvis.
- Internally rotate your arm more by moving your right elbow forwards.

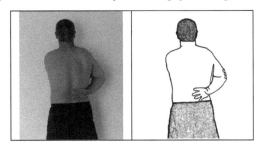

- Reach forwards and right with your left hand and grasp your right elbow.
- If you can't reach your elbow grasp it as near to your elbow as possible.
- Drop your right shoulder and keep it relaxed during the stretch.

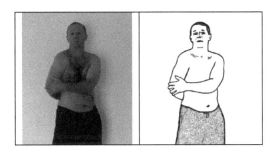

Technique

- Take a deep breath in.
- Exhale and pull your right elbow forwards and inwards with your left hand.
- Feel the stretch behind the right shoulder and the right side of your spine.
- Keep your pelvis still and make sure to move your arm and not your spine.
- Take another deep breath and hold it in.
- Push you wrist and forearm forwards and against you're the right side of your back and push your right elbow backwards.
- Resist any movement of your right elbow backwards with your left hand.
- After about 5 seconds cease the contraction, exhale and pull your right elbow forwards and inwards with your left hand to the new tension barrier.
- Repeat the stretch several times, increasing the stretch with each exhalation.
- Repeat the stretch on the left side.

5.0b Active shoulder external rotator stretch

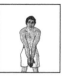

Starting position

- Stand up straight with your feet apart and arms at your sides.
- Internally rotate your arms and then flex them and bring the backs of your wrists, hands and fingers together in front of you.
- Keep your arms extended and keep your spine straight.

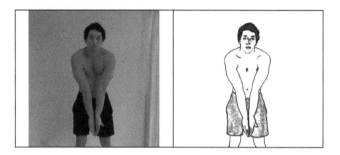

Technique

- Take a deep breath in.
- Exhale and roll your arms inwards and pull your shoulder forward and together.

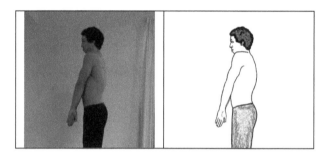

- Maintain full contact with the back of your wrist, hand and all fingers.
- Feel the stretch at the side of the shoulders and behind your back.
- Keep your spine straight.

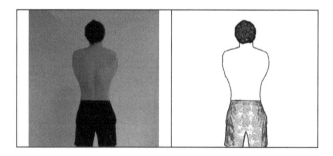

- Tuck your chin in and move your head into a posterior translation position.
- Repeat the stretch several times, increasing the stretch with each exhalation.

5.1 Shoulder flexor stretches - passive and post-isometric stretches for the shoulder flexor muscles

5.1a Shoulder flexor drop

Starting position

- Stand with your back to a low table or chair.
- Flex your hips and knees.
- Place your palms on the chair, shoulder width apart and with your fingers curled over the edge of the chair.
- Walk your heels away from the chair until your legs are straight.
- Flex your forearms and extend your arms and slowly lower your body towards the floor.
- Move your elbows backwards and towards each other.
- Relax your shoulders but stop the descent to the floor when you start to feel the initial stage of a stretch.

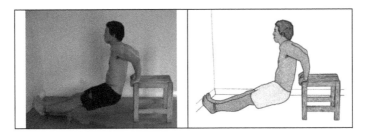

Technique

- Take a deep breath in.
- Exhale and allow your body to drop further towards the floor.
- Feel the stretch in front of your shoulders and down the side of your ribs.
- Keep your spine and legs straight and tuck your chin in.
- Your hands and elbows should remain shoulder width apart.

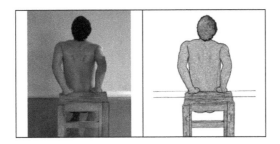

- Take in another deep breath and hold it in.
- Attempt to lift your body upward by pushing down on the chair for about five seconds but stop before there is any movement.
- Cease the isometric contraction, relax, exhale and allow your body to drop further towards the floor.
- Repeat the passive or post-isometric stretch several times.

5.1b Winged anterior deltoid stretch standing

Starting position

- Stand with your feet apart.
- Place your hands behind your back, palms down and with your fingers pointing down towards the floor.

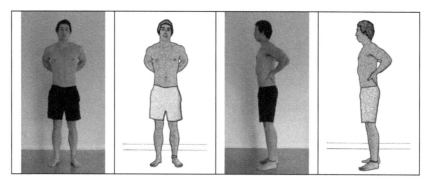

- Point your elbows backwards.
- Stand up straight.

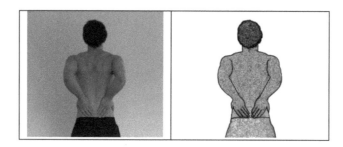

Technique

- Take a deep breath in.
- Exhale and combine the following movements:

  - Move your elbows backwards and towards each other.
  - Pull your shoulders backwards
  - Squeeze your shoulder blades together

- Feel the stretch in front of your shoulders and over your ribs.
- Repeat the stretch with each exhalation

5.2 Ledge squat stretches - passive and post-isometric stretches for the anterior shoulder muscles and fascia

5.2a Bilateral passive stretch against a ledge

Starting position

- Stand with your feet slightly apart and back towards a ledge or shelf.
- The ledge shoulder is about level with your lumbar spine.
- Flex your elbows and extend your shoulders and interlace the fingers of both hands behind your back.

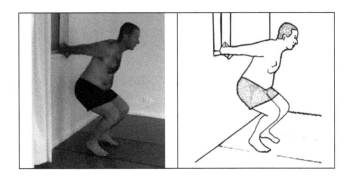

- Place your interlaced hands on the ledge.
- Your index fingers and thumbs are in contact with the ledge.
- Extend your forearms until your elbows are straight.
- Flex your knees until you feel a stretch across the front of your shoulders and down the front of your arms.

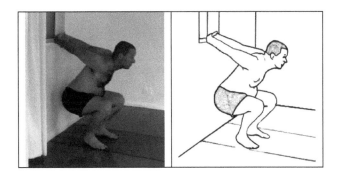

Technique

- Take a deep breath in.
- Exhale and extend your elbows, flex your hips and knees and lower your body to the floor.
- Feel the stretch down the front of your arms and shoulders.
- Your fingers should stay firmly clasped together.
- Keep your elbows and back straight and your head in line with your body.
- Allow your shoulders to relax.
- Repeat the passive stretch several times, each time with an exhalation.
- To also stretch your deep calf muscles keep your heels on the ground.

5.2b Bilateral post-isometric stretch against a ledge

Starting position

- Stand with your feet slightly apart and back towards a ledge or shelf.
- The ledge shoulder is about level with your lower lumbar spine.
- Flex your elbows and extend your shoulders and interlace the fingers of both hands behind your back.
- Place your interlaced hands on the ledge.
- Your index fingers and thumbs are in contact with the ledge.

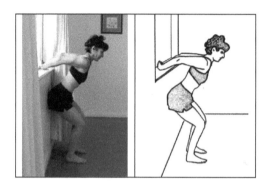

- Flex your knees until you feel a stretch across the front of your shoulders and down the front of your arms.
- Keep your elbows partially flexed.
- To stretch the deep calf muscles you must keep your heels on the ground.
- Or let your heels come off the ground and focus on the shoulder stretch.

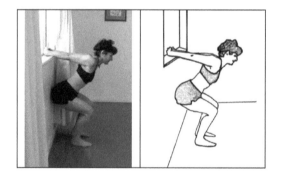

Technique

- Take a deep breath and hold it in.
- Attempt to simultaneous flex your arms and forearms by pushing downwards against the ledge.
- Hold the muscle contractions for about five seconds.
- Resist any movement of your body with a firm stance.
- Cease the muscle contractions, completely relax, exhale and then extend your elbows, flex your hips and knees and lower your body to the floor.
- Keep your fingers firmly clasped together, back straight and head in line with your body.
- Feel the stretch down the front of your arms and shoulders.
- Repeat the isometric stretch several times.

5.2c Unilateral passive and post-isometric stretch against a ledge

Starting position

- Stand with your feet apart and back towards a ledge or shelf.
- The ledge shoulder is about level with your lower lumbar spine.
- Extend your right arm and place the palm of your right hand on the ledge.
- Do not allow your arm to move into abduction.
- Rotating your thoracic spine to the left will help put your arm in extension.
- Your right hand should be behind your shoulder and your elbow straight.
- Flex your hips and knees until you feel a stretch across the front of your shoulder and down the front of your arms.

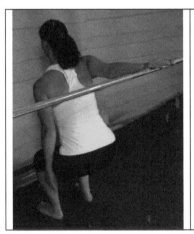 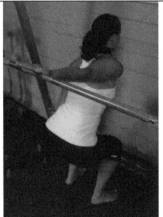 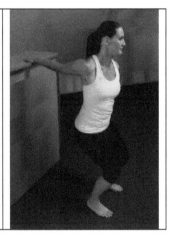

Technique

- Take a deep breath in.
- Exhale, extend your right elbow, flex your hips and knees and lower your body to the floor.
- Your palm should stay fixed on the ledge.
- Keep your elbow and back straight and your head in line with your body.
- Allow your right shoulder to relax.
- Feel the stretch down the front of your arm and shoulder.
- Take another deep inhalation and hold it in.
- Push your right arm down on the ledge for about five seconds.
- Resist any movement of your body with a firm stance.
- Cease the isometric muscle contraction, relax all the muscles across the front of your shoulder, then exhale and repeat the movement: extend your elbow and flex your hips and knees, so as to lower your body to further to the floor.
- Repeat the passive or post-isometric stretch several times.
- Repeat the stretch on the other side.

5.3 Elbow flexor stretches - passive and post-isometric stretches for muscles responsible for forearm flexion

5.3a Passive elbow flexor stretch

Starting position

- Stand under a doorframe or near the corner of a room with your feet apart.
- Your right leg and foot pass through the doorway or in front of the corner of the room and your left leg and foot remain outside the doorway.
- The right side of your back is towards the doorframe or corner of the room.
- Extend your right arm and place the palm of your right hand on the wall.
- Your arm and forearm are horizontal and level with your shoulder.
- The vertical edge of the doorframe or corner of the room is at right angles to your arm – crossing your arm about a third of the way from your elbow to your shoulder.
- Your fingers, palm, wrist, forearm, elbow and part of your arm remain in contact with the wall.
- Keep your right elbow straight

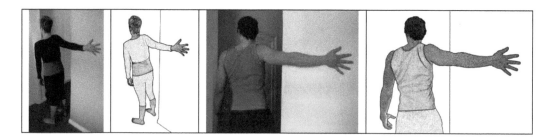

Technique

- Take in a deep breath and as you exhale:

  - Rotate your thoracic spine to the left
  - Rotate your left shoulder backwards.
  - Retract your scapula
  - Maintain elbow extension by contracting triceps.

- Localise the stretch at the elbow by allowing the elbow to move a few millimetres away from the wall.
- Relax the upper limb and increase the stretch with each exhalation.

  - increase thoracic and shoulder rotation and elbow extension
  - biceps include elbow supination and shoulder horizontal extension
  - brachialis and brachioradialis include pronation
  - anterior forearm muscles include wrist and finger flexion.

- Repeat the stretch on the right elbow several times and then stretch the left elbow flexor muscles.

148

5.3b Post-isometric elbow flexor stretch

Starting position

- Stand under a doorframe or near the corner of a room with your feet apart.
- Your right leg and foot pass through the doorway or in front of the corner of the room and your left leg and foot remain outside the doorway.
- The right side of your back is towards the doorframe or corner of the room.
- Extend your right arm and place the palm of your right hand on the wall.
- Your arm and forearm should be horizontal and level with your shoulder.
- The vertical edge of the doorframe or corner of the room should be at right angles to your arm – crossing your arm about a third of the way from your elbow to your shoulder.
- Your fingers, palm, wrist, forearm, elbow and part of your arm remain in contact with the wall.
- Keep your right elbow straight

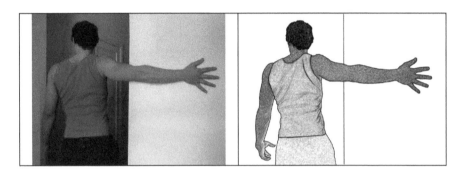

Technique

- Take in a deep breath and hold it in:

  - Flex your right elbow
  - For biceps include elbow supination and shoulder horizontal flexion 'Push against the wall with your hypothenar eminence'
  - Follow this by further extending and pronating your forearm
  - For the anterior forearm muscles, include wrist and finger flexion. Push against the wall with the palm of your hand.

- Exhale, relax and the increase thoracic and shoulder rotation to the left and increase elbow extension.
- Localise the stretch at the elbow by moving the body a few millimetres away from the plane of the wall.
- Repeat the stretch on the right elbow several times

5.4 Triceps stretch - passive stretch for the triceps and muscles responsible for shoulder adduction

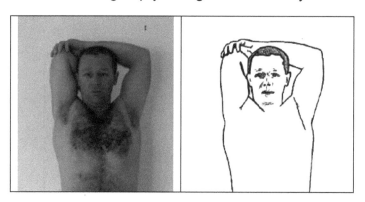

5.4 Triceps stretch

Starting position

- Stand with your feet apart and your arms at your sides.
- Flex your right forearm until it is fully flexed.
- Abduct your right arm to the fully abducted position.
- Your right elbow should now be near your right ear and the palm of your right hand should rest on your upper thoracic spine.
- Abduct your left arm and grasp your right elbow with your left hand.

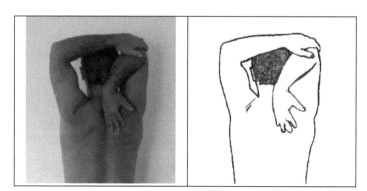

- Keep your arms and forearms back and slightly behind your head.
- Keep a straight spine and maintain spine and head alignment.
- Don't let your forearms push your head into a flexed position.
- Relax your shoulders.

Technique

- Take a deep breath in.
- Exhale and pull your right elbow medially and behind your head.
- Feel the stretch down the back of your right arm, down the outside of your shoulder and between your scapula and spine.
- Do not move your head or spine or pelvis.
- Move your arm but relax your shoulder.
- Increase the stretch with each exhalation.
- Repeat the stretch for the left shoulder.

5.5 Supinator stretch - active and post-isometric stretch for the muscles responsible for forearm supination

5.5 Supinator stretch

Starting position

- Stand with your feet are apart and with your right side opposite a doorframe or firmly anchored vertical pole.
- Lift your right arm and grasp the doorframe with your right hand.
- Grasp the doorframe at point just below the level of your shoulder.
- Your thumb should point upwards towards the ceiling.
- Keep your elbow extended.

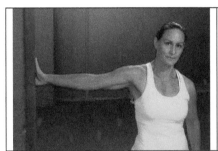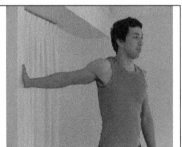

Technique

- Take a deep breath in.
- Exhale, while pronating your right forearm by rolling it forwards, inwards and downwards.
- Feel the stretch behind your right elbow and forearm.

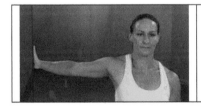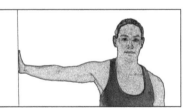

- Take another deep breath and hold it in.
- Attempt to supinate your right forearm by rolling it backwards, outwards and downwards against the doorframe.
- Maintain a firm stance and a firm hold of the doorframe.
- After about five seconds cease the isometric contraction, relax your elbow, exhale and then roll your right forearm forwards, inwards and downwards.
- Feel the stretch behind your right elbow and forearm.
- Keep your right elbow extended and shoulder relaxed.
- Repeat the stretch several times either actively or combined with a post-isometric contraction, increasing the stretch with each exhalation.
- Repeat the stretch for the left arm.

5.6 Pronator stretches - active, passive and post-isometric stretches for pronator teres and pronator quadratus

5.6a Pronator stretch using a doorframe

Starting position

- Stand with your feet apart and with your right side near to a doorframe or firmly anchored vertical pole.
- Lift your right arm and grasp the doorframe with your right hand at the point just below your shoulder level, and make sure your thumb points downwards.
- Straighten your right arm.
- Rotate your upper body to the left until you reach the point of minimum tension in the shoulder and arm muscles - somewhere between abduction and extension.
- You may need to readjust the height you grasp the doorframe.
- Also position your arm to make it easy for you to roll the forearm outwards.

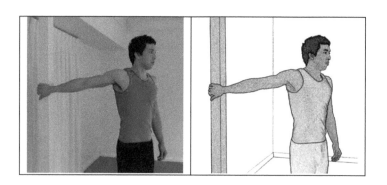

Technique

- Take a deep breath in.
- Exhale and supinate your right forearm by rolling it outwards and upwards.
- Feel the stretch down the front and inside of your right elbow and forearm.
- Take another deep breath and hold it in.
- Attempt to rotate your forearm inwards and downwards and push your hand downwards against the doorframe.
- Attempt to pronate your forearm by rolling it inwards and downwards - push your thumb and the radial side of your hand against the doorframe.
- Resist any movement with a firm stance of your body and by maintaining a firm hold of the doorframe with your right hand.
- After about five seconds cease the isometric contraction, relax your elbow, exhale and then increase supination by rolling your right forearm outwards.
- Feel the stretch down the front and inside of your right elbow and forearm.
- Keep your elbow extended.
- Repeat the active or post-isometric stretch several times, increasing the stretch with each exhalation.
- Repeat the stretch for the left arm.

5.6b Passive pronator stretch assisted by the other hand

Starting position

- Stand with your feet apart.
- Bend your right elbow 90 degrees.
- Rotate your right forearm outwards (supination) as far as possible.
- Grasp your right wrist with a firm hold of your left hand.

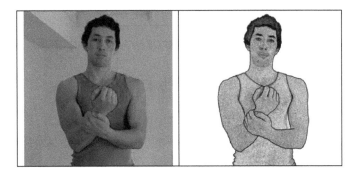

Technique

- Take a deep breath in.
- Exhale and increase right forearm supination by extending your left wrist.
- Introduce some extension in your right forearm to stretch pronator teres.

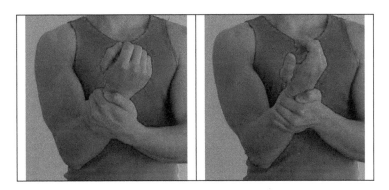

- Take another deep breath and hold it in.
- Attempt to roll your right forearm inwards and upwards by pushing the front and outside of your wrist against the pads of your fingers.
- Resist any rotation movement of your forearm (flexion and pronation) with a firm hold of your right wrist with your left hand.
- After about five seconds cease the isometric muscle contraction, relax, exhale and then supinate your forearm.
- Straighten your right elbow a little to increase the stretch in pronator teres.
- Repeat the passive or post-isometric stretch several times, increasing the stretch with each exhalation.
- Repeat the stretch for the left arm.

5.7 Wrist extensor stretches - passive and post-isometric stretches for the extensor muscles of the wrist and hand

5.7a Kneeling unilateral wrist extensor stretch

Starting position

- Kneel on the floor, preferably on a carpet or on a mat.
- Bend forwards at the hips and place your left hand, palm down on the floor in front of you.
- Flex your right arm, forearm and hand and place the back of your right hand on the floor, so your palm faces upwards.
- Your arms are straight and vertical and your hands are directly in line with and below your shoulders.
- Keep your knees and feet apart for easier balance.
- Your spine should be in a neutral position - neither flexed nor extended.

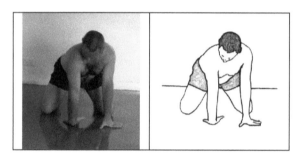

Technique

- Take a deep breath in.
- Exhale, flex your hips and knees and move your trunk in a straight line backwards, so your right shoulder passes over your right wrist and your buttocks move towards your feet.
- Keep your elbow extended and your wrist flexed.
- Do not allow the weight of your body to be taken by your right wrist.

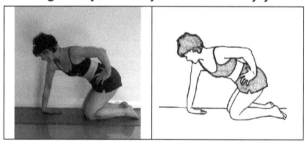

- Take another deep breath and hold it in.
- Push the back of your right hand into the floor for about five seconds.
- Resist any movement of your body with a firm stance.
- Cease the contraction, relax and exhale while moving your trunk backwards so your right shoulder passes over your right wrist.
- Repeat the passive or post-isometric stretch several times, increasing the stretch with each exhalation.
- Repeat the stretch for the left hand extensor muscles.

5.7b Kneeling bilateral wrist extensor stretch

Starting position

- Kneel on the floor, preferably on a carpet or on a mat.
- Bend forwards at the hips, flex your elbows and wrists and place the backs of your hands on the floor with your fingers pointing towards your knees.
- Extend your elbows so your arms are straight and vertical and your hands are directly in line with and below your shoulders.
- Keep your knees and feet apart for easier balance.
- Your spine should be in a neutral position - neither flexed nor extended.
- Do not take the weight of your upper body through your wrists.

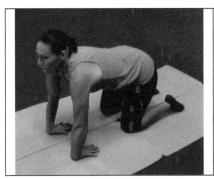 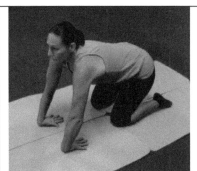

Technique

- Take a deep breath in.
- Exhale, flex your hips and knees and move your trunk in a straight line backwards, so your shoulders pass over your wrists and your buttocks move towards your feet.
- Keep your elbows extended, wrists flexed and the back of your hands and fingers flat on the floor.

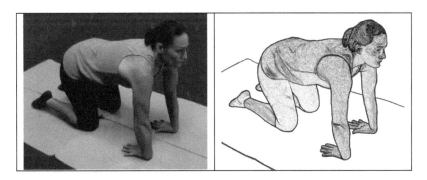

- Reposition your hands forwards if necessary to maintain good balance.
- The further your hands are in front of the knees the greater the stretch.
- Increase the stretch with each exhalation.

5.7c Kneeling wrist extensor and ulna deviator stretch

Starting position

- Kneel on the floor, preferably on a carpet or on a mat.
- Bend forwards at the hips, flex your wrists and internally rotate your arms and place the backs of your hands on the floor with your fingers pointing outwards, laterally and away from your body.
- Extend your elbows so your arms are straight and vertical.
- Keep your knees and feet apart for easier balance.
- Your spine should be in a neutral position - neither flexed nor extended.
- Keep the whole of the back of your hands and fingers flat on the floor.
- Your wrists are shoulder width apart.
- Do not take the weight of your upper body through your wrists.

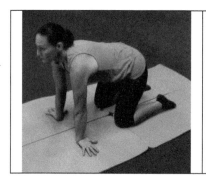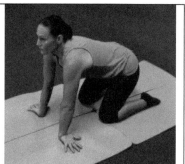

Technique

- Take a deep breath in.
- Exhale, flex your hips and knees and move your pelvis, trunk, head and neck backwards and towards your feet, almost horizontally with the floor.
- Keep your elbows straight, wrists extended and palms flat on the floor.
- Increase the stretch with each exhalation.

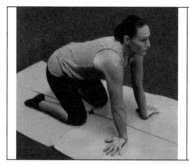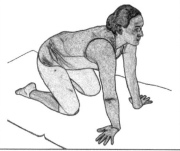

- This is a localised stretch for extensor carpi ulnaris and combines wrist flexion with radial deviation and forearm pronation.
- The further apart your hands and the further they are in front of the knees the greater the stretch on extensor carpi ulnaris

5.7d Kneeling wrist extensor and radial deviator stretch

Starting position

- Kneel on the floor, preferably on a carpet or on a mat.
- Bend forwards at the hips, flex your wrists and externally rotate your arms.
- Place the backs of your hands on the floor with your fingers pointing inwards, medially and towards each other.
- Extend your elbows so your arms are straight and vertical.
- Keep your knees and feet apart for easier balance.
- Your spine should be in a neutral position - neither flexed nor extended.
- Keep the whole of the back of your hands and fingers flat on the floor.
- Your wrists should be shoulder width apart.
- Do not take the weight of your upper body through your wrists.

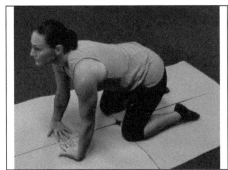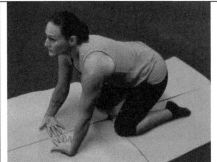

Technique

- Take a deep breath in.
- Exhale, flex your hips and knees and move your pelvis, trunk, head and neck approximately horizontally backwards and towards your feet.
- Keep your elbows straight, wrists extended and palms flat on the floor.
- Increase the stretch with each exhalation.

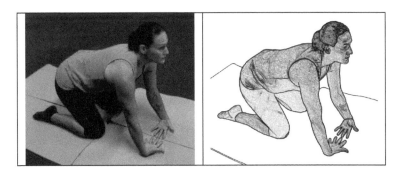

- This is a localised stretch for extensor carpi radialis longus and combines wrist flexion with ulna deviation and forearm supination.
- The further apart your hands are and the further they are in front of the knees the greater the stretch on extensor carpi radialis longus.

5.8 Wrist flexor stretch - passive and post-isometric stretches for the flexor muscles of the wrist and hand

5.8a Kneeling unilateral wrist flexor stretch

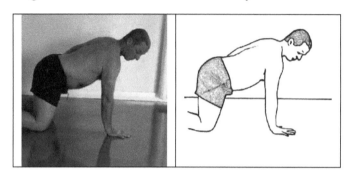

Starting position

- Kneel on the floor, preferably on a carpet or on a mat.
- Bend forwards at the hips, flex your right arm and forearm and place the palm of your right hand on the floor in front of you.

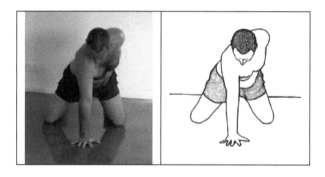

- Fully extend your right elbow so that your arm is straight.
- Your arm should be vertical and your wrist directly under your shoulder.
- Keep your knees and feet apart for balance.
- Your spine should be in a neutral position, neither flexed nor extended.

Technique

- Take a deep breath in.
- Exhale, while moving your trunk forwards, so your right shoulder passes over your right wrist.
- Keep your elbow and wrist extended, and palm flat on the floor.
- Take another deep breath and hold it in.
- Push the palm of your right hand into the floor for about five seconds.
- Resist any movement of your body with a firm stance.
- Cease the contraction, relax and exhale while moving your right shoulder in a straight line forwards and over your right wrist.
- Repeat the passive or post-isometric stretch several times, increasing the stretch with each exhalation.
- Repeat the stretch for the left hand flexor muscles.

5.8b Kneeling bilateral wrist flexor stretch

Starting position

- Kneel on the floor, preferably on a carpet or on a mat.
- Bend forwards at the hips, externally rotate your arms and place your palms on the floor with your fingers pointing backwards towards your knees.
- Extend your elbows so your arms are straight and vertical and your hands are directly in line with and below your shoulders.
- Keep your knees and feet apart for easier balance.
- Your spine should be in a neutral position - neither flexed nor extended.

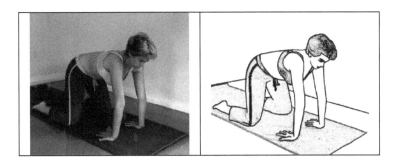

Technique

- Take a deep breath in.
- Exhale, while flexing your hips and knees, and moving your trunk backwards so your buttocks are closer to your feet.
- Keep your elbows and wrists extended and palms flat on the floor.
- Reposition your hands forwards if necessary to maintain good balance.

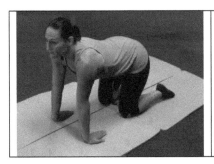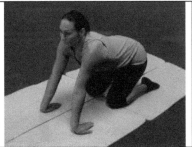

- The further your hands are in front of the knees the greater the stretch.
- Increase the stretch with each exhalation.
- This stretch combines wrist extension with forearm supination.

5.8c Kneeling wrist flexor and radial deviator stretch

Starting position

- Kneel on the floor, preferably on a carpet or on a mat.
- Bend forwards at the hips, externally rotate your arms and place your palms on the floor with your fingers pointing outwards, laterally and away from your body.
- Extend your elbows so your arms are straight and vertical.
- Keep your knees and feet apart for easier balance.
- Your spine should be in a neutral position - neither flexed nor extended.
- Keep the palms flat on the floor and wrists shoulder width apart.

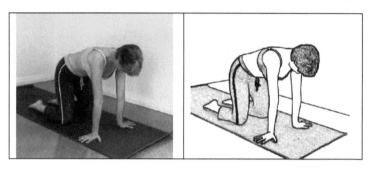

Technique

- Take a deep breath in.
- Exhale, flex your hips and knees and move your pelvis, trunk, head and neck approximately horizontally backwards and towards your feet.
- Keep your elbows straight, wrists extended and palms flat on the floor.
- Increase the stretch with each exhalation.

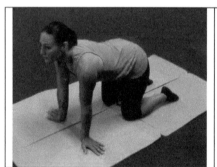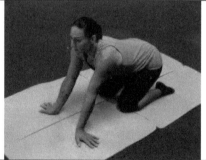

- This is a localised stretch for flexor carpi radialis and combines wrist extension with ulna deviation and forearm supination.
- The further apart your hands are and the further they are in front of your knees the greater the stretch.

5.8d Kneeling wrist flexor and ulna deviator stretch

Starting position

- Kneel on the floor, preferably on a carpet or on a mat.
- Bend forwards at the hips, internally rotate your arms and place your palms on the floor with your fingers pointing inwards, medially and towards each other.
- Extend your elbows so your arms are straight and vertical
- Keep your knees and feet apart for easier balance.
- Your spine should be in a neutral position - neither flexed nor extended.
- Keep the palms flat on the floor and wrists shoulder width apart.

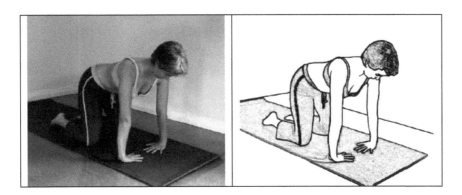

Technique

- Take a deep breath in.
- Exhale, flex your hips and knees and move your pelvis, trunk, head and neck approximately horizontally backwards and towards your feet.
- Keep your elbows straight, wrists extended and palms flat on the floor.
- Increase the stretch with each exhalation.

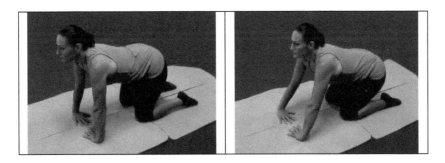

- This is a localised stretch for flexor carpi ulnaris and combines wrist extension with radial deviation and forearm pronation.
- The further the hands are apart and the further they are in front of the knees the greater the stretch.

5.8e Standing unilateral wrist flexor stretch

Starting position

- Stand next to a table with your feet apart.
- Place the palm of your right hand on the table in front of you.
- Place the palm of your left hand over the back of your right hand, perpendicular to it and covering the whole hand up to the wrist.
- Fully extend your elbows so that your arms are straight.
- Flex your hips and knees so that your spine remains straight.

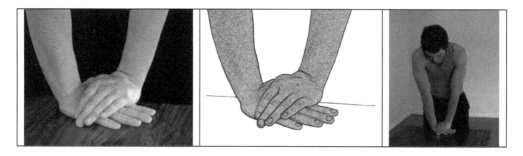

Technique

- Take a deep breath in.
- Exhale and move your hips, pelvis, spine and shoulders to your left, thereby moving your right shoulder over your right wrist.

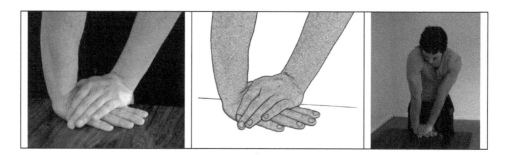

- Keep your right wrist and elbow extended, and palm flat on the table.
- Increase the stretch with each exhalation.
- Repeat the stretch for the left hand flexor muscles.
- The kneeling stretches 5.8a to 5.8d can also be done standing using a table in the way described here.

5.9 Finger flexor stretch - post-isometric and passive stretch for the forearm, wrist, hand and fingers

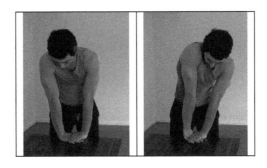

5.9 Standing finger flexor muscle stretch on a table

Starting position

- Stand with the palm of your right hand on the top of a table.
- Place your left hand across the back of your right hand, perpendicular to your hand and just distal to your metacarpophalangeal joints.

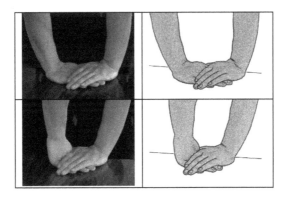

- The fingers of your left hand fix the fingers of the right hand to the table and act as a fulcrum around which joint movement can occur.
- Your shoulders sit directly above your wrists with your elbows extended.
- Sideshift your shoulders and upper thoracic spine to your left and allow your fingers to extend at the metacarpophalangeal joints.
- If the table is too high flex your left elbow to sideshift your trunk to the left.
- Stop when you feel the initial stages of a stretch in your fingers or forearm.

Technique

- Take in a deep breath and hold it in.
- Exhale, while moving your trunk to the left.
- Keep your right elbow extended.
- Feel the stretch in the fingers, hand and forearm but stop when you feel an increase in resistance.
- Repeat the stretch several times, increasing the stretch with each exhalation.
- Repeat the stretch for the left hand finger flexor muscles.

6.0 Iliopsoas stretches - passive and post-isometric stretches for iliacus, psoas and other hip flexor muscles

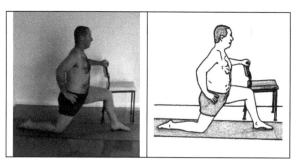

6.0a The lunge

Starting position

- Kneel on the floor with a chair at your side to help maintain balance.
- Place a small pillow or blanket under your right knee or use a mat.
- Flex your left hip and place the sole of your left foot on the mat about 50 cm in front of your body.

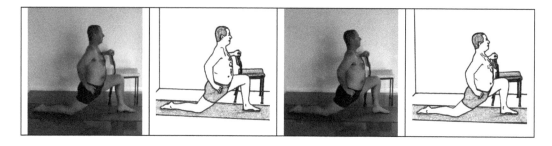

- Hold onto the chair with your left hand to maintain balance.
- Take your left knee forwards and allow your body will descend slightly.
- Stop when you feel the initial stages of a stretch in front of your right hip.
- Adjust the placement of your left foot so your thigh and leg form a right angle and your knee is directly over your foot.
- Your spine should be straight and vertical.

Technique

- Take a deep breath in.
- Exhale, while moving your left knee and pelvis forwards and allow your pelvis and upper body to descend towards the floor with a lunge action.
- Feel the stretch deep in your right groin.
- Use your right hand to control your pelvis to prevent it from rotating if necessary.
- Keep your spine straight, vertical and over the centre of your hips.
- Use the chair at the side of your body to maintain balance.
- Repeat the stretch several times moving your pelvis further forwards and downwards with each exhalation.
- Repeat the stretch for the left hip flexor muscles.

164

6.0b The forwards splits

Starting position

- Kneel on the floor.
- A chair may be placed at your left side to help maintain balance.
- Place a small pillow or blanket under your right knee or use a mat.
- Flex your left hip and place the heel of your left foot on the mat about 1 m in front of your body and your left knee on a foam roll.
- You will not need a roll under your knee or a chair for balance if you have good flexibility and can do this stretch comfortably.
- Slide your left heel forwards to extend your right thigh at the hip and extend your left leg at the knee.
- Allow your body to descend but stop as soon as you feel the initial stages of a stretch in front of your right hip or behind your left knee.
- Your spine should be straight and vertical.

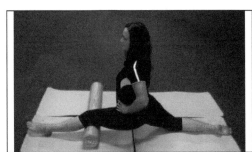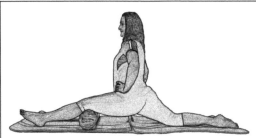

Technique

- Take a deep breath in.
- Exhale and move your left heel forwards and allow your body to descend towards the floor.
- Feel the stretch deep in your right groin and in the back of your left knee.

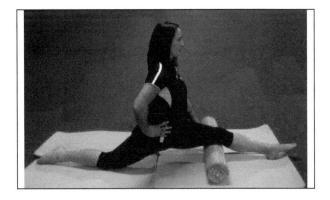

- Keep your spine straight and positioned vertically over your hips.
- Hold onto the chair to maintain balance.
- Move forwards and down and increase the stretch with each exhalation.
- Repeat the stretch for the left iliopsoas and right hamstrings.

6.0c The hanging hip stretch

Starting position

- Lay on your back on a strong and stable table.
- Move the right side of your pelvis as close as possible to the edge of the table but keep the rest of your body securely on the table.
- Use a small pillow under your head to help relax your cervical spine.
- Flex your left hip and knee, grasp your knee with both hands, pull it towards your body and hold your thigh against your chest.
- Lower your right leg over the side of the table.
- Hold your left thigh firmly against your chest with both hands.

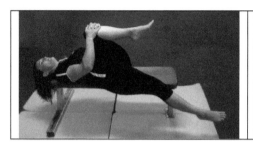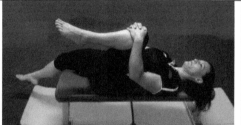

Technique

- Take a deep breath in.
- Exhale, let your hip muscles relax and allow your right thigh, leg and foot to drop towards the floor.
- Feel a stretch in front of your right hip and thigh as your lower limb hangs over the edge of the table.

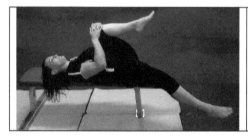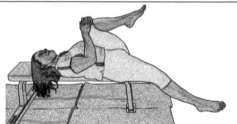

- Take another deep breath and hold it in.
- With a combined contraction of your right hip and knee lift your foot about 50 cm upwards towards the ceiling.
- Hold the position for about five seconds, then cease the muscle contraction, relax, exhale and allow your leg to drop towards the floor
- Repeat the passive or post-isometric stretch several times.
- Repeat the stretch on the left side.

6.1 Mixed Gluteus stretches - passive and post-isometric stretches for piriformis and gluteus minimus, medius and maximus in hip flexion and external rotation

6.1a Passive stretch for hip extensors and rotators

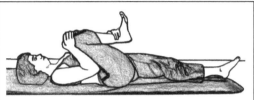

Starting position

- Lie on your back on a mat or carpet and flex your right hip and knee.
- Grasp your right knee with your right hand and grasp your right foot with your left hand.

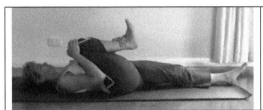

- Pull your right knee towards your right shoulder and flex your hip further.
- Pull your right foot towards your left shoulder to externally rotate your hip.
- Move your right knee across your chest and towards your left shoulder to adduct your hip but without losing the flexion and rotation.

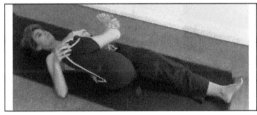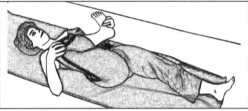

Technique

- Take a deep breath in and then exhale and perform the following actions:

  - Pull your right knee towards your right shoulder - flex your hip
  - Pull your right knee across your body and towards your left shoulder - horizontally adduct your hip
  - Pull your right foot towards your left shoulder - externally rotate your hip

- Hip flexion and external rotation may be combined and hip adduction and external rotation may be combined.
- Each variation will place a stretch on a different muscle or muscle group.
- Feel the stretch in your right buttock.
- Keep the back of your left thigh and leg in contact with the floor.
- Repeat the stretch in the left side.

6.1b Post-isometric stretch for hip extensors and rotators

Starting position

- Lie on your back on a mat or carpet and flex your right hip and knee.
- Grasp your right knee with your right hand and grasp your right foot with your left hand.

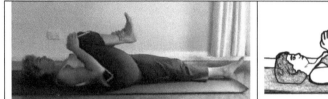

- Pull your right knee towards your right shoulder to flex your hip.
- Pull your right foot towards your left shoulder to externally rotate your hip.
- Move your right knee across your chest and towards your left shoulder.
- In other words flex, then externally rotate and then adduct your right hip

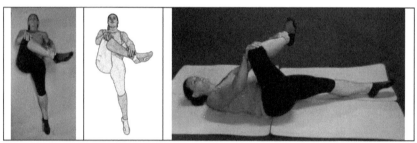

Technique

- Take a deep breath in hold it and perform the following actions:

  - Push your right knee upwards towards the ceiling but resist hip extension with a firm hold on your knee with your right hand
  - Push your foot upwards and outwards to your right but resist hip internal rotation with a firm hold on your foot with your left hand
  - Push your knee outwards to your right side but resist hip horizontal abduction with a firm hold on your knee with your right hand

- Resist all movement with an equal and opposite counterforce.
- After about five seconds cease the isometric contraction, relax your muscles, then exhale and bring your body to a new position.

  - Pull your right knee towards your right shoulder - flex your hip
  - Pull your right knee across your body and towards your left shoulder - horizontally adduct your hip
  - Pull your right foot to your left shoulder - externally rotate your hip

- Feel the stretch in your right buttock.
- Keep the back of your left thigh and leg in contact with the floor.
- Repeat the stretch in the left side.

6.1c Passive cross leg stretch for hip extensors and rotators

Starting position

- Lie on your back on a mat with your hips and knees partially flexed.
- Fully flex your right hip, then externally rotate it and place your right foot on your left thigh just above your knee.
- Reach through the space between your thighs and right leg with your right hand and grasp your left thigh and leg just below your knee.

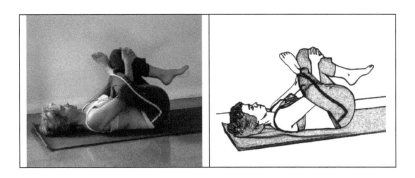

- Reach around the outside of your left thigh with your left hand and grasp your left thigh and leg just below your knee.
- Interlace the fingers of both hands around your left knee.
- Pull your left knee towards your chest.
- This flexes and externally rotates your right hip.

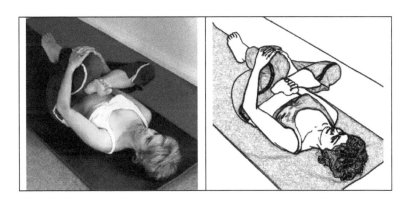

Technique

- Take a deep breath in.
- Exhale and pull your left knee towards your chest with both hands.
- Flexion of the left hip pushes the left thigh against the outside of your right foot which results in right hip flexion, external rotation and abduction.
- Allow your right knee to drop out to the side and down to the floor.
- Feel the stretch in the right buttock and hip.
- Repeat the stretch in the left side.

6.1d Post-isometric cross leg stretch for hip extensors and rotators

Starting position

- Lie on your back on a mat with your hips and knees partially flexed.
- Fully flex your right hip, then externally rotate it and place your right foot on your left thigh just above your knee.
- Reach through the space between your thighs and right leg with your right hand and grasp your left thigh and leg just below your knee.
- Reach around the outside of your left thigh with your left hand and grasp your left thigh and leg just below your knee.
- Interlace the fingers of both hands around your left knee.
- Pull your left knee towards your chest.
- This flexes and externally rotates your right hip.

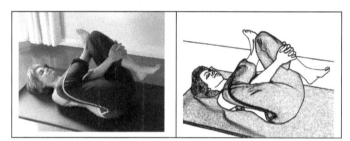

Technique

- Take a deep breath and hold it in.
- Push your right foot away from your body and against your left thigh but resist any movement of your right foot and hip with a firm hold of your left thigh and leg with both hands.
- After about five seconds cease the isometric contraction of your hip extensor and internal rotator muscles, relax, exhale and pull your left knee, thigh and leg towards your chest with both hands.
- Flexion of the left hip presses the left thigh against the outside of your right foot which results in right hip flexion, external rotation and abduction.

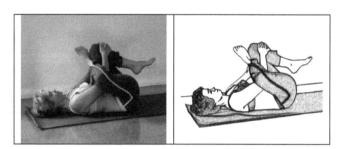

- Movement of the left leg is transferred to the right hip through the foot.
- Allow your right knee to drop out to the side and down to the floor.
- Feel the stretch in the right buttock and hip.
- Repeat the stretch in the left side.

6.1e Passive and post-isometric stretch for hip extensors and rotators on a table

Starting position

- Stand facing a table
- Place the outside of your right foot and ankle on the table in front of your left hip.
- Your right hip is flexed, externally rotated and abducted.
- Flex your spine and left hip and lean forwards taking your body weight over your right foot.

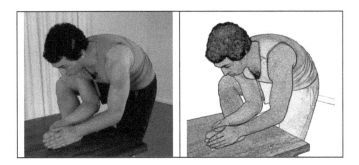

Technique

- Take a deep breath and hold it in.
- Exhale and rotate your spine to the right and lean forwards and downwards towards the table - spinal and left hip flexion.
- The force of your body weight is transferred to your right hip increasing hip flexion and external rotation.

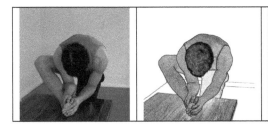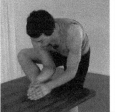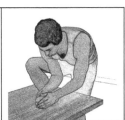

- Take another deep breath and hold it in.
- Push your right foot down and into the table and attempt to lift yourself up and off the table but resist any movement of your body with a firm stance.
- After about five seconds cease the isometric contraction of your hip extensor and internal rotator muscles, relax, exhale and lower your body over your right foot with flexion and a small amount of rotation to the right.
- Feel the stretch in your right buttock and hip.
- Allow your right knee to drop towards the table.
- Repeat the stretch in the left side.

6.1f Passive and post-isometric stretch for hip extensors, rotators and abductors on a table

Starting position

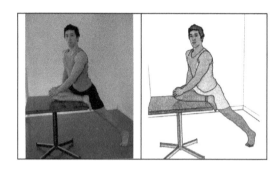

- Stand facing a table or bench
- Place the outside of your right thigh, knee and leg on the table.
- Your right hip is flexed, externally rotated and adducted.
- Grasp your right knee with both hands.
- Straighten your body by extending your spine and by pushing your hands against your knee and extending your elbows.
- Rotate your spine and pelvis to the right.

Technique

- Take a deep breath and hold it in.
- Exhale and combine the following actions:

  - Bend forwards - flex your spine and flex your pelvis on your hip
  - Use your body weight - lean over your hip.
  - Rotate your spine to the right
  - Rotate your pelvis to the right - pivoting around your right hip.

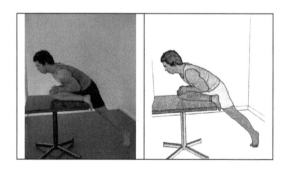

- Take another deep breath and hold it in.
- Push your right leg down and into the table and attempt to lift yourself up off the table but resist any movement of your body with a firm stance.
- After five seconds cease the isometric contraction of your hip extensor and internal rotator muscles, relax, exhale and adopt the actions above.
- Increase flexion and external rotation of your right hip by leaning over your hip and using your body weight.
- Feel the stretch in your right buttock and hip.
- Repeat the stretch in the left side.

6.1g Post-isometric stretch for gluteus minimus with your hips in flexion seated on a chair

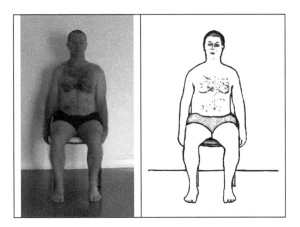

Starting position

- Sit on a chair with your back straight and your feet apart and firmly planted on the floor.
- Flex your right hip and knee and place the outside of your right ankle on your left thigh just above your knee.
- Allow your right knee to drop until you feel a mild stretch in your groin.
- Place your right hand on you right thigh just above your knee.

Technique

- Take a deep breath and hold it in.
- Push your right knee upwards and towards the ceiling.
- Resist any movement with an equal and opposite counterforce with your right hand.
- After about five seconds cease the isometric contraction, relax your hip muscles, exhale and push your right knee further towards the floor.

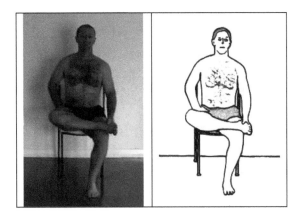

- Your hip moves into greater external rotation.
- Feel the stretch in the buttock and groin.
- Repeat the post-isometric contractions several times.
- Repeat the stretch on your left side.

6.2 Hip external rotator stretches - passive and post-isometric stretches for the hip external rotators and abductors

6.2a Hip external rotator stretch supine

Starting position

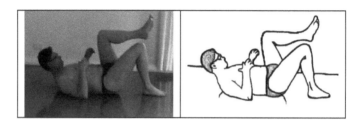

- Lie on your back on the floor.
- Flex your hips and knees and place your feet on the floor slightly apart.
- Lift your left leg, move it over the top of your right knee and hook it around your right thigh in a cross legged position.

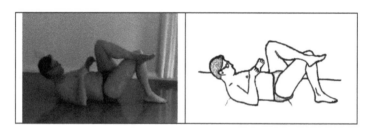

- Pull your right knee to the left and across your body with your left leg but stop when you feel the initial stages of hip tension.
- Keep your head, shoulders, arms, spine, pelvis and right foot on the floor.

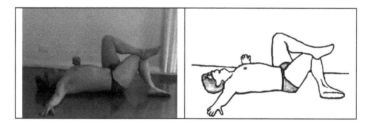

Technique

- Take a deep breath in.
- Exhale and push your right knee to the left with your left leg.
- Ideally do not allow your pelvis to rotate and lift off the floor.

- Take another deep breath and hold it in.
- Push your right knee to the right and push your right foot to the left and down into the floor but resist the movement with your left leg.
- After five seconds cease the isometric contraction, relax your hip muscles, exhale and pull your right knee further to the left with your left leg.
- Repeat the stretch several times and then repeat the stretch on the left.

6.2b Piriformis stretch supine

Starting position

- Lie on your back on the floor.
- Flex your right hip and knee and place the sole of your foot on the floor on the outside of your left leg just below your knee.
- Place the fingers of your left hand on the lateral side of your right knee.
- Place the fingers of your right hand on the top and right side of your pelvis.
- Push your right knee to the left with your left hand while holding your pelvis firmly down on the floor with your right hand.
- Stop when you feel the initial stages of a stretch in your right hip.

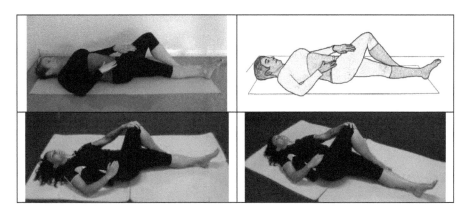

Technique

- Take a deep breath in.
- Exhale and push your right knee further to the left with your left hand while holding your pelvis against the floor with your right hand.
- Feel the stretch deep in the right buttock.
- Moving your right knee to the left results in right hip adduction and internal rotation.

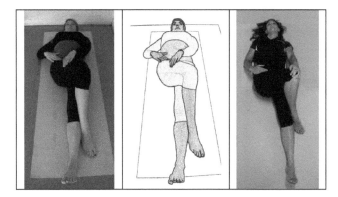

- Take another deep breath and hold it in.
- Push your right knee to the right but resist movement with your left hand.
- After five seconds cease the isometric contraction, relax your hip muscles, exhale and pull your right knee further to the left with your left hand.
- Repeat the passive or post-isometric stretch several times.
- Repeat the stretch on the left.

6.2c Hip external rotator stretch standing using a chair

Starting position

- Stand at the front of a chair with your feet together.
- Face the right side of the chair with the outside of your right leg touching the front of the chair.
- Grasp the back of the chair and stand up straight.
- Flex your right knee and internally rotate your right hip and place your right leg on the seat of chair with your foot poking out to the back of the chair.
- Your leg is supported by the seat of the chair and the inside of your right ankle rests against the inside of back of the chair on the left side.
- The chair seat needs to be the correct height for your body.
- Use a padded chair or a small pillow or towel on the seat for comfort.

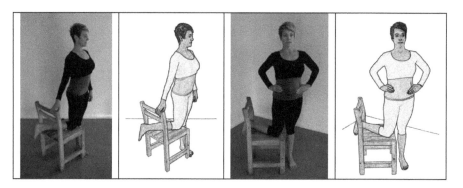

Technique

- Take a deep breath in.
- Exhale and rotate the left side of your pelvis and left hip to the right and forwards.
- Feel the stretch in your right buttock and hip.

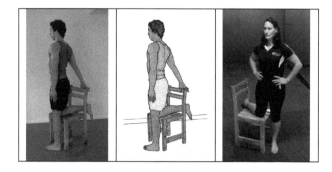

- Take another deep breath and hold it in.
- Push your right ankle inwards against the back of the chair.
- Resist this action by keeping a firm stance with your body.
- After about five seconds cease the isometric contraction, relax your hip muscles, exhale and rotate your left hip and left side of your pelvis to the right and forwards.
- Repeat passive or post-isometric stretch several times.
- Repeat the stretch on your left side.

6.3 Hip internal rotator stretch - active, passive and post-isometric for gluteus minimus and anterior gluteus medius

6.3a Gluteus minimus stretch supine

Starting position

- Lie on your back on a mat or carpet.
- Flex your right hip and knee.
- Place the outside of your right foot on your left leg just above your ankle.
- Lower your right knee towards the mat and externally rotate your right hip.

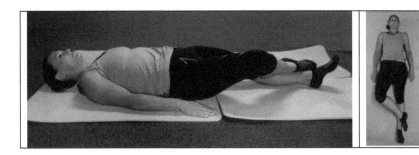

Technique

- Take a deep breath in.
- Exhale and move your right knee towards the floor.
- Contract your hip external rotators to actively stretch gluteus minimus.
- Take another deep breath in, then exhale and allow your right knee to drop towards the floor.
- Use the weight of your thigh and leg to passively stretch gluteus minimus.
- Place your right hand on your right thigh.

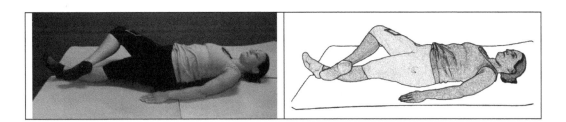

- Take another deep breath and hold it in.
- Push your right foot downwards against your left leg and push your right knee upwards towards the ceiling and resist the movement with an equal and opposite counterforce with your right hand.
- After about five seconds cease the isometric contraction, relax your hip muscles, exhale and allow your knee to drop further towards the floor.
- Feel the stretch in your right buttock and around the top of the hip joint.
- Repeat the active, passive or post-isometric stretch several times.
- Repeat the stretch on your left side.

6.3b Active and post-isometric stretches for gluteus minimus sidelying

Starting position

- Lie on your left side on a mat or carpet.
- Flex your right hip and knee.
- Place your right foot in front of your left leg, about half way between your knee and ankle.
- Lift your right knee and point it towards the ceiling but keep the sole of you right foot firmly planted on the mat - externally rotate your right hip.

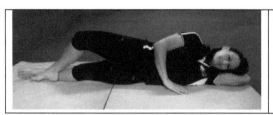

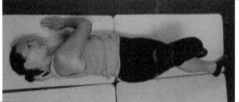

Technique

- Take a deep breath in.
- Exhale and move your right knee backwards by contracting the muscles that externally rotate your hip.
- Feel the stretch in your buttock and around the top of you hip joint.
- Place your right hand on your right thigh.

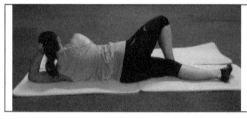

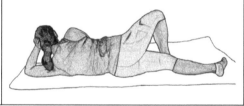

- Take another deep breath and hold it in.
- Push your right knee forwards and resist the movement with an equal and opposite counterforce with your right hand.
- After about five seconds cease the isometric contraction, relax your hip muscles, exhale and take your knee further backwards.
- Feel the stretch in your right buttock and around the top of the hip joint.
- Repeat the active or post-isometric stretch several times.
- Repeat the stretch on your left side.

6.3c Post-isometric stretch for gluteus minimus prone

Starting position

- Lie on your front on a mat or carpet.
- Flex your knee and abduct and externally rotate your right hip.
- Place the inside your right knee, leg and foot flat on the mat.
- Slide your right foot under your left leg at a point just above your ankle.
- The weight of your pelvis and right leg puts your hip into external rotation.

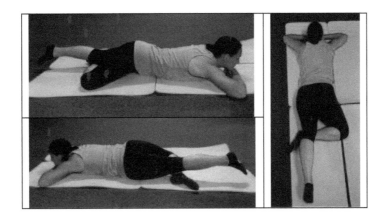

Technique

- Take a deep breath and hold it in.
- Push your right knee into the mat and push your right foot upwards and against the front of your left leg.
- Resist this action by contracting your left quadriceps and hip flexor muscles to keep your left knee and hip in extension - keep your leg firm.
- After about five seconds cease the isometric contraction, relax your hip muscles, exhale and take your right groin further towards the mat.

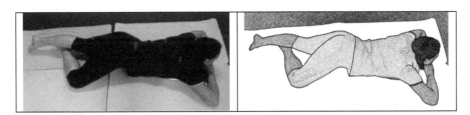

- Try and flatten your body at the hip and produce greater hip rotation.
- Feel the stretch in your right buttock and around the top of the hip joint.
- Repeat post-isometric stretch several times.
- Repeat the stretch on your left side.

6.3d Gluteus minimus stretch standing using a chair

Starting position

- Stand on the right side of chair near its back leg with your feet together.
- Face to the rear of the chair, with your body parallel to the back of the chair and with the outside of your right leg touching the side of the chair.
- Grasp the back of the chair and stand up straight.
- Flex your right knee and then flex and externally rotate your right hip.
- Place your right leg on the seat of chair so the inside of your knee is against the back of the chair, the outside of your ankle is against the front of your left leg and your leg is supported by the seat of the chair.
- The chair seat needs to be the correct height for your body.
- Use a padded chair or a small pillow or towel on the seat for comfort.

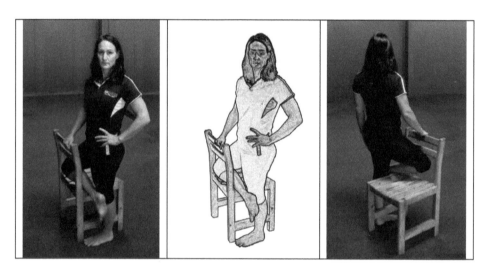

Technique

- Take a deep breath in.
- Exhale, rotate the left side of your pelvis and left hip outwards and to the left and move the right side of your pelvis and right hip forwards, pushing your right groin towards the back of the chair.
- Feel the stretch in your right buttock, the top of you hip and your groin.
- Take another deep breath and hold it in.
- Push your right knee forwards against the back of the chair and push your right foot backwards and against the front of your left leg.
- Resist this action by keeping a firm stance.
- After about five seconds cease the isometric contraction, relax your hip muscles, exhale and take your right groin further towards the back of the chair and rotate the left side of your pelvis and left hip outwards to the left.
- Repeat passive or post-isometric stretch several times.
- Repeat the stretch on your left side.

6.4 Hip abductor stretches - passive and post-isometric stretches for tensor fasciae latae, gluteus medius, minimus and the upper fibres of gluteus maximus

6.4a Passive stretch for tensor fasciae latae standing

Starting position

- Stand straight with your feet apart.
- Flex your hips and knees about 45 degrees.
- Move your right leg backwards, behind your left leg and to your left.
- Bend your left knee until it is in 90 degrees flexion.
- Lean forward and grasp your knee with both hands.
- Use your knee to support and stabilize your upper body with your arms.
- Adjust the left-right position of your right foot for optimum balance.
- Most of your body weight should be over your left knee and foot.

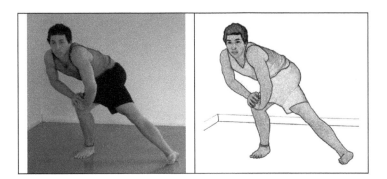

Technique

- Take a deep breath in.
- Exhale and lower your pelvis towards the floor.
- Increase the flexion of your left knee.

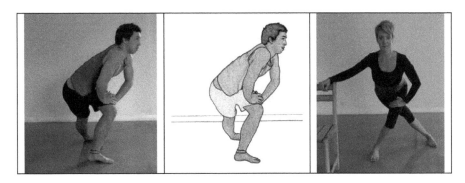

- Keep your spine straight.
- Keep your right knee straight and your right leg out to the side.
- Feel the stretch down the side of your right thigh.
- Repeat the technique for the left hip.
- This technique requires good quadriceps strength and body balance.
- If balance is a problem the body can be supported between two chairs.

6.4b Passive stretch for gluteus maximus and medius kneeling

Starting position

- Kneel on a small pillow or mat besides a chair or stool.
- Flex your left hip and place the outside of your left foot on the floor in front of you and to your right.
- Place your right hand on the chair for support.
- Slide your left foot diagonally forwards and away from your body and as you do so bend your right hip backwards and move your pelvis forwards.
- Slide your left foot as far as possible to your right and as you do so, sideshift your pelvis to the right and adduct your right hip.
- Keep your left knee partially flexed.
- Allow your spine to sidebend left but keep it well balanced on your pelvis.

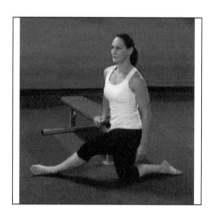

Technique

- Take a deep breath in.
- Exhale while sliding your left foot along the floor to the right, sideshifting your pelvis to the right and adducting your right hip.
- Feel the stretch down the outside of your right hip and thigh.

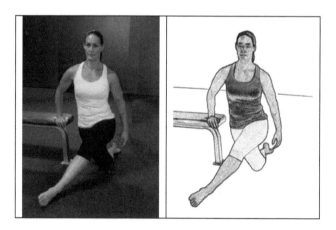

- Keep your left knee slightly flexed but do not put weight on it.
- Allow your spine to sidebend but keep it well balanced on your pelvis.
- Repeat the stretch several times, each time with an exhalation.
- Repeat the technique for the left hip.

182

6.4c Passive stretch for tensor fasciae latae standing

Starting position

- Stand straight with your feet together and the right side of your body opposite to and at arms length away from a wall or post.
- Abduct your right arm until it is level with your shoulder and place the palm of your hand on the wall.
- Extend your right hip and then adduct your hip and place your right foot on the floor behind and to the side of your left foot.
- Place your left hand on the left side of your pelvis.
- Sideshift your pelvis to the right and towards the wall.
- Make sure both of your knees remain straight and your spine is straight.
- Keep your pelvis in line with the frontal plane of your body.

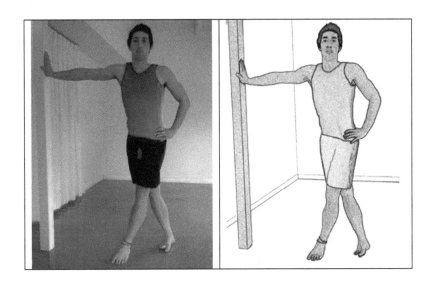

Technique

- Take a deep breath in.
- Exhale and move your pelvis right and towards the wall.
- Feel the stretch in your right hip and down the side of your thigh.
- Sideshifting your pelvis to the right produces sidebending to the left.
- Keep your spine, right arm and both knees straight.
- Repeat the stretch several times, each time with an exhalation.
- Repeat the technique for the left hip.

6.4d Passive or post-isometric hip abductor stretch supine

Starting position

- Lie on your back on a mat or carpet.
- Flex your left hip and knee and lift your left foot off the ground.
- Adduct your right leg to the left until you feel the initial stages of resistance from the muscles and fascia of the lateral thigh then place it on the mat.
- Place your left foot down on the mat against the outside of your right knee.
- This pins down the right leg in an adducted position.
- Flex your right hip and knee until the top of your right thigh presses against the bottom of the calf muscle of your left leg.

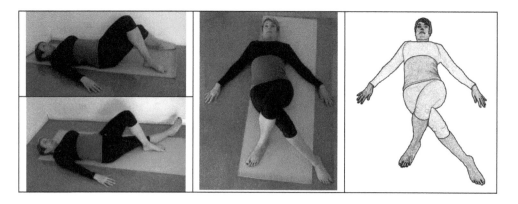

Technique

- Take a deep breath and hold it in.
- Push the outside of your right knee against the inside of your left leg by contracting your right hip abductor muscles, but resist the movement with an equal and opposite counter contraction from your left hip muscles.
- Keep your left foot fixed on the mat and a firm stance of your body.

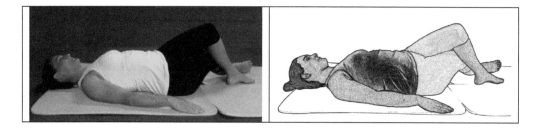

- After about five seconds cease the isometric contraction, exhale, and push your right thigh and knee to the left with your left leg.
- Reposition your right foot further to the left and then move your left foot to the left and pin down your right leg in a more adducted position.
- Repeat the manoeuvre several times, each time with an exhalation.
- This isometric stretch with the right knee flexed can be done as a passive stretch and with the right knee straight or the two may be combined.
- Repeat the stretch on the left side.

6.4e Passive stretch for quadratus lumborum, tensor fasciae latae and gluteus maximus sidelying on a table

Starting position

- Lie on your left side on a table or couch with a small pillow for your head.
- Move your shoulders forward and your pelvis backward so that you are lying diagonally across the table.
- Flex your left hip 90 degrees and flex your left knee 90 degrees.
- Move your right lower limb backwards and drop your right foot and leg over the side of the table and lower them towards the floor.
- Rest the inside of your right knee on the edge of the table or if the table is too hard on a small pillow on the table on the soft part of your left foot.
- One useful option is to grasp the end of the table with your right hand to stretch latissimus dorsi and use the tension to stabilise the pelvis and avoid unwanted lumbar sidebending.

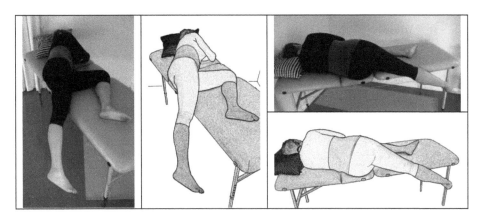

Technique

- Take a deep breath in.
- Exhale, drop your right knee off the edge of the table and lower your leg towards the floor.
- Feel the stretch down the right side of your body, especially down the outside of your right thigh.
- Keep your right knee straight.
- If you turn your leg so your toes point towards the floor you internally rotate your hip joint and this focuses the stretch on gluteus maximus.
- If you turn your leg so your toes point towards the ceiling you externally rotate your hip joint and this focuses the stretch on tensor fasciae latae.
- Repeat the stretch several times, each time with an exhalation.
- Repeat the stretch on the left side.

6.4f Post-isometric stretch for quadratus lumborum, tensor fasciae latae and gluteus maximus sidelying on a table

Starting position

- Lie on your left side on a table or couch with a small pillow for your head and adopt the starting position of the unilateral passive stretch sidelying.
- Hook your right foot under the table or hook your knee under your left foot.

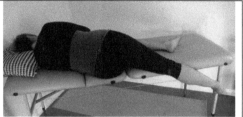

Technique

- Take a deep breath and hold it in.
- Push your right leg upwards against the table or the outside of your left foot.
- Use the underside of the table or the fixed position of your left foot to resist the contraction of your right hip abductor muscles.
- Maintain the isometric muscle contraction for about five seconds.

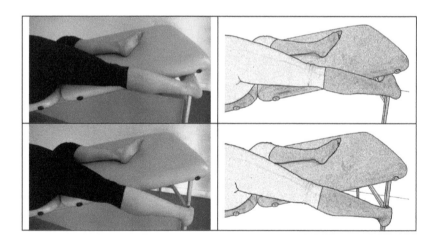

- Cease the contraction, exhale and then allow your right leg to drop further towards the floor and to a more adducted position.
- Repeat the manoeuvre several times, each time taking your leg further to the floor.
- Repeat the stretch on the left side.

6.4g Passive and post-isometric stretch for tensor fasciae latae and gluteus maximus sidelying with the knee straight

Starting position

- Lie on your right side with your legs straight and arms in front.
- Place your palms flat on the floor shoulder width apart.
- Push your hands into the floor and raise your upper body off the floor.
- Your shoulders are horizontal and level
- Your head, cervical and upper thoracic spine are vertical.
- Most of the sidebending is in your hips but with some in the lumbar spine.

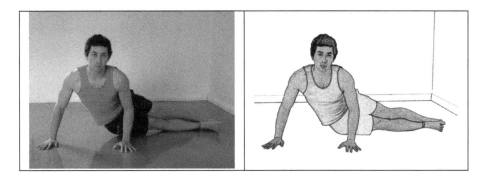

Technique

- Take a deep breath in.
- Exhale, push into the floor with both hands, extend your elbows and raise your shoulders higher off the floor.
- Feel the stretch down the right side of your hip and down your thigh.
- Repeat the passive stretch several times, raising your body further off the floor with each exhalation.
- Maintain the position.
- Take another deep breath and hold it in.
- Attempt to lift your pelvis off the floor and straighten your body at the hips.
- Do not allow your pelvis to actually come off the floor - only use enough muscle effort for an isometric contraction.
- After about five seconds cease the contraction, relax your hip muscles, exhale and raise your upper body further off the floor.
- To localise the stretch on tensor fasciae latae your hips should be in extension, and your knees between extension and 30 degrees flexion.
- Keep your pelvis and thighs vertical and in one plane.
- Repeat the post-isometric stretch several times.
- Repeat the stretch on the left side.

6.4h Passive and post-isometric stretch for gluteus medius and gluteus minimus sidelying with the knee bent

Starting position

- Lie on your right side with your legs flexed and arms in front.
- Place your palms flat on the floor shoulder width apart.
- Push your hands into the floor and raise your upper body off the floor.
- Your shoulders are horizontal and level.
- Your head, cervical and upper thoracic spine are vertical.
- Most of the sidebending is in your hips but with some in the lumbar spine.

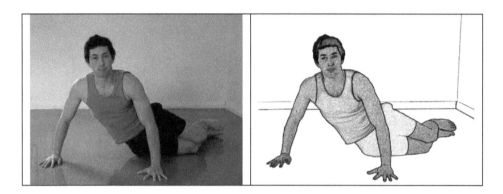

Technique

- Take a deep breath in.
- Exhale, push into the floor with both hands, extend your elbows and raise your shoulders higher off the floor.
- Feel the stretch in your right hip.
- Repeat the passive stretch several times, raising your body further off the floor with each exhalation.
- Maintain the position.
- Take another deep breath and hold it in.
- Push your feet into the floor and attempt to lift your pelvis off the floor and straighten your body at the hips.
- Do not allow your pelvis to actually come off the floor - only use enough muscle effort for an isometric contraction.
- After about five seconds cease the contraction, relax your hip muscles, exhale and raise your upper body further off the floor with your hands.
- To localise the stretch on gluteus minimus keep your pelvis and legs vertical and in one plane.
- Keep your knees flexed.
- Repeat the post-isometric stretch several times.
- Repeat the stretch on the left side.

6.5 Hip adductor stretches - active, passive and post-isometric stretches for the hip adductors, extensors and internal rotators

6.5a Bilateral stretch for hip adductors & internal rotators sitting

Starting position

- Sit on the floor with your pelvis and back vertical and against a wall.
- Push your sit bones as far back along the floor and against the wall as possible.
- Flex your hips and knees as much as possible but do not allow your sit bones to come away from the wall.

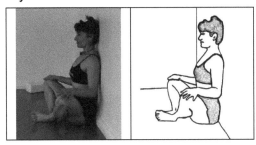

- Grasp your ankles and pull your feet as close as possible to your groins.
- Bring the soles of your feet together.
- Allow your knees to drop towards the floor.
- Place the palms of your hands on your knees.
- Keep your shoulders, spine and pelvis in contact with the wall.

Technique

- Take a deep breath then exhale and actively bring your knees to the floor.
- Repeat the active stretch several times.
- Take another deep breath in.
- Exhale and push your knees down towards the floor with your hands.
- Repeat the passive stretch several times.

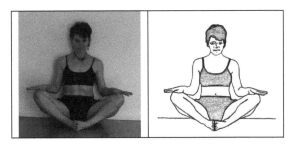

- Take another deep breath and hold it in.
- Push your knees toward the ceiling and apply an equal and opposite counterforce with your hands for about five seconds.
- Cease the isometric contraction, relax your hip muscles and then exhale and bring your knees further towards the floor.
- Repeat the post-isometric stretch several times.
- Feel the stretch down the inside of your thighs and into the groins.

6.5b Bilateral active stretch for the hip adductors, extensors and internal rotators sitting

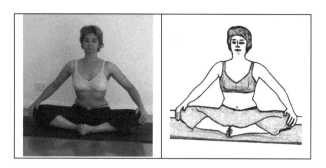

Starting position

- Only do this stretch if you can comfortably abduct your hips.
- See the starting position for stretch 6.5a for more details.
- Sit on the floor with your pelvis and back against a wall, knees flexed, hips abducted, heels to your groins and the soles of your feet together.

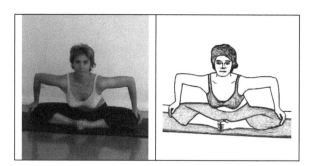

- Allow your knees to drop towards the floor.
- Place the palms of your hands on your knees.

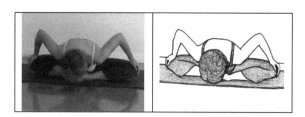

Technique

- Take a deep breath in.
- Exhale, lift your spine up and out of your pelvis and lengthen your spine.
- Take another deep breath in.

- Exhale and while maintaining the lift in your spine bend forwards.
- Flex in your hips, rather than in your spine.
- Keep your knees on the floor or as close to floor as is comfortable.
- Feel the stretch in the back, the inside of your thighs and into your groins.

6.5c Bilateral passive stretch for the hip adductors and extensors sitting

Starting position

- Sit on the floor with your pelvis and back vertical and against a wall.
- Push your sit bones back into the corner of the room.
- Grasp your knees and move your legs apart, but stop when you feel a stretch down the inside of one or both of your thighs.
- Keep your legs an equal distance apart and pelvis in contact with the wall.
- Walk your fingers across the floor and away from you until you feel a stretch in the groins and inside of your thighs.

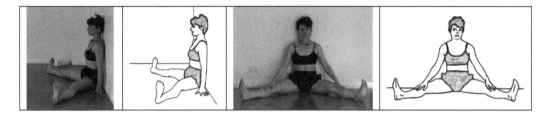

Technique

- Take a deep breath in.
- Exhale and walk your fingers across the floor and away from you.
- Feel a stretch down the inside of your thighs into your groins.
- Hold this position, and try and keep your lumbar spine extended.
- Take another deep breath, then exhale and perform the following actions:

  - Move your upper thoracic spine and shoulders forwards and parallel with the floor
  - Flex at the hips, tilt your pelvis forwards
  - Lift your spine up and out of your pelvis - feel it lengthening

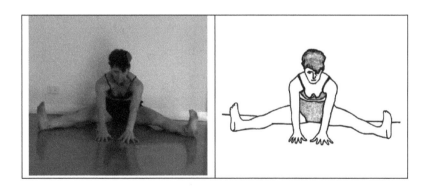

- Repeat the stretch several times, each time with an exhalation.
- After each stretch, reposition your hands and upper body and reposition your legs so they are further apart.
- Your lumbar may flex a little but aim to extend it or keep it straight by lifting out of the pelvis.

6.5d Bilateral post-isometric stretch for the hip adductors and extensors sitting

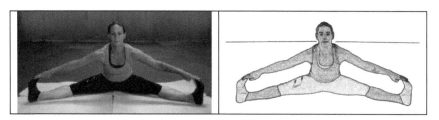

Starting position

- Sit on the floor, preferably on a mat, with your legs in front of your body.
- Grasp your knees and move your legs apart but stop when you feel a stretch down the inside of one or both of your thighs.
- Keep your legs an equal distance apart.

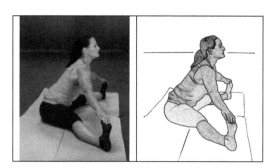

- Lean forwards and depending on your flexibility grasp the inside of your knees, legs, or toes.
- Flex at the hips - tilt your pelvis forwards.
- Maintain a firm hold of your knees, legs, or toes with both hands.
- Keep your arms straight and keep your spine and upper limbs firm.

Technique

- Take a deep breath and hold it in, and perform the following actions:

  o Push your legs inwards towards each other
  o Push your arms outwards against the inside of your knees, legs or feet
  o Push your arms down into the floor

- Resist all movement with an equal and opposite counterforce.
- After about five seconds cease the isometric contraction, relax your muscles, then exhale and bring your body to a new position

  o Flex your pelvis on the hip joints
  o Take your upper thoracic and shoulders forward and along the floor
  o Extend your lumbar spine
  o Abduct your hips so your legs are further apart.

- Repeat the stretch and each time reposition your hands and upper body.

192

6.5e Bilateral active and passive stretch for the hip adductors supine and with legs against a wall

Starting position

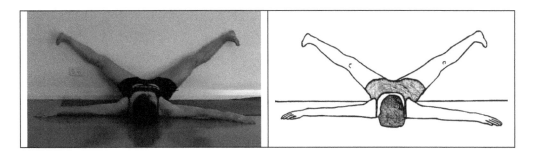

- Sit on the floor facing a wall and with your hips and knees flexed.
- Move as close as possible to the wall and place the bottom of your pelvis hard up against the wall.
- You may need to wriggle your body along the floor.
- Lean backwards and lay your head, spine, pelvis and arms on the floor.
- Straighten your knees and place the back of your legs against the wall.

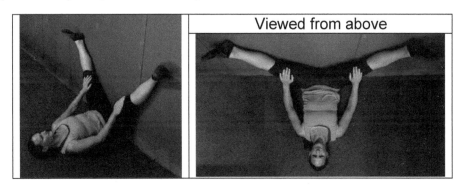

- Move your legs apart but stop when you feel the initial stages of a stretch down the inside of one or both of your thighs or groins.
- Keep your legs an equal distance apart and your pelvis in contact with the wall.
- Keep the back of your head, shoulders, spine and pelvis on the floor.
- A pillow may be placed under your head.

Viewed from above

Technique

- Take a deep breath in.
- Exhale and bring your legs apart, along the wall and towards the floor.
- Take another deep breath in.
- Exhale and now externally rotate your hips and take your toes down towards the floor.
- Internally rotate your hips, then lift your legs off the wall and place them back on the wall in a more abducted position.
- Repeat the stretch several times each time with an exhalation and then after each stretch move your legs further apart and along the wall.

6.5f Bilateral stretch for the hip adductors and internal rotators supine and with knees flexed and heels against a wall

Starting position

- Sit on the floor facing a wall and with your hips and knees flexed.
- Move as close as possible to the wall and place the bottom of your pelvis hard up against the wall.
- You may need to wriggle your body along the floor.
- Lean backwards and lay your head, spine, pelvis and arms on the floor.
- Move your legs apart.
- Flex your hips and flex your knees so only your heels are in contact with the wall and they become a pivot for hip movement.
- Move your knees apart and towards the wall and the floor.
- A pillow may be placed under your head for greater comfort.

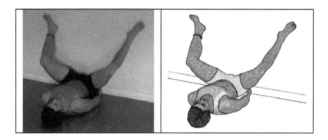

Technique

- Take a deep breath in.
- Exhale, contract your hip muscles and move your knees further apart.
- Rotate your hips outwards, pivoting around your heels.
- Reposition your heels further apart and along the wall.
- Repeat the active stretch several times with an exhalation.
- Place your hands on your thighs and take another deep breath in.
- Exhale, relax your hips and push your knees further apart.
- Repeat the passive stretch several times with an exhalation.

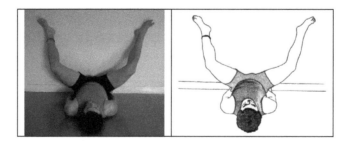

- Take a deep breath in and hold it.
- Attempt to push your knees together and away from the wall, against an unyielding resistance offered by your hands pushing against your thighs.
- After about five seconds cease the muscle contraction, relax your hips, exhale and allow your knees to drop towards the wall.
- Repeat the post-isometric stretch several times.
- Feel a stretch down the inside of your thighs and into your groins.

6.5g Bilateral stretch for the hip adductors and internal rotators supine with knees flexed and feet against a wall

Starting position

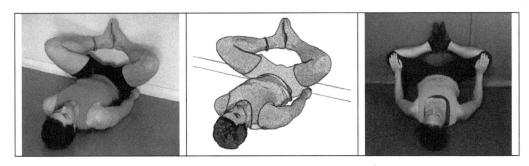

- Sit on the floor facing a wall and with your hips and knees flexed.
- Move as close as possible to the wall and place the bottom of your pelvis hard up against the wall.
- You may need to wriggle your body along the floor.
- Lean backwards and lay your head, spine, pelvis and arms on the floor.
- Flex your knees and bring your heels towards your groins.
- Bring the soles of your feet together so the outsides of your feet rest against the wall and allow your knees to move towards the wall.
- A pillow may be placed under your head for greater comfort.

Technique

- Take a deep breath in.
- Exhale, contract your hip muscles and move your knees towards the wall.
- Repeat the active stretch several times with an exhalation.
- Place your hands on your thighs and take another deep breath in.
- Exhale, relax your hips and push your knees towards the wall.
- Repeat the passive stretch several times with an exhalation.

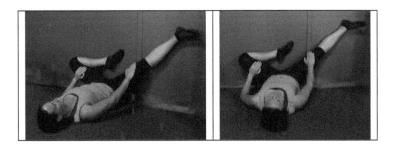

- Take a deep breath in and hold it.
- Attempt to push your knees away from the wall and against an unyielding resistance offered by your hands pushing against your thighs.
- After about five seconds cease the muscle contraction, relax your hips, exhale and allow your knees to drop towards the wall.
- Repeat the post-isometric stretch several times.
- Feel a stretch down the inside of your thighs and into your groins.
- This technique can be combined with either of the previous two stretches.

6.5h Bilateral stretch for the hip adductors standing

Starting position

- Stand facing a chair or low table with your feet wide apart.
- Bend forwards and place the palms of your hands on the chair.

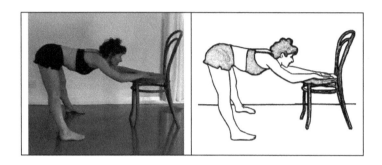

- Continue flexing your body at the hips until you feel the initial stages of a stretch down the inside your thighs.
- Discard the chair if you can easily touch the floor with both hands with your knees straight and spine in a neutral position.

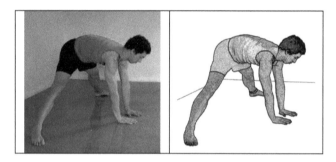

Technique

- Take a deep breath in.
- Exhale and drop the top of your pelvis towards the floor and lift your coccyx and the bottom of your pelvis up towards the ceiling.
- At the same time arch your spine and lift your head.

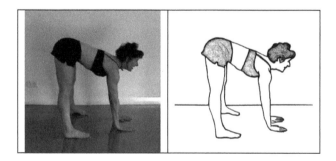

- Feel a stretch down the inside of your thigh and into your groins.
- Move your feet further apart and repeat the stretch with each exhalation.
- If you wear a pair of socks you can slide your feet apart on wooden floor.

6.5i Unilateral passive stretch for the hip adductors standing

Starting position

- Stand with your feet wide apart.
- Flex your left hip and knee but keep your right leg straight.
- Bend forwards and place the palms of your hands on the floor.
- If you are unable to reach the floor then grasp the edge of a table.
- Continue flexing your left hip and knee until you feel the initial stages of a stretch in your groin or down the inside your right thigh.
- Your spine should remain in a neutral position.

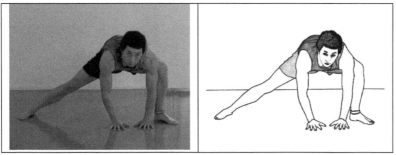

Technique

- Take a deep breath in.
- Exhale, move your left hip and knee in to a more flexed position and drop your pelvis towards the floor.
- Raise your head and try and extend your spine into an arched position.

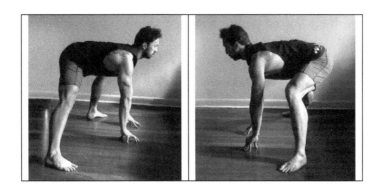

- Feel an increased stretch into your right groin and down the inside of your right thigh.
- Repeat the stretch several times, each time with an exhalation.
- Repeat the stretch on the other side.

6.5j Bilateral stretch for the hip adductors and internal rotators supine

Starting position

- Lie on your back on a carpet or mat on the floor.
- Flex your hips and knees so your feet are on the floor near your groins.
- Drop your knees out to the side and bring the soles of your feet together.
- Feel the initial stages of a stretch down the inside of your thighs.
- Keep your spine straight and body relaxed.
- Place pillows under your thighs if your hips are very stiff or if there is pain.
- A pillow may be placed under your head for greater comfort.

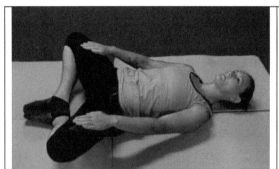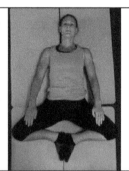

Technique

- Take a deep breath in.
- Exhale and allow your knees to drop towards the floor.
- Take another deep breath in.
- Exhale and pull your knees and thighs towards the floor by contracting your hip muscles.
- Feel a stretch down the inside of your thighs and into your groins.
- Repeat the active stretch several times, each time with an exhalation.
- Place your hands on your thighs and take another deep breath in.
- Exhale, relax your hips and push your knees to the floor with both hands.
- Repeat the passive stretch several times with an exhalation.

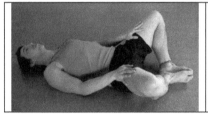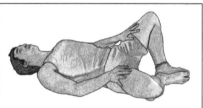

- Take a deep breath in and hold it.
- Attempt to push your thighs upwards against an unyielding resistance offered by your hands pressing down against your thighs.
- After about five seconds cease the muscle contraction, relax your hips, exhale and allow your knees to drop towards the floor.
- Repeat the post-isometric stretch several times.

6.5k Bilateral stretch for the hip adductors kneeling with knees flexed and hips externally rotated

Starting position

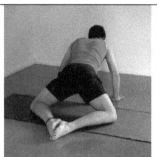

- Kneel on a mat on the floor and place your hands palms down on the floor just in front of your body, about shoulder distance apart.
- Two mats may be used which slide across the floor during the stretch.
- Your arms should be straight and vertical.
- Move your knees apart and then move your feet apart.
- Your spine should be straight and in a neutral position.

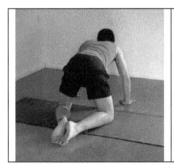

Technique

- Take a deep breath in.
- Exhale and move your pelvis backwards towards your feet.
- Reposition your body by first moving your knees apart and then moving your feet apart.
- With your knees apart and feet together there is more hip external rotation.
- With your feet more apart than your knees there is more internal rotation.
- Flex your elbows more as your hips drop further to the floor.

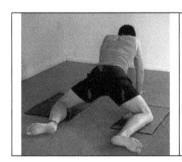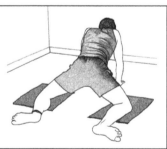

- Repeat the active stretch several times with a zig-zag action of the leg.
- Take another deep breath and hold it in.
- Push your knees down and into the floor.
- The floor acts as an unyielding resistance as you push against it.
- After about five seconds cease the isometric muscle contraction, relax, exhale and then move your knees further apart and move your feet apart.
- Repeat the post-isometric stretch several times.
- Keep your spine in neutral, and your shoulders and arms firm.
- Feel a stretch down the inside of your thighs and into your groins.

6.5l Bilateral stretch for the hip adductors kneeling with hips extended and knees flexed

Starting position

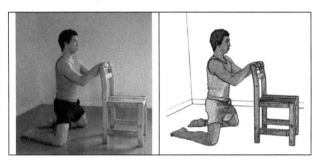

- Kneel on a mat on the floor and grasp the back of a chair.
- Place your arms at your sides extended with your elbows partly flexed.
- Move your knees apart and then move your feet apart.
- Your toes should be pointing backwards.
- Your spine should be straight, vertical and in a neutral position.

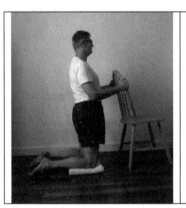

Technique

- Take a deep breath in.
- Exhale and move your knees apart and then move your feet apart.
- With the knees more apart than the feet there is more hip external rotation.
- With the feet more apart than the knees there is more internal rotation.
- Allow your elbows to flex as your body drops further to the floor.
- Keep your spine straight, vertical and in neutral.
- Repeat the active stretch several times with a zig-zag action of the leg.

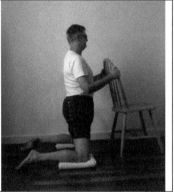

- Take a deep breath and hold it in.
- Push your knees together and downwards into the floor.
- The floor acts as an unyielding resistance as you push against it.
- After about five seconds cease the isometric muscle contraction, relax, exhale and then move your knees further apart and move your feet apart.
- Repeat the post-isometric stretch several times.
- Keep your spine, shoulders and arms firm.
- Feel a stretch down the inside of your thighs and into your groins.

6.5m Bilateral stretch for the hip adductors standing with hips and knees extended

Starting position

- Stand facing the back of a chair or low table with your feet wide apart.
- Grasp the back of the chair.
- Your arms should be extended at your sides and your elbows partly flexed.
- Move your feet further apart but keep your toes pointing forward.
- If your feet do not slide on the floor easily then wear a pair of socks.
- Your spine should be straight, vertical and in a neutral position.

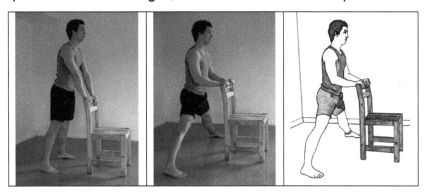

Technique

- Take a deep breath in.
- Exhale and move your feet further apart.
- Allow your elbows to flex as your body drops to the floor.
- Feel a stretch down the inside of your thighs and into your groins.
- Repeat the active stretch several times.

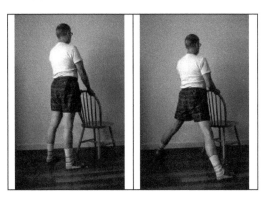

- Take a deep breath and hold it in.
- Pull your feet together, downwards and into the floor.
- The floor acts as an unyielding resistance to your muscle contraction.
- After about five seconds cease the isometric muscle contraction, relax, exhale and then move your feet further apart.
- Repeat the post-isometric stretch several times.
- Keep your spine straight, vertical and in a neutral position, and keep your spine, shoulders and arms firm.
- Feel a stretch down the inside of your thighs and into your groins.

6.5n Unilateral stretch for the hip adductors sidelying with your back against a wall and your hips and knees extended

Starting position

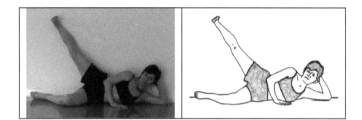

- Lay on your left side with your back against a wall.
- Flex your left hip and knee and find a comfortable stable sidelying position.
- Flex your left elbow and shoulder, and support your head with your hand.
- Flex your right elbow and shoulder, and place your palm flat on the floor.
- Lift your right leg as high up the wall as possible and fix it on the wall.

Technique

- Take a deep breath in.
- Exhale, turn your right leg outwards and lift it further up the wall.
- Lead with your toes and move your foot towards your head.
- After a five second muscle contraction move your heel away from the wall, turn your foot inwards and fix your leg further up the wall.
- Feel a stretch down the inside of your thighs and into your groins.
- Repeat the active stretch several times.

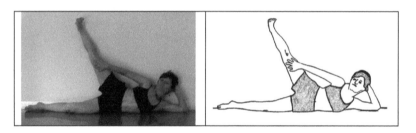

- Grasp your right knee, leg or foot depending on your flexibility.
- Do not allow your pelvis, back or shoulders to come away from the wall.
- Take another deep breath in.
- Exhale and pull your leg upwards and towards your head with your hand.
- Reposition your heel further up and along the wall.
- Repeat the passive stretch several times.
- Take a deep breath and hold it in.
- Push your right leg downwards, along the wall and towards the floor.
- Resist the push with your right hand.
- After about five seconds cease the isometric muscle contraction, relax, exhale and then move your foot further along the wall.
- Repeat the post-isometric stretch several times.

6.6 Quadriceps stretch - active and passive stretches for the quadriceps, tibialis anterior and the toe extensor muscles

6.6a Quadriceps stretch standing

Starting position

- Stand beside a chair or wall with your left side near to the chair.
- Grasp the back of the chair with your left hand.
- Flex your right hip and knee.
- Grasp the front of your right ankle with your right hand.
- Move your right knee and thigh backwards but keep your knee flexed.
- Hold your foot, and keep your spine and left leg straight and vertical.

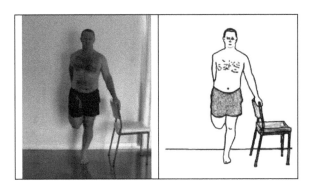

Technique

- Take a deep breath in.
- Exhale and move your right knee backwards while pulling the heel of your right foot into your buttock with your right hand.

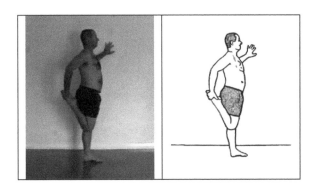

- As you move your right knee backward do not allow your body to go forwards - keep your pelvis and spine vertical.
- With each exhalation continue bringing your knee further backwards.
- Repeat the stretch on the left side.

6.6b Passive knee, ankle and toe stretch standing

Starting position

- Stand near a wall or fixed solid object with your left side near to the wall.
- Grasp the wall or object (i.e. a chair or post) with your left hand.
- Flex your right hip and knee.
- Grasp the front of your right foot and toes with your right hand.
- Move your right knee and thigh backwards but keep your right knee flexed.
- Hold your foot, and keep your spine and left leg straight and vertical.

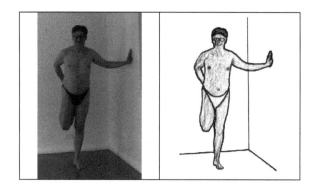

Technique

- Take a deep breath in.
- Exhale and push the palm of your right hand against the top of your foot and pull back on your toes with the fingers of your right hand.
- Bring your toes and the end of your foot closer towards your body.
- Plantarflex your foot, flex your toes and try to increase your longitudinal arches.
- Feel a stretch in the front of your leg and ankle and down your foot.
- Grasp around the top of your foot.

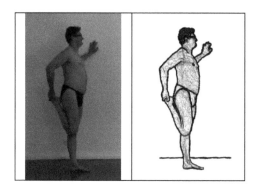

- Take another deep breath in.
- Exhale and squeeze your right foot with your right hand.
- Curl the sides of your foot and increase the transverse metatarsal arch.
- Feel a stretch on the top of your foot between the metatarsal bones.
- Keep your knees together, and your pelvis and spine vertical.
- Repeat each stretch several times with an exhalation.
- Repeat the stretch on the left side.

6.6c Post-isometric knee, ankle and toe stretch standing

Starting position

- Stand near a wall or fixed solid object with your left side near to the wall.
- Grasp the wall or object (i.e. a chair or post) with your left hand.
- Flex your right hip and knee.
- Grasp the front of your right ankle with your right hand.

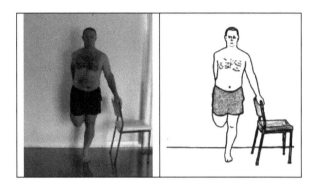

- Move your right knee backwards but keep your knee in full flexion.
- Hold your foot and keep your spine and left leg straight and vertical.

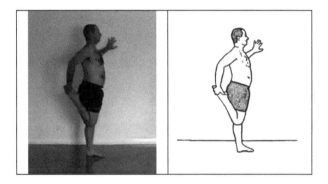

Technique

- Take in a deep breath and hold it in.
- Attempt to move your foot backwards and away from your body.
- Resist the movement with an equal and opposite counterforce of your right hand.
- After about five seconds cease the isometric contraction, relax, exhale and move your body to a new stretch position.
- Either move your right knee backwards or push the heel of your right foot forwards and into your buttock with your right hand.
- As you move your right knee backwards do not allow your body to go forwards - keep your pelvis and spine vertical.
- Repeat the stretch several times with an exhalation.
- Repeat the stretch on the left side.

6.6d Quadriceps stretch semi-supine

Starting position

- Sit on a mat with your legs straight and in front of you.
- Flex your right hip and knee.
- Grasp your right ankle with your right hand, lean to the left and take your foot under your thigh and place it to the side of your right hip and pelvis.
- You are now in a half kneeling position.

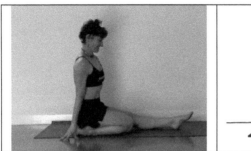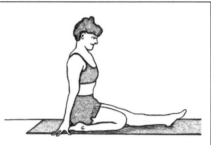

- Extend your shoulders and flex your elbows.
- Lean backwards and support your upper body on your bent elbows.
- Your right knee is now in full flexion.
- Your right foot remains beside your hip and your sole faces upwards.
- Keep your spine and left leg straight.

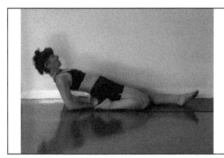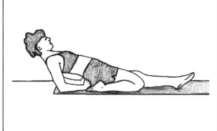

Technique

- Take in a deep breath and hold it in.
- Exhale and slide your elbows towards your feet.
- As you lean backwards, lower your spine towards the floor.
- Feel a stretch in front of your right thigh and in front of your ankle.
- Do not extend your back - keep your spine straight.
- With each exhalation bring your spine nearer to the floor.
- Repeat the stretch on the left side.

6.6e Passive and post-isometric quadriceps stretch prone

Starting position

- Lie on your front on the floor with your legs straight.
- Flex your right knee and bring your foot towards your buttocks.
- Lean backwards and grasp your right foot behind your ankle with your right hand or both hands.
- Pull your right foot nearer to your buttocks.
- Your left knee is in extension and your right knee is in full flexion.
- Lift your head off the floor but keep the rest of your spine straight.

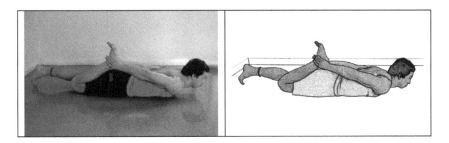

Technique

- Take a deep breath in.
- Exhale and pull the heel of your right foot into your right buttock or down the side of your buttock towards the floor.
- Feel a stretch in the front of your right thigh and knee.

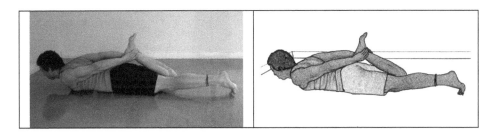

- Take in another deep breath and hold it in.
- Attempt to push your right foot backwards and away from your body.
- Resist the movement with an equal and opposite counterforce from your right hand.
- After about five seconds cease the isometric contraction, relax, exhale and move the heel of your right foot into your buttock with your right hand.
- You can extend your cervical and upper thoracic spine but do not arch your lower back - keep your lumbar and thoracic spine straight.
- With each exhalation bring your foot nearer to your buttock and the floor.
- Repeat the stretch on the left side.

6.6f Quadriceps stretch sidelying

Starting position

- Lay on your left side on the floor, using a mat for greater comfort.
- Flex your right hip and knee and grasp your right ankle or foot with your right hand.
- Extend your right hip but keep your knee flexed.

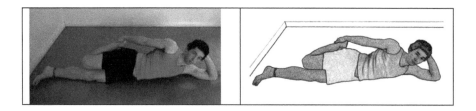

- Flex your left shoulder and elbow, and rest the left side of your head in the palm of your left hand.
- Straighten your spine and left leg.
- Pull your right foot towards your body and into your right buttock.

Technique

- Take a deep breath in.
- Exhale, move your right knee backwards and pull the heel of your right foot into your buttock with your right hand.
- Feel a stretch in the front of your right thigh and knee.

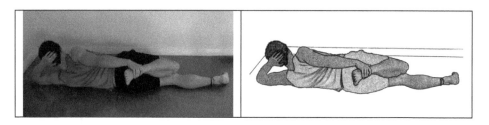

- Take in another deep breath and hold it in.
- Attempt to push your right foot backwards and away from your body.
- Resist the movement with an equal and opposite counterforce from your right hand.
- After about five seconds cease the isometric contraction, relax, exhale and move your right knee and heel to a new stretch position
- As you move your right knee backwards do not allow your spine to arch backwards - keep your pelvis and spine straight.
- Repeat the stretch several times with each exhalation.
- Repeat the stretch on the left side.

6.7 Hamstring stretches - active, passive and post-isometric stretches for semitendinosus, semimembranosus and biceps femoris

6.7a Easy passive and active stretch for the hamstrings standing

Starting position

- Stand on the floor facing a table or window ledge.
- Flex your right hip and put the heel of your right foot on the window ledge.
- Straighten your right leg at the knee.
- If you can maintain good balance hold the side of your hips, alternatively use the back of a chair for support.
- The table or window ledge should be high enough so that it provides a challenging stretch for the hamstrings.

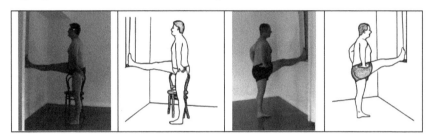

Technique

- Take a deep breath in.
- Exhale and straighten your spine and both legs.
- Feel the stretch down the back of your right thigh and knee.
- Place a book under the heel of your right foot, thereby raising it slightly.

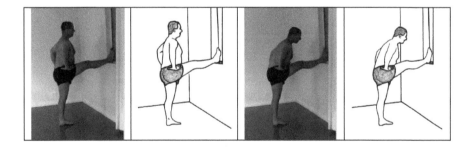

- Take another deep breath in, then exhale and repeat the stretch.
- Take another deep breath in.
- Exhale and bend forwards at the hips - tilt your pelvis forwards.
- Aim to lift your spine up and out of your pelvis, and to lengthen your spine.
- Keep your knees and spine straight.
- Feel the stretch down the back of your right thigh and behind your knee.
- Repeat the stretch with progressively higher foot positions.
- Repeat the stretch on the left side.

6.7b Combined active and passive stretch for the hamstrings standing

Starting position

- Stand with the heel of your right foot on a table or window ledge.
- Place the heel of your right foot on the window ledge with your leg straight.
- Hold the back of a chair with your left hand for support.

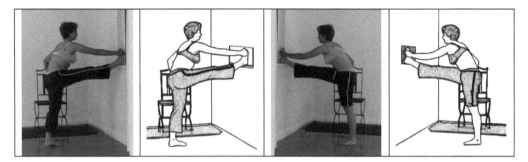

- Reach forward and grasp a point down your right leg with your right hand.
- Grasp your foot or toes if you have above average hamstring flexibility.
- Grasp your knee or ankle if you have below average hamstring flexibility.
- Keep your right arm in a fixed position.
- Depending on your flexibility it can either be straight or flexed at the elbow.
- Keep your spine and both legs straight throughout the stretch.

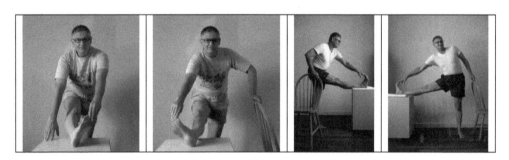

Technique

- Take a deep breath in.
- Exhale and while keeping the spine straight do the following passive and active stretches:

  - contract your shoulder and arm muscles and pull your trunk forwards
  - bend forwards at the hips and tilt the pelvis forwards.

- Combine these actions with any of the following options: rotate your right hip inwards; rotate your right hip outwards; rotate the left side of your pelvis outwards; point your right heel away and bring your toes towards you; grasp your right foot with your left hand and use a diagonal hold.
- Adjust your hand grip and body position after each stretch.
- Repeat the stretch several times, each time with an exhalation.
- Repeat the technique on the left side.

6.7c Passive stretch for the hamstrings supine

Starting position

- Lie on your back on a carpet or mat on the floor.
- Flex your hips and knees, and place your feet on the mat.

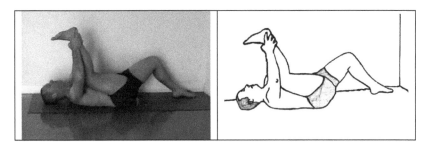

- Flex your right hip, lift your foot off the mat and move it towards your head.
- Flex your head and upper spine, and grasp your right foot behind your ankle with both hands.
- If you cannot reach your foot, flex your left hip and knee more.
- Pull your right foot up and over your head but stop when you feel the initial stages of tension in the back of your thigh or behind your knee.

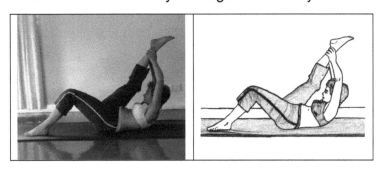

Technique

- Take a deep breath in.
- Exhale and pull your right foot up and over your head.
- Feel the stretch in the back of your right thigh or behind your right knee.
- Repeat this action several times, each time with an exhalation.
- Take another deep breath in.
- Exhale and slide your left foot along the mat and away from you, by extending your left hip and knee.
- Resist any movement of your right leg with a firm hold on your right ankle with both hands.
- Allow your pelvis to move back towards the floor, but do not allow your right thigh to move.
- Feel the stretch in your back of your right thigh or behind your right knee.
- Repeat this action several times, each time with an exhalation.
- Repeat the stretch on the left side.

6.7d Post-isometric stretch for the hamstrings supine

Starting position

- Lie on your back on a carpet or mat.
- Flex both hips and knees, and place your feet on the mat.

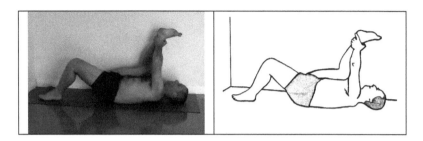

- Flex your right hip, lift your foot off the mat and move it towards your head.
- Flex your head and upper spine, and grasp your right foot behind your ankle with both hands.
- If you cannot reach your foot, flex your left hip and knee more.
- Pull your right foot up and over your head, but stop when you feel the initial stages of tension in the back of your thigh or behind your knee.

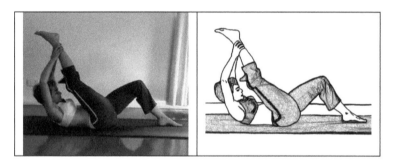

Technique

- Take a deep breath and hold it in.
- Attempt to push your right foot away from your head, and parallel with the mat by contracting the muscles that flex your knee and extend your hip.
- Resist the movement with an equal and opposite counterforce from your hands.
- After about five seconds cease the contraction, exhale and pull your right foot further up and over your head.
- Move to a new stretch position.
- Feel the stretch in your back of your right thigh.
- During the muscle contraction keep a firm hold on your ankle with both hands and hold your body in an almost rigid position.
- Repeat the post-isometric stretch several times.
- Repeat the stretch on the left side.

6.7e Active and post-isometric stretch for the hamstrings supine with one leg vertical and against a post

Starting position

- Lie on your back on a carpet or mat
- Position the inside your left thigh beside a vertical post or the outside corner of a wall.
- Flex your right hip and place the back of your heel against the post.
- Your right hip is flexed and your left hip is extended.
- Straighten your left leg and feel the initial stages of tension in the back of your right thigh or behind your right knee.

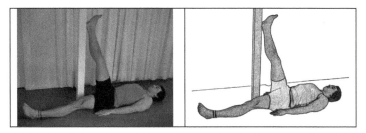

Technique

- Take a deep breath in.
- Exhale, push the back of your right knee towards the post and attempt to straighten your leg by contracting your quadriceps muscles.
- Repeat the active stretch and exhalation several times, each time bringing the back of your knee further towards the post.
- When your right knee is fully extended, slide your body along the mat and move your right ischial tuberosity nearer to the post.
- Allow your right knee to flex.
- Repeat the active stretch extending your right knee with each exhalation.

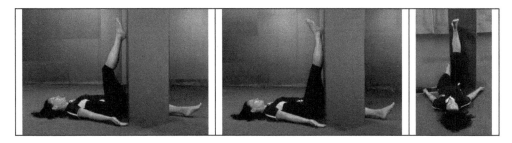

- Take another deep breath and hold it in.
- Attempt to push your right heel downwards and into the post by contracting the muscles that flex your right knee and extend your right hip.
- The post will act as an unyielding resistance against your movement.
- After about five seconds cease the contraction, exhale and move the back of your right knee further towards the post.
- Feel the stretch in the back of your right thigh and behind your right knee.
- Repeat the post-isometric stretch several times.
- Repeat the stretch on the left side.

6.7f Passive and post-isometric stretch for the hamstrings standing with hips flexed

Starting position

- Stand with your feet apart and facing a chair, blocks or empty floor.
- Use a chair if your hamstrings are short, blocks if they are moderately flexible, or the floor if they are very flexible.
- With increasing flexibility, progress from the chair to blocks to floor, and from fingertips to palms.
- Bend forwards at the hips and place your hands on a chair, blocks or floor.
- Flex your left hip and knee, then adduct your hip, then extend it and place the toes and balls of your left foot on the floor outside and behind your right foot so your left thigh and leg wrap around your right thigh and leg.

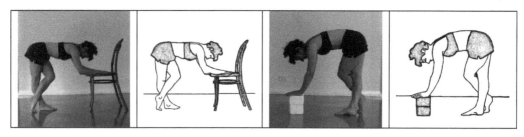

- Move your left foot backwards, sliding your toes along the floor until your left calf presses against the front of your right leg.
- Flex your elbows and lower your body towards the floor - bend at the hips.
- Stop when you feel the start of a stretch behind your thigh and knee.

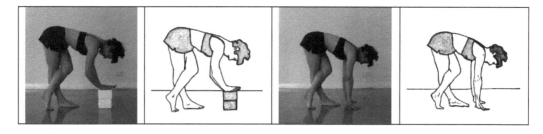

Technique

- Take a deep breath in.
- Exhale, flex your elbows and lower your body further towards the floor.
- Bend forwards at the hips, keeping your spine as straight as possible.
- Keep your right leg straight by pressing your left leg backwards against it.
- Take another deep breath and hold it in.
- Push your right knee forwards into the back of your left leg but resist the contraction with an equal and opposite pressure with your left leg.
- After five seconds cease the contraction, relax your muscles, exhale, and then flex your elbows and lower your body further towards the floor.
- Bend forwards at the hips and keep your spine straight.
- Feel the stretch in the back of your thigh or behind your knee.
- Repeat the passive or post-isometric stretch, each time with an exhalation.
- Repeat the stretch on the left side.

6.7g Active and passive stretch for the short head of biceps femoris standing with legs vertical

Starting position

- Adopt the starting position in technique 6.7f.
- In this technique there is no need to bend forwards at the hips because hip flexion does not influence the short head of biceps femoris which only passes over the knee joint. So the chair is only used for support.
- Internally rotate your right hip and place your right foot on the floor turned inwards about 45 degrees.

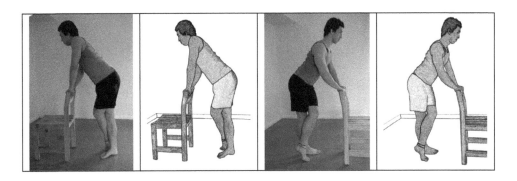

- Push your left knee backwards against your right leg and extend your right knee by contracting your quadriceps.
- Keep most of your weight on the right leg, but do not let your left foot slide on the floor.

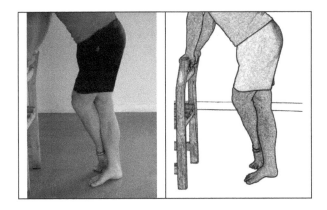

Technique

- Take a deep breath in.
- Exhale, pull up your right knee cap by contracting your quadriceps while simultaneously pushing back against your right knee with your left knee.
- You are trying to increase extension in your already extended right knee.
- This is an active stretch combined with a passive stretch.
- The active part of this stretch involves contracting the quadriceps in your right thigh to try to further straighten your already straight right leg.
- The passive part of this stretch involves contracting the quadriceps in your left thigh to push the back of your left knee against your right knee.
- Repeat the stretch several times with an exhalation then do the other leg.

6.8 Popliteus stretch - active, passive, and post-isometric stretches for popliteus

6.8a Active and passive stretch for the popliteus standing

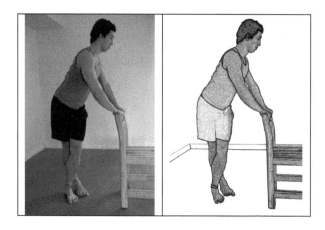

Starting position

- Stand with your feet apart facing a table or the back of a chair.
- Externally rotate your right hip and place your right foot on the floor pointing outwards about 45 degrees.
- Grasp the back of the chair with both hands and use it for support.
- Flex your left hip and knee and then adduct and externally rotate your left hip and take your left foot in front on your right leg.
- Extend your adducted hip and place the toes and balls of your left foot on the floor outside and just behind your right foot.
- Your left thigh and leg wraps around your right thigh and leg.
- Move your left foot backwards, sliding your toes along the floor until your left calf presses against the front of your right leg.
- Stop when your feel the initial stages of a stretch behind your right knee.
- Try to extend both knees.
- Your left knee is partially flexed but pressing back on your right leg and your right knee is straight.
- Keep most of your weight on the right leg but do not let your left foot move.

Technique

- Take a deep breath in.
- Exhale, pull up your right knee cap by contracting your right quadriceps and simultaneously push your left knee back against your right leg by contracting your left quadriceps, thus increasing extension in both knees.
- This is an active stretch of the right knee combined with a passive stretch from your left knee pushing on your right leg - both involve the quadriceps.
- Repeat the stretch several times with an exhalation
- Repeat the stretch for the other leg.

216

6.8b Post-isometric stretch for the popliteus standing

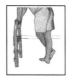

Starting position

- Stand with your feet apart facing a table or the back of a chair.
- Externally rotate your right hip and place your right foot on the floor pointing outwards about 45 degrees.
- Grasp the back of the chair with both hands and use it for support.
- Flex your left hip and knee and then adduct and externally rotate your left hip and take your left foot in front on your right leg.
- Extend your adducted hip and place the toes and balls of your left foot on the floor outside and just behind your right foot.
- Your left thigh and leg wraps around your right thigh and leg.
- Move your left foot backwards, sliding your toes along the floor until your left calf presses against the front of your right leg.
- Stop when you feel the initial stages of a stretch behind your right knee.
- Try to extend both knees.
- Your left knee is partially flexed but pressing back on your right leg and your right knee is straight.
- Keep most of your weight on the right leg but do not let your left foot move.

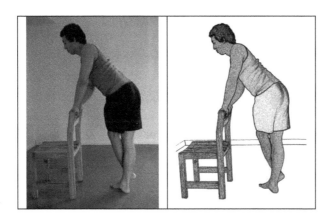

Technique

- Take a deep breath and hold it in.
- Attempt to flex your right knee by pushing your knee forwards against the back of your left leg.
- Resist contraction with an equal and opposite pressure with your left leg.
- After about 5 seconds cease the contraction, relax your muscles, exhale and then push your right leg into greater extension with your left leg.
- Repeat the post-isometric stretch several times for the right leg.
- Repeat the stretch for the left leg.

6.9 The Dog - active, passive and post-isometric stretches for the hamstrings, gastrocnemius and posterior fascia

6.9a Unilateral Lower Dog - an active and passive stretch

Starting position

- Stand on a mat or on the floor.
- Flex your hips and knees and place your hands, palms down on the mat, shoulder width apart, with the tips of your fingers touching a wall.
- Extend your right hip, take your right foot backwards and place the sole of your foot on the floor.
- Extend your right knee until it is nearly straight.

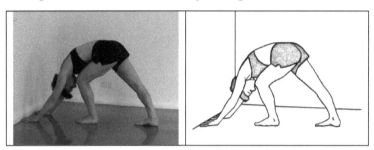

- Keep your left hip, knee and ankle flexed and relaxed.
- Place your left foot just in front of and to the side of your right foot.
- Keep your arms and spine straight and in line.
- Adjust your stance for optimum balance in preparation for the stretch.

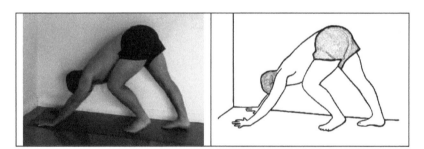

Technique

- Take a deep breath in.
- Exhale and perform the following actions individually or together:

  - Move your pelvis backwards and nearly parallel with the floor
  - Move the heel of your right foot down towards the floor
  - Extend your right knee
  - Extend your thoracic spine and move your chest towards the floor.

- Repeat the stretch several times with an exhalation.
- Feel the stretch behind your right thigh, knee, leg and ankle.
- Repeat the stretch for the left leg.

6.9b Unilateral Lower Dog - a post-isometric stretch for the posterior thigh and leg

Starting position

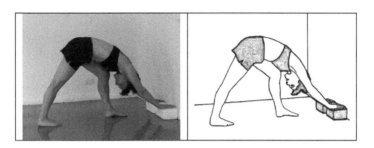

- Adopt the same starting position as in technique 6.9a.
- If the stretch is too difficult then it may be done with the palms on a block.

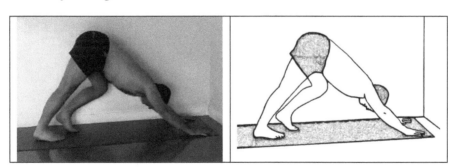

Technique

- Take a deep breath in and hold it.
- Push the palms of both hands, and the toes and ball of your right foot down and into the floor.
- Resist the effort with an equal and opposite counterforce from the muscles of your posterior thigh and leg, and anterior trunk.
- Do not allow your heel to lift off the floor - keep your whole body rigid.
- After about five seconds cease the isometric contraction, relax your muscles, exhale, and then perform the following actions:

  o Move your pelvis backwards and parallel with the floor
  o Move the heel of your right foot down towards the floor
  o Extend your right knee

- Extend your thoracic spine and move your chest towards the floor.
- Repeat the post-isometric stretch several times with an exhalation.
- Feel the stretch behind your right thigh, knee, leg and ankle.
- Repeat the stretch for the left leg.

6.9c The Dog

Starting position

Only do the bilateral stretch when you can do the unilateral technique easily. If you can do the stretch with blocks easily then the blocks may be discarded.

- Stand on a mat or floor with your feet apart.
- Flex your hips and knees, and place your hands, palms down on the floor or on two blocks on the floor in front of you about shoulder width apart.
- Walk your feet away from the blocks.
- Extend your knees until your legs are straight.
- Keep your arms and spine straight.

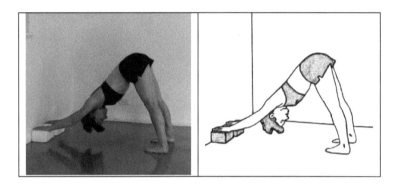

Technique

- Take a deep breath in.
- Exhale and perform the following actions, either individually or together:

    o Move your pelvis backwards and parallel with the floor
    o Move your heels down towards the floor
    o Extend both knees
    o Extend your thoracic spine and move your chest towards the floor.

- Keep your elbows and knees straight.
- Feel the stretch behind your thighs, knees, legs and ankles.
- Take another deep breath and hold it in.
- Push the palms of both hands and the toes and balls of both feet down and into the floor.
- Resist the effort with an equal and opposite counterforce, from the muscles of your posterior thigh and leg and anterior trunk.
- Do not allow your heels to lift off the floor - keep your whole body rigid.
- After about five seconds cease the isometric contraction, relax your muscles, exhale, and then perform the actions listed above.
- Repeat the stretch several times with each exhalation.

220

7.0 Forward bends - active, passive and post-isometric stretches for the hamstrings, hip adductors and external rotators and gastrocnemius and strengthening trunk muscles

7.0a Active forward bend sitting

Starting position

- Sit on a mat with your legs straight out in front and your feet together.
- Flex your left hip and knee, and place the sole of your left foot against the inside of your right thigh, as near as possible to your groin.
- Place your left hand on the mat behind you and lift your body off the mat.
- Move your anterior superior iliac spines forwards and the ischial tuberosities of your pelvis backwards.
- Grasp the toes of your right foot or right knee with both hands.
- Hamstring flexibility plays a major role in determining the starting position.

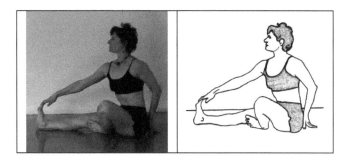

Technique

- Take a deep breath in, then exhale and perform the following actions:

  - Take the top of your pelvis forwards
  - Extend your the lumbar spine and increase the lordosis
  - Move your lumbar, lower thoracic and lower ribs forwards with the ilium
  - Move your left knee downwards and towards the floor
  - Point your right heel away, pull up your foot and dorsiflex your ankle

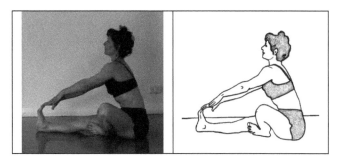

- With each muscle contraction and movement, either flex your elbows more, reposition the grip on your foot or move your hands down your leg.
- Maintain or try to produce a concavity in your lumbar spine by actively extending your lumbar and lower thoracic spine.
- Feel the stretch in your left groin and the back of your right thigh.
- Repeat the stretch on the other side.

7.0b Passive forward bend sitting

Starting position

- Sit on a mat with your legs straight out in front and your feet together.
- Flex your left hip and knee and place the sole of your left foot against the inside of your right thigh as near as possible to your groin.
- Place your left hand on the mat behind you and lift your body off the mat.
- Move your anterior superior iliac spines forwards and the ischial tuberosities of your pelvis backwards.
- Grasp the toes of your right foot or right knee with both hands.
- Hamstring flexibility plays a major role in determining the starting position.

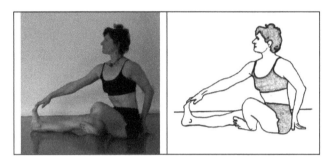

Technique

- Take a deep breath in, then exhale and perform the following actions:

  o Flex your elbows and retract your scapula to pull your spine, lower ribs and the top of your ilium forwards
  o Use your arms to flex your hip and extend your lumbar spine
  o Allow your left knee to drop downwards and towards the mat.
  o Pull up on your foot with your fingers, and dorsiflex your right ankle.

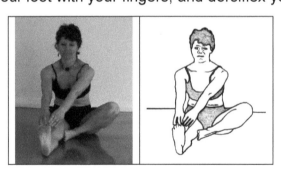

- Keep a firm hold on your foot or leg below your knee.
- Use your shoulders and elbows as levers to pull your body forwards.
- After each stretch, either flex your elbows more, reposition the grip on your feet or move your hands further down your legs.
- Maintain as much concavity in your lumbar spine as possible.
- Feel the stretch in your left groin and behind your right knee.
- Repeat the stretch on the other side.

7.0c Post-isometric forward bend sitting

Starting position

- Sit on a mat with your legs straight out in front and your feet together.
- Flex your left hip and knee and place the sole of your left foot against the inside of your right thigh as near as possible to your groin.
- Place your left hand on the mat behind you and lift your body off the mat.
- Move your anterior superior iliac spines forwards and the ischial tuberosities of your pelvis backwards.
- Grasp the toes of your right foot or right knee with both hands.

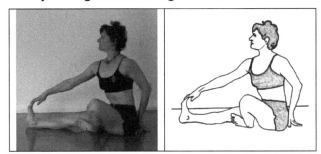

Technique

- Take a deep breath, hold it in and then perform the following actions:

    - Push your right heel downwards into the floor with a light force
    - Resist knee flexion with a firm hold of your foot with your hands.
    - After five seconds cease the isometric contraction, relax, exhale and then pull your hips into progressively increasing flexion with your arms.

    - Push forward and downward on your foot or leg with a light force
    - Resist spinal flexion with an unyielding rigidity of spine and upper limbs
    - After five seconds cease the isometric contraction, relax, exhale and then pull on your foot or leg with your arms to move your body forwards and extend your lumbar spine.

    - Push your right foot and toes downwards with a light force
    - Resist the plantar flexion with a firm hold of your hands or towel.
    - After five seconds cease the isometric contraction, relax, exhale and then pull your foot into greater dorsiflexion with your arms.

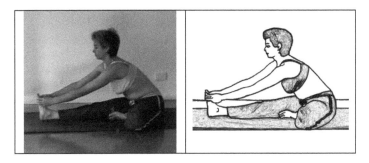

- Feel the stretch behind your right knee.
- Repeat the stretch on the other side.

7.0d Bilateral forward bend sitting

Starting position

- Sit on a mat with your legs straight out in front and your feet together.
- Place one hand on the mat behind you, lift your body off the mat and then move your anterior superior iliac spines forwards and the ischial tuberosities of your pelvis backwards.
- Hamstrings play a major role in determining your starting position and depending on their flexibility grasp your toes or legs with both hands.

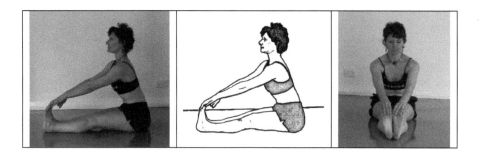

Technique

- Take a deep breath in, then exhale and perform the following actions:

  o Take the top of your ilium forwards
  o Extend your the lumbar spine and increase the lordosis
  o Move your lumbar, lower thoracic and lower ribs forwards with the ilium
  o Push the backs of your knees downwards and towards the floor
  o Point your heels away and pull back on your feet with your hands.

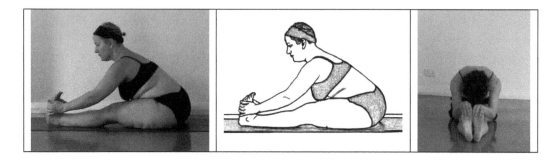

- Feel the stretch down the back of your thighs and behind your knees.
- With each exhalation flex your elbows, flex your hips and extend your lumbar spine.
- At the end of the exhalation reposition your hand hold further down your legs or around the soles of your feet.
- Elongate your spine - do not try and bring your head to your knees.

224

7.1 Calf stretches - active, passive and post-isometric stretches for gastrocnemius, soleus and posterior leg muscles

7.1a Unilateral passive stretch for gastrocnemius

Starting position

- Stand facing a wall and with your feet slightly apart.
- Interlace your fingers and bend your elbows so that your arms and forearms make a 90 degree angle.
- Place your elbows and ulna side of forearms and hands against the wall.
- Your elbows should be shoulder width apart and your arms are parallel.

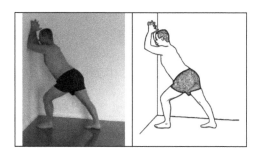

- Flex your left hip and knee and put your left foot down near the wall.
- Extend your right hip and place your right foot on the floor behind you.
- Extend your right knee and bring your right heel to the floor.

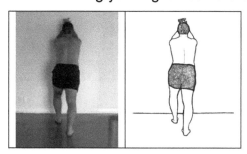

Technique

- Take a deep breath in, then exhale and perform the following actions:

  - Relax your right ankle and calf muscles, and allow your right heel to drop towards the floor
  - Lean against the wall and use your body weight to stretch the calf
  - Pull your knee cap up and push your knee backwards
  - Flex your left hip and knee, lunge forwards and take your pelvis and hips towards the wall.

- Do not push against the wall - allow your ankle to dorsiflex.
- Keep your spine and right leg straight, and allow the force from the weight of your body to be transferred down the spine and leg to your right ankle.
- Feel the stretch behind your right knee, leg and ankle.
- Repeat the stretch several times with an exhalation.
- Repeat the stretch for your left leg.

7.1b Unilateral post-isometric stretch and variations for gastrocnemius

Starting position

- Adopt the same starting position as in technique 7.1a.
- Alternatively keep both feet together and bend the left hip and knee.

Technique

- Take a deep breath and hold it in.
- Push the toes and ball of your right foot, down and into the floor.
- Resist the contraction of your calf muscles with an equal and opposite counterforce from your shoulders, elbows and forearms pressing against the wall.
- Do not allow your heel to lift off the floor - keep your body in a fixed stance.
- After about five seconds cease the isometric contraction, relax your calf muscles, exhale, and then allow your heel to drop towards the floor.
- Move your pelvis nearer the wall but keep your spine and right leg straight.
- Feel the stretch behind your right knee, leg and ankle.
- Repeat the post-isometric stretch several times.
- Repeat the stretch for your left leg.

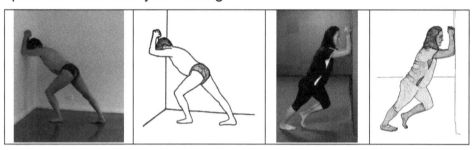

The passive stretch described above can be converted into an active stretch by contracting tibialis anterior and actively dorsiflexing your right ankle. To increase the intensity of the stretch, move your left foot backwards and place it next to your right foot, thereby changing your centre of gravity.

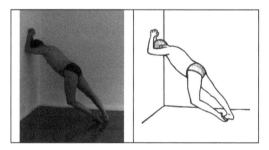

Turning your right foot outwards increases the stretch on popliteus and the medial head of gastrocnemius, while turning it inwards increases the stretch on the short head of biceps femoris and the lateral head of gastrocnemius. Sideshifting your pelvis right increases the stretch on tensor fasciae latae and the lateral head of gastrocnemius, while sideshifting your pelvis left increases the stretch on gracilis, sartorius and the medial head of gastrocnemius.

7.1c Bilateral passive stretch for gastrocnemius

Starting position

- Stand facing a wall with your feet slightly apart.
- Interlace your fingers and make an angle with your arms and forearms.
- Place your elbows, and ulna side of forearms and hands against the wall.
- Your elbows should be shoulder width apart and your arms parallel.
- Extend your knees and bring your heels to the floor.
- Your feet should be hip width apart and parallel, and your spine and legs straight.

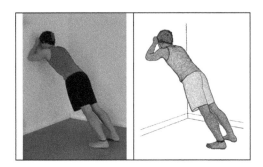

Technique

- Take a deep breath in.
- Exhale, relax your ankles and calf muscles, and allow your heels to drop towards the floor and your ankles to dorsiflex.
- Keep your spine and legs straight and in line.
- Lean against the wall and allow the force from the weight of your body to be transferred down your legs to your ankles - do not push on the wall.
- Feel the stretch behind your knees, legs and ankles.

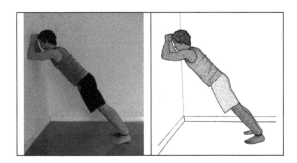

- Take another deep breath and hold it in.
- Push the toes and ball of your feet down and into the floor.
- Resist the contraction of your calf muscles with an equal and opposite counterforce from your upper limb muscles pressing against the wall.
- Do not let your heels lift off the floor - keep your body in a fixed stance.
- After about five seconds, cease the isometric contraction, relax your calf muscles, exhale, and then allow your heel to drop towards the floor.
- Repeat the stretches several times with an exhalation.

7.1d Bilateral stretch for gastrocnemius using a block

Starting position

- Stand facing two small blocks or bricks and a wall.
- Using the wall for support, place your feet on the edge of the blocks.
- The blocks edge crosses your forefoot at the distal end of the metatarsals.
- Extend your hips and knees.
- Your heels should hang over the side of the blocks without touching the floor.
- Keep your knees and body straight.
- Push against the wall and slowly move your body backwards to bring your centre of gravity further over your ankles.
- Stop when your body weight falls mid-point between your ankles.

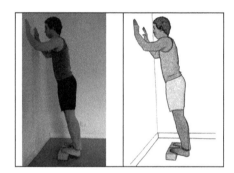

Technique

- Take a deep breath in.
- Exhale, relax, and allow your heels to drop over the back of the block, as your body descends to the floor by increasing dorsiflexion at your ankles.
- Repeat the stretch several times with each exhalation.
- Take another deep breath and hold it in.
- Push the toes and ball of your feet down and onto the blocks.

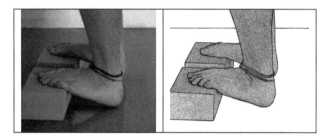

- Resist the contraction of your calf muscles with an equal and opposite counterforce from your upper limb muscles pressing against the wall.
- Do not let your heels move away from the floor - keep a fixed stance.
- After about five seconds, cease the isometric contraction, relax your calf muscles, exhale, and then allow your heels to drop towards the floor.
- Repeat the stretches several times with an exhalation.

This can be done with shoes on or off, on a doorway step while holding a doorframe or over the edge of a pavement using a parked car for support.

7.1e Unilateral stretch for soleus and other posterior leg muscles, ankle ligaments and the Achilles tendon

Starting position

- Stand facing a chair or wall, holding the chair or wall for support.
- Place your left foot in front of your right foot, and nearer to the wall.
- Flex your hips and knees.
- Stop when your right ankle joint is fully dorsiflexed but make sure your right heel remains in contact with the floor.

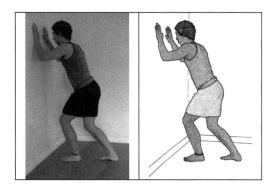

Technique

- Take a deep breath in.
- Exhale, move your right knee forwards and over your right foot, by flexing your hips and knees.
- When you get to full ankle dorsiflexion, make small circles with your knee.
- Move your knee in a plane horizontal with the floor.
- Use hip and knee leverage and your body weight to increase dorsiflexion.
- Take another deep breath in.
- Move your right knee forward and 20 - 30 degrees to the right of your foot.
- Exhale and make small horizontal circles over the floor with your knee.
- Maintain dorsiflexion and do not allow your heel to come off the floor.

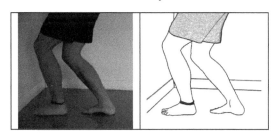

- Take another deep breath in.
- Move your right knee forward and 20 - 30 degrees to the left of your foot.
- Exhale and make small horizontal circles over the floor with your knee.
- Try to increase ankle dorsiflexion.
- Your heel should remain in contact with the floor at all times.
- Keep your body's centre of gravity over your right ankle.
- Repeat the stretches several times, each time with an exhalation.
- Repeat the stretch for your left leg.

7.1f Unilateral stretch for peroneus muscles, tibialis posterior, flexor digitorum longus and flexor hallucis longus on a sloping floor

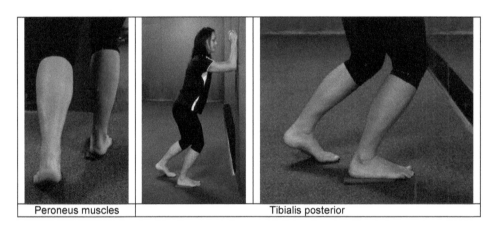

Starting position

- Stand facing a chair or wall, holding the chair or wall for support.
- Place your left foot in front of your right foot and nearer to the wall.
- Place your right foot along the right edge of a thin block of wood.
- Make sure the sharp edge of the block passes down the middle of your foot and heel so that it makes your ankle tilt outwards.
- As an alternative to the edge of a thin block of wood, use a board slanting downwards to the right.
- Flex your hips and knees.
- Stop when your right ankle joint is fully dorsiflexed but make sure your right heel remains in contact with the block or board on the floor.

Peroneus muscles	Tibialis posterior

Technique

- Take a deep breath in.
- Exhale, move your right knee forwards and lower your body to the floor.
- Flex your right hip and knee, and dorsiflex your right ankle.
- Feel the stretch down the back and lateral side of your leg and ankle.
- Maintain your body's centre of gravity over your right ankle.
- Repeat the stretch several times with each exhalation.
- With the edge of the block facing right or the board slanting right, there will be more stretch in peroneus longus and brevis, and lateral fibres of soleus.
- Now place your right foot along the left edge of a thin block of wood or a board slanting downwards to the left.
- Take another deep breath in and then exhale and repeat the stretch.
- Feel the stretch down the back and medial side of your leg and ankle.
- With the edge of the block facing left or the board slanting left, there will be greater stretch in tibialis posterior, Flexor hallucis longus and flexor hallucis longus and the medial fibres of soleus.
- Repeat the stretch for your left leg.

7.1g Unilateral stretch for soleus using a block or wall

Starting position

- Stand next to a small block or brick between 3 cm and 8 cm thick.
- Flex your hips and knees.
- Lift your right foot and place your forefoot on the block in front of you.

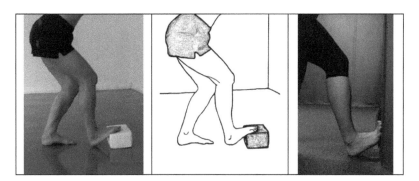

- The distal ends of your metatarsal bones rest on the edge of the block.
- Your heel remains in contact with the floor.
- Flex your right knee until you feel the initial stages of a stretch in the back of the leg and ankle.
- Grasp a table, the back of a chair or a nearby wall for support.
- This stretch can be done with shoes on or off, or with the ball of your toes against a wall.

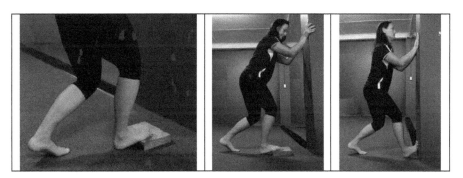

Technique

- Take a deep breath in.
- Exhale and take your right knee forwards and over the block.
- This involves flexing your right hip and knee, and dorsiflexing your right ankle.
- Keep your balance by maintaining your body's centre of gravity over the mid-point between your feet.
- This will involve leaning your upper body further forwards as you increase the stretch.
- Repeat the stretch several times with each exhalation.
- Repeat the stretch for your left leg.

7.1h Bilateral or unilateral active stretch for gastrocnemius and soleus

Starting position

- Sit or lie on the floor or a mat with your legs straight.

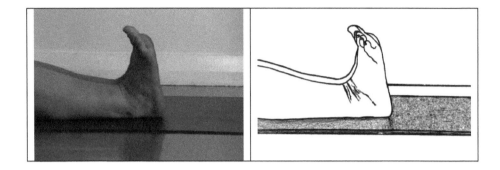

Technique

- Take a deep breath in.
- Exhale and move your heels down and away from you, and move your feet and toes, up and towards you.
- Keep your knees extended, as you dorsiflex your ankles and extend your toes.
- Feel the gastrocnemius stretch behind your legs and knees.
- Repeat the stretch several times, each time with an exhalation.
- Place a pillow under your knees and relax your legs in a flexed position.

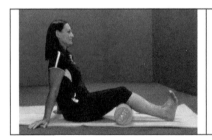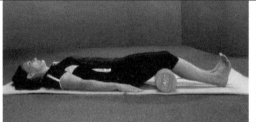

- Take another deep breath in.
- Exhale and move your heels down and away from you, and move your feet and toes, up and towards you.
- Keep your knees flexed as you dorsiflex your ankles and extend your toes.
- Feel the soleus stretch in the back of your legs.
- Repeat the stretch several times, each time with an exhalation.

7.2 Tibialis anterior stretches - active and passive stretches for tibialis anterior and the toe extensor muscles

7.2a Bilateral active stretch for the ankle dorsiflexor and toe extensor muscles

Starting position

- Sit or lie on the floor or a mat with your legs straight.
- Bring your feet together and bring your big toes together.

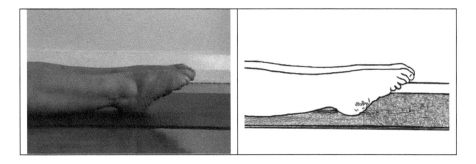

Technique

- Take a deep breath in.
- Exhale and point your feet and toes down and away from you.
- Actively plantarflex your ankles and flex your toes.

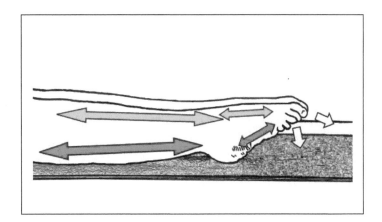

- Keep your knees extended
- Feel the stretch in the front of your legs and ankles.
- Repeat the stretch several times.

7.2b Unilateral passive stretch for the ankle dorsiflexor and toe extensor muscles standing

Starting position

- Stand facing a wall and hold the wall for support.
- Place your left foot in front of your right foot, and closer to the wall.
- Flex your hips and knees.
- Lift your right foot off the floor, extend your hip and then place it back on the floor with the sole of your foot facing upwards and your toes pointing backwards.

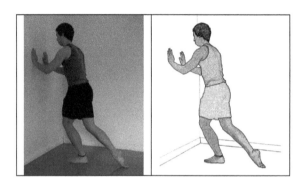

Technique

- Take a deep breath in.
- Exhale and actively flex your left hip and knee, and move your left knee forwards and over your right ankle, and lower your body towards the floor.
- Keep your body in a fixed position with your spine straight, your right hip extended and your right knee flexed.
- Allow movement in your right ankle and foot.
- Use the leverage of your leg and your body weight to increase dorsiflexion.

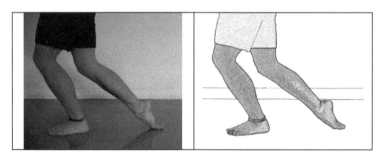

- Take another deep breath and hold it in.
- Push the dorsum of your foot and toes down into the floor for five second.
- Maintain a rigid stance with your body – do not allow any movement.
- Cease the isometric contraction, exhale, relax and then lower your body towards the floor as outlined above for the passive stretch.
- Feel the stretch down the front of your leg and ankle, over the dorsum of your foot and top of your toes.
- Keep your body's centre of gravity back towards your right ankle.
- Repeat the stretch several times each time with an exhalation.
- Repeat the stretch for your left foot.

7.3 Foot and toe stretches - passive and post-isometric stretches for the long and short foot and toe muscles

7.3a Toe flexor stretch standing

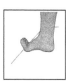

Starting position

- Stand facing a wall.
- Place your palms on the wall about shoulder height for support.
- Extend the toes of your right foot and place your foot against the wall, so that your toes are against to the wall, the balls of your feet are in the corner of the room and your heel and metatarsal are on the floor.
- Flex your hips and knees slightly.
- Stop when you feel the initial stages of a stretch under your toes.
- Make sure your heel and metatarsals remains in contact with the floor.

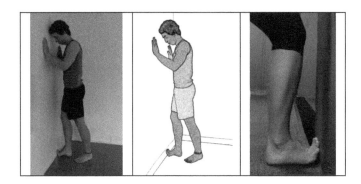

Technique

- Take a deep breath in.
- Exhale, move your right knee forwards and over your right foot by flexing your hips and knees.
- Hip and knee leverage and your body weight increase toe extension.
- Reposition your foot with your toes higher up the wall

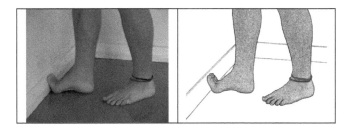

- Take another deep breath and hold it in.
- Push your toes against the wall for about five seconds.
- Resist any movement of your foot with a firm stance.
- Cease the contraction, relax, exhale and move your right knee forwards and over your right foot by flexing your hips and knees.
- Keep your body's centre of gravity over your right ankle.
- Repeat the passive or post-isometric stretch several times.
- Repeat the stretch for your left foot.

7.3b Toe flexor stretch seated

Starting position

- Sit in a chair with your feet apart and planted on the floor.
- Flex your right hip and knee and place the outside of your right ankle on your left thigh just above your knee.
- Allow your right knee to drop into a comfortable abducted position.
- Grasp the heel of your right foot with your left hand and hold it steady.
- Reach under your toes and the bottom of your right foot with your right hand and grasp your toes and the end of your foot.
- Hook your thumb over your big toe and fingers over your other toes.
- Flex your right elbow, wrist and fingers and pull up your toes.
- Stop when you feel the initial stages of a stretch under your toes.

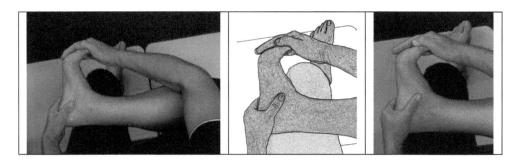

Technique

- Take a deep breath in.
- Exhale and pull your toes upwards to stretch the toe flexor muscles.
- Feel the stretch under your foot and deep in the back of your leg.

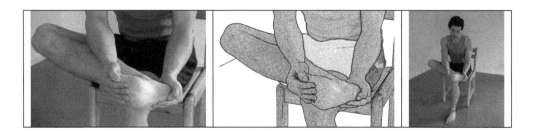

- Take another deep breath and hold it in.
- Attempt to curl your toes downwards and away from you but resist this action with the fingers of your right hand.
- After about five seconds cease the contraction, relax your toe muscles, exhale and pull your toes further upwards and into extension.
- Repeat the passive or post-isometric contractions several times.
- Repeat the stretches on the left foot.

7.3c Foot evertor or foot invertor stretch seated

Starting position

- Sit in a chair, flex your right hip and knee and place the outside of your right ankle on your left thigh just above your knee.
- Grasp the heel of your right foot with your left hand and hold it steady.
- Reach under your toes and the bottom of your right foot with your right hand and grasp the distal ends of your metatarsals.
- Pull on the fourth and fifth metacarpal heads to dorsiflex and evert the foot to stretch the foot invertor muscles and pull on the first metacarpal head to dorsiflex and invert the foot to stretch the foot evertor muscles.

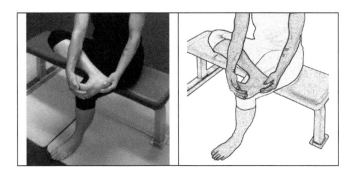

Technique

- Take a deep breath in.
- Exhale and pull up on the distal ends of your first metacarpal bone to stretch the foot evertor muscles or pull up on the distal ends of your fourth and fifth metacarpal bone to stretch the foot invertor muscles.
- Feel the stretch under your foot and down the back and sides of your leg.

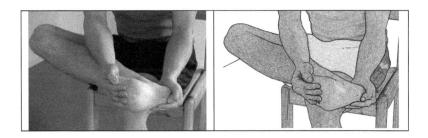

- Take another deep breath and hold it in.
- Attempt to curl your foot downwards and inwards into plantar flexion and inversion but resist this action with the fingers of your right hand.
- After about five seconds cease the contraction, relax your foot muscles, exhale and pull your foot into dorsi flexion and eversion.
- Similarly attempt to curl your foot downwards and outwards into plantar flexion and eversion but resist this with the fingers of your right hand.
- After about five seconds cease the contraction, relax your foot muscles, exhale and pull your foot into dorsi flexion and inversion.
- Repeat the passive or post-isometric contractions several times.
- Repeat the stretches on the left foot.

7.3d Toe extensor stretch seated

Starting position

- Sit in a chair with your feet apart and planted on the floor.
- Flex your right hip and knee and place the outside of your right ankle on your left thigh just above your knee.
- Allow your right knee to drop into a comfortable abducted position.
- Grasp your right ankle with your right hand and hold your foot steady.
- Reach over your toes and the dorsum of your right foot with your left hand and grasp your toes and the end of your foot
- Place your thumb over your big toe and your fingers over your toes.
- Extend your left shoulder and flex your left wrist and fingers and pull your toes downwards and towards you.
- Stop when you feel the initial stages of a stretch over the top of your foot.

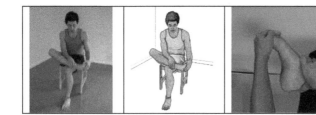

Technique

- Take a deep breath in.
- Exhale and pull your toes downwards, and increase flexion at the metacarpophalangeal joints or interphalangeal joints.
- Feel the stretch over the top of your foot and toes.

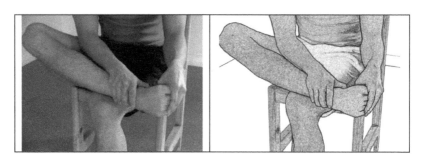

- Take another deep breath and hold it in.
- Attempt to curl your toes upwards and away from you but resist this action with the fingers of your left hand.
- Contract your toe extensor muscles for about five seconds, then cease the contraction, relax your toe muscles, exhale and pull your toes further downwards and into flexion.
- Stretch the metacarpophalangeal joints or interphalangeal joints.
- Repeat the passive or post-isometric contractions several times.
- Repeat the stretch on the toes of the left foot.

7.4 Hip and back stretches - active, passive and post-isometric stretches for the hamstrings, piriformis, gluteus medius, gluteus maximus, abdominal and lumbar muscles

7.4a Hip and back active and passive straight leg stretch

Starting position

- Lie on your back on the floor with your arms abducted about 90 degrees.
- Flex your right hip and then extend your knee so that your leg is straight.
- Keep your right leg vertical, and keep your left leg straight, horizontal and as close to the ground as possible throughout the stretch.

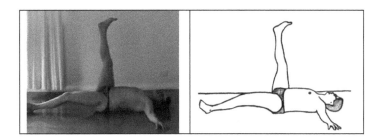

Technique

- Take a deep breath in, then exhale and perform the following actions:

  o Take your right hip further into flexion to stretch the hamstrings.
  o Point your heel upwards and draw your toes downward to stretch gastrocnemius and the posterior fascia.
  o Move your right leg across your body towards your left, keeping it level with your pelvis to stretch gluteal muscles and piriformis.
  o Continue moving your right leg to the left, but this time allow your pelvis to come off the floor to stretch the rotator muscles of the lumbar spine.

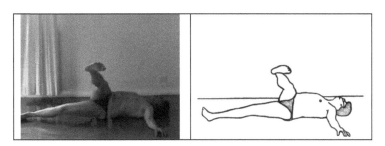

- At the final stage of the technique your foot may come into contact with the floor or myofascial tension may prevent further movement.
- Feel the stretch down the right side of your abdomen, spine and ribs, right buttocks, behind your right knee and down the back and side of your thigh.
- Throughout all stages of the stretch keep your head, arms, shoulders, thoracic spine and left leg on the floor, and keep both legs straight.
- If necessary to maintain your balance grasp the leg of a table with your right hand and use the table for stability.
- Repeat the stretch on the left side.

7.4b Hip and back passive and isometric stretch for hip abductors and external rotators and muscles in the lumber spine

Starting position

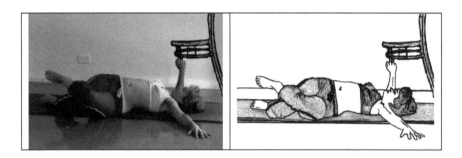

- Lie on your back on the floor.
- Flex your hips and knees, and place your feet on the floor slightly apart.
- Lift your left leg, move it over the top of your right knee and hook it around your right thigh in a cross legged position.
- Pull your right knee to the left with your left leg to adduct the hip and rotate the pelvis but stop when you feel the initial stages of back muscle tension.
- Keep your shoulders on the floor.

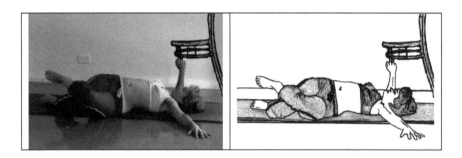

Technique

- Take a deep breath in.
- Exhale and push your right knee to the left with your left leg.
- Do not allow either shoulder to lift off the floor.

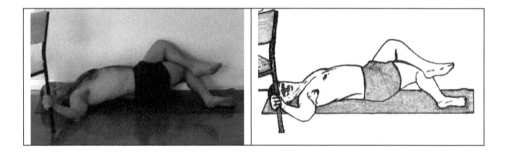

- Take another deep breath and hold it in.
- Push your right knee up and to the right, and push your right foot down into the floor and to the left but resist the movement with your left leg.
- After five seconds cease the isometric contraction, relax your hip and back muscles, exhale and pull your right knee further down into the floor and to the left with your left leg.
- Feel the stretch deep in the right buttock and across the lumbar spine.
- Repeat the passive or isometric stretch several times.
- Repeat the stretch on the left side.

7.5 Squats - active stretches and strengthening exercises for the whole body

7.5a Squat with palms together above head

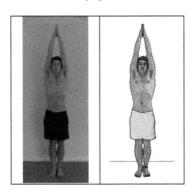

Starting position

- Stand straight with your feet together or apart and arms at your sides.
- Abduct your arms until your hands are above your head.
- Bring your palms together but keep your elbows straight.

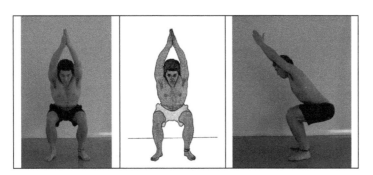

Technique

- Take a deep breath in.
- Exhale and take your hands further away from your head.
- Reach towards the ceiling and feel the stretch in your thoracic spine, ribs, shoulders, arms, forearms, hands and fingers, through to the fingertips.
- Keep your elbows straight.
- Repeat the stretch several times, each time with an exhalation.

- Take another deep breath in.
- Exhale and flex your hips and knees and lower your body towards the floor until your thighs are horizontal.
- Hold the position, keeping your elbows straight and your palms together.
- Your arms and forearms should be in line with your spine.
- Maintain a straight spine and keep your head in line with your spine.
- Do not allow your heels to come off the floor or your feet to splay out.
- Inhale and return to the straight standing position.
- Repeat the stretch several times, each time with an exhalation.

7.5b Squat with arms in front of body

Starting position

- Stand straight with your feet parallel and approximately hip width apart.
- Flex your arms until they are level with your shoulders and horizontal.
- Keep your elbows straight.
- Bend both hips and knees, and lower your body towards the floor.
- Stop before your heels come off the floor and before there is any strain on your body.
- Hold this easy squatting position.

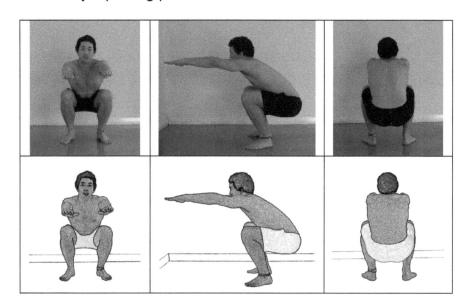

Technique

- Take a deep breath in.
- Exhale and increase the flexion of your hips and knees.
- Lower your body towards the floor.
- Reach forward with your arms and use them to keep balanced.
- Maintain a straight spine and keep your head in line with your body.
- Do not allow your heels to come off the floor.
- Keep your toes pointing forwards - don't let them splay outwards too far.
- Hold the position for five to 10 seconds.
- Inhale and return to the straight standing position.
- Allow the limbs to relax for a few of seconds and then repeat the technique aiming to flex your hips and knees further each time until you are in the full squatting position.

7.6 Pelvic tilt - active stretch for posterior muscles of the lumbar and cervical spine and strengthening exercise for the abdomen

7.6 Pelvic tilt supine

Starting position

- Lie on the floor, preferably on a carpet or mat, with your hips and knees flexed, and your arms on the floor at your side about shoulder height.
- If after you lie down your head drops backwards into extension, tuck your chin in, flatten the arch and lengthen the back of your neck.
- If you have an exaggerated and inflexible forward curvature in your thoracic spine, then you may need to place your head on a pillow or book.

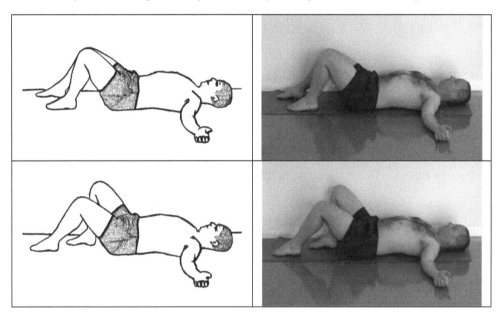

Technique

- Tilt your pelvis backwards until your lumbar spine presses on the floor or the concavity of your lumbar spine is as flat as possible against the floor.
- Hold the pelvic tilt and lumbar flattening while you slide your feet up and down along the floor in an unbroken cyclic manner.
- Slide one foot away from you while simultaneously bringing the other foot towards you and then repeat this up down movement with the feet in the other direction.
- Maintain your lumbar spine in a flattened position with a continuous contraction of your abdominal muscles.
- Also try and keep your cervical spine in a flattened position by contracting your anterior neck muscles and tucking in your chin.

8.1 Nerve stretches

These stretches improving their ability of nerves to slide and glide through the joints and muscles. With inactivity muscles can become tight and compress and restrict the free movement of nerves, and joints can become stiff and irritate nerves as they pass over them. This can lead to inflammation and pain. Scar tissue or adhesions can also build up around nerves and trap them.

Nerve stretches that involve movement are called neural glides of neural flossing. For the lower limb this may involve movement of the shoulder, elbow or wrist or sideways movement of the head and neck. For the lower limb this involves movement or the knee, ankle or toes or flexion of the head and trunk.

Upper or lower limb nerve roots may be affected by a disc bulge (herniation) or osteophytes in the spine. In the cervical spine the C7 nerve root between vertebrae C6 and C7 is the most commonly affected, followed by C6, C5 and C8. In the lumbar spine the L5 and S1 nerve roots are the most commonly affected by disc herniation. Herniation of the L4/L5 disc damages the L5 nerve root and herniation of the L5/S1 disc damages the S1 nerve root.

8.1a Median nerve stretch

To stretch the median nerve abduct your arm about 90 degrees and place your palm on a wall with finger tips pointing back and away from your trunk and parallel to the floor. Rotate your trunk away from the wall keeping your elbow straight and sidebend your head and neck away from the side you are stretching.

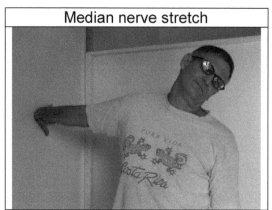
Median nerve stretch

The median nerve arises from all five roots of the brachial plexus but chiefly from C6, C7, C8 and T1 roots. From the axilla it runs down the front of the arm, deep and medial to biceps. It enters the medial side of the cubital fossa and passes under the bicipital aponeurosis and later pronator teres. It runs down the middle of the forearm supplying some flexor muscles and through the carpal tunnel to supply the thenar muscles and skin of the lateral palm. The nerve may be affected by inflammation and swelling of the wrist or trauma to the front of the wrist. Compression within the wrist may result in carpal tunnel syndrome.

Techniques 3.6, 3.8a, 3.8b, 3.8c, 4.0a, 4.0b, 4.0e, 5.3a, 5.3b, 5.5 and 5.6 stretch the median nerve.

8.1b Radial nerve stretch

The radial nerve arises from all five roots of the brachial plexus but especially from C6, C7 and C8 nerve roots. From the posterior axilla it winds around posterior humerus over the spiral groove to an anterior position. In front of the lateral epicondyle it splits into deep and superficial branches.

The superficial nerve runs down anterolateral forearm over the anatomical snuffbox to supply the skin on the radial side of the dorsum of the hand especially between the thumb and index finger (web space).

It supplies the triceps, supinator, brachioradialis and extensor muscles of the wrist and hand. The nerve may be affected by pressure to the back of the arm or trauma to the triceps muscle.

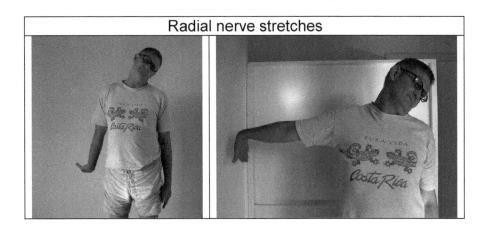

Radial nerve stretches

To stretch the radial nerve abduct your arm about 90 degrees and place the back of your hand on a wall. Internally rotate your arm so your fingers point backwards and away from your trunk and are parallel to the floor. Rotate your trunk away from the wall keeping your elbow straight, and sidebend your head and neck away from the side you are stretching.

An alternative way to stretch the radial nerve is to keep your arm beside your body, internally rotate your arm and then flex your wrist. Sidebend your head and neck away from the side you are stretching. Neural flossing of the radial nerve involves the abduction and internal rotation of your arm. Maintain a straight elbow and sidebend your head away from the side you are stretching. Then move your wrist upwards and downwards into flexion and extension.

Techniques 3.8d, 3.8e, 5.2a and 5.2b stretch the radial nerve.

8.1c Ulnar nerve stretch

To stretch the nerve abduct your arm about 90 degrees and rotate your forearm so your palm is faces upward like a waiter carrying a plate above their shoulder. Sidebend your head away from the side of the bent arm.

For a stronger wrist stretch place the tip of your thumb and index finger together to form a circle while keeping the other fingers straight. Place your straight fingers, palm up, down and around your chin and bring your circled finger-thumb up to your eyes to form a mask.

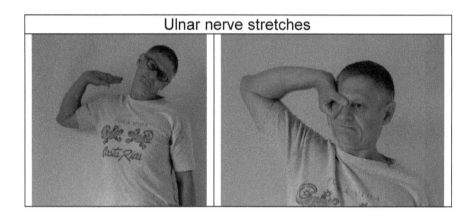

Ulnar nerve stretches

The ulnar nerve arises from vertebral levels C8 and T1 and sometimes from C7. From the axilla it runs down the medial arm with the brachial artery. It passes behind the medial epicondyle of humerus and then under flexor carpi ulnaris which it supplies with part of flexor digitorum profundus. It continues down the anteromedial forearm and passes between the pisiform and the hook of the hamate bone into the hand where it supplies the hypothenar muscles, medial lumbricals and interossei and skin on the medial side of the hand, especially the tip of your little finger.

The nerve may be affected by pressure or trauma to the medial side of the elbow or forearm or the medial side and front of the wrist.

Techniques 4.8 and 5.4 stretch the ulnar nerve.

8.1d Sciatic nerve stretch

To stretch the sciatic nerve, lie on your back, flex one hip, grasp behind the knee and pull your thigh to your chest. Straighten your knee until you feel an initial pull in the back of the thigh. Dorsiflex your foot until you feel a stretch in the calf.

An alternative way to stretch the sciatic nerve is to sit on a chair or table, flex one hip and extend the knee so it is straight, then dorsiflex your foot and extend your toes. Increase the stretch by flexing your head and spine.

Take care not to overstretch the spine. Do not do the seated stretch if you have a history of disc pathology or suspect disc pathology. Neural flossing involves moving your ankle and toes up and down into flexion and extension.

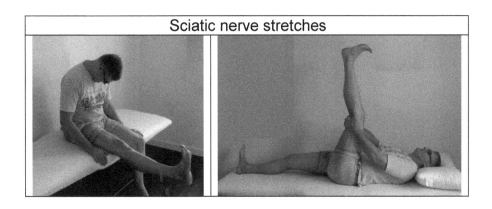

Sciatic nerve stretches

The sciatic nerve arises from the lumbosacral plexus L4, L5, S1, 2 and 3. It leaves the pelvis through the greater sciatic foramen, passes midway between greater trochanter and ischial tuberosity, then descends down back of thigh under cover of biceps femoris. It divides into the tibial nerve and common peroneal nerve. The common peroneal nerve supplies the short head of biceps femoris and splits into deep and superficial branches suppling muscles in the leg and foot. The tibial nerve supplies semimembranosus, semitendinosus and the long head of biceps femoris, some of the fibres of adductor magnus and muscles in the leg and foot.

Irritation to the sciatic nerve anywhere along its length can result in symptoms of numbness, pain or pins and needles. Prolonged sitting, especially slouching can lead to disc degeneration and herniation.

The piriformis muscle is located deep in the hip in close proximity to the sciatic nerve and if the piriformis muscle becomes tight or inflamed, it can irritate the sciatic nerve and causes sciatic symptoms such as pain, tingling and numbness in the buttock, down back of thigh and leg and into the foot. This is piriformis syndrome. Prolonged sitting on an object such as a large wallet in the back pocket can sometimes cause problems with the sciatic nerve.

Technique 6.7a to 6.7f, 6.9a to 6.9c and 7.0a to 7.0d stretch the sciatic nerve.

8.1e Femoral nerve stretch

To stretch the femoral nerve, stand straight, flex one knee and grasp your foot. Pull your foot further towards your buttock then move your knee backwards by extending your hip but keep your body straight.

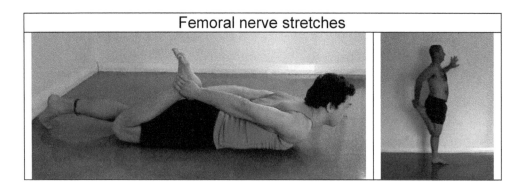

Femoral nerve stretches

The femoral nerve arises from the lumbar plexus L2, L3 and L4. It runs downward through the substance of psoas major and supplies iliacus before passing under the inguinal ligament into the front of the thigh where it supplies the quadriceps, sartorius and pectineus muscles, the skin of anterior thigh and medial leg and foot.

Techniques 6.6a to 6.6f stretch the femoral nerve.

Part B. Anatomy, Biomechanics and Safety

1.1 The Lion - active stretches for the face, tongue, jaw, shoulders, cervical and thoracic spine

1.1a, 1.1b & 1.1c Lion stretches

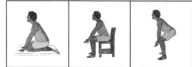

1.1a Lion stretch kneeling

Starting Position: Kneeling with your hips flexed and abducted, knees flexed and ankles plantarflexed. Your elbows are extended, wrists resting on your knees and palms downwards. Your shoulders are internally rotated, forearms pronated, fingers spread, scapulae depressed, cervical and thoracic spine extended, eyes open and mouth open, and tongue protruded. The lion stretch may also be done seated or standing.

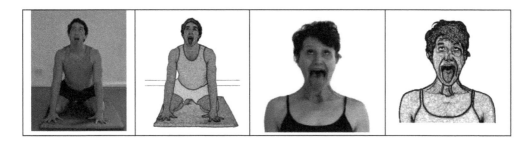

Technique: See Part A. Page 49, 50 and 51.

Direction and range of movement

This is an active stretch involving multiple movements: extension of the head and spine down to the middle thoracic, opening of the mouth and jaw, protrusion of the tongue, elevation of the eyelids, upwards movement of the eyes, depression of the shoulders, extension of the elbows and abduction and extension of the fingers.

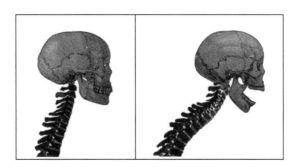

In the lion stretch there is partial extension of the head, cervical spine and upper and middle thoracic spine. Total extension of the head and cervical spine (occiput to T1) is about 80 degrees. Total extension of the upper and middle thoracic (T1 -T10) is about 20 degrees.

In the upper limb there is depression of the shoulders, extension of the elbows and abduction of the fingers. There are between 1 and 2 cm of depression at the shoulders. When the elbows are fully extended, the arm and forearm should be in a straight line - except in hypermobile individuals where there may be up to 10 degrees hyperextension at the elbows.

In the kneeling variation of the lion stretch there is partial hip flexion, full knee flexion and full ankle plantarflexion. During this stretch one would expect partial hip flexion of about 100 degrees, full passive knee flexion of about 160 degrees, and full passive ankle plantar flexion which is about 60 degrees.

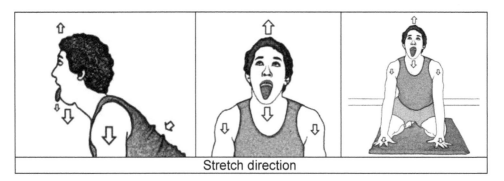
Stretch direction

The temporomandibular joint facilitates full opening of the mouth. Incisal opening is between 40 and 50 mm, measured from the upper incisal edge to the lower. That is approximately the width of the three middle fingers. Protrusion of the jaw is about 10 mm and there is about 10 mm lateral movement each side. During opening, the condyles of the mandible roll and then slide anteriorly on a disc situated between them and the temporal bones of the skull. There is some overlap between rolling and sliding, but just under half of the opening is as result of rotation and the rest is as a result of sliding.

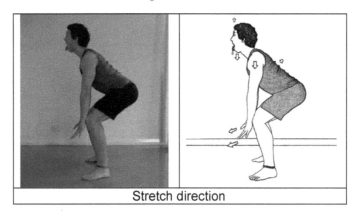
Stretch direction

The lateral pterygoid muscle is made up of two heads, a superior head which acts to pull the disc forwards and an inferior head which pulls the condyle of the mandible forward on the mandibular fossa. The muscle also acts to protrude the jaw and works with gravity and a large number of hyoid muscles to open the jaw.

Target tissues

Stretching primarily occurs in the muscles of the face, jaw, tongue, shoulders and anterior cervical spine. Specifically this is a stretch for upper trapezius, levator scapulae, temporalis, masseter, zygomaticus, depressor, orbicularis oris, orbicularis oculi, the tongue and prevertebral cervical muscles.

There is also secondary stretching of the arms, hands, thighs, legs, feet and eyes.
In generating the stretch, the following muscles are contracted: frontalis, occipitalis, sternocleidomastoid, subclavius, pectoralis minor, lower trapezius, lateral pterygoid, digastric, geniohyoid, mylohyoid, platysma, suboccipital and posterior cervical muscles, intrinsic and extrinsic muscles of the tongue and upper fibres of erector spinae.

The suboccipital muscles responsible for active extension of the head include rectus capitis posterior major and minor and obliquus capitis superior.

250

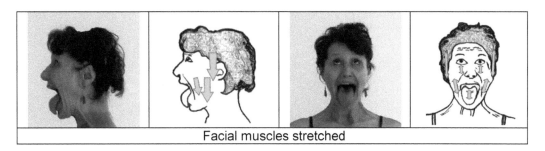

Facial muscles stretched

The posterior cervical muscles, sternocleidomastoid and the erector spinae muscles are responsible for extension of the lower cervical spine and thoracic fibres of erector spinae are responsible for extension in the upper thoracic spine.

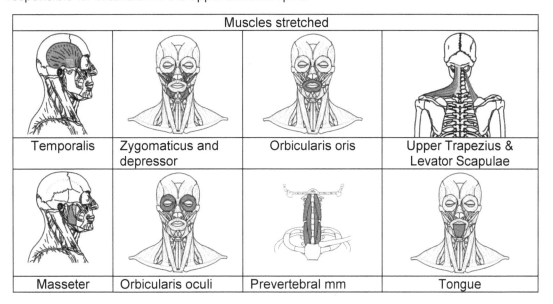

Muscles stretched			
Temporalis	Zygomaticus and depressor	Orbicularis oris	Upper Trapezius & Levator Scapulae
Masseter	Orbicularis oculi	Prevertebral mm	Tongue

Active opening of the jaw or depressing the mandible is produced by contracting the lateral pterygoid and the hyoid muscles - digastric, mylohyoid and geniohyoid.

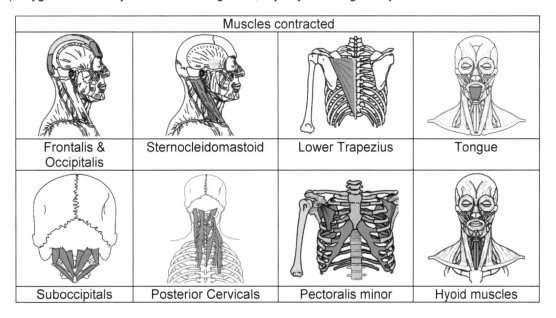

Muscles contracted			
Frontalis & Occipitalis	Sternocleidomastoid	Lower Trapezius	Tongue
Suboccipitals	Posterior Cervicals	Pectoralis minor	Hyoid muscles

Upwards movement of the eye is due to contraction of the extraocular muscles – the superior rectus and inferior oblique muscles. Tongue protrusion occurs as a result of contracting genioglossus and the combined action of the transverse and vertical intrinsic muscle fibres.

Tongue depression is as a result of contracting hyoglossus and the inferior longitudinal intrinsic muscle fibres pull the tip of the tongue downwards. The eyelids are raised by contracting muscles of the forehead and at the back of the scalp - frontalis and occipitalis. The shoulders are depressed by contracting subclavius, pectoralis minor and lower trapezius.

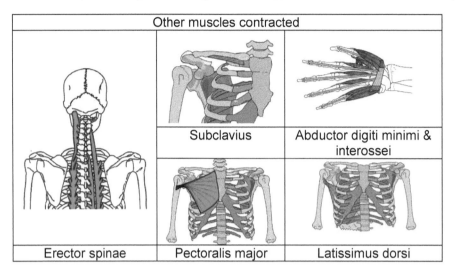

Other muscles contracted		
	Subclavius	Abductor digiti minimi & interossei
Erector spinae	Pectoralis major	Latissimus dorsi

Pectoralis major and latissimus dorsi exert force on the scapula via their attachment to the humerus; thus indirectly depressing the shoulder. Finger abduction is produced by contracting the dorsal interossei and abductor digiti minimi muscles of the hands.

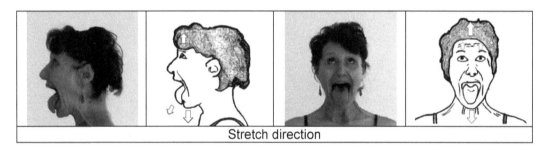

Stretch direction

In the kneeling variation of the stretch, tibialis anterior and three of the quadriceps muscles are stretched. In the sitting and standing variations gluteus maximus, quadriceps and the calf muscles are contracted.

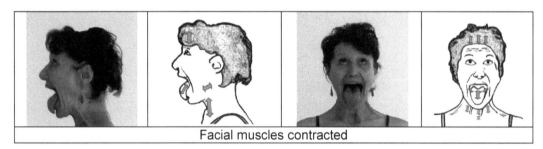

Facial muscles contracted

Safety

Do not over-extend the spine, especially the joints at the base of the skull, at or near to T4 or the thoracolumbar spine. These areas may be in an extended position and do not need more. Focus on stretching the most restricted areas of the spine and avoid stretching any extended areas. Do not overstretch and strain ligaments which support the joints in the jaw. The mandible can be dislocated anteriorly. People with congenital hypermobility are most at risk.

If the discs and joints of the lower cervical spine have been subject to degenerative changes, the resulting arthritic changes will make this area vulnerable to overstretching. Degenerative joint disease (osteoarthritis) can also affect the surfaces of the temporomandibular joint.

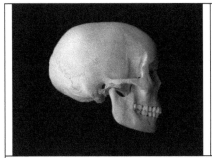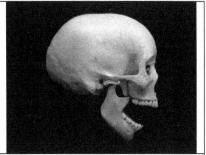

Temporomandibular joint movement

Vulnerable areas

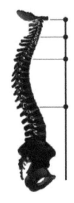

Occiput, C1 & C2

C6 & C7

T4

T12 & L1

	Region	Level of risk
1.	Sub-occipital spine Occiput, C1 & C2	Low
2.	Lower cervical spine and cervico-thoracic junction C6, C7 & T1	Low
3.	Temporomandibular joints (TMJ / Jaw)	Medium
4.	Joints at or near to T4	Medium
5.	Thoraco-lumbar spine (T11, T12 & L1)	Low

Key:

1.1a The Lion stretch kneeling	
1.1b The Lion stretch seated	
1.1c The Lion stretch standing	

Related stretches			
2.8 Extended cat		4.0b Easy pectoralis stretch standing	
4.3 Active scapular elevator stretch		6.5h Bilateral stretch for the hip adductors standing	

1.2 The Shrug - an active, post-isometric and passive stretch for the face, jaw, shoulders, arms and hands

1.2 Shrug

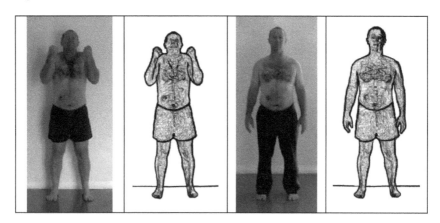

Starting position: Standing with your feet apart and arms at your sides. Fully flex both elbows and clench your fists. Elevate both shoulders. Close your eyes and carefully clench your teeth together.

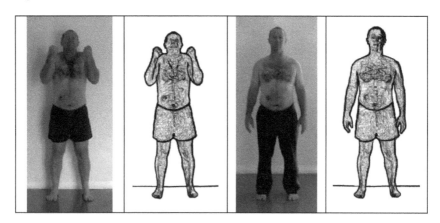

Technique: See Part A. Page 52

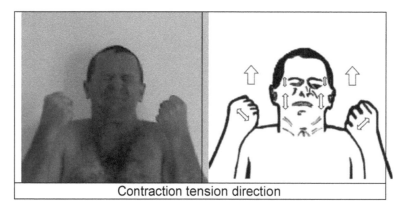

Contraction tension direction

Direction and range of movement

This is an active post-isometric and passive stretch involving many joints in a combination of different movements: closing of the jaw, elevation of the scapula and clavicle and flexion of the forearms and fingers.

Elevation of the scapula is between 8 cm and 12 cm depending on the size and flexibility of the individual. Active forearm flexion is about 145 degrees and is limited by the contact between the anterior muscles of the arm and forearm.

Flexion of the metacarpophalangeal joints is about 90 degrees at the index finger and increases progressively to the little finger. Flexion of the proximal interphalangeal joints is about 100 degrees and flexion of the distal interphalangeal joints is about 90 degrees.

Two temporomandibular joints (TMJs), one on each side of the head, work in unison to allow the opening and closing of the mouth; additionally the TMJ also allows protrusion, retraction and side to side movement of the jaw. Each joint is formed between a right and left mandibular condyle that sit within a shallow concave depression or mandibular fossa on the lower surface of the temporal bone. The condyles and fossa are separated by a fibrocartilagenous articular disc which divides each joint into two compartments.

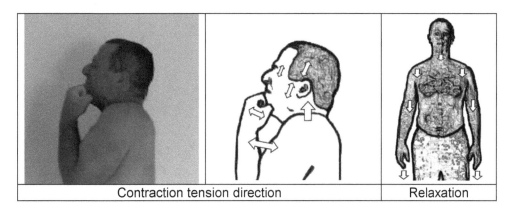

| Contraction tension direction | Relaxation |

The superior surface of the disc articulate with the temporal bone and the inferior surface of the disc articulate with the condyles. The inferior compartment between the condyle of the mandible and disc is involved in rotational movement, which is the initial movement of the jaw when the mouth begins to open. The superior compartment of the temporomandibular joint between the temporal bone and disc is involved in an anterior and slightly inferior gliding movement as the mouth opens wider.

Target tissues

Stretching primarily occurs in muscles, fascia and ligaments attached to the skull, jaw, scapula, arm, forearm, fingers, ribs and cervical and thoracic spine.

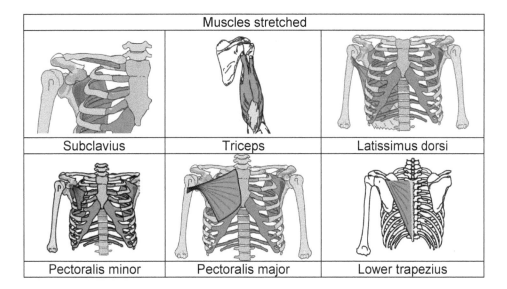

Muscles stretched		
Subclavius	Triceps	Latissimus dorsi
Pectoralis minor	Pectoralis major	Lower trapezius

Stretching occurs by two mechanisms: through the internal tension generated within a muscle during its contraction, and through the force exerted by a muscle or group of muscles on a bone, stretching another muscle or group of muscles attached to the opposite side of that bone - its antagonist.

Movement ceases when the elastic limit of the soft tissue is reached, or a muscle reaches maximum contraction, or the anatomical limit of the body part is reached with soft tissue compression, or there is bone on bone contact.

The increase of internal muscle tension generated by the muscle contraction stretches the facia within the muscle. When the muscles are relaxed there is a net reduction in resting muscle tension.

Stretching occurs in the following muscles: subclavius, triceps, latissimus dorsi, pectoralis minor and the lower fibres of pectoralis major and trapezius.

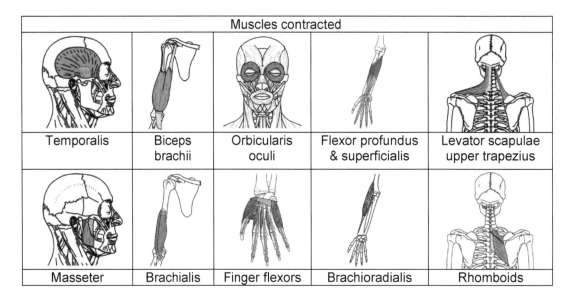

Muscles contracted				
Temporalis	Biceps brachii	Orbicularis oculi	Flexor profundus & superficialis	Levator scapulae upper trapezius
Masseter	Brachialis	Finger flexors	Brachioradialis	Rhomboids

Stretching occurs through the internal tension is generated by the contraction of the following muscles: upper trapezius, levator scapulae, rhomboid major and minor, temporalis, masseter, biceps, brachialis, brachioradialis, flexor digitorum superficialis, flexor digitorum profundus, finger flexor muscles in the hand, orbicularis oculi and other muscles of the face.

When relaxing your contracted muscles make sure you relax them in a natural way. Be careful that you do not just lower your arms by slowly reversing the contraction of your muscles - eccentric contraction. As soon as you stop contracting your muscles, let go of your arms and shoulders. Allow your arms to drop to your sides - completely let go of them. In contrast to unnatural reverse contraction is the explosive method. Both are incorrect ways of letting go. When relaxing your contracted muscles make sure you don't throw your arms down to your sides with a forceful ballistic or explosive movement.

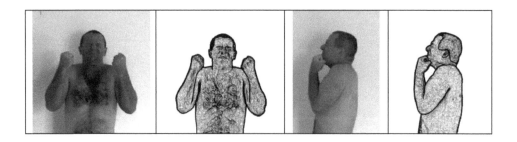

The standing shrug is the recommended way of performing this technique. The shrug can also be done lying on your back on a soft mat or blanket. The standing shrug has one important advantage over the supine shrug in that it uses gravity, and the weight of the arms and shoulders to pull the shoulders down to stretch the muscles.

The technique of tensing and then relaxing a muscle or group of muscles is an effective way to reduce anxiety. It may be done in any part of the body but is most useful for the upper body where people tend to hold most tension. When applied to different and more localised parts of the body, it is known as progressive muscle relaxation (PMR).

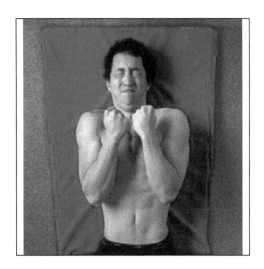

Safety

The shrug should be done well away from any hard objects such as furniture. When you relax after holding the shrug position, your arms should just drop down to your sides and your hands should safely bounce off the sides of your body. For this reason, do not do this seated on a chair with a hard wooden or plastic side. When you relax you do not want your hands to drop and hit the side of the chair. You need to be confident that you can do let go of your arms without hurting yourself. If you are using a chair, place a large pillow on your lap for your hands to land comfortably, or sit on a soft sofa.

Do not do this technique if you have high blood pressure, blood vessel problems, ocular hypertension or eye disorders relating to high intraocular pressure, a heart problem or a history of strokes. From a joint and muscle perspective this is a relatively safe technique. While contracting your muscles keep your head in line with the plane of your body. Do not push your chin forwards into the anterior occiput position, and do not extend your neck or flex your thoracic spine. Keep your posture straight vertically and in neutral plane.

Only clench your jaw if you have good integrity in your teeth and jaw. If you have dental decay, malocclusion problems (your teeth do not fit together) or have a temporomandibular joint dysfunction such as a damaged disc then leave out jaw clenching part of the technique.

Key:

1.2 The Shrug	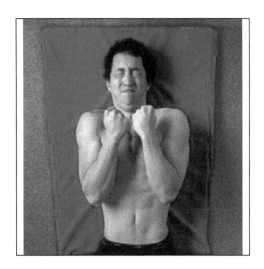

Related stretches	
4.2 The shoulder drop	

For more detailed anatomy of the head, face and jaw 1.1 – 1.2 see page 538.

1.3 Chin tuck - active stretches for the suboccipital, cervical and upper thoracic spine

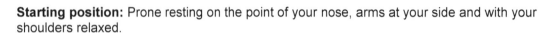

1.3a, 1.3b & 1.3c Chin tucks

1.3a Chin tuck prone

Starting position: Prone resting on the point of your nose, arms at your side and with your shoulders relaxed.

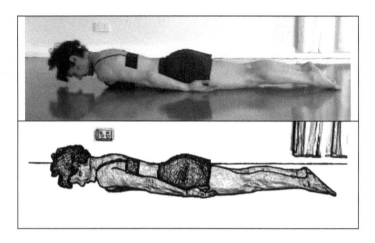

Technique: See Part A. Page 53, 54 and 55

Careful execution of this technique is necessary for it to be effective. Do not allow scapula retraction or extension of the head, cervical, lumbar or lower thoracic spine, or let anything except your head to lift off the floor.

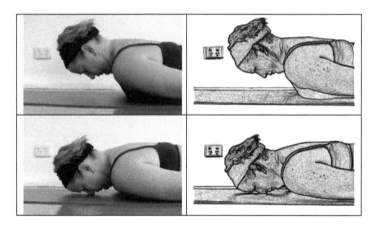

The chin tuck prone is the most useful of the chin tuck variations because it works against gravity. The chin tuck can however be done seated, standing or supine; they are described as individual stretches in the first part of this book. As the principles of these variations are the same therefore they will not be repeated in this section.

Direction and range of movement

This technique combines head and neck flexion, with upper and middle thoracic extension. The head and cervical spine translate posteriorly and the head remains parallel with the top-bottom axis of the body at all times.

Total head, cervical and upper thoracic flexion is about 45 degrees. This technique however involves a combination of flexion (nutation) of the occiput, partial cervical flexion and partial upper thoracic extension. Flexion increases from T1 to the occiput and extension increases from T3 to about T6 in the middle of the thoracic spine.

Cervical flexion is neutralised by thoracic extension. Although the head flexes on the atlas and moves (translates) posteriorly, there is no net flexion or extension of the head relative to the spine and the body as a whole. The head remains parallel with the body throughout the technique. At about T2 vertebral level there is a neutral point where there is neither flexion nor extension of the vertebra on the one below.

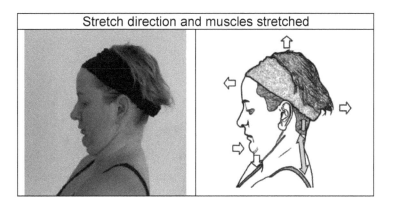

Stretch direction and muscles stretched

There should be no extension of the spine below the middle thoracic. In most people the apex of the thoracic kyphosis is at about T6, but the shape of the spine and the apex will vary between individuals.

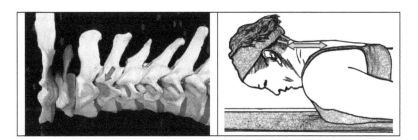

Target tissues

This is an active stretch for the superficial muscles, fascia and ligaments of the posterior cervical and upper thoracic spine and the sub-occipital muscles. The lower origins of these soft tissues are anchored to the posterior part of a vertebra or rib, and the upper ends are attached to the occiput, or another vertebra or rib above. This is also a stretch for sternocleidomastoid and the anterior scalene.

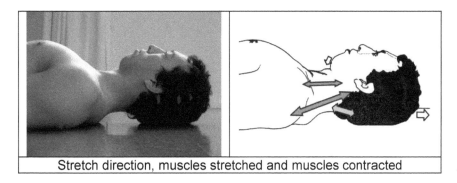

Stretch direction, muscles stretched and muscles contracted

Contraction of the cervical prevertebral muscles produces head and neck flexion. Rectus capitis anterior and longus capitis flex the head, and longus colli flexes the cervical spine.

Contraction of erector spinae and levator scapulae produces posterior translation of the head and neck relative to the rest of the body, lifting the head and neck off the floor when the chin tuck is done prone.

This is a good stretch and a good strengthening exercise. It serves a dual purpose of lengthening short muscles and strengthening key postural muscles, which act against gravity and are subject to postural fatigue. It is a useful technique for correcting common bad posture patterns such as the chin forward posture. In this posture, the occiput is fixed in a bilateral or unilateral anterior position and the cervical spine is fixed in extension.

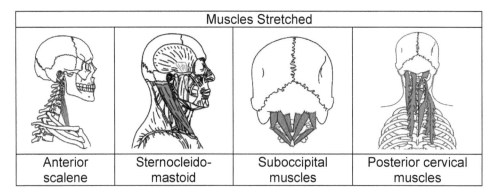

Muscles Stretched			
Anterior scalene	Sternocleido-mastoid	Suboccipital muscles	Posterior cervical muscles

The anterior occiput is more commonly found on the right side and to correct a right sided anterior occiput it is necessary to introduce head rotation right and sidebending left as you tuck in your chin. The prone chin tuck is the most effective of the chin tuck stretches in strengthening muscles because it requires muscle contraction against gravity.

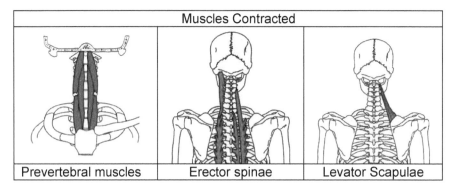

Muscles Contracted		
Prevertebral muscles	Erector spinae	Levator Scapulae

Safety

If your upper thoracic and cervical spine is very stiff, or if you have an exaggerated thoracic kyphosis or cervical lordosis there may be problems with this technique. When attempting the standing chin tuck you may not be able to touch the wall with the back of your head. When attempting the chin tuck prone you may not be able to lift your head off the floor. When attempting the chin tuck supine you may need a pillow or book under your head to stop your head tilting backwards. After stretching for a while and gaining some flexibility in your upper thoracic spine you may be able to discard the pillow.

It is important that you do not allow your head to tilt backwards and put strain on your suboccipital spine. Thus ensure you tuck in your chin and keep your head in a vertical plane. Work with your current level of flexibility.

Do not allow movement below the mid thoracic spine. This is more of a problem in the prone chin tuck, where you can more easily lift your shoulder and upper thoracic off the floor. Use a prop to prevent movement - a straight back chair, a wall or the floor. If you do not use a prop then be sure to keep your pelvis upright. When sitting, keep your pelvis perpendicular to the seat and your spine firm, straight and vertical. Keep the stretch localised to the head, neck and upper thoracic spine. The lumbar, lower thoracic spine and pelvis should not move.

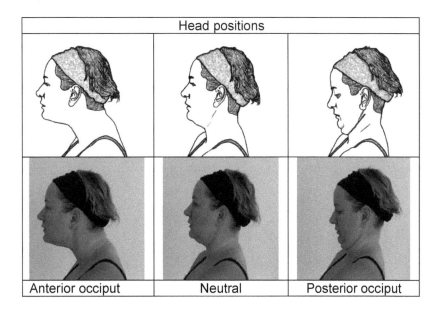

Head positions		
Anterior occiput	Neutral	Posterior occiput

If there are degenerative changes in the discs and joints of the lower cervical spine this part of the spine may be sensitive to extension movement and caution may be required when doing this stretch. Use a pillow when attempting the supine chin tuck if there is any degeneration.

Vulnerable areas

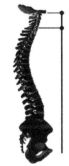

Occiput, C1 & C2

C6 & C7

	Region	Level of risk
1.	Sub-occipital spine Occiput, C1 & C2	Low
2.	Lower cervical spine C5, 6 & C7	Medium

Key:

1.3a Chin tuck prone	
1.3b Chin tuck standing or sitting	
1.3c Chin tuck supine	

Related stretches			
1.4b Head & neck post-isometric flexion stretch supine		1.9 Atlanto-occipital post-isometric technique seated	

1.4 Neck flexion stretches - active, passive and post-isometric flexion stretches for the suboccipital, posterior cervical and upper thoracic spine

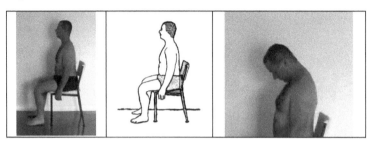

1.4a Head & neck active flexion stretch seated

Starting position: Seated upright with your feet apart and planted on the floor, arms hanging at your sides and your shoulders relaxed.

Technique: See Part A. Page 56

1.4b Head & neck post-isometric flexion stretch supine

Starting position: Supine with your hips and knees flexed, feet apart and feet firmly planted on the floor. Interlace your fingers behind your head.

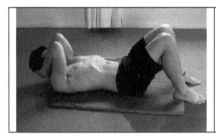
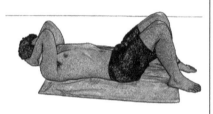

Technique: See Part A. Page 57

1.4c Head & neck localised post-isometric flexion, sidebending and rotation stretch supine using eye muscle contraction

Starting position: Supine on a mat on the floor. Lift your head off the floor. Flex your left arm and forearm, reach behind your head and wrap your left hand around your suboccipital spine. The fingers of your left hand point towards your right ear. Rotate your head to the left and into your left arm and forearm. Flex your right arm and forearm, reach behind your head with your hand and wrap your hand around the back of your cervical spine with your fingers over the vertebra you want to stretch.

Carefully sidebend your head and neck to the left by moving your left arm to the left and your right arm to the right. Your left hand supports your head, protects the suboccipital area against overstretching, and helps sidebend your neck. Use the forefinger of your right hand to localise the stretch to the desired vertebral level. Do not pull on the head or neck – stop when you feel muscle resistance in each plane of movement, flexion, rotation and sidebending.

Technique: See Part A. Page 58

Stop moving when you feel the initial stages of muscle resistance. Work through each plane of movement - flexion, rotation and sidebending. Do not let your thoracic spine, rib cage or shoulders to come off the floor; they serve as anchors for the muscles. Do not move your head and suboccipital spine - localise the stretch to your cervical spine.

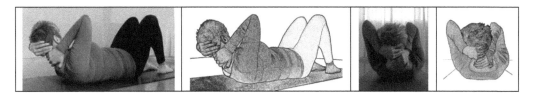

Direction and range of movement

These are active stretches combining muscle contraction with gravity or against gravity, and involve full flexion of the cervical and upper thoracic spine, and flexion of the head (nutation of occiput on the atlas).

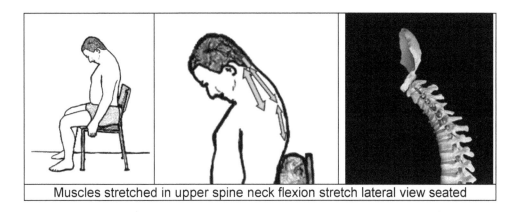

Muscles stretched in upper spine neck flexion stretch lateral view seated

Flexion of the head, neck and upper thoracic spine (occiput to T4) is about 45 degrees. Approximately 15 degrees of flexion occurs between the occiput and C2 and 30 degrees between the C2 and T1.

Target tissues

This is primarily a stretch for the muscles, fascia and ligaments of the posterior suboccipital, cervical and upper thoracic spine. The lower origins of these tissues are attached to the posterior part of a vertebra or rib and anchored there by the weight of the body. They are stretched with flexion of the head and neck.

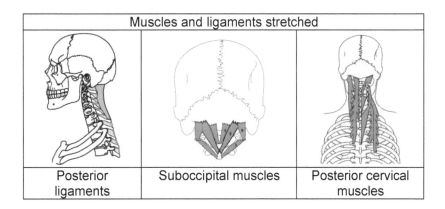

Muscles and ligaments stretched		
Posterior ligaments	Suboccipital muscles	Posterior cervical muscles

This is also a stretch for the cervical and upper thoracic fibres of erector spinae. When both scapulae are actively depressed or held down by grasping the chair with both hands, this is also a stretch for the upper trapezius, levator scapulae and rhomboids.

The seated and supine flexion stretches are both active techniques where muscles in the front of neck are contracted to flex the head and neck.

Sternocleidomastoid, the prevertebral muscles - longus coli and capitis, and rectus capitis anterior, plus the hyoid and anterior scalene muscles are the prime movers involved in head and neck flexion.

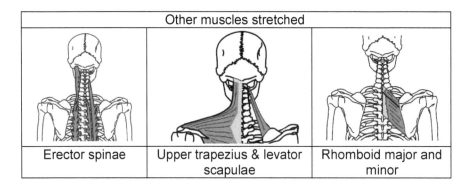

Other muscles stretched		
Erector spinae	Upper trapezius & levator scapulae	Rhomboid major and minor

The seated and supine stretches differ in one major respect – in the seated stretch gravity is acting with the anterior neck muscles, whereas in the supine stretch the head and neck muscles are contracting against gravity. In the supine stretch the arms should only be supporting the head against dropping backward and protecting the suboccipital spine, they should not be pulling on the head. Movement of the head in the supine stretch should be solely due to the contraction of anterior neck muscle. In this respect the supine stretch is more useful because it helps strengthen the anterior neck muscles.

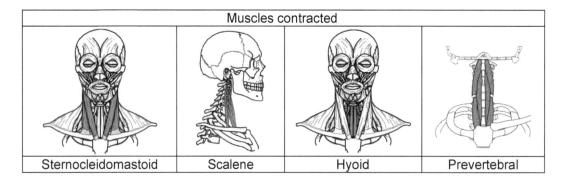

Muscles contracted			
Sternocleidomastoid	Scalene	Hyoid	Prevertebral

The seated stretch can be done as a passive stretch which means that head and neck flexion is solely the result of gravity acting on the head and neck and there is no assistance from the anterior neck muscles. At no time in the seated stretch should there be any involved of the arms pulling on the head as this could result in overstretch and strain to the muscles and ligament.

Variations

This stretch can also be done kneeling or standing. It can also be done sitting on the floor if your hips are flexible enough so you can maintain your pelvis and lower spine in a vertical position and sit up straight.

The supine flexion stretch can be done with one arm supporting and controlling the head. One arm is safer than with both arms because there is less danger of accidentally overstretching the neck. The one arm stretch may provide better control of the cervical spine for introducing sidebending and rotation. Shoulder depression can also be introduced to localise the stretch to the upper trapezius, levator scapulae and rhomboid muscles.

By modifying the amount of flexion introduced in the technique you can influence the amount of movement available for sidebending and rotation and influence which areas in the cervical spine are stretched the most in sidebending and rotation.

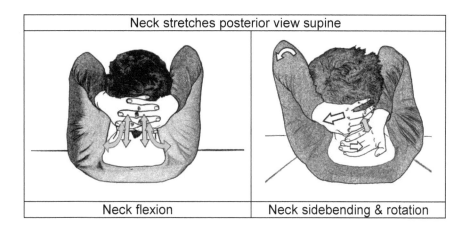

Neck stretches posterior view supine	
Neck flexion	Neck sidebending & rotation

When the neck is in neutral (i.e. there is no flexion or extension), sidebending and rotation occur relatively evenly throughout the cervical spine. But when the neck is fully flexed this reduces sidebending or rotation in the lower cervical spine but allows some sidebending or rotation to occur in the upper cervical spine. Sticking your chin out a bit also helps free up some movement in the upper cervical spine. So by locking up the lower cervical spine in flexion this can be a useful way to localise sidebending and rotation in the suboccipital spine. Sidebending mainly stretches rectus capitis lateralis and rotation mainly stretches the obliquus capitis inferior.

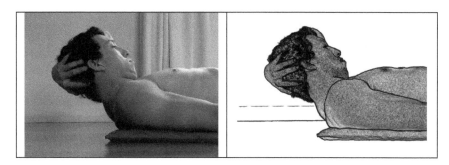

To increase flexion in the suboccipital spine tuck in your chin and take your forehead forwards and downwards with a forwards nodding action.

By making your eye muscles look in a particular direction this causes the muscles which move the head in that direction to contract.

Safety

In the seated stretch make sure you sit up straight or use a support to keep your pelvis, lumbar and lower thoracic spine vertical. Flex the cervical and upper thoracic spine but not the middle thoracic spine. In the seated stretch place your middle thoracic against the back of the seat and in the standing stretch place your back against a wall.

Do not circumduct your head and neck. Circumduction is moving your head around in a circle using a combination of flexion, extension, sidebending and rotation. This movement is not recommended because during circumduction the upper cervical joints have to compensate for the complex sidebending rotation coupling of the lower cervical spine, and this puts strain on the ligaments and cartilage in the joints in the neck.

As with any stretch the speed of the movement is an important factor in determining if there is any strain placed on a joint. If circumduction is done slowly there is less danger of injury.
 The neck flexion stretches are safe techniques if done correctly and if there is no underlying pathology. They are unsafe if they are executed incorrectly for example by pulling on the neck with force - and they are unsafe if there is an underlying pathology like osteoarthritis, which is relatively common after age 40 years.

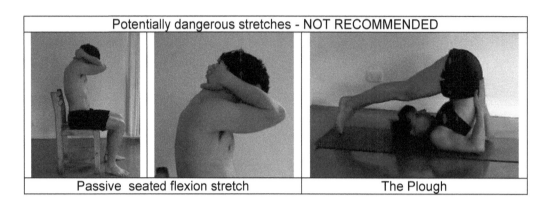

Potentially dangerous stretches - NOT RECOMMENDED	
Passive seated flexion stretch	The Plough

 The seated and standing neck flexion stretches carry the most risk because it is during these stretches that gravity pulls the most on the head and where there is greatest pressure on the discs. If there is history of ligament laxity and joint hypermobility (usually in the suboccipital region) or disc pathology (usually in the lower cervical spine) then the neck flexion stretches should be done with caution and ceased if there are symptoms such as pain or any abnormal sensations in the upper limb.

Avoid pulling on the head and overstretching the suboccipital muscles. Avoid pushing down on the head and compressing the lower cervical, upper thoracic and ribs. Avoid exaggerating an increased kyphosis.

Problems are more likely to occur with the passive stretch than with the active stretch, because the relatively powerful arm muscles and leverage acting through the arms and shoulder can overwhelm the less powerful spinal muscles. Problems are also more likely to occur with the seated passive stretch than with the supine passive stretch, because with the seated stretch there is the additional force of gravity acting to pull down the head and because thoracic spine is less supported.

Vulnerable areas

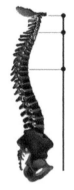

Occiput, C1 & C2

C6 & C7

T6-8

	Region	Level of Risk
1.	Occiput, C1 & C2	Low
2.	C6 & C7	Low
3.	T6 to T8	Low

1. Occiput, C1 and C2 - occipito-atlanto-axial joints of the sub-occipital region.

Care should be taken not to over-stretch the muscles and ligaments of the suboccipital region. These are vulnerable to over-pressure and can be strained with excessive force. This stretch is best achieved using the weight of head, combined with a small amount of pressure from the muscles at the front of the neck. Strains to the ligaments of the sub-occipital region mostly occur if you pull on the head with a strong force of both arms.

2. C6 & C7 - the lower cervical spine and cervicothoracic junction

Care should be taken not to put excessive pressure on the lower cervical spine if the discs and joints in this region have degenerative changes. Cervical arthritis commonly begins by about 40 years and increases with age. The degenerated tissues are vulnerable to further tissue damage and overstretching may precipitate pain.

Cervical arthritis results in increased stiffness. In other respects the lower cervical spine may be without symptoms. A reduced range of movement in the lower cervical spine may result in hypermobility in the upper cervical spine so care should be taken not to overstretch this area.

3. T6 to T8 - the middle of the thoracic spine

The neck flexion stretch should be localised to the cervical and upper thoracic spine and the middle thoracic should remain neutral. If the stretch is done seated then sit upright and do not slouch. In particular do not flex the joints in the middle thoracic spine between about T6 and T8 and do not stretch the muscles or ligaments in this region. This is especially important if you have a stooping posture - an increased kyphosis.

Use a wall to keep the back straight when you do the stretch standing or when sitting on the floor. Overstretching the middle thoracic is easier if the back is not supported. Doing the stretch supine has benefits – the floor keeps the back straight and the anterior neck muscles are strengthened by having to work against gravity.

Key:

1.4a Head & neck active flexion stretch seated	
1.4b Head & neck post-isometric flexion stretch supine	
1.4c Head & neck post-isometric flexion, sidebending and rotation stretch supine	

Related stretches					
1.3a Chin tuck prone		1.3b Chin tuck standing or seated		1.3c Chin tuck supine	
1.9 Atlanto-occipital post-isometric technique seated		2.9a Flexed cat kneeling		2.9b Flexed cat standing	

1.5 Neck extension stretch - active and passive stretch for the suboccipital, cervical and upper thoracic spine

1.5 Head & neck extension stretch seated

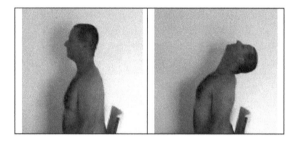

Starting position: Seated upright with your feet apart and firmly planted on the floor, arms hanging at your sides and your shoulders relaxed.

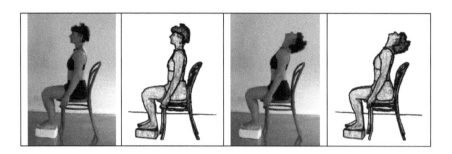

Technique: See Part A. Page 59

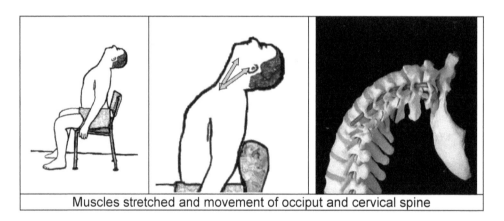

Direction and range of movement

This technique involves full extension of the cervical and upper thoracic spine, and extension of the head (counter nutation of occiput on the atlas). Extension of the head, neck and upper thoracic spine (occiput to T4) is about 90 degrees.

| Muscles stretched and movement of occiput and cervical spine |

The first part of this technique involves eccentric muscle contraction of the sternocleidomastoid, hyoid and cervical prevertebral muscles, which lower the head to a comfortable extended position. During eccentric muscle contraction the anterior neck muscles elongate while under tension from the weight of the head. This can be seen as a reverse muscle contraction with the opposing force of the head greater than the force generated by the muscle contraction.

The second part of this technique, the active stretch, involves eye movement combined with gravity and concentric muscle contraction of the neck extensor muscles. It can also be done as a passive stretch, which is solely the result of gravity acting on the weight of the head and with no muscle contraction.

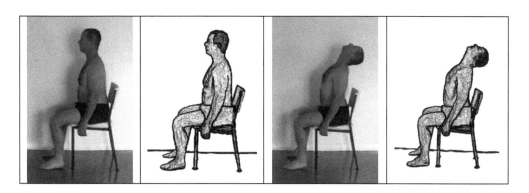

Target tissue

This mainly stretches the muscles, fascia and ligaments of the anterior cervical spine and upper ribs, including the sternocleidomastoid, the prevertebral muscles - longus capitis and colli, and the hyoid muscles. The lower ends of these tissues are anchored to the sternum, clavicle or to the anterior part of a vertebra or rib.

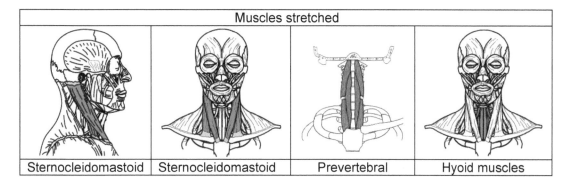

Muscles stretched			
Sternocleidomastoid	Sternocleidomastoid	Prevertebral	Hyoid muscles

If the jaw is closed by clenching the teeth, then the platysma, inferior and superior hyoid muscle will also be stretched.

This is also a mild stretch for the clavicular fibres of pectoralis major, the clavipectoral fascia and intercostal muscles attaching to the upper ribs. When both scapulae are actively depressed this increases the stretch on the clavicular part of sternocleidomastoid.

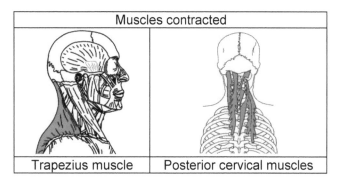

Muscles contracted	
Trapezius muscle	Posterior cervical muscles

In the passive neck extension stretch gravity is the primary factor acting on the head to stretch the anterior neck muscles. Active extension in the seated stretch should be limited to a mild muscle contraction activated by eye movement. The trapezius can act as a powerful head extensor and should not be forcefully contracted. Instead the relatively less powerful posterior cervical muscles should be the prime mover extending the head; these should be moderated by eccentric muscle contraction of the anterior antagonists.

Variations

This can be done as an active stretch, preferably standing, flexed at the hips or in a kneeling position such as in the cat. In both these positions the spine is horizontal and by lifting your head against gravity you with be strengthening muscles of the posterior spine.

This can be done as an isometric stretch or in a variety of positions, sitting, standing, kneeling or lying on your front; and with the mouth open or closed.

Safety

This is best done as a passive stretch using gravity and allowing the weight of the head to stretch the tissues at the front of the neck. If it is done as an active stretch in the seated position then you will be combining gravity (the weight of the head), with the contraction of powerful head extensor muscles such as trapezius, erector spinae, splenius and semispinalis capitis on both sides of the spine. This can take the stretch beyond safe limits, overstretching and straining prevertebral muscles and ligaments in the front of the neck and compress suboccipital tissues or muscles and ligaments.

If you have degenerative changes in the lower cervical spine or hypermobility in the upper cervical spine then you should avoid this technique. And it should be avoided if there are adverse symptoms when you do the technique.

If your neck is structurally healthy then this stretch should be done carefully, especially if this is your first attempt at doing it. The stretch should be done slowly; done as pure extension; and not involve circumduction - combinations of extension, sidebending and rotation – as this may cause or accelerate disc or cartilage damage.

Do not extend the middle thoracic spine near to T4, or the thoracolumbar spine. If done as an isometric stretch care should be taken not to pull the head back and down.

Vulnerable areas

This is a relatively benign technique and carries few risks. Avoid pulling the head backward. Avoid increasing extension in already extended regions of the spine: the atlanto-occipital joint, T4 and the thoracolumbar spine.

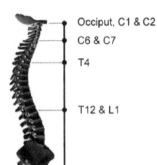

Occiput, C1 & C2

C6 & C7

T4

T12 & L1

	Region	Level of Risk
1.	Occiput, C1 & C2	Low
2.	C6 & C7	Low
3.	T4	Low
4.	T12 & L1	Low

1. Occiput, C1 and C2 - the occipito-atlanto-axial joints of the sub-occipital region.

Care should be taken not to hyperextend the head, over-stretch ligaments and force an anterior occiput into a further anterior position. Hyperextension of the head can irritate or

270

compromise the vertebral arteries which pass through the suboccipital region from the cervical spine into the skull.

In the elderly and in where there is arterial disease, ligament laxity or joint instability forceful extension can result in arterial irritation or tearing. People who are congenitally hypermobile should be cautious when extending the head on the neck. The stretch is best achieved solely using the weight of head. The stretch should be localised to the cervical and upper thoracic spine. The rest of the spine should remain straight. Do not bend backwards in the middle thoracic or lumbar spine. Care should be taken not to put excessive pressure on the joints in the lower cervical vertebra if they have been subject to degenerative changes.

2. C6 & C7 - the lower cervical spine and cervicothoracic junction.

Care should be taken not to put excessive pressure on the lower cervical spine if the discs and joints have undergone degenerative changes. These tissues are vulnerable to injury and overstretching may cause further tissue damage.

3. Any of the vertebrae in the thoracolumbar spine T11, T12 or L1 may be fixed in an extended position. The key to preventing further extension at T4 and in the thoracolumbar region is to keep the thoracic spine relatively straight and rigid with the stabilising action of muscles in the hips and abdomen or with the support of the back of a chair or pillow.

4. The middle thoracic spine near to T4 is sometimes fixed in an extended position. Care should be taken not to push T4 into further extension.

Key:

1.5 Head & neck extension stretch seated	

Related stretches					
1.1a, b & c The Lion kneeling, seated & standing		2.6b Full Cobra		2.8 Extended cat	
6.5d Bilateral post- isometric stretch for hip adductors and extensors sitting		6.5h Bilateral stretch for the hip adductors standing		7.0a to 7.0d Forward bend sitting	

1.6 Neck rotation stretch - active stretch for the suboccipital, cervical and upper thoracic spine

1.6 Head & neck active rotation stretch seated

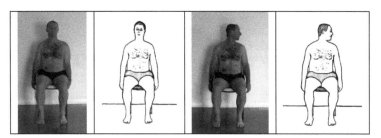

Starting position: Seated with your feet apart and firmly planted on the floor, arms hanging at your sides and your shoulders relaxed. Turn your head left until it is in a comfortable fully rotated position.

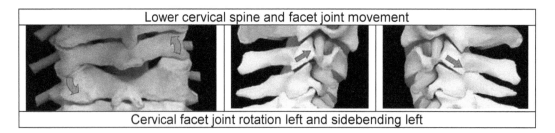

Technique: See Part A. Page 60

Direction and range of movement

Rotation of the head, neck and upper thoracic spine (occiput to T2) is about 90 degrees each side. About 50% of total rotation occurs in the suboccipital spine, mainly between C1 and C2.

Lower cervical spine and facet joint movement

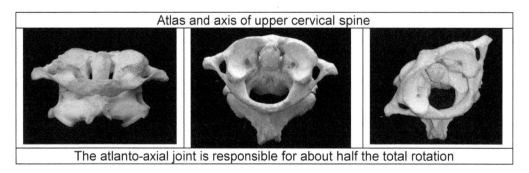

Cervical facet joint rotation left and sidebending left

In the cervical spine rotation is coupled with sidebending. In the atlanto-occipital joints rotation to the left is coupled with sidebending to the right and vice versa for rotation right. In the rest of the joints of the cervical spine from below C2, rotation to the left is coupled with sidebending to the left and vice versa for rotation right.

Atlas and axis of upper cervical spine

The atlanto-axial joint is responsible for about half the total rotation

Target tissues

This is an active stretch for the sub-occipital muscles, and the superficial and deep cervical rotator muscles. The suboccipital muscles that are most stretched with rotation are the rectus capitis posterior major and obliquus capitis inferior. Of the deep cervical group of muscles, multifidus is stretched the most with rotation.

Rotatores may be absent in the cervical spine but would be stretched in the upper thoracic spine. Other posterior cervical muscles stretched with rotation include semispinalis capitis, semispinalis cervicis, splenius cervicis and splenius capitis, and of the erector spinae group the longissimus capitis is the most stretched. This is a weak stretch for sternocleidomastoid and levator scapulae but will lengthen these muscles when they are very short.

Some of these muscles are anchored to a ribs but the majority attach to the vertebra, running between one to several vertebral levels.

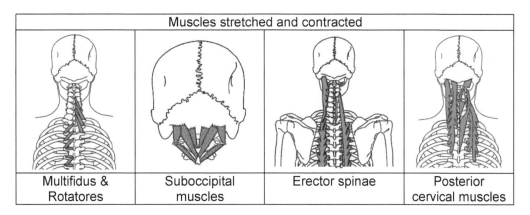

Muscles stretched and contracted			
Multifidus & Rotatores	Suboccipital muscles	Erector spinae	Posterior cervical muscles

The active stretch involves the contraction of muscles responsible for rotating the head and neck. The muscles on one side of the cervical spine are used to stretch the muscles on the opposite side.

The following muscles contract to produce head and neck rotation: rectus capitis posterior major and obliquus capitis inferior of the sub-occipital group; multifidus, splenius capitis and splenius cervicis of the deep cervical rotator group; and levator scapulae and sternocleidomastoid are the superficial muscles.

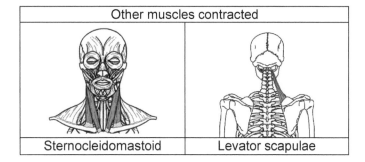

Other muscles contracted	
Sternocleidomastoid	Levator scapulae

Variations

This can also be done standing, kneeling or supine or prone. This can be done as a post-isometric technique but care should be taken not to pull on the head, straining the suboccipital muscles and ligaments. The post-isometric technique is done by placing the palm of one hand against the side of the face and applying a rotation muscle contraction against the hand.

The hand offers an equal and opposite counterforce, an unyielding resistance to the rotation of the head. After about five seconds exhale, cease the isometric muscle contraction, then relax and rotate the head further to the side. The muscles responsible for diagonal eye movement can also be used to increase cervical rotation. The eye technique is described above in the active stretch. Increase head rotation after each eye movement.

Safety

Occiput, C1 and C2 - the occipito-atlanto-axial joints of the sub-occipital region. Care should be taken not to over-stretch the muscles and ligaments of the suboccipital region. These are vulnerable and can be strained with excessive force. The upper cervical spine may be hypermobile and this stretch is best achieved using active muscle contraction. Strains to the sub-occipital region mostly occur if you pull on the head.

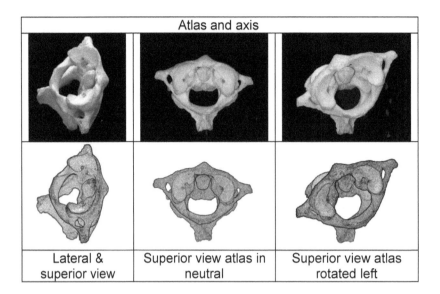

Atlas and axis		
Lateral & superior view	Superior view atlas in neutral	Superior view atlas rotated left

Vulnerable areas

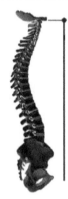

Occiput, C1 & C2

	Region	Level of Risk
1.	Occiput, C1 & C2	Low

Key:

1.6 Neck Rotation stretch	

Related stretches					
2.6d Rotation Cobra		3.1a Passive spinal twist seated		3.1b Active spinal twist seated	
3.1c Spinal twist sitting on the floor		3.2b Active spinal twist standing		3.5 Passive and active spinal twist prone	

1.7 Neck sidebending stretches - active, passive and isometric for the suboccipital, cervical, upper thoracic and shoulders

*Head & neck **active** sidebending stretch with both shoulders relaxed and both arms **free** to hang at your side. Stretch for the lateral neck muscles.*

1.7a & 1.7e Free shoulder

Starting position: Seated with both feet planted on the floor, both shoulders relaxed and both arms hanging freely at your side. In this position there is less pull on trapezius and greater stretch can be applied to the lateral cervical muscles. Other movements may be combined with sidebending to localise the stretch to different muscles and muscle fibres: rotation, anterior or posterior translation, flexion or extension. Different amounts of sideshifting of the upper thoracic spine can be used to localise the stretch to different areas of the cervical and upper thoracic spine. The free shoulder stretch can also be done standing.

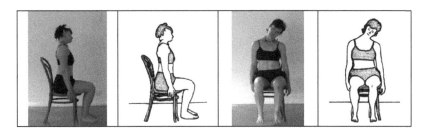

To localise the stretch to different cervical rotator muscles combine sidebending with greater amounts of rotation to the left. To localise the stretch to different areas of the cervical or upper thoracic spine combine sidebending with sideshifting (lateral translation). Move your body weight onto your right buttock to sideshift to the right. Greater amounts of sideshifting localises the stretch further down the thoracic spine. Also to localise the stretch to other cervical muscles combine sidebending with different combinations of rotation, anterior translation or posterior translation, flexion or extension.

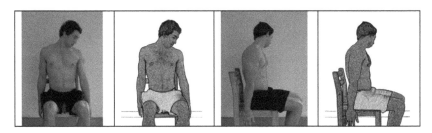

Technique: See Part A. Pages 61 and 65

*Head & neck **active** sidebending stretch with one shoulder **fixed** in a depressed position and serving as an anchor for the localised stretching of trapezius & other muscles.*

Fixed shoulder
1.7b, 1.7c, 1.7d, & 1.7f.

Starting position: Seated with both feet planted on the floor. Sideshift your body to one side, reach down to the floor with your hand and grasp the side of the chair. This fixes one shoulder in a descended position. Keep the other shoulder relaxed. As an alternative to grasping a chair the shoulder can be held in a descended position by contracting shoulder depressor muscles.

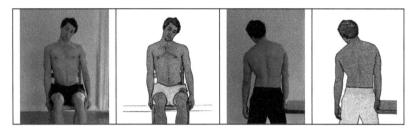

Sidebend your head away from the side of the fixed depressed shoulder. Feel the stretch in trapezius which is anchored to the fixed shoulder. The lateral cervical muscles will be less stretched. To localise the stretch to different shoulder muscles and muscle fibres other movements may be combined with sidebending. Upper thoracic sideshifting can be introduced to localise the stretch down the upper thoracic spine. The fixed shoulder stretch can also be done standing.

Technique: See Part A. Pages 62, 63, 64 and 66

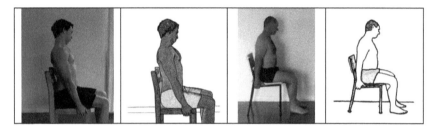

Posterior translation combined with sidebending, localises the stretch to sternocleidomastoid and the clavicular fibres of upper trapezius. The more rotation you introduce during sidebending the more you stretch levator scapulae and the less you stretch upper trapezius.

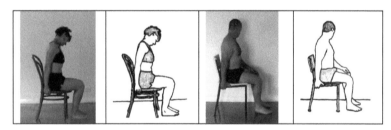

Sidebending combined with flexion stretches rhomboid minor, posterior fascia and the fibres of trapezius, which attach on the spine of the scapula. If you also tuck your chin in, you will increase the stretch to the occipital fibres of trapezius. Combine sidebending with different combinations of rotation, anterior translation, posterior translation, flexion or extension to vary the stretch. Localise the stretch down the thoracic spine with greater amounts of sideshifting.

*Head & neck **post-isometric** sidebending technique with one shoulder **fixed** in a depressed position, and serving as an anchor for the localised stretching of trapezius and other neck and shoulder muscles.*

1.7g & 1.7h Fixed post-isometric

Starting position: Seated with both feet planted on the floor. Sideshift your body to one side, reach down to the floor with your hand and grasp the side of the chair; this fixes the shoulder in a descended position. Raise your other arm, reach over your head with your hand to grasp your head and suboccipital spine on the side of the fixed shoulder.

Sidebend your head away from the side of the fixed depressed shoulder but stop before you feel a stretch in trapezius, which is anchored to the fixed shoulder. To localise the lengthening

276

effect of the technique to specific shoulder muscles and muscle fibres, other movements may be combined with sidebending. Upper thoracic sideshifting can be introduced to localise sidebending further down the upper thoracic spine. The fixed post-isometric shoulder technique can also be done standing.

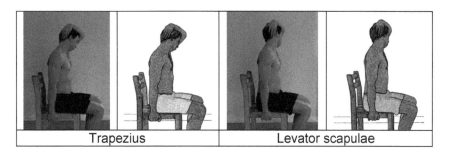

Trapezius | Levator scapulae

Technique: Sidebend your head to the left. Take in a deep breath and hold it in. Attempt to push your head to the right but resist the movement with your left hand using an equal and opposite counterforce. After about 5 seconds cease the contraction, exhale and sidebend your head left to the new tension barrier - do not pull on the head.

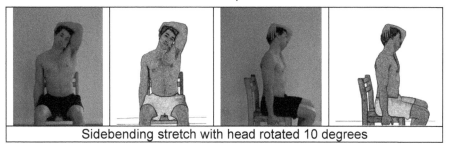

Sidebending stretch with head rotated 10 degrees

To localise the technique to middle scalene and the fibres of trapezius attached to the acromion process keep your head and neck in neutral; do not allow your head to rotate left. To localise muscle lengthening to the occipital fibres of trapezius tuck your chin in and flex your head. To localise muscle lengthening to the clavicular fibres of trapezius move your head backwards without tilting it (posterior translation), while holding the chair near the front leg.

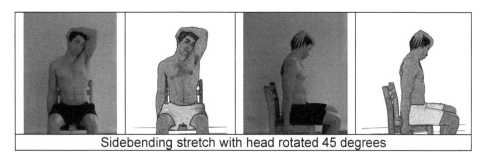

Sidebending stretch with head rotated 45 degrees

To localise the technique to anterior scalene use posterior translation but allow your chin to poke out a bit. To localise muscle lengthening to the scapular fibres of trapezius and the posterior neck muscles flex your head and neck and hold the chair near the back leg.

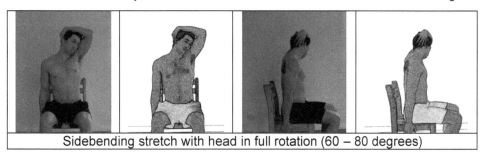

Sidebending stretch with head in full rotation (60 – 80 degrees)

By rotating your head and cervical spine to the left you will localise the technique on the levator scapulae. Combine sidebending with different combinations of rotation, anterior translation, posterior translation, flexion or extension to vary the stretch. Localise the stretch down the thoracic spine with greater amounts of sideshifting of your upper body.

1.7i Levator scapulae active, passive or post-isometric stretch sidelying

Starting position: Lying on your left side on the floor. Rest on your left shoulder with your left arm straight out in front of you, or bent at the elbow and tucked under your rib cage. Position your body so your shoulders and ribs are perpendicular to the floor. Reach down your right side with your right hand and place your palm flat on your right hip. Allow your head to drop to the floor into a left sidebent position. Rotate your head as far as possible to the left so the left side of your forehead rests on the floor.

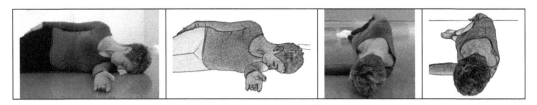

Technique: See Part A. Page 69

Direction and range of movement

The upper cervical spine is that part of the spine between the C2 and the occiput, and includes the axis articulating with the atlas at the atlanto-axial joints and the atlas articulating with the occiput at the atlanto-occipital joints. The lower cervical spine is that part of the spine between the C2 and T1 of the thoracic spine.

Full sidebending of the head, cervical and upper thoracic spine (Occiput to T4) is about 45 degrees each side. Full rotation of the head and cervical spine is about 90 degrees each side. About half of the rotation is between C1 (atlas) and C2 (axis).The other half is fairly evenly distributed down the rest of the cervical spine.

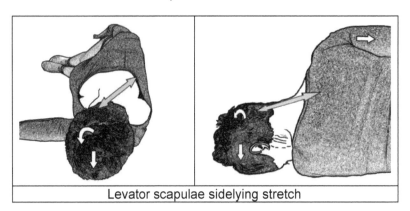

Levator scapulae sidelying stretch

Sidebending and rotation are coupled movements. The more movement taken up by one, the less there is available for the other. At the atlanto-occipital joint sidebending occurs in the opposite direction to rotation whereas in the rest of the cervical spine sidebending occurs in the same direction as rotation.

In addition to the sidebending and rotation coupling, there is also some automatic extension in the lower cervical spine during sidebending. This is compensated for in the upper cervical spine with increased flexion.

During sidebending the facet joints on one side of the lower cervical spine slide upwards and the facet joint on the other side slides downwards. It is a consequence to this sliding movement of the lower cervical spine that sidebending, rotation and extension are composite

278

movements, linked together; during sidebending left there is always some rotation to the left and some extension of the facet on the side of sidebending.

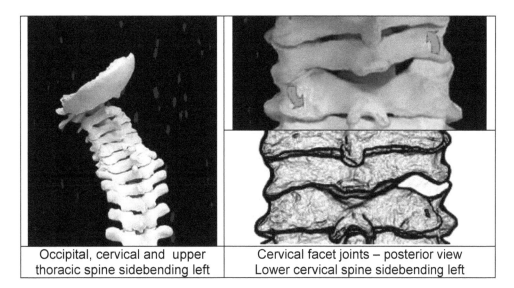

Occipital, cervical and upper thoracic spine sidebending left	Cervical facet joints – posterior view Lower cervical spine sidebending left

The upper cervical spine needs to compensate for the lower cervical sidebending, rotation and extension combined movements to maintain the head in a neutral position. This is achieved by the suboccipital muscles, which finely tune the position of the head so that it remains pointing to the front, by removing the unwanted rotation and extension components.

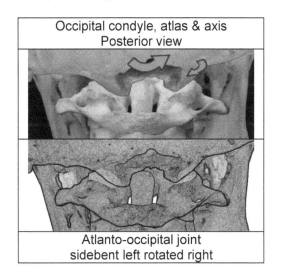

Occipital condyle, atlas & axis
Posterior view

Atlanto-occipital joint
sidebent left rotated right

Sidebending is greatest while the head and neck remains in the coronal plane, and decreases as other movements are introduced. Sidebending progressively decreases with increasing levels of rotation, flexion, extension or anterior or posterior translation. The more there is of each individual movement, and the more combinations of movements are introduced, the less movement will be available for sidebending.

Target tissues

The sidebending techniques primarily stretch the lateral muscles of the shoulders, cervical and upper thoracic spines. With the introduction of additional movements the sidebending techniques also stretch anterolateral and posterolateral muscles.

The shoulders muscles most stretched are trapezius and levator scapulae and the muscles least stretched are sternocleidomastoid and the rhomboid muscles. In the cervical region the muscles stretched include: the suboccipital muscles (rectus capitis lateralis, rectus capitis anterior, rectus capitis posterior major, obliquus capitis superior and obliquus capitis inferior), intertransversarii, multifidus, the prevertebral muscles (longus capitis and longus colli), the posterior cervical muscles (semispinalis capitis, semispinalis cervicis, splenius cervicis and splenius capitis), anterior, middle and posterior scalene muscles and erector spinae (iliocostalis cervicis, longissimus cervicis, longissimus capitis and spinalis cervicis). To a lesser extent the sidebending also stretches platysma and lateral cervical fascia.

The lower attachment of all these muscles includes the posterior and lateral parts of a vertebra, the middle shaft of a rib, the scapula and clavicle.

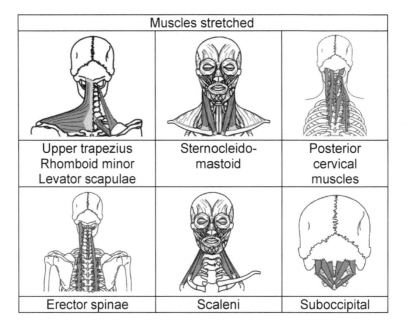

Muscles stretched		
Upper trapezius Rhomboid minor Levator scapulae	Sternocleido-mastoid	Posterior cervical muscles
Erector spinae	Scaleni	Suboccipital

During active sidebending of the head and neck the muscles that are stretched on one side of the neck are the same muscles, by name - but on the opposite side of the neck - as those that contract to produce the movement. In other words the muscles (agonists) on one side of the neck contract to stretch their paired mirror counterpart muscles (antagonists) on the other side of the neck. The list of muscles stretched (above) is therefore identical to the list of muscles contracted in the performance of the active stretch.

There are 8 sidebending techniques described in chapter 1.7 - a mixture of sidebending, sidebending with flexion, sidebending with translation (usually posterior translation, occasionally anterior translation) and sidebending with rotation.

Within the group of sidebending techniques there are four main variables that influence which parts of the spine and which muscles are stretched:

1. One shoulder fixed in a depressed position or both shoulders free.
2. The head and neck in neutral, flexion, extension, anterior translation or posterior translation during sidebending.
3. Rotation combined with head and neck sidebending.
4. Lateral translation or sideshifting of the upper thoracic spine.

Sidebending variables

1. One shoulder fixed in a depressed position or both shoulders free

One shoulder is fixed in a depressed position by reaching down towards the floor, hooking your fingers around the side of a chair or table and grasping under it. The scapula and clavicle then become anchor points for two major shoulder muscles; the levator scapulae and upper trapezius, which can be stretched and lengthened, by sidebending the head and neck. By combining sidebending with other movements the stretch can be localised to target specific muscles and muscle fibres.

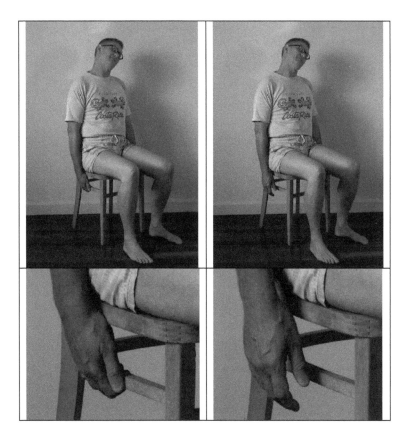

When the shoulder is fixed in the depressed position, and the head and neck sidebent away from the fixed shoulder, the stretch will be greater in the upper trapezius and levator scapulae muscles than in the lateral cervical muscles because the lateral cervical muscles have no scapular or clavicular attachment. The rhomboid minor and sternocleidomastoid are attached to the medial sides of the scapula and clavicle, and so when the head and neck are sidebent they will also be stretched - but to a much lesser extent.

Muscles stretched	
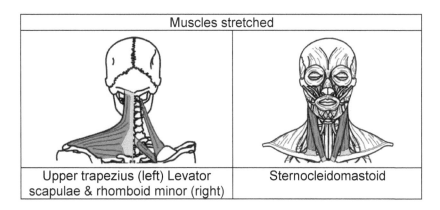	
Upper trapezius (left) Levator scapulae & rhomboid minor (right)	Sternocleidomastoid

When the shoulder is fixed, upper trapezius is stretched the most, levator scapulae is moderately stretched, while sternocleidomastoid and rhomboid minor are mildly stretched. The lateral cervical muscles are least stretched.

As an alternative to grasping under a chair or table specific shoulder muscles can be contracted to hold the scapula and clavicle in the depressed position. These muscles include: pectoralis minor, lower trapezius (part IV), latissimus dorsi, subclavius and inferior fibres of pectoralis major and serratus anterior.

When the shoulder is free the muscles are relaxed and the arm is allowed to naturally hang down at the side of the body. The weight of the scapula, clavicle and upper limb depresses the shoulder. The total weight of these pulling on trapezius is not great, but adds mild resistance to the muscle when there is head and neck sidebending stretch away from the depressed arm.

In the seated position, if you place your forearm on your thigh you will relax and shorten the trapezius. The shoulder will be free to lift off the rib cage. The shoulder is not held in a depressed position nor is it pulled down by gravity.

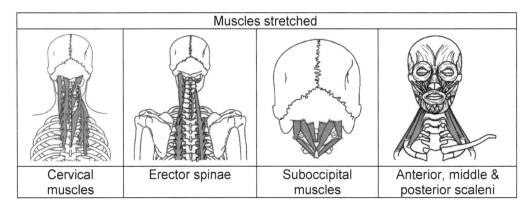

Muscles stretched			
Cervical muscles	Erector spinae	Suboccipital muscles	Anterior, middle & posterior scaleni

When the head and neck are sidebent in the relaxed position the upper trapezius and levator scapulae muscles are shortened and they are stretched less stretch, especially when compared with the lateral cervical muscles.

The following cervical muscles are stretched when the shoulder is free:
rectus capitis lateralis, rectus capitis anterior, rectus capitis posterior major and minor, obliquus capitis superior and inferior, intertransversarii, multifidus, longus capitis, longus colli, semispinalis capitis and cervicis, splenius capitis and cervicis, anterior, middle and posterior scalene, iliocostalis cervicis, longissimus cervicis and spinalis cervicis. The more lateral the muscle, the greater the stretch. So during head side bending, rectus capitis posterior major will be stretched more than rectus capitis posterior minor.

2. The head and neck in neutral, flexion, extension, anterior translation or posterior translation during sidebending

Neutral
A neutral cervical spine is where the overall tissue tension is lowest and the vertebrae are in a balanced state, at or near the midpoint position between flexion and extension, and anterior and posterior translation. In the neutral position the ligaments and muscles are in their most relaxed state, the facet joints are idling and there is symmetrical and minimal disc compression.

As explained earlier, sidebending and rotation are coupled movements. During sidebending, rotation automatically occurs with sidebending and in the same direction. In addition to rotation, extension also plays a role in sidebending. So from a biomechanical perspective there is no neutral cervical spine during sidebending; neutral only exists for the head. The head is in neutral when it is in the vertical anatomical position and as a result of complex compensatory mechanisms which keep it from tilting during sidebending. By neutral, I am therefore only referring to the head; specifically to the absence of flexion or extension or anterior or posterior translation of the head during sidebending.

For the head to maintain a neutral stance during sidebending, ipsilateral rotation and extension in the lower cervical spine, is compensated for in the upper cervical spine with contralateral rotation and flexion.

When there is head and neck sidebending in the neutral position, the cervical muscles stretched the most are: rectus capitis lateralis, obliquus capitis superior and inferior, intertransversarii, semispinalis capitis and cervicis, splenius capitis and cervicis, anterior, middle and posterior scalene and iliocostalis cervicis.

282

The cervical muscles stretched the least with neutral sidebending include: rectus capitis anterior, rectus capitis posterior major, longus capitis, longus colli, longissimus cervicis and spinalis cervicis.

Posterior translation
Posterior translation is a combination of head flexion, cervical flexion and upper thoracic extension. It is achieved by taking your head backwards, while tucking your chin in and maintaining your head in vertical position.

Combining sidebending with posterior translation is useful when you want to stretch short muscles associated with an anterior translation posture – head extension, cervical extension and upper thoracic flexion. The anteriorly translated head posture is by far the most common form of bad posture - the classical dowager hump between C7 and T2, the chin poking out, while the head slumps forwards and down. Posterior translation with sidebending is the most appropriate stretch when an anterior translation posture coexists with a dowager hump.

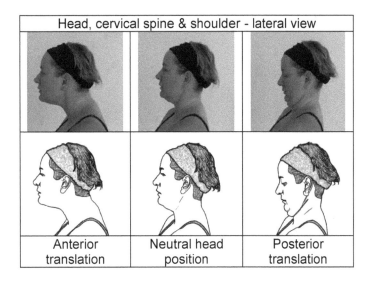

Head, cervical spine & shoulder - lateral view

| Anterior translation | Neutral head position | Posterior translation |

When head and neck sidebending is combined with posterior translation this becomes a unilateral stretch for sternocleidomastoid, the clavicular and acromial fibres of upper trapezius, and in the cervical spine rectus capitis lateralis, rectus capitis posterior major, obliquus capitis superior and inferior, splenius capitis and cervicis, anterior scalene, semispinalis capitis, and the most superior cervical fibres of intertransversarii, multifidus, spinalis cervicis, semispinalis cervicis, longissimus cervicis and iliocostalis cervicis.

As the previous paragraph indicates many muscles are responsible for maintaining the anterior head translation posture. But in terms of its contribution to this poor posture and its effect on respiration and the arterial and nerve supply to the upper limb the anterior scalene muscle stands out as being the most significant of these muscles.

In addition to challenging an anterior translation posture with sidebending and posterior translation, the anterior translation posture can be challenged using the bilateral stretch described as the Chin tuck in chapter 1.3.

Anterior translation
Anterior translation is a combination of head extension, upper cervical extension and lower cervical and upper thoracic flexion – an exaggeration of the cervical lordosis, especially in the upper cervical spine. Anterior translation is achieved by taking your head forwards while poking your chin out and maintaining your head in vertical position.

Combining sidebending with anterior translation is useful when you want to stretch short muscles associated with a posterior translation posture – head flexion, cervical flexion and upper thoracic extension – the reversed cervical lordosis. And it may be useful in the rare situation where the head is fixed in a bilateral flexed position.

When head and neck sidebending is combined with anterior translation this becomes a unilateral stretch for rectus capitis anterior, longus capitis, longus colli and posterior scalene.

Head and neck flexion
Head and neck flexion is a combination of head flexion (also known as nutation), cervical flexion and upper thoracic flexion. It is achieved by tilting your head forwards and downwards.

Combining sidebending with head and neck flexion is useful when you want to stretch short upper cervical muscles associated with an anterior head translation posture. It is also useful when you want to stretch short erector spinae associated with an extended upper thoracic spine between T3 and T5. Head and neck flexion should not be used if there is an acutely flexed upper thoracic between C7 and T2, known as a dowager hump, as flexion will tend to exaggerate the hump. Whenever a dowager hump is present use posterior head translation, either alone or combined with the sidebending.

Occiput, cervical & thoracic spine - lateral view	
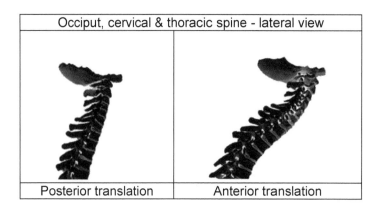	
Posterior translation	Anterior translation

Head flexion can be useful for localising the stretch to the most posterior cervical muscles, the occipital fibres of upper trapezius and the posterior suboccipital muscles, especially rectus capitis posterior major. It is particularly helpful for relieving tension in antigravity muscles of the upper thoracic spine including the rhomboid and middle trapezius.

When head and neck sidebending is combined with flexion this becomes a unilateral stretch for the fibres of upper and middle trapezius. It is also a mild stretch for levator scapulae, rhomboid minor and to a lesser extent rhomboid major. In the cervical spine it is a stretch for rectus capitis lateralis, rectus capitis posterior major, obliquus capitis superior, obliquus capitis inferior, intertransversarii, multifidus, semispinalis capitis, semispinalis cervicis, splenius cervicis, splenius capitis, posterior scalene, iliocostalis cervicis, longissimus cervicis and spinalis cervicis.

Head and neck extension
Head and neck extension is a combination of head extension (also known as counter-nutation), cervical extension and upper thoracic extension. It is achieved by tilting your head backwards and downwards.

Combining sidebending with head and neck extension, is useful when you want to stretch short muscles associated with a posterior head translation posture and a dowager hump – head flexion, cervical flexion and upper thoracic flexion. It can be used to counter the flexion rigidity of a reversed cervical lordosis.

When head and neck sidebending is combined with extension this becomes a unilateral stretch for sternocleidomastoid, anterior scalene, rectus capitis anterior and the prevertebral muscles - longus colli and longus capitis. When the jaw is closed this will also stretch platysma and the inferior and superior hyoid muscles.

Each combination of stretches - sidebending with posterior translation, sidebending with anterior translation, sidebending with flexion and sidebending with extension is useful for a specific type of posture. The stretches that you use depend on your unique posture. It is important to improve posture by stretching the right muscles and to avoid making a bad posture worse.

Although generalised stretching is good for all muscles, targeted localised stretches such as these require that you have a reasonable knowledge of your own posture. It may be helpful to have your posture evaluated by a qualified therapist who will then be able to prescribe the correct exercises. Spinal X-rays are useful if you want to know the shape of your spine and be sure you are doing the right stretches.

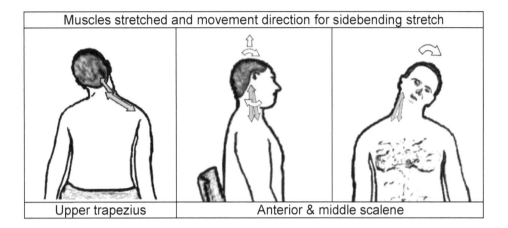

Muscles stretched and movement direction for sidebending stretch		
Upper trapezius	Anterior & middle scalene	

Here are some generalisations about the cervical and upper thoracic spine and human posture that may be useful.

The neutral cervical spine has a smooth even posterior facing concave curvature - a cervical lordosis. But this is the typical text book view of the cervical spine and in reality it doesn't look like this.

In humans there is a range of postures with extremes of anterior translation and posterior translation at each end and neutral in the middle. Individual humans may lie anywhere along this spectrum but a mild to moderate anterior head translation posture is by far the most common postural variation, with the majority of people lying between neutral and extreme anterior translation.

The neutral cervical posture and the exaggerated upper cervical lordosis associated with the anterior head translation posture and are the most common postures found in the adult human population. The decreased or reversed cervical lordosis exists but it is rare. The neutral upper thoracic posture and the flexed upper thoracic (dowager hump) are common, as is the extended upper thoracic posture between T2 or T3 and T5. The number of vertebra involved does vary but the extended posture is part of the universal posture found in most people.

In the anterior translation posture the head can be extended bilaterally with both occipital condyles fixed anteriorly, or it can be extended unilaterally with only one occipital condyle fixed anteriorly. More commonly, only the right occiput is fixed anteriorly at the atlanto-occipital joint. When this occurs the head will also be rotated to the left and sidebent to the right. The head doesn't actually rotate to the left or sidebend to the right because vertebra below the atlanto-occipital joint compensate by rotating and sidebending in the opposite direction. The head is kept straight and vertical. In addition to compensating for rotation and sidebending, lower cervical spine also compensate for head extension by increasing flexion. The end result is usually extension in the upper half of the cervical spine and progressively greater levels of flexion below; especially at the cervicothoracic junction between C7 and T2, which becomes the characteristic dowager hump. Below this the thoracic usually extends. The extension can be at one vertebral level (usually T4) or over a range of vertebral levels (usually T2 to T5). Below this extended area the thoracic is usually moderately flexed but any variation is possible from an extremely convex increased thoracic kyphosis to a flat 'poker' back posture or even on rare occasions there may be a reversed thoracic kyphosis.

Our posture is influenced by three main factors: our genes, gravity and muscle tone, including muscle and ligament elasticity. We cannot change our genetic programming but we can counter its effects with postural management skills such as maintaining a good sitting posture, and appropriate stretching and strengthening exercises done regularly. Stress management skills may also be necessary as high stress levels increases muscle tone, and this can affect posture.

Gravity acts on our body all the time but is particularly problematic when we are sitting or standing. It pushes down on our structures, especially when they stray away from our centre of gravity. Postural muscles at the back of our neck, upper thoracic and shoulders are subject to the effects of gravity when we are slouching over a desk. Over time, gravity causes postural fatigue, which results in structural changes in muscles and ligaments and ultimately the exaggeration of our genetically determined structures. The dowager hump for example becomes progressively more pronounced with age.

The posterior translated posture is also known as a fixed flexion posture or reversed cervical lordosis. This posture is less flexible than the neutral concave cervical lordosis because the facet joints are in flexion and the ligaments are permanently stretched. An inflexible cervical spine is a problem for the obvious reason that it reduces mobility of the head, but also because it compromises the functionality of nerves and blood vessels and over time results in increased wear on the intervertebral discs and facet joints.

While generalised spinal rigidity or hypomobility is an unwanted characteristic of a posteriorly translated cervical spine, localised areas of hypomobility and hypermobility are unwanted characteristics of an anteriorly translated cervical spine.

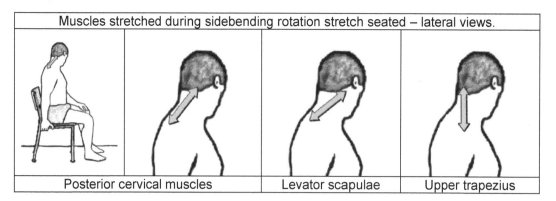

Muscles stretched during sidebending rotation stretch seated – lateral views.		
Posterior cervical muscles	Levator scapulae	Upper trapezius

3. Rotation combined with head and neck sidebending

When sidebending is combined with rotation to the same side this increases the stretch to levator scapulae. In the cervical spine it increases the stretch of rectus capitis posterior major, obliquus capitis inferior, splenius cervicis, splenius capitis, iliocostalis cervicis, longissimus cervicis and spinalis cervicis.
When sidebending is combined with rotation to the opposite side this increases the stretch to upper trapezius, sternocleidomastoid and rhomboid minor, while in the cervical spine it increases the stretch to rectus capitis lateralis, rectus capitis anterior, obliquus capitis superior, intertransversarii, longus capitis, longus colli, semispinalis capitis, semispinalis cervicis, anterior scalene, middle scalene, posterior scalene and multifidus.

With low levels of rotation during sidebending the stretch is more localised to: rectus capitis lateralis, rectus capitis anterior, longus capitis, longus colli, semispinalis capitis and semispinalis cervicis.

With high levels of rotation during sidebending the stretch is more localised to: rectus capitis posterior major and obliquus capitis inferior, splenius capitis and cervicis, iliocostalis cervicis and to a lesser extent longissimus cervicis, spinalis cervicis and the scalenes.

In contrast to sidebending which mainly stretches the fibres of muscles and ligaments that run in a vertical plane, especially the most lateral fibres, rotation mainly stretches the fibres of muscles and ligaments that run in a horizontal or transverse plane.

During rotation in the lower cervical spine the facet joint on one side of the spine slides upwards while the facet joint on the other side slides downwards.

Rotation, sidebending and extension are composite movements - in other words extension and sidebending are always linked with rotation and during rotation there is always some sidebending and some extension. In the lower cervical spine rotation left results in sidebending to the left, and extension of the facet on the side of rotation. This sidebending and extension in the lower cervical spine is compensated for with flexion and sidebending in the opposite direction of the upper cervical spine. The suboccipital muscles act to finely tune the position of the head so that it remains upright by removing the unwanted sidebending and extension components.

4. Lateral translation or sideshifting of the upper thoracic spine.

Sideshifting or lateral translation of the upper thoracic spine and shoulders, influences which part of the cervical and upper thoracic spine you will stretch. Sideshifting is achieved by moving the weight of your body towards one of your ischial tuberosities. Depending how far you move, you can localise the apex of the sidebending curve to your lower cervical spine, cervicothoracic junction, upper thoracic spine or middle thoracic spine.

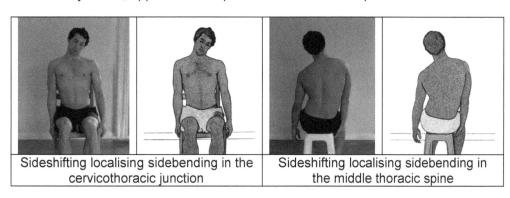

Sideshifting localising sidebending in the cervicothoracic junction	Sideshifting localising sidebending in the middle thoracic spine

Tilting your pelvis at different angles changes your centre of gravity and forces your spine to sidebend in different parts of the spine, it localises the apex of the sidebending curve to one area in the spine. The cervical or thoracic spinal muscles are maximally stretched at the apex of the curve and by altering the pelvic tilt you can focus the stretch. Once the correct sideshifting sidebending posture has been found then the position can be fixed by holding the side of the chair at the nearest available point.

When your body is equally balanced on both buttocks and your spine is upright, then when you sidebend your head, the apex of the sidebending curve will be localised near to the middle of your cervical spine. With a small amount of sideshifting, the apex of the sidebending curve, and the greatest level of stretch, will be localised near the lower cervical spine.

With moderate amounts of sideshifting the apex will localised the stretch to the cervicothoracic junction. If you tilt the pelvis so there is maximum sideshifting, the apex of sidebending curve will localise to the upper or middle thoracic spine. In general as you take more weight onto one ischial tuberosity the apex shifts lower down the spine and the stretch is greater lower down the spine.

The further you sidebend your head and cervical spine the further down the spine the apex of the sidebending curve will be. Combine head and cervical sidebending with sideshifting to fine tune the stretch to different area of the spine. Also the further you sideshift your upper thoracic spine the more emphasis there is on stretching trapezius compared with other muscles.

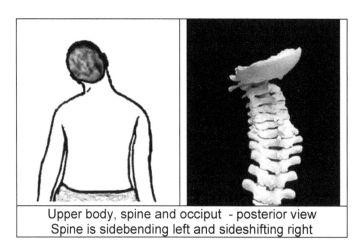

Upper body, spine and occiput - posterior view
Spine is sidebending left and sideshifting right

Variations

In addition to the seated and standing stretches described, the sidebending stretches can also be done kneeling, supine or sidelying. If done kneeling, reach down towards the floor with one hand and grasp your ankle. Holding under your ankle as far as possible will fix your shoulder in the depressed position. Sidebend your head and neck away from the fixed shoulder to stretch your cervical and shoulder muscles.

If done supine, reach down one side of your body with one arm to depress your scapula, then fix your scapula in the depressed position by placing your hand under your buttock. Use the weight of your pelvis to pin down your arm, then sidebend your head and neck to stretch your cervical and shoulder muscles. A small pillow under your head may be useful to prevent over extension and ligament strain in the upper cervical spine.

Seated is arguably the most useful of the positions available for doing the active and post-isometric sidebending techniques. This is because in the seated position, the ischial tuberosities can be used as pivot points around which the pelvis can be tilted. In addition, and sidebending can be combined with sideshifting to localise the stretch in different areas of the spine (see 4).

Seated is not however a good position for doing passive sidebending stretches for the cervical spine. Although the adult head weighs about 5 kg, when you attempt to sidebend the head in the seated position, the head does not move far enough beyond its centre of gravity to exert sufficient force to passively stretch the lateral cervical and shoulder muscles. In the seated or standing positions passive sidebending stretching is not effective. The passive sidebending stretches can only be done when the body is in a sidelying position or when the spine is in a partially sidebent position.

Safety

Post-isometric techniques are safe when done correctly. They do however have potential dangers in the cervical spine; especially for cervical sidebending.

The active stretches require the contraction of intrinsic lateral neck muscles to create sidebending of the head and neck. The intrinsic muscles are paired opposites, with the agonists on one side of the cervical spine contracting and stretching the antagonists on the other. These cervical muscles are relatively weak compared with the muscles of the upper or lower limb. Also the paired opposites are equal in power. As a result of these two facts it is fair to say that contraction of the intrinsic muscles is unlikely to cause over-stretching, thus the active stretches are relatively safe techniques.

In contrast, the post-isometric techniques use extrinsic muscles of the upper limb to sidebend the head and neck. These upper limb muscles are powerful and can overwhelm the relatively weak neck muscles. They should not be used to stretch the lateral neck muscles because there is the potential for straining them, including the suboccipital muscles and ligaments.

The post-isometric technique may be combined with the active or passive stretch but it is not an active or a passive stretch. It is a relocalisation of joint position after isometric contraction. After isometrically contracting the lateral cervical muscles the correct response should be to just take up the slack gained by the muscle contraction. Do not pull on the head. In some situations and for some joints and muscles the post-isometric technique can be followed with a passive stretch. But this is not true for cervical sidebending.

Do not place your hands on the side of the head and use your arm to pull your head to one side; the passive stretch, assisted by the upper limb is potentially dangerous. The lateral ligaments and cervical muscles are relatively weak when compared with the shoulder and arm muscles. They are more vulnerable to strain and can easily be injured by pulling with the arm. The force coming from the hand and leverage on the neck created due to the position of the arm, could strain the muscles or ligaments on the side of the neck, causing disc damage or irritating the nerves of the brachial plexus.

With age and trauma the lower cervical spine is subjected to degenerative changes and stiffness. There may also be hypermobility in the joints above or below the areas of restriction; hypermobility is especially common in the sub-occipital area of the spine.

The active stretches are the safest of the sidebending techniques. The passive stretches and the post-isometric techniques are safe provided no external force is applied to the head. In particular excessive force from upper limb muscle contraction, as well as leverage, should be avoided. Be especially careful with the sidebending techniques if there is cervical spine pathology such as osteoarthritis.

<u>Vulnerable areas</u>

1. The sub-occipital region - occipito-atlanto-axial joints (Occiput, C1 & C2)
2. The lower cervical spine and cervico-thoracic junction (C6, C7 & T1) if there is disc disease and arthritic changes.

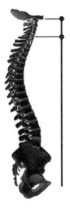
Occiput, C1 & C2
C6 & C7

	Region	Level of Risk
1.	Occiput, C1 & C2	Medium
2.	C6 & C7	Medium

Key:

1.7a Head & neck active sidebending stretch seated. Free shoulders	
1.7b Head, neck & shoulder active sidebending stretch seated. Fixed shoulder	
1.7c Head, neck & shoulder active sidebending and flexion stretch for trapezius seated. Fixed shoulder	
1.7d Head, neck & shoulder active sidebending stretch standing. Fixed shoulder	
1.7e Head & neck active sidebending and rotation stretch seated. Free shoulders	
1.7f Head, neck & shoulder active sidebending and rotation stretch for levator scapulae seated. Fixed shoulder	
1.7g Head, neck & shoulder post-isometric sidebending and rotation stretch seated. Fixed shoulder	
1.7h Post-isometric stretch for trapezius and levator scapulae seated. Fixed shoulder	
1.7i Active, passive and post-isometric stretch for levator scapulae sidelying	

Sidebending options for muscles stretched on the right side

Sidebending left	Sideshifting right	Head and cervical spine neutral	Scapular free	Middle scalene
Sidebending left	Sideshifting right	Head translated posteriorly	Scapular free	Anterior scalene
Sidebending left	Sideshifting right	Head translated anteriorly	Scapular free	Posterior scalene
Sidebending left	No sideshifting	Head and cervical spine rotated 10 degrees	Scapular free	Posterior upper and middle cervical muscles responsible for sidebending
Sidebending left	No sideshifting	Head and cervical spine rotated 45 degrees	Scapular free	Posterior upper and middle cervical muscles responsible for sidebending & rotation
Sidebending left	No sideshifting	Scapular free Head and cervical spine rotated 80 degrees	Scapular free	Posterior upper and middle cervical muscles responsible for rotation
Sidebending left	No sideshifting	Head neutral cervical spine flexed	Scapular free	Posterior upper and middle cervical muscles responsible for extension
Sidebending left	Sideshifting right	Head and cervical spine rotated 10 degrees left	Scapular free	Posterior lower cervical and upper thoracic muscles responsible for sidebending
Sidebending left	Sideshifting right	Head and cervical spine rotated 45 degrees left	Scapular free	Posterior lower cervical and upper thoracic muscles responsible for sidebending & rotation
Sidebending left	Sideshifting right	Head and cervical spine rotated 80 degrees left	Scapular free	Posterior lower cervical and upper thoracic muscles responsible for rotation
Sidebending left	Sideshifting right	Head neutral cervical spine flexed	Scapular free	Posterior lower cervical and upper thoracic muscles responsible for extension
Sidebending left	Sideshifting right	Head translated posteriorly	Scapular fixed	Upper trapezius (Part 1)
Sidebending left	Sideshifting right	Head and cervical spine neutral	Scapular fixed	Upper trapezius (Part 2)
Sidebending left	Sideshifting right	Head neutral cervical spine flexed	Scapular fixed	Upper trapezius (Part 3) & Rhomboid minor
Sidebending left	Sideshifting right	Head neutral & fully rotated left	Scapular fixed	Levator scapulae
Sidebending left	Sideshifting right	Head extended & cervical spine extended	Scapular fixed	Sternocleidomastoid

1.8 Sternocleidomastoid stretch - an active stretch for sternocleidomastoid and the cervical spine

1.8 Head & neck extension, sidebending and reverse rotation stretch kneeling, seated or standing for sternocleidomastoid

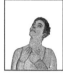

Starting position: Kneeling on the floor, seated in a chair or standing. Flex your elbows and place the fingertips of your left hand over the lower part of your right sternocleidomastoid just above the clavicle, reinforced them with the fingertips of your right hand. Partially extend your head and cervical spine, then sidebend your head to the left and slightly rotate it to the right.

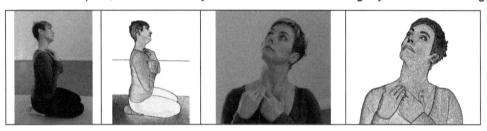

Technique: See Part A. Page 70.

Direction and range of movement

This technique involves partial extension of the head and cervical spine, partial sidebending of the head and cervical spine away from the side being stretched, and partial rotation of the head towards the side being stretched. During this technique there is partial movement of the head, cervical spine and upper two thoracic vertebrae.

The sternocleidomastoid muscle needs pining, so the stretch uses a combination of lateral and transverse forces. Full head and cervical extension is about 90 degrees, full sidebending is about 45 degrees, and full rotation is about 90 degrees.

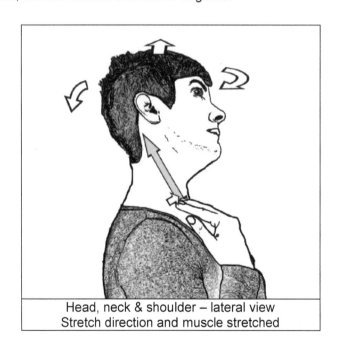

Head, neck & shoulder – lateral view
Stretch direction and muscle stretched

The first part of this technique, moving into the starting position, involves eccentric muscle contraction of the sternocleidomastoid, as well as the hyoid and cervical prevertebral muscles. During eccentric muscle contraction these muscles elongate while under tension from the weight of the head and the head is lowered into an extended position. This is a reverse muscle contraction with the opposing force of the head greater than the force generated by the muscle contraction.

The second part of this technique is the active stretch which combines concentric muscle contraction of the neck extensor muscles with gravity and transverse pressure on the sternocleidomastoid muscle with the fingertips. Pinning the sternocleidomastoid with the fingertips is necessary because it is a long muscle and it is difficult to stretch the muscle effectively without the addition of a transverse force.

Target tissues

This mainly stretches the sternocleidomastoid. It also stretches the muscles, fascia and ligaments of the anterior and lateral cervical spine, including the prevertebral muscles - longus capitis and colli, and the hyoid muscles. The lower ends of these tissues are anchored to the sternum, clavicle or to the anterior part of a vertebra or rib while the upper ends are moved.

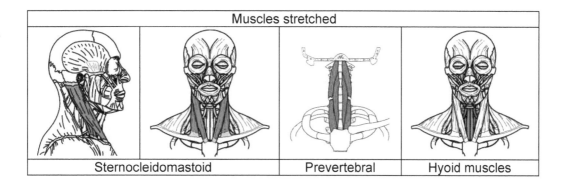

Muscles stretched		
Sternocleidomastoid	Prevertebral	Hyoid muscles

Safety

This is an active stretch combining muscle contraction with gravity. Care should be taken with this stretch because the posterior neck muscles are powerful and they can overstretch ligaments and muscles in the front of the neck. If you have degenerative changes in the lower cervical spine or hypermobility in the upper cervical spine then you should avoid this technique.

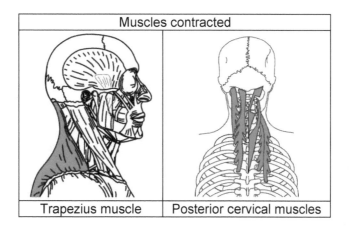

Muscles contracted	
Trapezius muscle	Posterior cervical muscles

Vulnerable areas

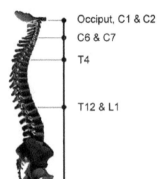

Occiput, C1 & C2

C6 & C7

T4

T12 & L1

	Region	Level of Risk
1.	Occiput, C1 & C2	Low
2.	C6 & C7	Low

Cease the stretch if there are adverse symptoms such as light headedness, dizziness or pain. This is a relatively safe technique and carries few risks. Avoid taking the head too far backward as hyperextension of the head can irritate or compromise the vertebral arteries which pass through the suboccipital region from the cervical spine into the skull.

Where there is arterial disease, ligament laxity or joint instability forceful extension can result in arterial irritation or tearing. Both the elderly and people who are congenitally hypermobile should be cautious when extending the head on the neck.

Care should be taken not to put excessive pressure on the joints in the lower cervical vertebra, especially if they have been subject to degenerative changes. The discs and joints are vulnerable to injury; overstretching may cause further tissue damage.

Key:

1.8 Head & neck extension, sidebending and reverse rotation stretch seated or standing for sternocleidomastoid	

Related stretches			
2.1b Extended Cat		1.5 Head & neck active extension stretch seated	

1.9 Post-isometric technique for the atlanto-occipital joints

1.9 Atlanto-occipital post-isometric technique seated

Starting position: Sitting upright with your pelvis vertical and your back resting against the back of a chair. Your feet are apart and firmly planted on the floor.

Place your right hand behind your neck with your little finger over the occiput, ring finger over the atlas (C1), middle finger over the axis (C2) and index finger and thumb over the vertebrae below. Your right elbow points forward. Grasp the back and right side of your head with your left hand, just above your right hand. Your left elbow points forward and slightly to the left.

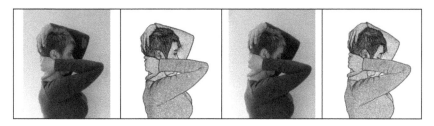

Introduce posterior translation of your head by flexing your head, tucking in your chin and taking your head backwards. Stop if you feel your atlas push backwards against your fingers. Introduce sidebending left and then introduce rotation right but maintain flexion and do not allow your atlas to move backwards against your fingers.

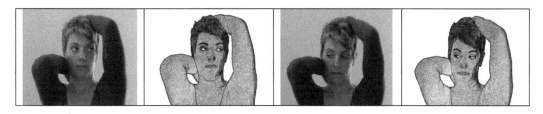

This technique uses eye movement to generate contraction in the suboccipital muscles: Look upwards, feel your head attempt to move backwards - but resist the movement with your left hand. Then after a few seconds, exhale, look downwards and move to the new flexion barrier.

Technique: See Part A. Page 71.

Direction and range of movement

This is a unilateral post-isometric technique involving sidebending of the head to one side, rotation of the head to the other side and head flexion (nutation of the occiput on the atlas). Sidebending and rotation are mechanically interconnected and move in opposite directions so that sidebending on one side automatically causes rotation to the other and rotation on one side automatically causes sidebending to the other.

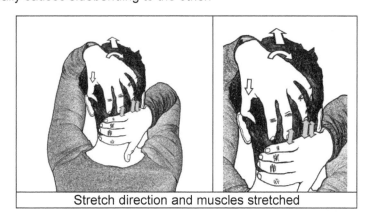

Stretch direction and muscles stretched

Flexion of the head (occiput) on the atlas is about 10 degrees. Extension of the head on the atlas is about 15 degrees. Sidebending of the occiput on the atlas is about 5 degrees. Rotation of the occiput on the atlas is about 10 degrees.

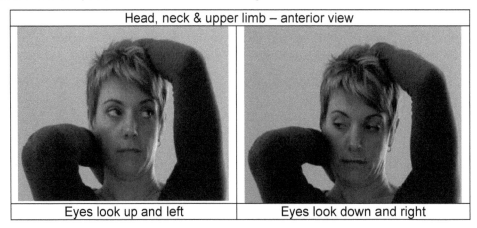

Head, neck & upper limb – anterior view	
Eyes look up and left	Eyes look down and right

The technique localises movement on one atlanto-occipital joint, right or left. If restricted the joint may be fixed in extension, sidebending and reverse rotation. For example if the right occiput is fixed on the atlas in a position of extension, sidebending right and rotation left it will be restricted in flexion, right rotation and left sidebending.

Use this technique to flex, right rotate and left sidebend the right condyle of the occiput on the right superior facet of the atlas. Focus on muscles that tilt the head backwards on the atlas on one side of the spine. The technique is repeated on the other side if the restriction is bilateral.

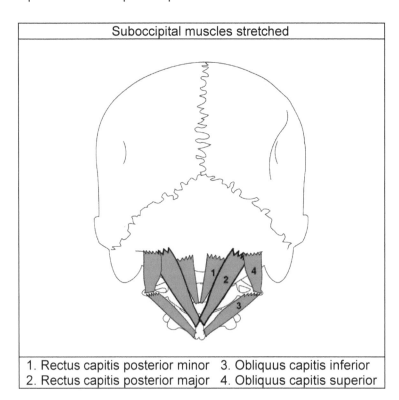

Suboccipital muscles stretched	
1. Rectus capitis posterior minor	3. Obliquus capitis inferior
2. Rectus capitis posterior major	4. Obliquus capitis superior

The most useful bony landmark for the localisation of this technique is the spinous process of the axis (C2), which is the most prominent bump in the midline just below the occiput. Use this landmark and use the subtle pressure of the posterior tubercle of the atlas pushing back through the fascia and skin during head flexion to localise the stretch to the atlanto-occipital joint. Some atlantoaxial movement is unavoidable due to the interconnected arrangement of the atlanto-occipital-axial complex but focus on the atlanto-occipital joint.

Target tissues

This is primarily a technique for lengthening the muscles of the posterior and lateral suboccipital spine, and in particular at the atlanto-occipital joints. These muscle pass between the axis, atlas and occiput.

Although other suboccipital muscles attaching on the axis such as rectus capitis posterior major and obliquus capitis inferior are also involved in head movement, in this technique we are mainly concerned with movement of the atlanto-occipital joint.

The primary muscles lengthened with this technique are rectus capitis posterior minor, obliquus capitis superior and rectus capitis lateralis, which pass between atlas and occiput; and rectus capitis posterior major, which passes between axis and occiput; and obliquus capitis inferior, which passes between axis and atlas. Some muscle pass over one joint and some pass over two.

Rectus capitis posterior minor and obliquus capitis superior are involved in head extension. Rectus capitis lateralis produce ipsilateral sidebending. Obliquus capitis superior produces ipsilateral sidebending and contralateral rotation. This means the right superior oblique produces rotation of the head to the left and the left superior oblique produces rotation of the head to the right. Flexion of the head is produced by the contraction of the most superior cervical prevertebral muscles, rectus capitis anterior and rectus capitis lateralis.

The anterior occiput is one of the most common postural fixations in the spine. It can exist bilaterally, but it is more commonly found unilaterally on the right side with the occiput fixed in extension, sidebent right and rotated left. This technique counters this with flexion, sidebending left and rotation right.

Variations

This technique can also be done kneeling, standing or supine. In all of the upright variations it is essential that you sit up straight. In the standing variation, a useful option is to place the back of your spine and rib cage against a wall.

This technique is based on certain characteristics of the suboccipital muscles. They have a high density of muscle spindles, which makes them highly responsive to sensory and motor control of the head and upper cervical spine. The suboccipital muscles are also connected to the muscles that move the eyes via the tectospinal tract. This nerve pathway coordinates head and eye movements and mediates reflex postural movements of the head in response to visual and auditory stimuli. When the eyes receive information about space and movement, this information is sent to the suboccipital muscles and then to the rest of the spine.

In the example described above, contraction of the superior rectus muscle of the left eye and the inferior oblique muscle of the right eye causes the simultaneous contraction of the suboccipital muscles responsible for moving the head into extension, sidebending right and rotation left. Specifically, these eye muscles cause the contraction of rectus capitis posterior major and minor to produces head extension, obliquus capitis inferior on the left to produce head rotation to the left and obliquus capitis superior on the right to produce head extension, sidebending to the right and rotation to the left. This head movement has great complexity and unwanted actions of some muscles are neutralised by the contraction of other muscles.

The suboccipital contraction is isometric because head movement in resisted by the left hand. After about five seconds the isometric contraction ceases and contraction of the inferior rectus muscle of the right eye and the superior oblique muscle of the left eye causes the simultaneous contraction of anterior and lateral upper cervical muscles to move the head into flexion, rotation right and sidebending left. In this technique the isometric contraction is followed by an active stretch, thus benefiting from reciprocal innervation relaxing the suboccipital muscles. In contrast this technique can be done as a passive stretch by following the isometric contraction with a subtle movement of the head to the new flexion, rotation, sidebending barrier with the left hand.

Safety

The suboccipital region between the occiput, C1 and C2, the occipito-atlanto-axial joints is vulnerable to strain because unlike the rest of the cervical spine it remains relatively flexible even into late life. In contrast the region between C5, C6 and C7 is prone to degenerative changes, which commonly begins by about 40 years and increases with age. In extreme cases it can result in neurological problems in an upper limb, but usually it results in neck and shoulder muscle pain or there may be no symptoms other than increased stiffness. Loss of movement in the lower cervical spine can result in hypermobility in the upper cervical spine and special care should be taken not to overstretch the upper spine when degenerative changes exist in the spine below.

Overstretching hypermobile suboccipital joints with excessive force may result in strain to the muscles and ligaments in this region. Avoid pulling on the head or pushing down and compressing the joints. If you feel pain in the head, neck, throat or arms during this technique or any similar exercise where the head is used as a lever then cease the activity immediately.

Care should be taken not to put excessive pressure on the lower cervical spine if there are pre-existing degenerative changes in the joints or if there is a history of disc problems such as prolapse or herniation which would leave them vulnerable to damage from overstretching. To prevent these type of problems avoid slouching. Prolonged sitting will eventually lead to stiffness and exaggerate poor posture. An increased thoracic kyphosis or dowager hump may cause the head forwards posture, which can be helped with this technique.

Vulnerable areas

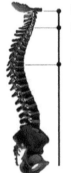

Occiput, C1 & C2

C6 & C7

T6-8

	Region	Level of Risk
1.	Occiput, C1 & C2	Medium
2.	C6 & C7	Low

Key:

1.9 Head post-isometric flexion stretch seated	

Related stretches					
1.3a Chin tuck prone		1.3b Chin tuck sitting or standing		1.3c Chin tuck supine	
1.4b Head & neck post-isometric flexion stretch supine					

For more detailed anatomy of the suboccipital and cervical spine 1.3 – 1.9 see page 543.

2.0 Chair supported thoracic, lumbar and hip active sidebends

2.0a & 2.0b Thoracic, lumbar and hip sidebending stretches standing

Starting position: Standing and grasping the back of a chair with your left hand. Use the chair as a pivot and for support and control. Raise your right arm to the vertical position. Keep your legs straight, your weight evenly balanced on both feet and your body in the coronal plane. Flex your left elbow to sidebend your spine left but stop when you start to feel a stretch down your right side.

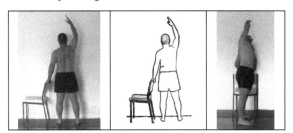

Technique: Take a deep breath in. For a localised stretch of your right lumbar spine: sideshift your pelvis to the right (away from the chair); exhale and reach 45 degrees up and to the left with your right arm; keep your right arm straight and reach with your fingertips.

For a localised stretch of your right thoracic spine: sideshift your pelvis to the left (towards the chair); flex your right forearm 90 degrees; point the tip of your right elbow 45 degrees up and to the right; exhale and sidebend your thoracic spine and ribs to the left by sideshifting your upper thoracic spine and ribs to the right (away from the chair).

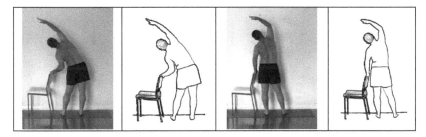

Hold the stretch for about 5 seconds or the length of a full exhalation. Flex your left elbow to sidebend your spine further to the left. Hold this position and then repeat the stretch several times for the right side of your body. Repeat the stretch for the left side of the spine.

Direction and range of movement

Thoracic sidebending to one side is about 20 degrees. Lumbar sidebending to one side is about 30 degrees. Most sidebending in the lumbar occurs in the middle lumbar and the least sidebending occurs at the lumbar sacral spine.

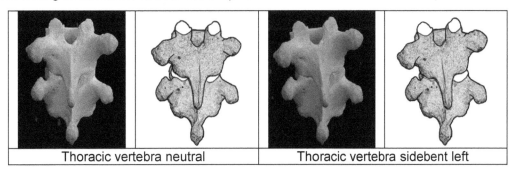

Thoracic vertebra neutral	Thoracic vertebra sidebent left

The back of the chair is important for enabling you to have control over the stretch. It supports your body weight and also acts as a pivot. By adjusting the amount of sidebending of the spine and sideshifting of the pelvis and/or the upper torso the sidebending stretch can localised to different areas of the spine.

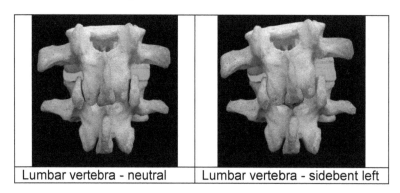

| Lumbar vertebra - neutral | Lumbar vertebra - sidebent left |

Sidebending is produced by increasing the amount of flexion of the elbow closest to the chair, while sideshifting is produced by moving the pelvis way from or toward the chair. Sideshifting the upper torso in the opposite direction to the sideshifting of the pelvis can be useful for more emphatic localisation.

Increasing the amount of lateral pelvic movement or sideshifting away from the chair (as in stretch 2.0a) results in greater lower lumbar sidebending and less thoracic sidebending - the thoracic spine remains relatively straight (see image 2).
With little to no sideshifting, greater emphasis is placed on sidebending of the upper lumbar spine or the thoracolumbar region (see image 3).

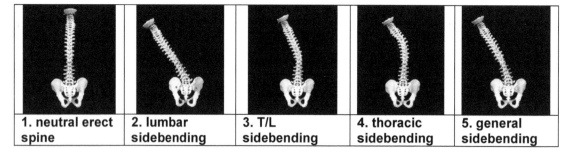

| 1. neutral erect spine | 2. lumbar sidebending | 3. T/L sidebending | 4. thoracic sidebending | 5. general sidebending |

Increasing lateral pelvic movement or sideshifting towards the chair (as in stretch 2.0b) results in greater middle and lower thoracic sidebending and less lumbar sidebending - the lumbar spine remains relatively straight. Even greater thoracic sidebending is achieved by combining this lateral pelvic movement with upper torso sideshifting away from the chair (see image 4).

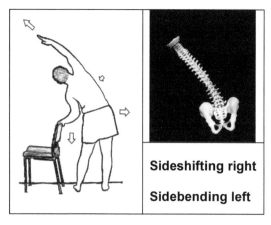

Sideshifting right

Sidebending left

A generalised sidebending of the spine is possible with moderate amounts of sideshifting away from the chair (see image 5). Generalised sidebending or targeted sidebending is recommended to avoid exaggerating areas of hypermobility in the thoracic or lumbar spine.

If you know the state of your spine, with regard to its structure and mobility, then you should targeted those areas in the spine where there is restricted sidebending and avoid overstretching area where there is hypermobility.

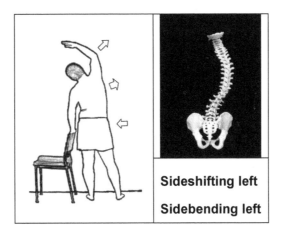

Sideshifting left

Sidebending left

If you don't know the state of your spine then focus on generalised sidebending, placing greater emphasis on lengthening the spine and less emphasis on increasing sidebending.

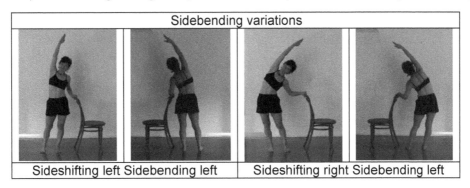

Sidebending variations	
Sideshifting left Sidebending left	Sideshifting right Sidebending left

Target tissues

Stretching primarily occurs in the lateral abdominal muscles, quadratus lumborum, and the lateral fibres of the erector spinae - the iliocostalis lumborum and thoracis. These muscles are anchored onto the iliac crest and attach on ribs above.

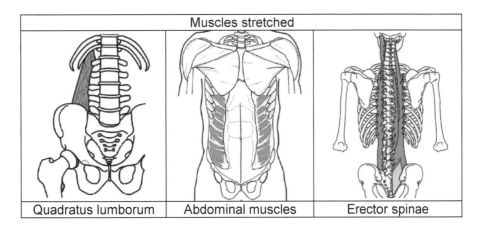

Muscles stretched		
Quadratus lumborum	Abdominal muscles	Erector spinae

This is also a good stretch for the intercostal muscles, psoas, latissimus dorsi, thoracolumbar fascia, teres major, lower fibres of pectoralis major, lateral fascia of the hip, lateral ligaments of the spine, tensor fasciae latae, gluteus medius and the upper fibres of gluteus maximus. This is a mild stretch for teres minor, the lower fibres of posterior deltoid and the long heads of biceps and triceps.

Although there is a passive component to this technique this is mainly an active stretch. The passive component uses gravity and the weight of the upper body, which is controlled by flexing the elbow nearest the chair and lowering the upper body to the side.

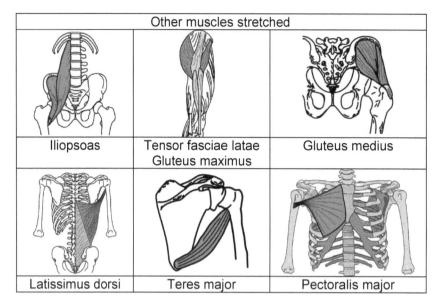

Other muscles stretched		
Iliopsoas	Tensor fasciae latae Gluteus maximus	Gluteus medius
Latissimus dorsi	Teres major	Pectoralis major

This is a very dynamic stretch with the active component of the technique involving shoulder muscle contraction to increase the intensity of the stretch, thus increasing the number of muscles stretched. The shoulder muscles are also engaged so that the stretch occurs broadly across many vertebral levels and does not focus solely on small single spinal muscles such as the deep rotators. For safety reasons the stretch should be spread across many muscles and tissues, including lower trapezius, latissimus dorsi, quadratus lumborum and the thoracolumbar fascia.

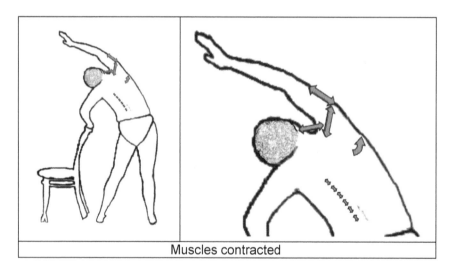

Muscles contracted

Supraspinatus, middle deltoid, trapezius and serratus anterior actively contract to abduct the scapula and shoulder, thereby stretching muscles such as latissimus dorsi and lower fibres of pectoralis major.

Variations

As an alternative to using a chair other objects can be used for support. These include a table, bench, wall, gate or a fence. A wire mesh fence, such as is used at a tennis court provides a very useful support because you can grasp the wire mesh with both hands and use it to localise sidebending.

This technique can be also done with your back in contact with a wall, which provides postural feedback to enable you to keep your body squarely in the coronal plane (also known as the frontal plane), assisting in maintaining better alignment during the stretch.

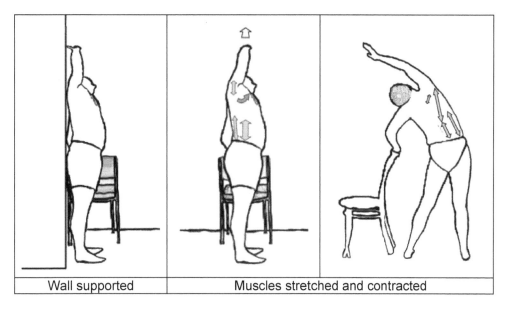

| Wall supported | Muscles stretched and contracted |

Technique

- Stand with your buttocks, back of your spine and rib cage against a wall.
- Place the backs of your heels 3 cm away from the wall for optimal balance.
- Grasp the back of a chair with your left hand and sideshift your pelvis (to the right for stretching the lumbar or to the left for stretching the lower thoracic), while sidebending your spine to the left to localise your stretch.
- Raise your right arm above your head and reach over your head.
- Keep the tip of your right thumb in contact with the wall during the stretch.
- Keep your back and other contact points in contact with the wall.

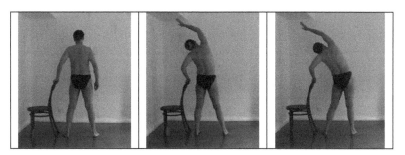

Another option is to stand near the corner of a room with your back against one wall for feedback and use the other wall for support and control.

Safety

If you have a scoliosis and know where in the spine it is and which direction it is sidebent, you can use this stretch to counter the scoliosis. Also if you have areas in your spine that are either stiff (hypomobile) and/or hypermobile you can taylor the stretch to the situation with greater and more focused stretching in the stiff areas and avoiding stretching the hypermobile areas.

If you are not aware of the structure of your thoracic and lumbar spine then you should do this technique as a generalised stretch, and not try to force sidebending in any single part of your spine.

Down each side of the vertebral column are many small muscles traversing one to three vertebral segments. Individually these muscles are relatively weak and can be strained if strong forces are used to sidebend the spine. You should try to spread the stretch across many vertebrae, thereby including larger muscle groups, as well as multiple muscle layers.

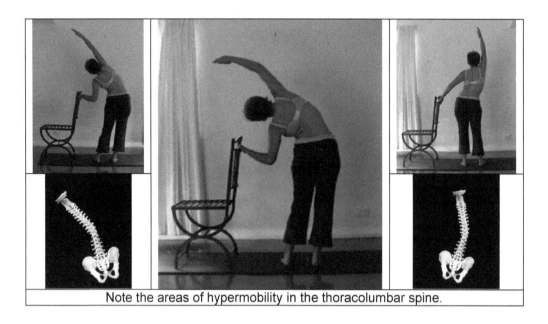
Note the areas of hypermobility in the thoracolumbar spine.

By stretching through the shoulder and involving lower trapezius, latissimus dorsi, quadratus lumborum and the thoracolumbar fascia, this technique is made much safer. You should feel like you are pulling your arm out of its socket, thereby lengthening the spine with traction, rather than squashing it with compression.

A safer stretch will cause less strain on vulnerable muscles and ligaments and less compression on intervertebral discs. Intervertebral discs are able to withstand normal sidebending movements; in fact healthy intervertebral discs will benefit from moderate lateral compression forces. But the combination of overstretching and pre-existing disc disease may result in a disc bulge and nerve root irritation. As one cannot predict the outcome of any stretching exercise, safety is always the best option.

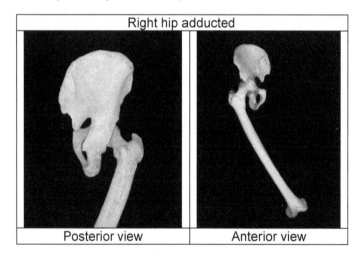
Right hip adducted

| Posterior view | Anterior view |

Care should be taken not to overstretch the spine if areas of localised hypermobility are identified. Hypermobility can exist in any area of the body, but more commonly it exists in the spine, particularly in the suboccipital, lower thoracic, thoracolumbar and sacroiliac spine. Stretching hypermobile areas may exaggerate the hypermobility, leading to muscle and ligament strain.

Vulnerable areas

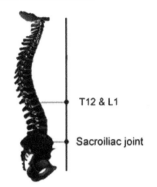

T12 & L1

Sacroiliac joint

	Region	Level of Risk
1.	Thoracolumbar	Low
2.	Sacroiliac joint	Medium

Key:

2.0a Lumbar and hip sidebending stretch standing	
2.0b Thoracic and thoracolumbar sidebending stretch standing	

Related stretches					
2.1a & 2.1c Wall supported sidebend stretch		2.1b Thoracic and rib sidebending seated		2.2a & 2.2b Thoracic and rib sidebending stretch seated	
2.3 Kneeling lateral side stretch		2.4a Hanging stretch erect		2.4 d Hanging passive stretch unilateral sidebending	
2.6c Sidebending Cobra		3.9a & 3.9b Supine spine & hip stretch over a rolled towel		7.4b Unilateral stretch for hip abductors and lumber spine	

2.1 Wall supported sidebend - passive sidebending stretch for the thoracic, lumbar and hip

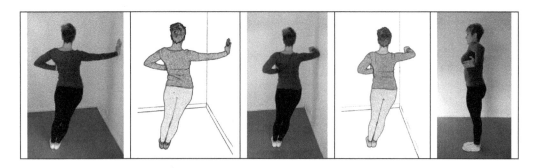

2.1a, 2.1b & 2.1c Wall supported sidebend stretches

Starting position: Standing with your feet together and the right side of your body opposite a wall. Abduct your right arm to 90 degrees and place your palm against the wall. Keep your right arm straight, horizontal and level with your shoulder. Alternatively place your forearm against the wall. In this position your forearm should be parallel with the floor, and both your arm and forearm should be level with your shoulder. Place your left hand against the side of your rib cage or pelvis, depending on whether you want to focus the stretch on the thoracic spine or hip.

Technique: See Part A. Pages 74. 75 and 76.

Direction and range of movement

Thoracic sidebending to one side is about 20 degrees. Lumbar sidebending to one side is about 30 degrees. Hip adduction is between 30 and 40 degrees. Hip abduction is about 45 degrees. Most sidebending in the lumbar occurs in the middle lumbar and the least occurs at the lumbar sacral spine.

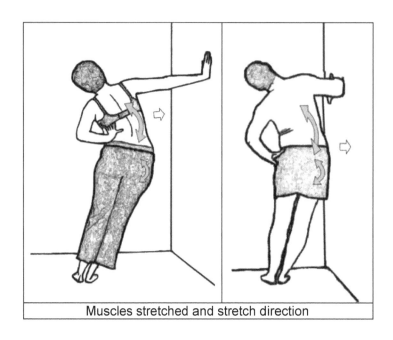

Muscles stretched and stretch direction

Target tissues

These are primarily for stretching the lateral abdominal muscles, quadratus lumborum, and the lateral fibres of the erector spinae; the iliocostalis lumborum and thoracis. These muscles are anchored on the iliac crest and attach on ribs above.

In addition these stretches may also be used to stretch the intercostal muscles, psoas, latissimus dorsi, thoracolumbar fascia and lateral fascia of the hip, lateral ligaments of the spine, tensor fasciae latae, gluteus medius and the upper fibres of gluteus maximus. By moving the pelvis forwards, greater emphasis is placed on stretching tensor fasciae latae.

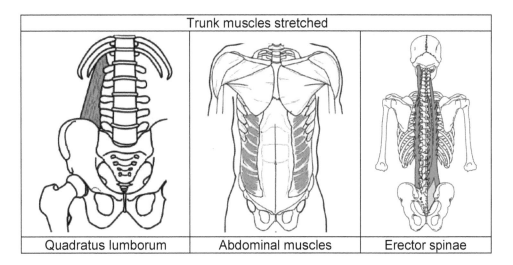

Trunk muscles stretched		
Quadratus lumborum	Abdominal muscles	Erector spinae

Techniques 2.1a and 2.1b are passive stretches using gravity and the weight of the body, combined with pressure from one hand against the side of the body and a sidebending directed effort towards the wall. The placement of your hand and the direction of force determine where the sidebending is focused – the thoracic or lumbar and hip. Technique 2.1c is a post-isometric stretch where an attempt to return to the straight standing position is resisted by pressure from the hand and the weight of the body.

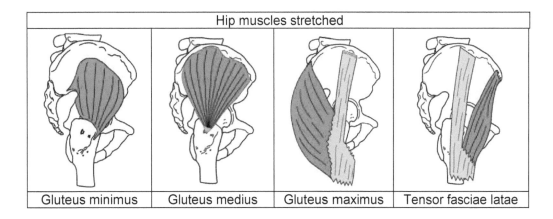

Hip muscles stretched			
Gluteus minimus	Gluteus medius	Gluteus maximus	Tensor fasciae latae

These stretches can also be done with the back of your pelvis and rib cage against a wall, and with the point of your elbow in the corner of a room. The wall provides support and useful postural feedback to help you keep your body in the frontal plane.

Safety

Greater levels of sidebending can be achieved with the elbow straight than with the elbow bent, but there is the danger of overstretching hypermobile areas of the spine. Do not flex the spine and allow it to drop into a forward slouching position or extend the spine by arching backward.

Vulnerable areas

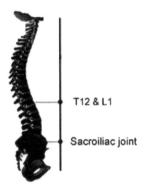

T12 & L1

Sacroiliac joint

	Region	Level of Risk
1.	Thoracolumbar	Low
2.	Sacroiliac joint	Low

The thoracolumbar and sacroiliac regions may have pre-existing hypermobility and further stretching of these areas may be cause problems such as ligament strains and increased hypermobility.

Key:

2.1a & c Wall supported sidebend stretch	
2.1b Wall supported sidebend stretch	

Related stretches					
2.0a Thoracic, lumbar and hip sidebending stretch standing		2.0b Thoracic, lumbar and hip sidebending stretch standing		2.2a & b Thoracic and rib sidebending stretch seated	
2.3 Kneeling lateral stretch / Kneeling side stretch		2.4a Hanging stretch erect		2.4 d Hanging passive stretch unilateral sidebending	

2.2 Thoracic and rib active sidebending stretches

2.2a & 2.2b Thoracic and rib sidebending stretch seated on a chair or kneeling on the floor

Starting position: Seated in a chair or kneeling on the floor. Flex your left elbow and place the palm of your left hand against the left side of your rib cage with your fingers pointing forwards and down the ribs. Sideshift your upper body to the right, so that more of your weight is on your right buttock. Fix your eyes forwards and sidebend your head to the left.

Keep your pelvis in a vertical position and your body in a frontal plane - no rotation. Raise your right arm until it is vertical and then reach over your head and to the left. Stop when you feel the initial stages of a stretch down your right side.

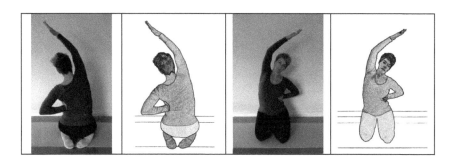

Technique: See Part A. Pages 77 and 78.

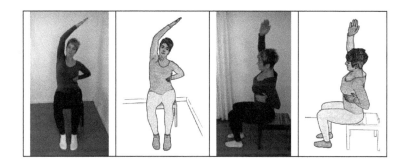

Direction and range of movement

Thoracic sidebending to one side is about 20 degrees. Supraspinatus and middle deltoid abduct the shoulder, while trapezius and serratus anterior actively contract to anchor the scapula and tilt it so the glenoid fossa faces upwards. The erector spinae assist in sidebending the spine.

Target tissues

This is primarily a stretch for the intercostal muscles and the lateral muscles of the middle thoracic spine, especially the lateral fibres of the erector spinae - the iliocostalis lumborum and thoracis.

These muscles are attached on the iliac crest and ribs, while the intercostal muscles connect adjacent ribs.

Secondarily stretching the teres major, latissimus dorsi, and the lower fibres of pectoralis major.

Safety

This is a relatively safe technique because the rib cage keeps the thoracic spine relatively firm and stable. Seated sidebending, if done correctly, does not place a lot of stress on the spine.

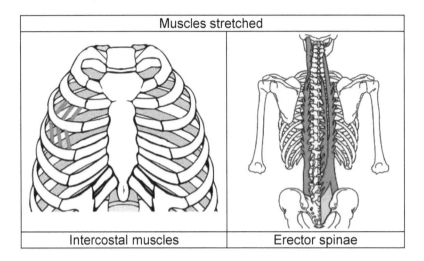

Muscles stretched	
Intercostal muscles	Erector spinae

Problems may arise if the pelvis is allowed to tilt backwards and the lumbar spine is allowed to flex. A slouching posture when combined with sidebending may place excessive compression forces on an intervertebral disc and if this is repeated over time may result in a disc prolapse, disc herniation, disc bulge, nerve root irritation and painful symptoms. If there is a known disc problem the seated sidebending stretch is contraindicated. A modified standing sidebending stretch is a more appropriate alternative.

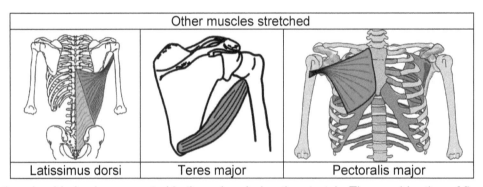

Other muscles stretched		
Latissimus dorsi	Teres major	Pectoralis major

Rotation should also be prevented in the spine during the stretch. The combination of flexion, sidebending and rotation in the seated position is particularly problematic for vulnerable intervertebral discs.

If a neutral posture is not maintained during seated sidebending then ligament strains are also possible, particularly in the sacroiliac joint. In addition, muscle strains are possible anywhere in the lumbar or thoracic spine, if an erect posture is not maintained during the execution of the technique.

If you have a scoliosis in the thoracic spine then it is particularly useful to focus on countering the scoliosis by stretching in the opposite direction to the sidebending.

Target the areas in the spine where stiffness is greatest and avoid stretching any areas that are hypermobile. Ribs 1 to 10 articulate with the sternum anteriorly, thus naturally offer the most resistance to movement in the thoracic spine. Vertebrae T11 and T12, linked with the floating ribs 11 and 12 and the first lumbar vertebra L1, form the thoracolumbar spine, and allow the most movement in this part of the spine. As a consequence, this is where you may find hypermobility.

Vulnerable areas

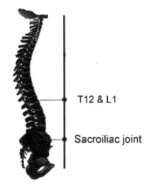

T12 & L1

Sacroiliac joint

	Region	Level of Risk
1.	Thoracolumbar	Low
2.	Sacroiliac joint	Medium

Key:

2.2a Thoracic and rib sidebending stretch seated	
2.2b Thoracic and rib sidebending stretch kneeling	

Related stretches					
2.0a Thoracic, lumbar and hip sidebending stretch standing		2.0b Thoracic, lumbar and hip sidebending stretch standing		2.1 Wall supported sidebend stretch	
2.1b Wall supported sidebend stretch		2.3 Kneeling lateral stretch / Kneeling side stretch		2.4a Hanging stretch erect	
2.4 d Hanging passive stretch unilateral sidebending		3.9a Supine hip and spine stretch over a rolled towel		3.9b Supine lumbar and thoracic spine stretch over a rolled towel	

2.3 Kneeling lateral stretch - active stretch for the shoulder, trunk and hip

2.3 Kneeling lateral stretch

Starting position: Kneeling with your right leg straight and your foot out to the right. Place your left hand on a block and then straighten your arm - keep it vertical. Keep your pelvis and thigh in a vertical plane and your left hip directly above your left knee.

Take your right arm over your head, keeping it in line with your body. Keep your spine and the side of your body that you are stretching in a frontal plane. Keep your pelvis and the thigh joined to your flexed knee, in a vertical plane. Avoid pelvic or spinal rotation.

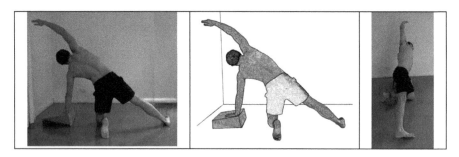

Technique: See Part A. Page 79.

Direction and range of movement

This is an active longitudinal stretch down one side of the body. It primarily involves shoulder abduction and elevation, a small amount of thoracic and lumbar sidebending and a very small amount of hip adduction. Sidebending is minimal.

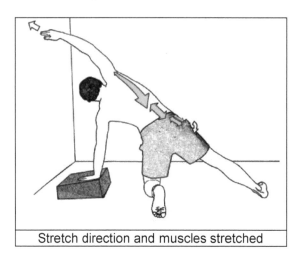

Stretch direction and muscles stretched

Target tissues

This is primarily a stretch for the lateral abdominal muscles - the external and internal obliques, plus quadratus lumborum and latissimus dorsi. Which other muscles are stretched depends on: the direction of movement; the intensity of the stretch; the height of the block; if a block is used; your current level of muscle tightness; and which muscle groups are short.

This may also stretch your hip flexors, internal rotators, abductors or hip adductors. Other muscles stretch may include tensor fasciae latae, sartorius, gluteus minimus, the anterior part of gluteus medius and gluteus maximus.

312

Latissimus dorsi attaches on the humerus and pulls on the thoracolumbar fascia to which it attaches inferiorly. The most posterior fibres of the external and internal obliques attach on the iliac crest and lower four ribs.

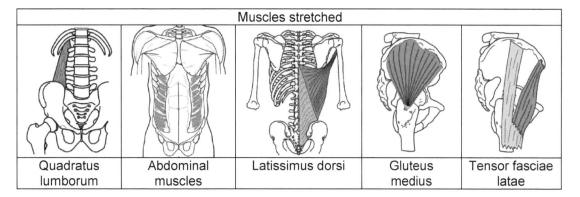

Muscles stretched				
Quadratus lumborum	Abdominal muscles	Latissimus dorsi	Gluteus medius	Tensor fasciae latae

Quadratus lumborum attaches on the iliac crest, lumbar spine and rib 12. Tensor fasciae latae and gluteus medius are lateral hip muscles.

To a lesser extent this technique also stretches teres major, pectoralis minor, lower fibres of trapezius, lower fibres of pectoralis major, upper fibres of gluteus maximus, the iliotibial band, the lateral intercostal muscles and the lateral fibres of the erector spinae - the iliocostalis lumborum and thoracis. If the foot is inverted peroneus longus and brevis are also stretched.

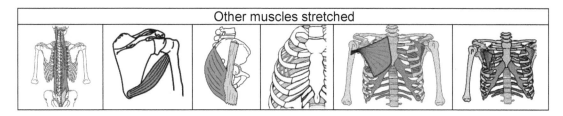

Other muscles stretched

Supraspinatus, middle deltoid, trapezius and serratus anterior actively contract to abduct the scapula and arm. Supraspinatus and middle deltoid abduct the shoulder, while trapezius and serratus anterior anchor and tilt the scapula it so the glenoid fossa faces upwards.

Safety

Vulnerable areas

This technique is safe because there is greater emphasis on lengthening the spine and less on sidebending. As sidebending in the thoracic and lumbar is minimal this is a good technique for hypermobile individuals who want a mild stretch for the side of the body. Problems may arise if a person is inflexible and does not use a block of a stool. This will result in rotation or flexion of the pelvis and spine, thus potential strain to the vertebral ligaments or muscles.

Key:

2.3 Kneeling lateral stretch	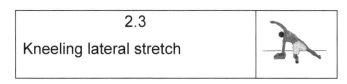

Related stretches					
2.0a Standing lumbar and hip sidebending stretch		3.9a & b Supine hip and spine stretch over a rolled towel		2.4a, b & d Hanging by the arm	

2.4 Hanging stretches - passive and post-isometric stretches for latissimus dorsi, the thoracolumbar fascia, quadratus lumborum and the lateral fibres of erector spinae

2.4a Hanging stretch erect

Starting position: Standing below a strong wooden pole or metal bar. Raise your right arm and grasp the pole with your right hand. Bend both hips and knees and lower your body towards the floor until your right arm is straight and you feel the initial stages of tension down the right side of your body.

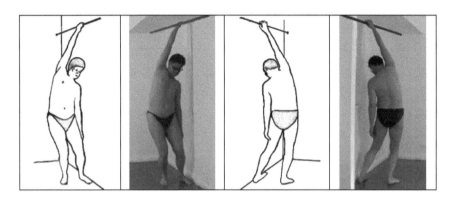

Technique: See Part A. Page 80.

2.4b & 2.4c Hanging stretches flexed

Starting position: Standing in front of a strong wooden pole or metal bar. Flex both hips and grasp the pole with your right hand. Keep your right arm straight and in line with your body.
Your knees are straight or slightly flexed. Lean backwards until you feel the initial stages of tension down the right side of your body. Alternatively grasp the pole with both hands, lean back and use your body weight to stretch both shoulders and both sides of your trunk.

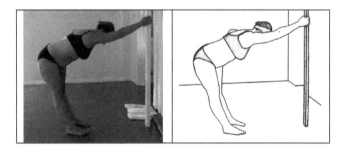

Technique: See Part A. Pages 81 and 82.

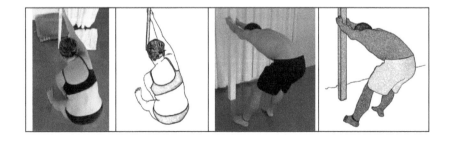

2.4d Hanging passive stretch unilateral sidebending

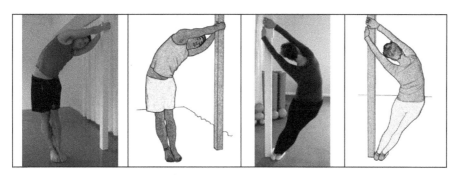

Starting position: Standing with your left side next to a post or pole with your feet together and knees straight. Make sure the post is firmly attached to the floor and ceiling. Abduct your arms until your hands are directly above your head. Sidebend your body at the hips, grasping the post with both hands. Keep your body in a coronal plane by adjusting your shoulders and pelvis – do not allow any flexion, extension or rotation.

Technique: See Part A. Page 83.

Direction and range of movement

This is a passive stretch and uses the weight of the body to stretch the muscles down one side of the body. Although moderate force is applied down the side of the body, there is very little joint movement in the spine. Most of the force is transmitted longitudinally.

This technique involves partial thoracic and lumbar sidebending, partial hip adduction, and full shoulder abduction – a combination of scapula abduction, elevation and upward rotation.

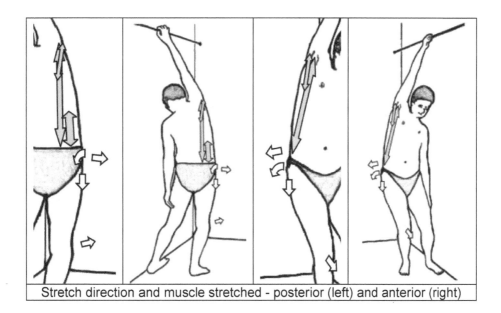

Stretch direction and muscle stretched - posterior (left) and anterior (right)

Full shoulder abduction is 180 degrees. Full thoracic sidebending is 20 degrees and full lumbar sidebending is 30 degrees. But only about half of the sidebending is involved in taking up tissue tension in this technique. The remainder of the tissue tension is taken up by a longitudinal stretch or traction as a result of dropping the pelvis.

Full hip adduction is 30 degrees but only about 10 degrees adduction is possible with the feet apart as described in this technique. A larger range of adduction can be achieved by placing your left foot in front of and to the right of your right foot, then sideshifting your pelvis to right.

Target tissues

These mainly stretch the muscles and fascia down one side of the body: shoulder, hip, ribs, thoracic and lumbar spine.

During the erect hanging stretch the pelvis is lowered and relaxed. The weight of the body produces a longitudinal passive stretch down one side. Grasping the pole with your hand fixes all the upper attachments of the muscles down the side of the body. The arm must be straight.

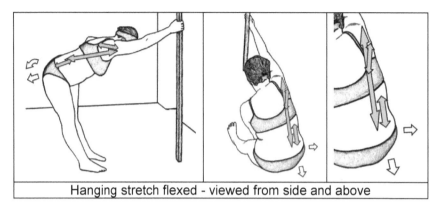

Hanging stretch flexed - viewed from side and above

To localise the stretch to one side of the body, the pelvis is moved in a specific direction. Sideshifting the pelvis to the right stretches the most lateral tissues: the lateral fibres of quadratus lumborum, latissimus dorsi and erector spinae (mainly iliocostalis lumborum), gluteus medius and gluteus minimus; the inferior fibres of serratus anterior; superior fibres of gluteus maximus, plus tensor fascia latae, and the iliotibial band (ITB).

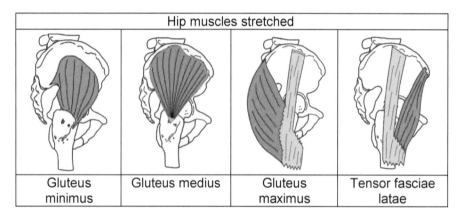

Hip muscles stretched			
Gluteus minimus	Gluteus medius	Gluteus maximus	Tensor fasciae latae

Tilting your pelvis backwards and tucking in the coccyx, stretches the most posterior tissues of the back and hip: the superficial fibres of erector spinae, the thoracolumbar fascia and superior fibres of gluteus maximus.

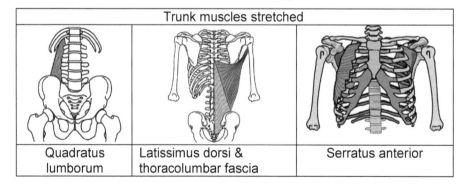

Trunk muscles stretched		
Quadratus lumborum	Latissimus dorsi & thoracolumbar fascia	Serratus anterior

Translating your pelvis forwards, tilting your pelvis forwards and taking the coccyx and the apex of your sacrum backwards stretches the most anterior tissues of your hip and lower

316

abdomen: Sartorius, rectus femoris, tensor fasciae latae, rectus abdominis and the abdominal fascia, psoas major and minor, iliacus, pectineus and adductor longus and brevis.

Sideshifting your shoulders and upper thoracic spine to the right stretches the most lateral muscles in your right shoulder: latissimus dorsi (especially the lower fibres), teres major, lower trapezius, and to a lesser extent the triceps, infraspinatus and teres minor.

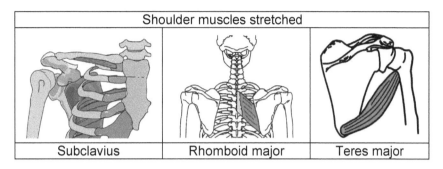

Shoulder muscles stretched		
Subclavius	Rhomboid major	Teres major

Translating your upper thoracic spine and shoulders backwards stretches the most posterior muscles in your right shoulder and upper thoracic spine: lower and middle trapezius, posterior deltoid, rhomboid major, latissimus dorsi including the upper fibres, serratus posterior inferior and the posterior fibres of erector spinae in the thoracic region; the iliocostalis and spinalis thoracis, and to a lesser extent infraspinatus and teres minor.

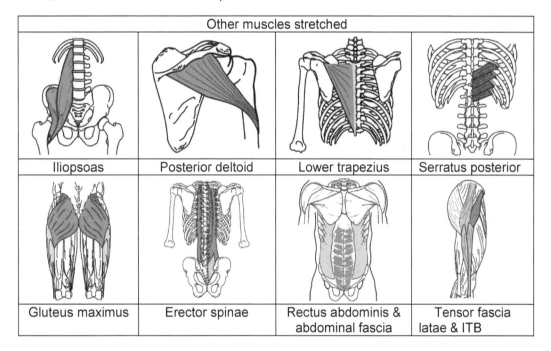

Other muscles stretched			
Iliopsoas	Posterior deltoid	Lower trapezius	Serratus posterior
Gluteus maximus	Erector spinae	Rectus abdominis & abdominal fascia	Tensor fascia latae & ITB

Translating your upper thoracic spine and shoulders forwards stretches the most anterior muscles of your right shoulder and upper thoracic spine: subclavius, pectoralis minor, anterior deltoid, the inferior fibres of pectoralis major and the anterior intercostal muscles.

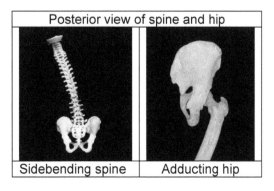

Posterior view of spine and hip	
Sidebending spine	Adducting hip

During the second phase of active shoulder abduction, the lower trapezius contracts to pull the scapular downwards and rotate it upwards so the glenoid cavity faces superiorly; however as this is a passive stretch involving shoulder elevation, lower trapezius is also stretched.

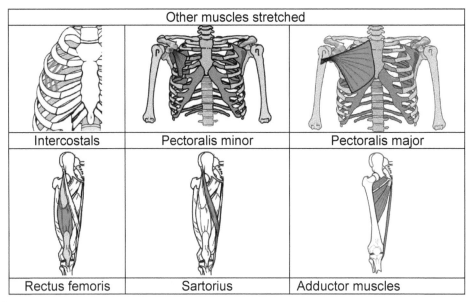

Other muscles stretched		
Intercostals	Pectoralis minor	Pectoralis major
Rectus femoris	Sartorius	Adductor muscles

Safety

This is a relatively safe technique. It may be painful to hang by the arm if the rotator cuff tendon is torn or compromised in any way. Caution should be taken if there is a known history of sacroiliac ligament laxity and strain but this technique is unlikely to over stretch muscles.

Key:

2.4a Hanging stretch erect	
2.4b Hanging stretch flexed unilateral	
2.4c Hanging stretch flexed bilateral	
2.4d Hanging stretch flexed bilateral	

Related stretches					
2.0a Standing lumbar and hip sidebending stretch		2.1b Thoracic and rib sidebending seated		2.2a & b Thoracic and rib sidebending stretch seated	
2.3 Kneeling lateral stretch / Kneeling side stretch		2.5a & b Upper Dog extension stretch kneeling		3.9a & b Supine hip and spine stretch over a rolled towel	

2.5 Upper Dog - active extension stretches for the shoulders, thoracic and lumbar spine

2.5a Upper Dog extension stretch kneeling

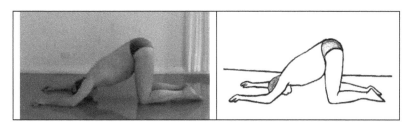

Starting position: Kneeling with your forehead, elbows, forearms and hands on the floor shoulder distance apart. Your palms are down flat on the floor. Your knees and feet are slightly apart and your hips should be directly over your knees and your thighs vertical.

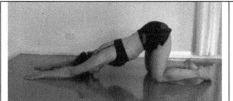

Technique: See Part A. Page 84.

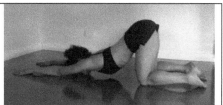

2.5b Upper Dog extension stretch standing

Starting position: Standing facing a wall with your feet apart. Place your palms on the wall above your head shoulder distance apart. Take a step back with one foot and flex your knees slightly. Extend your elbows until your arms are straight. Place your forehead on the wall and extend your thoracic spine.

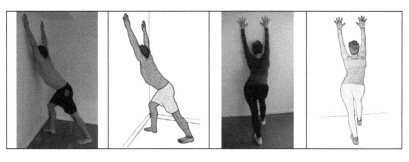

Technique: See Part A. Page 85.

2.5c Latissimus dorsi stretch kneeling

Starting position: Kneeling on the floor facing a stool. Bring your elbows, forearms and palms together. This will externally rotate your arms and separate your shoulder blades. Lean forwards and place your elbows on the stool. Your knees and feet are slightly apart for better balance.

Technique: See Part A. Page 86.

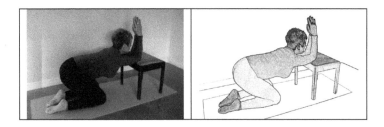

Direction and range of movement

This is primarily a stretch involving extension of the thoracic spine and hyperflexion of the shoulders. Sidebending of the thoracic spine can also be introduced into the technique.

Most of the thoracic spine is in the naturally flexed position, which is known as a thoracic kyphosis. Some areas of the thoracic spine deviate from this overall flexed position and much variation exists between individuals.

In the thoracic spine (T1 to T12) total extension is about 25 degrees. Much of the extension is usually between T10 and T12 and significant extension may be found around T4 or over several vertebrae between T3 and T6.

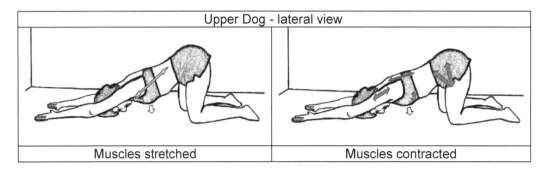

Upper Dog - lateral view	
Muscles stretched	Muscles contracted

Due to the shape of the vertebra and the discs in the spine there will be more extension in some part of the spine and less in others. In general areas of the spine that are in an extended position (lordosis) will have more extension and less flexion, and areas of the spine that are in a flexed position (kyphosis) will have more flexion and less extension. In this stretch it is important to identify the areas of flexion and extension, so as to extend the flexed areas and avoid further extending areas that are already extended.

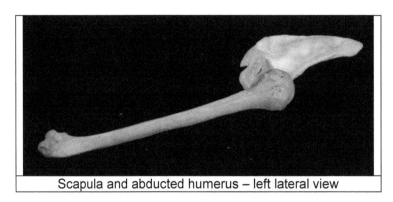

Scapula and abducted humerus – left lateral view

Shoulder flexion is 180 degrees but will be greater in hypermobile individuals. Shoulder flexion is movement of the arm forward and upwards to the vertical position. It is a combination of glenohumeral joint and scapulothoracic joint movement. Movement of the humerus is checked when the greater tuberosity comes in contact with the acromion process and area above the glenoid fossa. Movement continues as scapular protraction and upward rotation.

Target tissues

The upper dog stretches the muscles, fascia and ligaments attached to the clavicle, sternum, anterior ribs and the humerus.

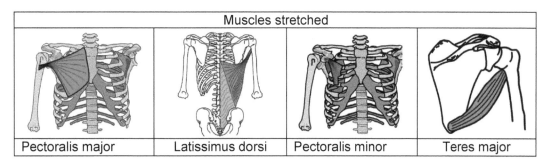

Muscles stretched			
Pectoralis major	Latissimus dorsi	Pectoralis minor	Teres major

This is mainly a stretch for latissimus dorsi, teres major, pectoralis minor and the sternocostal fibres of pectoralis major. To a lesser extent this is also a stretch for posterior deltoid, the long head of triceps and the most anterior intercostal muscles.

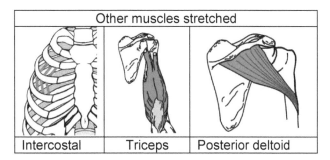

Other muscles stretched		
Intercostal	Triceps	Posterior deltoid

Stretching occurs as a result of muscle contraction from serratus anterior, lower trapezius, erector spinae and anterior deltoid and the assistance of gravity.

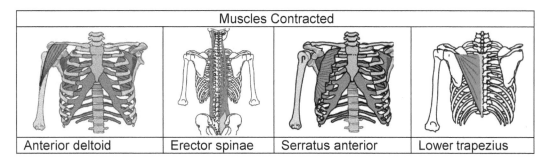

Muscles Contracted			
Anterior deltoid	Erector spinae	Serratus anterior	Lower trapezius

This technique should be done with the forehead resting on the floor. If this is uncomfortable because it puts pressure on your nose, then try resting your forehead on a small pillow. Do not allow your head to be pushed backwards and the weight of your body to be taken through your chin and strain muscles or ligament in the suboccipital spine. Keep the head and neck as close as possible to a neutral position – do not allow hyperextension.

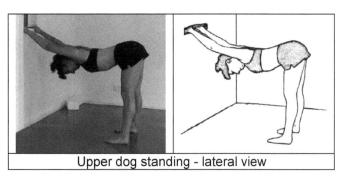

Upper dog standing - lateral view

Determine where your thoracic spine is most restricted and focus on this area. Vary how far the arms are apart by varying the placement of the hand. They can be close to the side of the head or wider apart. This will change, very slightly, which fibres of the muscle are stretched. This can be done as an active, passive or post-isometric technique. During the passive stretch relax and use the weight of the upper body to assistance with this stretch.

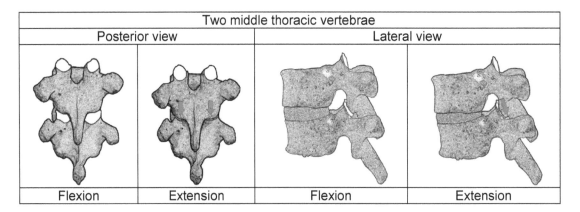

Two middle thoracic vertebrae			
Posterior view		Lateral view	
Flexion	Extension	Flexion	Extension

Other factors

The shape of the spine differs between individuals and this should influence the way different individuals do the upper dog.

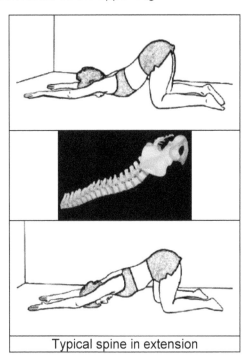

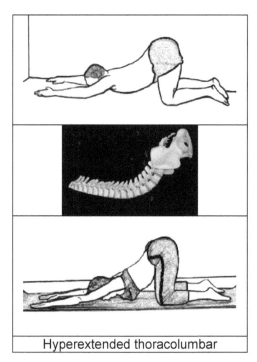

Typical spine in extension	Hyperextended thoracolumbar

This technique has benefits for individuals with slouched and round shoulders, who also may have fixed flexed areas within the thoracic spine, an increased kyphosis, a dowager hump, or a reverse lordosis in the thoracolumbar or lumbar region. Postural changes are associated with muscles in front of the shoulders becoming short, thus this technique counters the shortness well.

Safety

Care should be taken not to over extend the thoracolumbar spine. If the area is hypermobile then pressure on the joints may cause ligaments or muscles to be over stretched which may result in strain and injury.

The rotator cuff tendons are vulnerable to tearing in individuals with an exaggerated kyphosis, short pectoralis muscles, and inflexibility within the thoracic spine, ribs and shoulders.

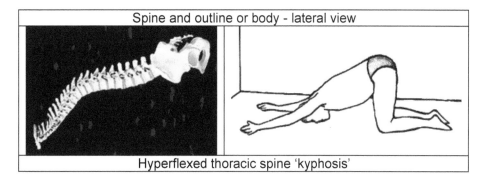

Spine and outline or body - lateral view

Hyperflexed thoracic spine 'kyphosis'

If you fit this profile then it is advisable that you stretch each shoulder separately before attempting to stretch both shoulders. Insufficient warming up prior to stretching, or moving into the stretch too quickly may result in a rotator cuff injury.

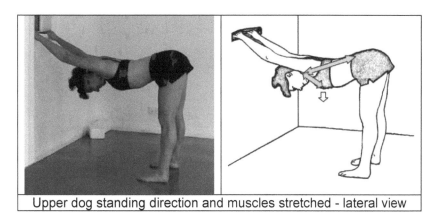

Upper dog standing direction and muscles stretched - lateral view

Do not do this stretch if you have a pre-existing bursitis or rotator cuff tear. Fix the problem with treatment (manual therapy or surgery) and build up the structural integrity of the cuff tendon with strengthening exercises before attempting the upper dog stretch. Always take your time to warm up your body before doing this stretch.

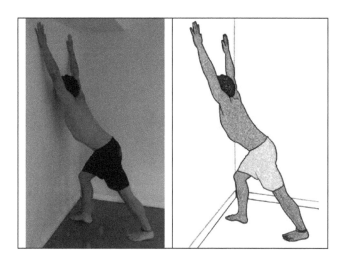

<u>Vulnerable areas</u>

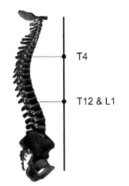

	Region	Level of Risk
1.	T4	Medium
2.	T10 to T12	Medium
3.	Rotator cuff	Low

Key:

2.5a Upper Dog extension stretch kneeling	
2.5b Upper Dog extension stretch standing	
2.5c Latissimus dorsi stretch kneeling	

Related stretches					
2.0a Standing lumbar and hip sidebending stretch		2.4b Hanging stretch flexed unilateral		2.4c Hanging stretch flexed bilateral	
2.6b Full Cobra		2.7a Diagonal locust		2.8 Extended cat	
4.0f & g Bilateral pectoralis stretch standing		6.9c Bilateral stretch for the hamstrings and gastrocnemius		7.5a Squat with palms together above head	

2.6 The Cobra - active and passive extension stretches for the shoulders, cervical, thoracic, lumbar spine and hips

2.6a Half Cobra

Starting position: Prone on the floor with your feet apart and your toes pointing backwards. Flex your elbows 90 degrees and place them at the side of your body directly under your shoulders so that your arms are vertical. Place your palms downwards, flat on the floor. Keep your spine straight so the tension on each side of your spine is even. Adjust your body so that the tissues are in their most relaxed state.

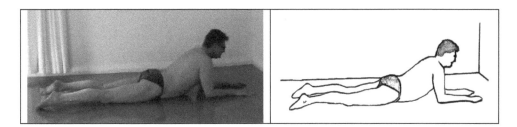

Technique: See Part A. Page 87

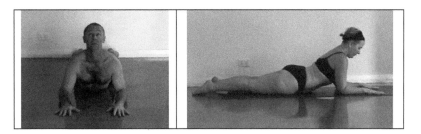

2.6b Full Cobra

Starting position: Prone on the floor with your feet apart, toes pointing backwards and your arm in the half cobra position described above. Slide your palms a few centimetres forward along the floor so they are in line with and directly in front of your shoulders. Straighten your elbows until you are in a mild backward bending position.

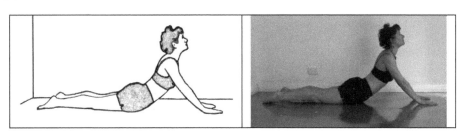

Technique: See Part A. Page 88.

2.6c Sidebending Cobra

Starting position: Prone on the floor with your feet apart and your toes pointing backwards and your arm in the half cobra positon described above. Sidebend your thoracic or lumbar spine or hip. Localise sidebending in the thoracic or lumbar spine or hip or adopt a generalised sidebending.

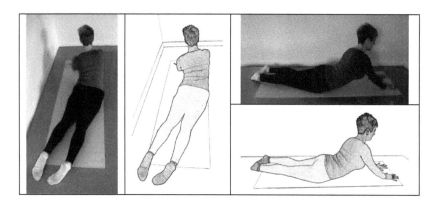

Technique: See Part A. Page 89.

2.6d Rotation Cobra

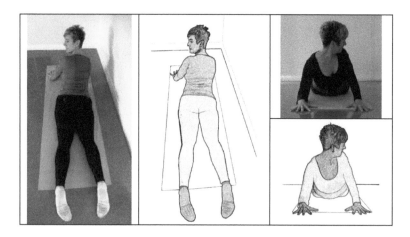

Starting position: Prone on the floor with your feet apart and your toes pointing backwards and your arm in the half cobra. Straighten your left elbow, allowing your shoulder, spine and rib cage to rotate to the left in the backward bending position.

Technique: See Part A. Page 90

Direction and range of movement

Active hip extension is between 10 and 20 degrees. Passive hip extension is between 15 and 30 degrees. Thoracic extension is about 25 degrees, with the greatest proportion usually between T10 and T12. Lumbar extension is about 35 degrees. Sacroiliac extension is between one and two degrees.

Active and passive spinal extension varies significantly between different individuals and depends on: genetics, past levels of activity or inactivity, age, and the presence of hypomobile or hypermobile areas and degeneration.

Target tissues

This is a stretch with an active and a passive component. In the active component muscle contraction from serratus anterior and pectoralis minor protracts the scapula, indirectly raising the thoracic spine and ribs off the floor, in turn allowing the spine and hips to extend. Scapula protraction mainly stretches the rhomboids and middle trapezius, while spinal extension stretches anterior muscles of the rib cage and abdomen.

As both arms are in a fixed stable position on the floor, scapula protraction dragging the ribs, and hence spine forward, may also produce distraction and longitudinal elongation of the spine, stretching deep spinal muscles such as multifidus, rotatores, intertransversarii and levator costarum, especially when there is a sidebending or rotation component in the cobra stretch.

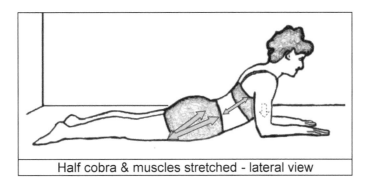
Half cobra & muscles stretched - lateral view

The passive component follows a cessation of muscle contraction and allows the weight of the upper body to stretch the spine, hips and shoulder muscles. By immediately following the active stretch with the passive stretch, muscle relaxation is greater than would have occurred if the muscle was simply allowed to relax on command.

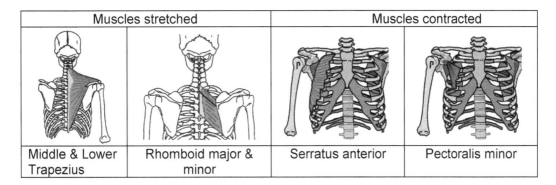

Muscles stretched		Muscles contracted	
Middle & Lower Trapezius	Rhomboid major & minor	Serratus anterior	Pectoralis minor

The passive part of the technique stretches serratus anterior, pectoralis minor and fibres of erector spinae involved with extension. Both active and passive components stretch the Iliopsoas, tensor faciae latae and abdominal muscles.

In addition to the shoulder movement, the upper thoracic fibres of erector spinae and posterior cervical muscles, contract to extend the thoracic spine and translate the cervical spine into a more posterior position, while gluteus maximus and the lumbar and sacral fibres of erector spinae contracts to push the pelvis into the floor. The gluteus maximus is assisted by the hamstrings and adductor magnus in extending the lower limb.

This is a good stretch for iliopsoas, and anterior fibres of the abdominal muscles. It also assists in stretching tensor faciae latae and the anterior intercostal muscles.

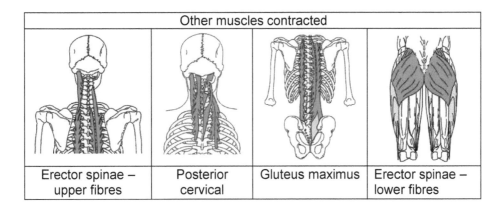

Other muscles contracted			
Erector spinae – upper fibres	Posterior cervical	Gluteus maximus	Erector spinae – lower fibres

Variations

The half and full cobra uses scapula protraction to stretch scapula retractor and anterior trunk muscles. However an alternative method could use scapula retraction combined with gravity to stretch scapula protractor muscles.

Take a deep breath in and squeeze the shoulder blades together. After a 5 second contraction, exhale and totally relax. As the upper body is supported on the elbows or hands, the weight of the thoracic spine and ribs will cause the thoracic spine to drop between the scapular, closer towards the floor and further into extension and the scapula will move closer together.

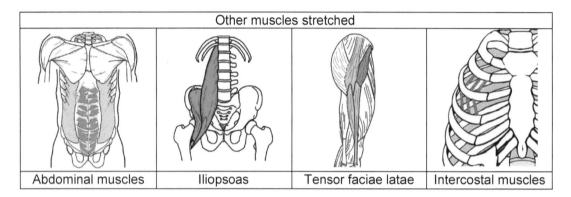

Other muscles stretched			
Abdominal muscles	Iliopsoas	Tensor faciae latae	Intercostal muscles

This is an active and passive stretch for serratus anterior and pectoralis minor, involving contraction of middle trapezius, rhomboid major and rhomboid minor.

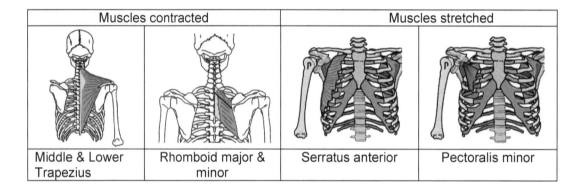

Muscles contracted		Muscles stretched	
Middle & Lower Trapezius	Rhomboid major & minor	Serratus anterior	Pectoralis minor

Full head and cervical extension can be used providing there are no known cervical problems or diseases, and there are no adverse reactions after doing the stretch. Extension can also be combined with sidebending or rotation.

Safety

The structure of our body - the shape, strength and elasticity of our bones, joints, ligaments and muscles is a key factor influencing how we do the cobra. If we were evenly flexible over our whole body, then there would be less of a safety issue for cobra. But flexibility is not evenly distributed over our whole body - joints are shaped differently in different parts of the spine, people are different, and environmental factors all act to influence flexibility, usually contributing to produce uneven flexibility.

Some people have stiffness in one area and over-flexibility in another, in other words combinations of hypermobile and hypomobile joints. When this occurs there is the danger that strong backward stretching increase hypermobility in already hypermobile joints but fail to stretch the hypomobile joints.

Hypermobility is a particular problem for stretches that produce movement in the spine by combining the weight of the body (gravity) with leverage and muscle contraction. This is the case with the full cobra where the weight of the pelvis plus leverage from the upper limb through to the spine, combine with muscle contraction from the muscles of the shoulders and spine to increase backward bending. When adjacent areas of hypermobility and hypomobility coexist in the spine there is the danger that stretching will amplify the hypermobility but not stretch the stiffness.

Ligaments provide stability to the spine and when they are forced to stretch beyond their anatomical elastic limits, either from repeated stretching or from a single overwhelming force then they may become lax and the joint become hypermobile. It is therefore important not to extend too far into the full cobra.

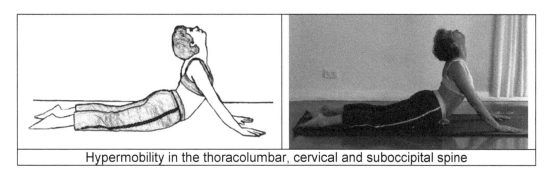

Hypermobility in the thoracolumbar, cervical and suboccipital spine

Before attempting backbends that use levers and strong muscle contraction it is important to work out if there are areas of your spine that are hypermobile and hypomobile, as well as where they are.

The half cobra is generally safe and can be done by anyone. In contrast the full cobra may be inappropriate for people with extreme hypermobility, hence may need to be dropped from the stretching program in favour of the half cobra or active extension techniques. If mild to moderate hypermobility exists, the full cobra may need to be modified by moving your hands away from your body, focusing the stretching to the areas of restriction.

Several months of mild stretching, may be required before overstretched ligaments can return to an optimum level of tightness. Areas of hypermobility in the spine may need to be protected while only the stiff areas are stretched. The hypermobile joints in the spine will yield to stretching before those in the hypomobile areas, therefore it is important to stop stretching before you get to this point.

The areas most vulnerable to hypermobility, that can be pushed further into extension with the full cobra are the: atlanto-occipital joint, lower cervical spine, middle thoracic near T4, the thoracolumbar spine, lumbosacral junction, and sacroiliac joints.

The cobra is a gravity assisted stretch involving leverage and strong muscle contraction. The risk of overstretching the spine is even greater if there is an underlying pathology such disc disease, osteoarthritis or a defect in the spine such as a spondylolisthesis. Extreme care should therefore be taken not to stretch too strongly by pushing so hard with the arms that you force the body into extension.

Vulnerable areas

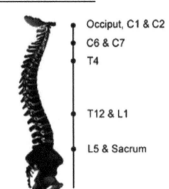

Occiput, C1 & C2

C6 & C7

T4

T12 & L1

L5 & Sacrum

	Region	Level of Risk
1.	Atlanto-occipital	Medium
2.	C6 to C7	Medium
3.	T4	Medium
4.	T12	Medium
5.	L5	Medium
6.	Sacroiliac	Medium

Key:

2.6a The Half Cobra	
2.6b The Full Cobra	
2.6c The Sidebending Cobra	
2.6d The Rotation Cobra	

Related stretches					
1.1a, b & c Lion stretch		1.5 Head & neck extension stretch seated		2.5a & b Upper Dog extension stretch	
2.7a, b & c The locust		2.8 Extended cat		6.5d Bilateral post-isometric stretch for the hip adductors and extensors sitting	
6.5h Bilateral stretch for the hip adductors standing		6.9c Bilateral stretch for the hamstrings and gastrocnemius		7.5a Squat with palms together above head	

2.7 The Locust - active stretches for the shoulders, thoracic, lumbar spine and hips

2.7a Diagonal Locust

Starting position: Prone on the floor with your feet slightly apart and your toes pointing backwards. Abduct both arms until they rest beside your head. Your hands are palms down on the floor above your head. Your head is straight, face down and resting on your nose or chin.

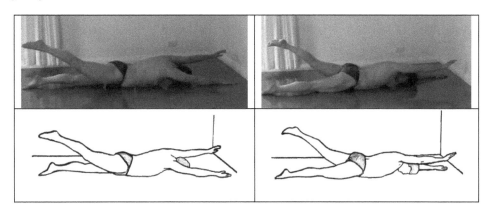

Technique: See Part A. Page 91.

2.7b Full Locust arms at side

Starting position: Prone on the floor with your arms at your side, palms upwards, feet apart and your toes pointing backwards. Keep your head straight, face down and rest on your nose or chin.

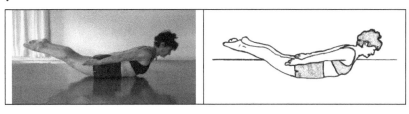

Technique: See Part A. Page 92.

2.7c Full Locust arms abducted

Starting position: Prone on the floor with your arms at your side, feet apart and your toes pointing backwards. Abduct both arms until they are in contact with the side of your head and your hands are together above your head. Alternatively abduct both arms 90 degrees and flex your elbows 90 degrees. Keep your head straight, face down, resting on your nose or chin, and your hands palms down facing the floor.

Technique: See Part A. Page 93.

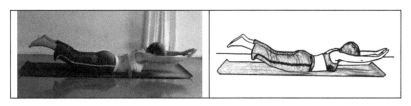

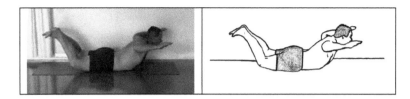

Direction and range of movement

Shoulder flexion is 180 degrees and is a combination of glenohumeral and scapulothoracic joint movement.

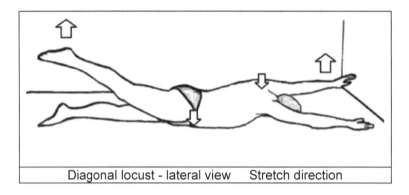

Diagonal locust - lateral view   Stretch direction

Active hip extension is about 20 degrees. Thoracic extension is about 25 degrees with the greatest proportion usually between T10 and T12. Lumbar extension is about 35 degrees and sacroiliac extension is between one and two degrees. Extension varies between individuals and depends on genetics, age, level of activity, history of stretching and injury, as well as if degeneration exists.

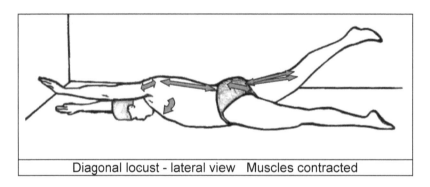

Diagonal locust - lateral view   Muscles contracted

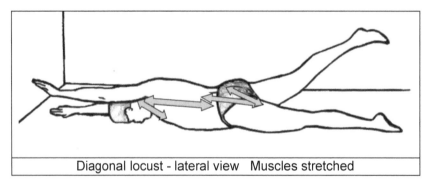

Diagonal locust - lateral view   Muscles stretched

Target tissues

This is an active stretch which strengthens muscles which are important for the maintenance of good posture.

332

The trapezius, rhomboids, serratus anterior muscles are contracted in flexing the upper limb. They are supported by supraspinatus, middle deltoid and the clavicular part of pectoralis major. Other muscles act as stabilisers and assist arm flexion including coracobrachialis and biceps brachii.

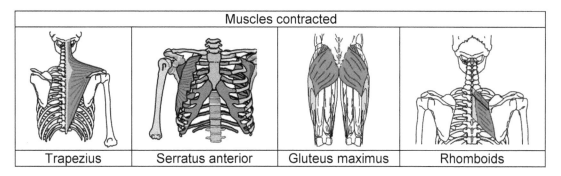

Muscles contracted			
Trapezius	Serratus anterior	Gluteus maximus	Rhomboids

The erector spinae muscles contract to extend the spine, while gluteus maximus is the primary muscle acting to extend the lower limb. It is assisted by the hamstrings and adductor magnus.

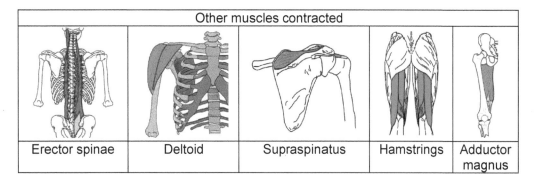

Other muscles contracted				
Erector spinae	Deltoid	Supraspinatus	Hamstrings	Adductor magnus

The locust is primarily a stretch for iliacus, psoas, latissimus dorsi and the sternocostal fibres of pectoralis major.

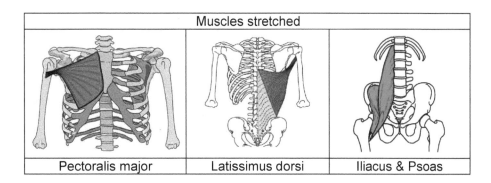

Muscles stretched		
Pectoralis major	Latissimus dorsi	Iliacus & Psoas

It also assists in stretching pectoralis minor, teres major, tensor faciae latae, pectineus, adductor brevis and the anterior fibres of the intercostal and abdominal muscles. With the knees flexed it assists in stretching rectus femoris and with the knees extended it has a mild stretch on sartorius

Safety

The locust strengthens and tones muscles in the shoulders, spine, pelvis and hips. Indirectly it also helps strengthen the muscles of the abdomen and helps tone internal organs.

The diagonal locust is a relatively safe stretch. When lifting your arm off the floor during the diagonal locust it is important that your thoracic spine does not rotate and your rib cage does not lift off the floor. Similarly when lifting your leg off the floor, it is important that your lumbar spine does not rotate and your pelvis does not lift off the floor.

People who are physical unfit, have a history of spinal problems or suspect they have spinal problems should not do the locust. Even people with moderate levels of fitness may find lifting one limb off the floor challenging.

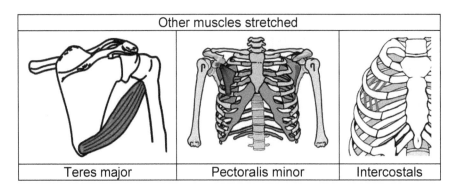

Other muscles stretched		
Teres major	Pectoralis minor	Intercostals

Beginners should start with a simplified version of the diagonal locus – by only attempting to lift one arm or one leg off the floor at a time. If this is impossible initially then continue trying. With practice the muscles will get stronger and eventually you will be able to oppose gravity and lift the limb off the floor. It will be worth the effort.

If after a few weeks of lifting one limb there are no problems then attempt the diagonal locust. If a few weeks of doing the diagonal locust there are no problems then attempt the full locust.

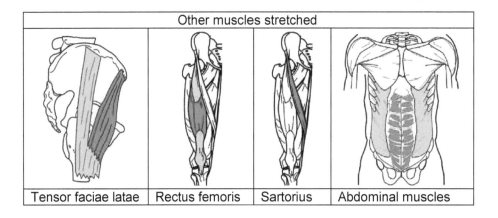

Other muscles stretched			
Tensor faciae latae	Rectus femoris	Sartorius	Abdominal muscles

The full locust has the most significant safety issues. This is due to the strong forces generated by the shoulder and hip muscles, as well as the leverage generated from the limbs, tending to multiply the forces. Strong forces are transferred from the limbs to the spine when lifting the limbs off the floor. In addition to extending the spine there is considerable compression placed on the spine. This is particularly strong when the arm is fully abducted, due to the pull of latissimus dorsi on the lumbodorsal fascia and the lumbar spine.

Caution should be applied if there is a weakness as a result of a hernia or any pre-existing congenital or degenerative problems such as ligament laxity, disc disease, a spondylolisthesis or osteoarthritis in the spine. The locust should not be done by women during pregnancy.

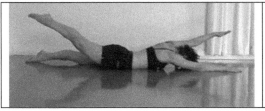 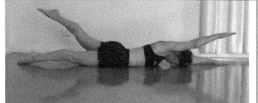

Vulnerable areas

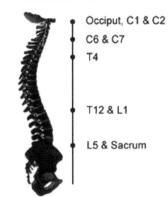

Occiput, C1 & C2

C6 & C7

T4

T12 & L1

L5 & Sacrum

	Region	Level of Risk
1.	C6 to C7	Medium
2.	T4	Low
3.	T12	Medium
4.	L5	Medium
5.	Sacroiliac	Medium

Key:

2.7a The diagonal Locust	
2.7b The full Locust arms at side	
2.7c The full Locust arms abducted	

Related stretches					
1.3a, b & c Chin tucks		2.5a & b Upper Dog extension stretch		2.6a & 2.6b The Half Cobra & Full Cobra	
2.8 Extended cat		4.0c & 4.0d Pectoralis stretches		6.0a The Lunge	
6.5d & 6.5h Bilateral stretches for the hip adductors		6.9c Bilateral stretch for the hamstrings and gastrocnemius		7.5a Squat with palms together above head	

2.8 The Extended Cat - an active extension stretch for the shoulders, hips, and cervical, thoracic and lumbar spine

2.8 Extended Cat

Starting position: Kneeling with your arms straight, palms down on the floor directly under your shoulders and fingers pointing forwards. Your knees are apart and directly under your hips, while your feet and toes point backwards. You head and spine are straight, in a neutral position and approximately horizontal with the floor.

Technique: See Part A. Page 94.

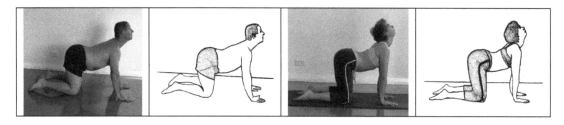

Direction and range of movement

The extend cat requires hip flexion, sacroiliac counter-nutation and extension of the spine and head.

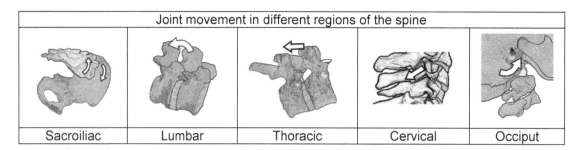

Joint movement in different regions of the spine				
Sacroiliac	Lumbar	Thoracic	Cervical	Occiput

Extension of the head, cervical, thoracic and lumbar spine (Occiput to L5) is about 150 degrees. Of that 90 degrees is in the head and neck, 25 degrees is in the thoracic and 35 degrees is in the lumbar. In the extended cat there is between one and two degrees sacroiliac joint extension and there is partial hip flexion of between 10 and 20 degrees.

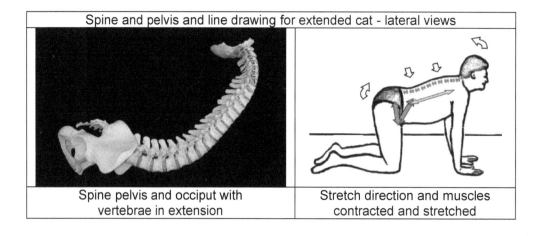

Spine and pelvis and line drawing for extended cat - lateral views	
Spine pelvis and occiput with vertebrae in extension	Stretch direction and muscles contracted and stretched

Target tissues

The extended cat is an active stretch. The suboccipital muscles, posterior cervical muscles, erector spinae and upper trapezius, extend the head and neck. The sternocleidomastoid assists in extending the head if there is simultaneous relaxation of the cervical prevertebral muscles.

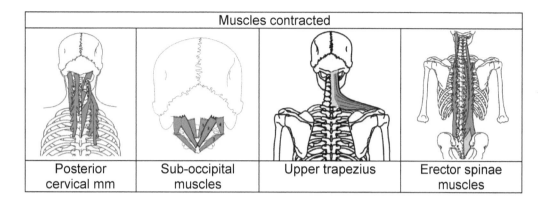

Muscles contracted			
Posterior cervical mm	Sub-occipital muscles	Upper trapezius	Erector spinae muscles

The erector spinae extends the spine. Iliacus, rectus femoris and tensor fascia latae produce hip flexion. Psoas major is also a hip flexor, but it can act as either a flexor or extensor of the lumbar spine, depending on the level of lumbar lordosis or reverse lordosis, the synergic action of other muscles and the degree of hip flexion at the start of movement. In the extended cat situation, psoas major acts as an extensor of the lumbar spine.

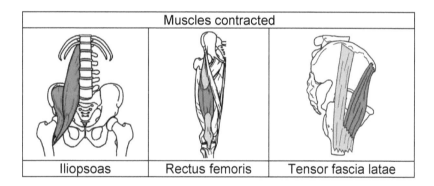

Muscles contracted		
Iliopsoas	Rectus femoris	Tensor fascia latae

The extended cat primarily stretches the muscles, fascia and ligaments of the ribs, abdomen and anterior cervical, thoracic and lumbar spine.

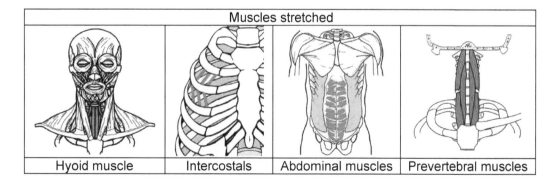

Muscles stretched			
Hyoid muscle	Intercostals	Abdominal muscles	Prevertebral muscles

These soft tissues arise on the sternum, pelvis, a vertebra or rib below and attach to the sternum, occiput, mandible, hyoid or a vertebra or rib above.

Safety

The extended cat is a relatively safe stretch. Movement into extension should be done slowly, with controlled breathing and without excessive force.

Caution should be applied if there are degenerative changes in the spine such as disc disease or osteoarthritis, or if there are congenital defects present such as a spondylolisthesis.

Care should be taken not to hyperextend the cervical spine and put pressure on the suboccipital joints when there is ligament laxity present.

If there is a pre-existing exaggerated posture such as an anterior occiput, increased thoracic kyphosis, dowager hump, thoracolumbar lordosis or reversed lumbar lordosis then the emphasis should be on countering the exaggeration.

Every person is unique, therefore it is important that each person be made aware of their unique structure by getting their posture professionally assessed. With this knowledge you will be able to apply the best emphasis to the stretch.

Vulnerable areas

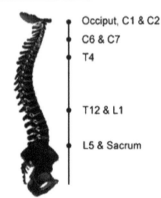

	Region	Level of Risk
1.	Occiput, C1 & C2	Low
2.	C6 to C7	Low
3.	T4	Low
4.	T12	Low
5.	L5	Low

Key:

2.8 Extended Cat	

Related stretches					
1.1a, b & c Lion stretches		1.5 Head & neck extension stretch seated		2.5a & 2.5b Upper Dog extension stretches	
2.6a & 2.6b Half Cobra & Full Cobra		2.7a, b & c Locust stretches		6.0a The Lunge	
6.5d & 6.5h Bilateral stretches for the hip adductors		6.9c Bilateral stretch for the hamstrings and gastrocnemius		7.5a Squat with palms together above head	

338

2.9 The Flexed Cat - active flexion stretches for the shoulders, hips, and cervical, thoracic and lumbar spine

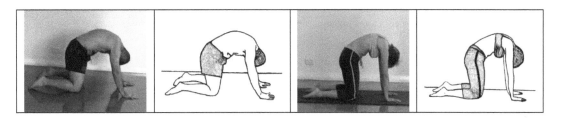

2.9a and 2.9b Flexed Cat

Starting position: Kneeling with your forearms extended, palms down on the floor, wrists directly under your shoulders and fingers pointing forwards. Abduct your hips so your knees are apart and rest directly under your hips. Your feet and toes point backwards. Your spine is straight, in a neutral position and approximately horizontal with the floor. Your head is also in a neutral position.

Technique: See Part A. Pages 95 and 96.

Direction and range of movement

The flexed cat requires hip extension, sacroiliac nutation and flexion of the spine and head.

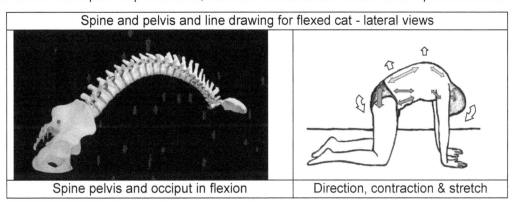

Spine and pelvis and line drawing for flexed cat - lateral views	
Spine pelvis and occiput in flexion	Direction, contraction & stretch

Flexion of the head, cervical, thoracic and lumbar spine (Occiput to L5) is about 150 degrees. There is a total of 45 degrees flexion in the head and neck, of which 15 degrees occurs between the occiput and C2, and 30 degrees between C2 and T1. There is 45 degrees flexion in the thoracic and 60 degrees in the lumbar. Thoracolumbar flexion (T10 – L1) is about 20 degrees. In the flexed cat there is between one and two degrees sacroiliac joint flexion, and there is partial hip flexion of between 10 and 20 degrees.

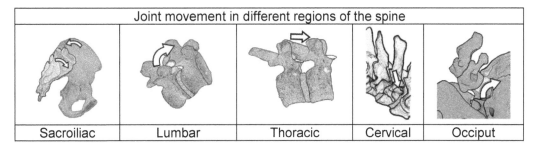

Joint movement in different regions of the spine				
Sacroiliac	Lumbar	Thoracic	Cervical	Occiput

Target tissues

The flexed cat is an active stretch. There is a small amount of assistance from gravity acting on the head but most of the movement is as a result of muscle contraction. Muscles of the anterior cervical spine, shoulders, hips, ribs and abdomen are contracted to flex the head and spine, and extend the hips.

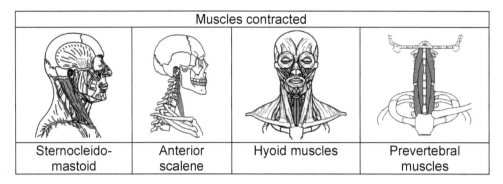

Muscles contracted			
Sternocleido-mastoid	Anterior scalene	Hyoid muscles	Prevertebral muscles

The sternocleidomastoid flexes the head and cervical spine providing there is simultaneous contraction of the cervical prevertebral muscles; this flexion is also assisted by the rectus capitis anterior, anterior scalene and some of the hyoid muscles.

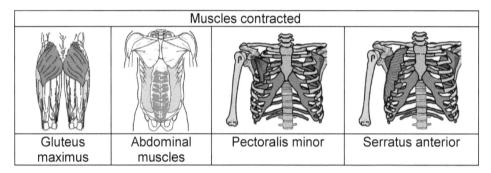

Muscles contracted			
Gluteus maximus	Abdominal muscles	Pectoralis minor	Serratus anterior

Rectus abdominis is the primary flexor of the lumbar and thoracolumbar spine. It is assisted by the internal and external abdominal obliques muscles and requires the relaxation of the iliopsoas. The anterior intercostal muscles act through the ribs in flexing the thoracic spine.

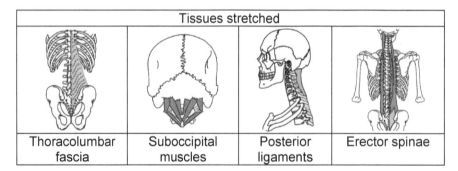

Tissues stretched			
Thoracolumbar fascia	Suboccipital muscles	Posterior ligaments	Erector spinae

Serratus anterior protracts the scapula, aided by pectoralis minor. The upper fibres protract most, with the lower fibres mainly working as upward rotators. Gluteus maximus produces hip extension; acting by tilting the pelvis posteriorly on the fixed hips. The flexed cat primarily stretches the muscles, fascia and ligaments of the posterior shoulders, ribs, suboccipital, cervical, thoracic and lumbar spines. These tissues arise on the pelvis, scapula, or on a vertebra or rib, and insert on the occiput. This is primarily a stretch for the posterior suboccipital and cervical muscles, the thoracic and lumbar fibres of erector spinae, trapezius, rhomboids, posterior spinal ligaments and thoracolumbar fascia.

Safety

The flexed cat is a relatively safe stretch. Caution should be applied if there is disc disease, or the potential for a disc prolapse or herniation in the spine, or pre-existing degeneration, most commonly in the lower cervical and lower lumbar spine.

340

Care should be taken not to over flex the spine. The posterior spinal muscles and ligaments, can be strained by excessive force and leverage generated by the arms, especially in area of the spine that are hypermobile. Movement should proceed slowly, with a focus on breathing, and the force should be mild.

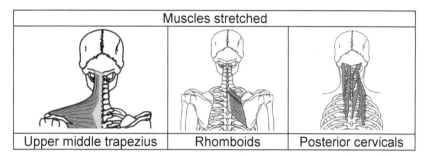

Muscles stretched		
Upper middle trapezius	Rhomboids	Posterior cervicals

If there is a pre-existing flexion posture such as an increased thoracic kyphosis, then you should avoid stretching this area of the spine.

Vulnerable areas

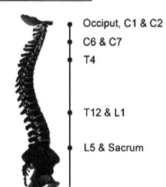

Occiput, C1 & C2
C6 & C7
T4
T12 & L1
L5 & Sacrum

	Region	Level of Risk
1.	Occiput, C1 & C2	Low
2.	C6 to C7	Low
3.	T4	Low
4.	T12	Low
5.	L5	Low

Key:

2.9a Flexed Cat kneeling	
2.9b Flexed Cat standing	

Related stretches					
1.3a Chin tuck prone		1.3b Chin tuck standing or seated		1.3c Chin tuck supine	
1.4a Head & neck active flexion stretch seated		1.4b Head & neck post-isometric flexion stretch supine		1.9 Atlanto-occipital post-isometric technique seated	
3.0a, b & c Knees to chest stretches supine		4.9a, b, c, d & e Scapula retractor stretches		7.5b Squat with arms in front of body	

3.0 Knees to chest - active, passive and post-isometric flexion stretches for the lower thoracic, lumbar and hips

3.0a & 3.0b Passive & post-isometric back stretch - knees to chest supine

Starting position: Supine on a carpet or mat, perhaps with a pillow under your head. Flex your hips and knees. Grasp around your knees with both hands, pull your flexed knees towards your chest.

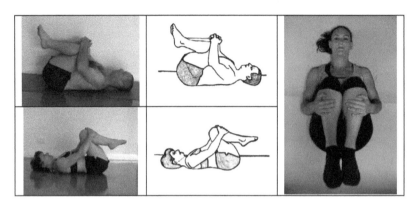

Technique: See Part A. Pages 97 and 98.

3.0c & 3.0d Active back stretches - knees to chest, with or without rotation

Starting position: Supine on a carpet or mat, perhaps with a pillow under your head. Flex your hips and knees, and bring your flexed knees towards your chest.

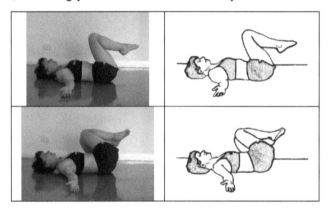

Technique: See Part A. Pages 99 and 100.

3.0e Unilateral stretch for the lumbar and gluteus maximus

Starting position: Supine on a carpet or mat, with a pillow under your head if you have a stiff flexed thoracic spine. Flex your right hip and knee. Grasp around your right knee and leg with both hands, and bring your knee towards your chest.

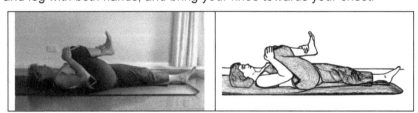

Technique: See Part A. Page 101.

Direction and range of movement

During the knees to chest stretches, the hips, sacrum and lumbar spine flex.

Lumbar flexion is about 45 degrees. Most lumbar flexion occurs in the middle lumbar between L4 and L5 and less occurs in the upper lumbar and between L5 and the sacrum. Active hip flexion with the knee bent is about 120 degrees and passive hip flexion is 150 degrees. People with hypermobile hip joints can sometimes bring their knees to the floor, creating 170 degrees or more of hip flexion.

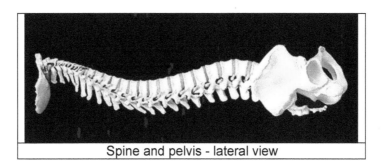

Spine and pelvis - lateral view

Flexion of the sacrum, also called nutation, occurs when the top of the sacrum moves forwards and downwards between the two innominate bones. In contrast extension or counter-nutation occurs when the top of the sacrum moves backwards between the two innominate bones. The sacrum articulates with the ilium at the right and left sacroiliac joints about a transverse axis.

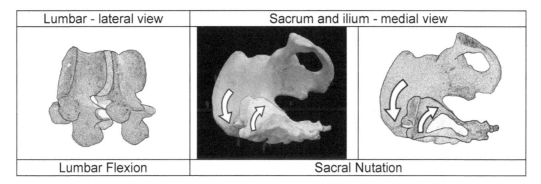

Lumbar - lateral view	Sacrum and ilium - medial view
Lumbar Flexion	Sacral Nutation

The total range of movement of nutation and counter nutation in the sacroiliac joint is about 2 degrees. This decreases with age and is greater in females, especially during pregnancy.

The passive knee to chest stretch 3.0a uses the upper limbs to pull on the lower limbs, exerting leverage through the hip to the ilium, sacrum, lumbar and lower thoracic spine. The active knees to chest stretch 3.0c uses abdominal and iliopsoas contraction to flex the hip, sacrum and lumbar spine.

The active stretch with rotation 3.0d uses abdominal and iliopsoas muscle contraction, but also involves gravity and the eccentric muscle contraction of the rotator muscles of the lumbar and thoracolumbar spine, gluteus medius, piriformis and the lowest fibres of gluteus maximus. The post-isometric technique 3.0b involves the isometric contraction of gluteus maximus and erector spinae.

Target tissues

This is primarily a stretch for quadratus lumborum and erector spinae. These muscles are anchored to the sacrum or iliac crest, and attach on ribs or vertebrae above.
This is also a stretch for the thoracolumbar fascia and gluteus maximus.

Muscles stretched	
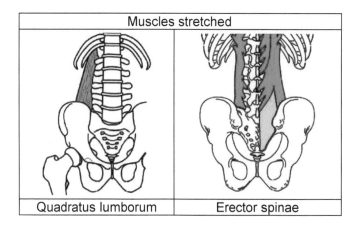	
Quadratus lumborum	Erector spinae

In the active variation of the stretch the rectus abdominis and iliopsoas are contracted and therefore strengthened.

Muscles stretched	
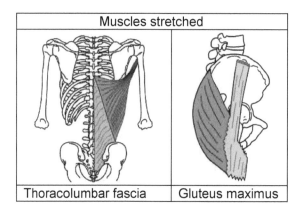	
Thoracolumbar fascia	Gluteus maximus

Variations

People with hypermobility and who have greater than average hip flexion will need to modify the knees to chest technique. To get a good stretch in the lumbar they will need to abduct their hips, and take their knees apart and around the sides of their rib cage and towards the floor. Only when their hip ligaments are sufficiently tight they will be able to move their pelvis backwards and stretch their lumbar spine.

Muscles contracted	
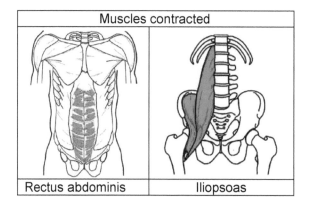	
Rectus abdominis	Iliopsoas

The knees to chest techniques stretch the lower back muscles and gluteus maximus. These muscles are frequently short, tight and have undergone fibrous structural changes, as a result of excessive loading and poor posture. The stretch is easy and offers great benefits for countering shortness and changes in these muscles. The active variation also has additional benefits, in that it helps strengthen the abdominal muscles, which are important in maintaining core strength and good posture.

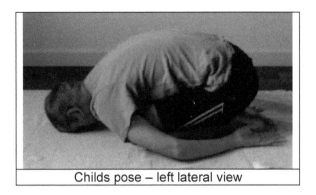
Childs pose – left lateral view

The passive knees to chest stretch can be done kneeling, with the spine and ribs folded over thighs. This 'chest to knees' stretch as it is an inverted variation of the knees to chest stretch. In yoga it is called the 'child's pose' and it is one of the relaxing yoga postures.

Safety

This is a relatively safe technique but there are some safety issues, contraindications and modifications which should be made to the stretches.

 The main disadvantage in all variations of the knees to chest stretch, is that bringing the knees to the chest, contracts the hip flexor muscles, the iliopsoas. The repeated contraction of any muscle potentially leads to shortness in that muscle.

Shortness of the iliopsoas is particularly undesirable because in the standing erect position a short iliopsoas pulls the lumbar and pelvis forward and downward, causing, perpetuating or exaggerating a lumbar lordosis, and it may also increase extension in the thoracolumbar or lumbosacral spine, all characteristics of the sway back posture.

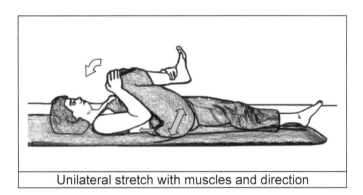
Unilateral stretch with muscles and direction

Ultimately ongoing iliopsoas shortness may lead to lower back pain. It is therefore important that in combination with the knees to chest stretch the iliopsoas muscles are stretched. The lunge 6.0a is the recommended technique for lengthening these muscles. If the structural integrity of the facet joints and the intervertebral discs of the spine, have been compromised by injury, postural stresses or years of overuse then this technique has risks.

Degeneration of the lower lumbar spine is a relatively common finding in people of middle age. It can be seen on X-ray. Spondylosis or degenerative osteoarthritis of the joints is associated with disc disease; a diseased disc being vulnerable to bulging. Nobody can predict exactly the probability of a disc bulge appearing, but if disc disease is present this technique should be done with care or not at all.

Over-enthusiastic application of the active or passive variation of this stretch poses the greatest danger in cases of disc degeneration. Caution should be taken in regards to how hard and how quickly you pull on the knees, in the passive stretch and in the post-isometric stretch.

Exercise is a double edge sword with the power to heal and the power to harm; the paradox is that this technique while having the potential to damage a disc, also helps protects against degeneration by stretching back muscles, and in the active stretch by also strengthening the abdominal muscles.

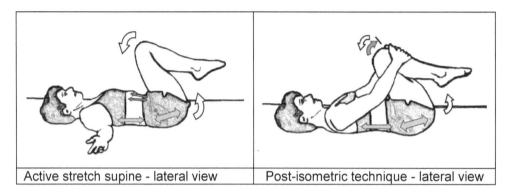

| Active stretch supine - lateral view | Post-isometric technique - lateral view |

Ligament strain is possible if hypermobility and associated ligament laxity exists in the spine. Loss of mobility in one area of the spine, may lead to compensatory hypermobility in another area. Genetically inherited or congenital hypermobility also predisposes to ligament strain.

Hypermobility can exist in the thoracolumbar, lumbosacral or sacroiliac spine, and when it does, over-stretching of the spine should be avoided. Strains are also possible when there is a lack of fitness or warm up prior to the stretch. Combined flexion-rotation stretches should be done with caution or avoided, if there is a history of ligament strain or known hypermobility.

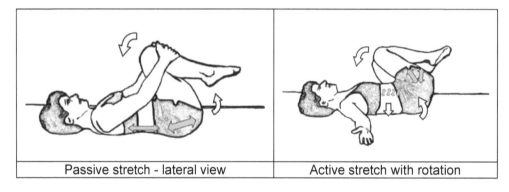

| Passive stretch - lateral view | Active stretch with rotation |

Where there is a known spondylolisthesis (defect in the bone) or spondylosis (osteoarthritis of the spine) caution should be taken. It would be prudent to avoid fast movements, particularly during the combined flexion and rotation stretches.

The kneeling variation of the stretch is usually safe but caution should be applied where there are problems with either of the knees. Cartilage or meniscus tears, cruciate ligament or collateral ligament tears and laxity, knee joint instability and hypermobility, and osteoarthritis may make the knee vulnerable during full flexion, especially in the kneeling variation. If there are problems with the knees, particularly in full flexion, then this stretch should be avoided or modified to avoid unwanted stress on the knees.

If you have groin pain, perhaps as a result of a muscle, tendon or ligament strain, then the knees to chest stretch may be contraindicated. Compression of the inguinal region during this stretch can be uncomfortable if there is a problem, and the stretch is best avoided until the problem is fixed.

Vulnerable areas

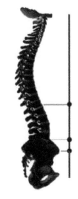

T12 & L1

L5 & Sacrum
Sacroiliac joint

	Region	Level of Risk
1.	Thoracolumbar	Low
2.	Lumbosacral	Low
3.	Sacroiliac joint	Low

Key:

3.0a Passive knees to chest stretch supine	
3.0b Post-isometric knees to chest stretch supine	
3.0c Active knees to chest stretch supine	
3.0d Active knees to chest stretch with rotation supine	
3.0e Unilateral stretch for the lumbar and gluteus maximus	

Related stretches					
4.9b & 4.9c Scapula retractor stretches squatting		6.0c The hanging hip stretch		6.1a - 6.1f Unilateral stretches for hip extensors	
6.5b Bilateral active stretch for hip adductors & extensors		7.5b Squat with arms in front of body			

3.1 - 3.5 Spinal twist sitting, standing, kneeling and prone - active and passive rotation stretches for the shoulders and the cervical, thoracic and lumbar spine

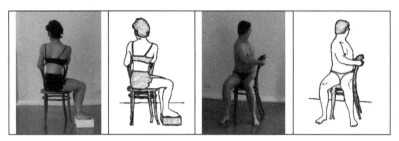

3.1a Passive spinal twist seated

Starting position: Seated with your back straight and your body at right angles to the back of the chair, so the side of one thigh is in contact with the back of the chair. Ensure both feet are planted on the floor or blocks so your body is grounded and spine upright. Rotate your head, neck, shoulders and spine towards the **back** of the chair, and grasp it with both hands.

Technique: See Part A. Page 102.

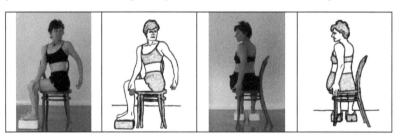

3.1b Active spinal twist seated

Starting position: Seated with your back straight and your body at right angles to the back of the chair, with the side of your thigh resting against the back of the chair. Ensure both feet are planted on the floor or blocks, and your spine is upright. Rotate your head, neck, shoulders and spine towards the **front** of the chair. Place the wrist of the hand nearest to your knee, against the side of your thigh and fully extend your forearm at the elbow. Allow your other arm to hang freely from the shoulder down at your side.

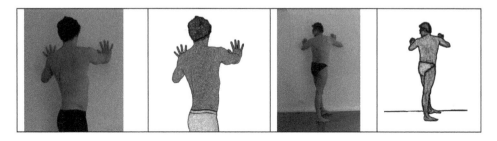

Technique: See Part A. Page 103.

3.2a Passive spinal twist standing wall supported

Starting position: Standing with your feet apart and the left side of your body about 20 cm from a wall. Flex your forearms about 90 degrees and flex your arms 45 degrees. Rotate your head, shoulders and spine to the left, so that your upper body faces the wall, but keep your pelvis fixed. Place your palms flat against a wall or intermesh your fingers in a wire fence about shoulder height.

Technique: See Part A. Page 105.

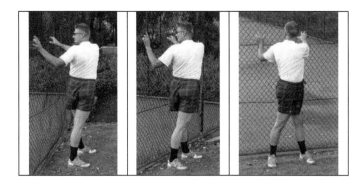

3.2b Active spinal twist standing

Starting position: Standing with your feet apart and your arms at your sides. Rotate your head, neck, shoulders and spine to the left but keep your pelvis and lower limbs in a fixed position. Relax your shoulders so they are dropped and your arms hang freely at your sides.

Technique: See Part A. Page 106.

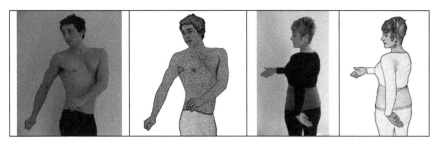

3.3 Active spinal twist standing flexed at the hips

Starting position: Standing with your feet 30 to 50 cm apart, about 1 m from a chair or table. Flex about 90 degrees at the hips and grasp the back of the chair. Lean backwards, away from the chair and drop your upper thoracic spine towards the floor. Keep your spine, legs and arms straight. Rotate your spine to the left, so that your upper body faces sideways. As an alternative to using a chair for support grasp a wire fence.

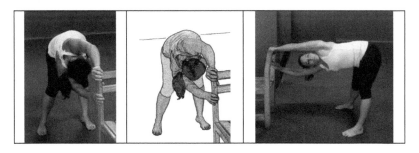

Technique: See Part A. Page 107.

3.4 Active spinal twist kneeling

Starting position: Kneeling with your hands palms down on the floor in front of you - as in the cat position. Move your left hand a few centimetres forward and flex your left elbow. Lift your right hand off the floor, then slide it along the floor and under your body to the left. This will rotate your spine to the left. The back of your right hand and arm rests on the floor, and your left elbow is flexed about 90 degrees.

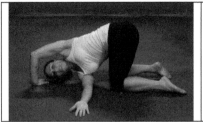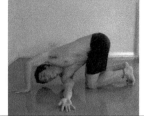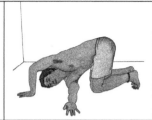

Technique: See Part A. Page 108.

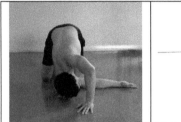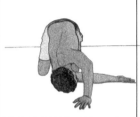

3.5 Passive and active spinal twist prone

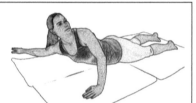

Starting position: Prone with your feet apart and your toes pointing backwards. Abduct your arms until your hands are level with your shoulders. Flex your left elbow and place your hand, palm down, nearer to your side. Raise your head and left shoulder and left elbow off the floor. This will rotate your spine to the left. Keep your pelvis on the floor.

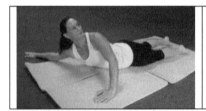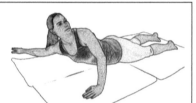

Technique: See Part A. Page 109.

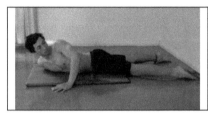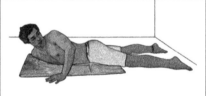

Direction and range of movement

Total spinal rotation to one side is about 130 degrees. Rotation of the head and neck (Occiput to C7) is about 90 degrees; rotation of the thoracic (T1 to T12) is about 35 degrees; and rotation of the lumbar (L1 to Sacrum) is about 5 degrees.

During trunk rotation there is about 14 cm of medial to lateral movement of the scapula along the rib cage (10 cm abduction and 4 cm adduction). During rotation one scapula moves away from the spine and around the chest wall (protraction or abduction) while the other scapula moves towards the spine (retraction or adduction).

Most spinal rotation occurs in the cervical spine, mid thoracic spine and at the junction of the thoracic and lumbar spine.

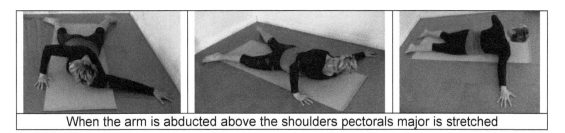

| When the arm is abducted above the shoulders pectorals major is stretched |

The passive spinal twist standing wall supported and the active spinal twist standing 3.2b also involve internal hip rotation on one side and external hip rotation on the other side.

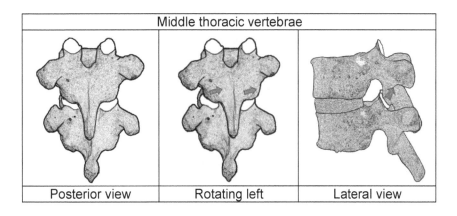

Middle thoracic vertebrae		
Posterior view	Rotating left	Lateral view

Target tissues

The spinal twist is primarily a stretch for the deep rotator muscles of the spine - the semispinalis thoracis, rotatores and multifidus. The lower origins of these muscles are anchored to a vertebra or rib by the weight of the body, while the upper ends attach to a vertebra or rib, one to six levels above.

This is also a stretch for the middle trapezius, rhomboid major and minor, abdominal obliques, intercostal muscles, serratus posterior inferior, spinal ligaments and thoracolumbar fascia.

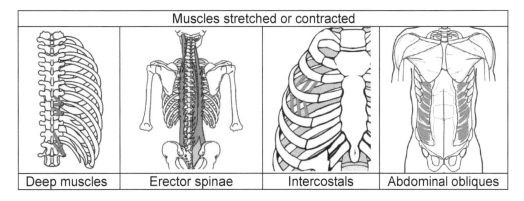

Muscles stretched or contracted			
Deep muscles	Erector spinae	Intercostals	Abdominal obliques

This is also a mild stretch for pectoralis minor and serratus anterior. If the arm is abducted above 90 degrees, for example during the spinal twist prone 3.5, then it becomes a good stretch for pectoralis major and its surrounding fascia.

When the head is rotated this is also a stretch for the suboccipital muscles - mainly rectus capitis posterior major and obliquus capitis inferior; the deep cervical rotator muscles -

multifidus; and the superficial posterior cervical muscles - semispinalis capitis, semispinalis cervicis, splenius cervicis and splenius capitis; and longissimus capitis and iliocostalis cervicis in the erector spinae group.

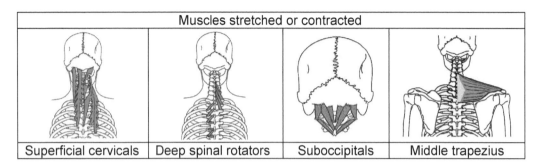

Muscles stretched or contracted			
Superficial cervicals	Deep spinal rotators	Suboccipitals	Middle trapezius

Greater rotation is achieved with the passive stretch, however more muscles are strengthened with the active stretch; these muscles being the antagonists to the muscles being stretched. They reside on the opposite side of the body and are the same by name as those listed above.

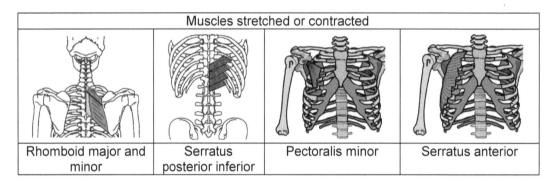

Muscles stretched or contracted			
Rhomboid major and minor	Serratus posterior inferior	Pectoralis minor	Serratus anterior

Other factors

The range of rotation is not the same at each vertebral level throughout the spine. Rotation is coupled with flexion and sidebending towards the same side as rotation. There is greater rotation in the thoracic compared with the lumbar spine. The range of rotation increases as you descend the spine and peeks at T7. It decreases between T8 and T10 and peaks again at T12. Rotation decreases considerably in the lumbar region.

Although rotation is limited by the rib cage it is the freest of all movements in the thoracic spine. Rotation increases from T1 to T7 because the ribs increase in length and decrease in curvature and because of the plane and shape of the costotransverse joints.

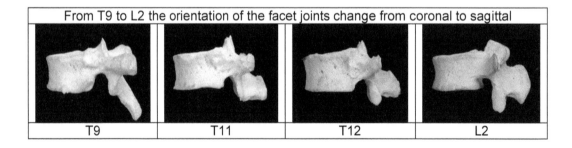

From T9 to L2 the orientation of the facet joints change from coronal to sagittal			
T9	T11	T12	L2

Rotation is less between T7 to T10 because the ribs get shorter and more curved and because they are part of a more rigid structure, a ring of cartilage, bone, ligaments and joints, serving as an anchor for the diaphragm and abdominal muscles.

Ribs 11 and 12 give the thoracic greater flexibility because they are free at their anterior ends, and do not attach on costal cartilage or the sternum.

The range of rotation is determined by the shape and orientation of the facet joints. The sagittal orientation of the facet joints in the lumbar spine significantly limits the range of rotation to only one degree per vertebra. In contrast the coronal orientation of the thoracic facet joints permits three times as much rotation per vertebra.

The transition from a coronal orientation of the facet joints in the thoracic to a sagittal orientation of the facet joints in the lumbar is shown below. In the lumbar sacral spine (L5/S1) the orientation of the facet joints can vary from slightly sagittal to slightly coronal and may be asymmetrical. The range of rotation between individual will vary. Movement in the lumbar and sacral spine is also limited by strong iliolumbar ligaments.

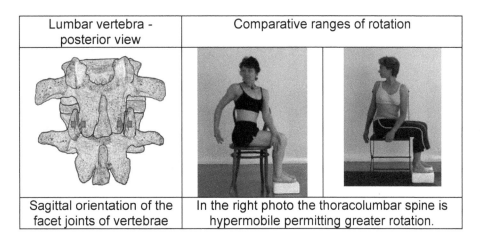

Lumbar vertebra - posterior view	Comparative ranges of rotation
Sagittal orientation of the facet joints of vertebrae	In the right photo the thoracolumbar spine is hypermobile permitting greater rotation.

Safety

The spinal twist seated in a chair is a relatively safe technique and carries few risks unless there is an underlying pathology or congenital deformity.

Avoid slouching during the rotation stretch. If the spine is kept in neutral - in other words neither in flexion or extension - then this will result in optimum rotation. This will maximise the overall range of rotation and the rotation will be distributed throughout the spine, appropriate to the anatomy of each vertebra.

Do not allow the pelvis tilt backward, the lumbar lordosis to flatten out or reverse, and do not allow the mid thoracic spine to flex or the thoracic kyphosis to become exaggerated.
This stretch should only be done sitting on the floor, if your hips joints are flexible enough and your hamstrings long enough to allow you to sit up straight, and maintain a comfortable upright position. People who have spent their whole lives sitting on chairs may not have sufficient flexibility to do the spinal twist while sitting on the floor and keep an erect spine.

Doing this stretch with a stooping posture restricts rotation, reduces it benefits and can cause injury. Until you have gained sufficient flexibility in your hips you should only do the chair technique. If you have healthy knee joints, another option is to do the active spinal twist kneeling.

Care should be taken not to over stretch the thoracolumbar part of the spine. If the area is hypermobile further stretching may result in increased hypermobility, ligament strain and injury.

Vulnerable areas

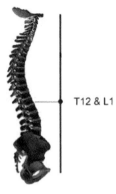

T12 & L1

	Region	Level of Risk
1.	Thoracolumbar	Low

Key:

3.1a Passive spinal twist seated in a chair		3.1b Active spinal twist seated on a chair	
3.1c Spinal twist sitting on the floor		3.2a Passive spinal twist standing wall supported	
3.2b Active spinal twist standing		3.3 Active spinal twist standing flexed at the hips	
3.4 Active spinal twist kneeling		3.5 Passive and active spinal twist prone	

Related stretches					
1.6 Head & neck active rotation stretch seated		2.6d Rotation Cobra		7.4a & 7.4b Unilateral passive, active & isometric stretches	

3.6 Rolled towel - active, post-isometric and passive stretch for pectoralis major, the ribs, thoracic and cervical spine

3.6 Pectoralis stretch supine over a rolled towel

Starting position: Sitting on the floor. Place a tightly rolled up towel behind your back and then lie over the towel with your feet apart and your palms upwards. The towel should be across your spine where your thoracic curve is most flexed. Bring your arms apart until you are in a cross position. Tuck your chin in and relax over the towel.

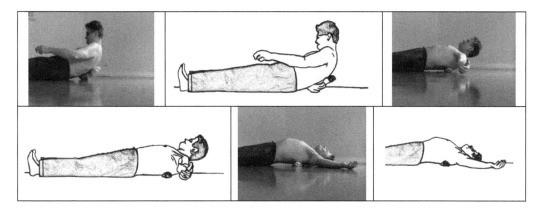

Technique: See Part A. Page 110.

Direction and Range of Movement

In the next four techniques the spine and rib cage are raised above the floor by a rolled up towel, resulting in increased extension through the thoracic spine and increased horizontal extension in the shoulder.

The rolled up towel should be between 4 cm and 6 cm in diameter. Use an old towel that has lost its fluffiness. Iron it flat and roll it up tightly. The rolled-up towel should be placed across the spine, perpendicular to the spine - not along it.

In this, the first of the rolled up towel techniques, the arms are abducted to 90 degrees, allowing both left and right pectoralis major muscles to be stretched.
In abduction and mild horizontal extension a person with normal flexibility should have full contact on the floor with their elbows, forearms and hands.

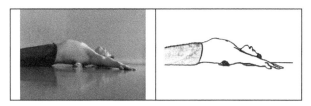

There is approximately 30 degrees horizontal extension at the shoulder which includes several centimetres of medial movement of the scapula on the thorax – scapula adduction or retraction. Between T1 and T12 in the thoracic spine there should be about 25 degrees extension.

The shape of the thoracic varies between individuals. It ranges from a reverse kyphosis, to a straight spine or 'poker back', to a normal kyphosis, to an exaggerated kyphosis.

If the person also has a scoliosis this will mean the sidebending interacting with the various flexion or extension curvatures listed above, and the introduction of a rotation component, because sidebending is biomechanically linked with rotation.

When there is a simple exaggerated kyphosis the rolled-up towel should be placed at, or near to, the apex of the kyphosis. This can be anywhere between T4 and T12 but is usually near T7, which is level with the inferior angle of the scapula.

When there is a scoliosis with a kyphosis, then the rolled up towel should be placed under the side the thoracic spine is rotated towards. This is the point the spine is most posterior and where the ribs are most pronounced. The towel is always across the spine, but when there is a scoliosis then moving the towel one or two centimetres towards the side the spine is rotated will help counter the rotation part of the scoliosis.

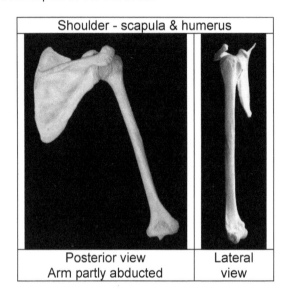

Shoulder - scapula & humerus	
Posterior view Arm partly abducted	Lateral view

The degree of abduction of the arm will also influence the effectiveness of the technique. At 90 degrees abduction, maximum leverage will be applied in the middle of the thoracic spine and between both scapulae. Above 90 degrees the leverage point moves towards the upper thoracic spine. Below 90 degrees it moves towards the lower thoracic, and as there is less pull on the ribs by the pectoralis major muscles the leverage quickly decreases in intensity.

Target tissue

This is primarily a stretch for pectoralis major, as well as the fascia of the anterior chest. It has particular benefit for any person with an increased kyphosis and round shoulders.

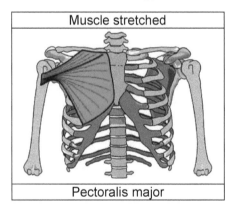

Muscle stretched
Pectoralis major

This is also a stretch for pectoralis minor, subscapularis, anterior deltoid and the anterior intercostal muscles.

This is a mild stretch for latissimus dorsi, teres major, lower trapezius, iliopsoas, rectus abdominis, anterior scalene and the abdominal facia.

When the palms are facing upwards towards the ceiling, the arms are externally rotated and the middle and lower fibres of pectoralis major are stretched. The lowest fibres can be stretched more strongly by flexing your elbows 90 degrees and then either actively moving your forearms towards the floor, or allowing the weight of the forearms to pull them back. External rotation also increases the stretch on latissimus dorsi and teres major.

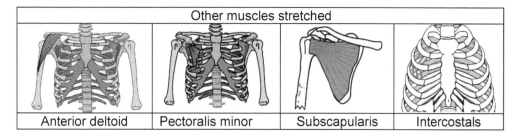

Other muscles stretched			
Anterior deltoid	Pectoralis minor	Subscapularis	Intercostals

When the palms are facing downwards into the floor, the arms are in an internally rotated position, which increases the stretch on infraspinatus, teres minor and posterior deltoid. The technique stretches the most anterior tissues or the spine and rib cage. It mainly stretches the anterior longitudinal ligaments in front of the thoracic vertebral bodies and the anterior fascia. To a lesser extent it stretches the capsular ligament supporting facet joints.

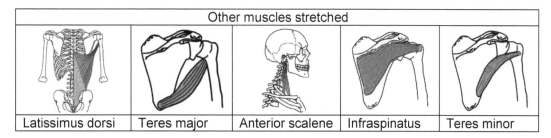

Other muscles stretched				
Latissimus dorsi	Teres major	Anterior scalene	Infraspinatus	Teres minor

The passive part of the stretch uses the weight of the arms and shoulders (gravity) to lengthen the anteriorly positioned tissues. The post-isometric part of the stretch involves contracting various muscles, tensing and then relaxing them to facilitate further lengthening of the anteriorly located tissues.

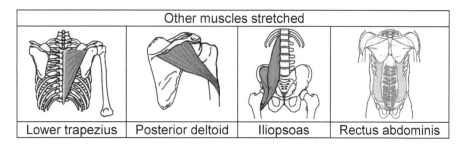

Other muscles stretched			
Lower trapezius	Posterior deltoid	Iliopsoas	Rectus abdominis

There is a mild active component in the stretch when the isometric contraction of muscles pulls against the resistance offered by ligaments, fascia and antagonist muscles, but this is mainly a post-isometric and passive stretch.

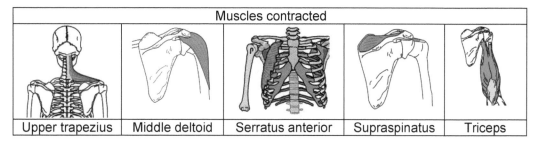

Muscles contracted				
Upper trapezius	Middle deltoid	Serratus anterior	Supraspinatus	Triceps

In actively stretching the upper limb the following muscles are contracted: triceps, supraspinatus, middle deltoid, upper trapezius and serratus anterior.

Safety

This is applicable to all the rolled towel stretches 3.6, 3.7, 3.8 and 3.9.

When lying across the rolled-up towel, do not to allow the head to drop back into hyperextension, placing strain on vulnerable tissues around the suboccipital joints. The occipito-atlanto-axial joints between the occiput, C1 and C2 are supported by relatively small muscles and ligaments which can be overstretched with too much extension. The weight of the head can force facet joints into extreme locked-in extension positions, potentially irritating structures such as the vertebral arteries.

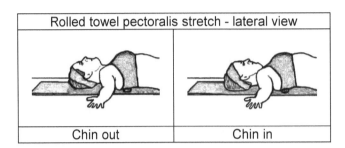

Rolled towel pectoralis stretch - lateral view	
Chin out	Chin in

Similarly do not allow the neck to over extend, putting pressure on the facet joints and intervertebral discs of the lower cervical spine. Particular caution should be applied if there is known degeneration in the lower cervical spine. Cervical or suboccipital hyperextension is more likely to occur when there is an increased thoracic kyphosis, including a dowager hump, as well as inflexibility in the thoracic spine.

Tuck in your chin when you initially lay over the rolled-up towel. As your body relaxes over the rolled up towel it will be necessary to periodically continue to tuck in your chin, thereby repositioning your head in progressively greater amounts of flexion. Repositioning your head helps protect the suboccipital and cervical joints from strain and helps counter the classical 'bad head posture' - the anterior occiput with an extended upper cervical spine, also known as an increased cervical lordosis.

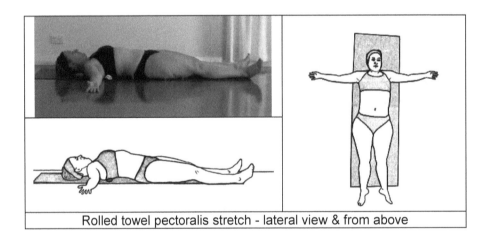

Rolled towel pectoralis stretch - lateral view & from above

If you are unable to correct for the hyperextension of the head with the tuck-in chin movement because the thoracic kyphosis is too great or there is too much inflexibility then there are two options: either place a small pillow under your head or reduce the thickness of the rolled-up towel. In some people the rigidity and increased flexion of the kyphosis may be so great that a rolled-up towel is inappropriate. In this case the person should simply lie on the floor, perhaps with a small pillow under the head. Over time, as flexibility in the thoracic spine increases, the pillow can be removed from under the head, and later still a small rolled-up towel placed under the thoracic spine.

Care should also be taken not to strain the rotator cuff tendons or aggravate a pre-existing rotator cuff injury while lying over a rolled up towel with arms at various ranges of abduction. Warm up exercises for the shoulders may be used to prepare for the rolled-up towel stretches, for example in the standing position, moving the shoulders in progressively wider circles. If you have an exaggerated and/or rigid kyphosis, or if there is history of rotator cuff strain, it may also be a good idea to move slowly into the roller-up towel stretches.

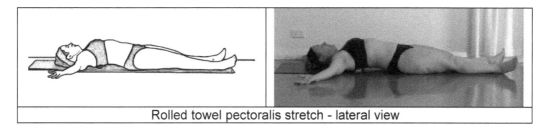

Rolled towel pectoralis stretch - lateral view

Make sure the rolled up towel is between 4 and 6 cm in diameter, or smaller, depending on the size of the person using it and the state of the spine.

Do not place the rolled towel under thoracic vertebrae that are in extension - in other words vertebrae that are fixed in a backward bent position. This most common occurs in the thoracic at or near T4. It may involve one vertebra, several vertebrae or in rare situations the whole of the thoracic spine may form a reversed kyphosis. The logic of this technique is to address parts of the thoracic spine that are in excess flexion, not to add to or create extra extension in areas that may already be in extension.

Vulnerable areas

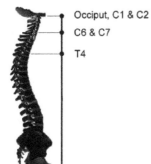

Occiput, C1 & C2
C6 & C7
T4

	Region	Level of Risk
1.	Occiput, C1 & C2	Medium
2.	Cervical spine	Low
3.	T4	Low
4.	Rotator cuff	Medium

Key:

3.6 Rolled towel stretch for pectoralis major	

Related stretches					
1.3a, b & c Chin tuck stretches		2.5a & b Upper Dog extension stretches		2.6a Half Cobra	
2.8 Extended cat		3.7, 3.8 & 3.9 Supine rolled towel stretches		4.0a to 4.0h Pectoralis stretches	
5.3a & 5.3b Elbow flexor stretches		5.5 Supinator stretch		5.6a Pronator stretch using a doorframe	

3.7 Rolled towel - active, passive and post-isometric stretch for the shoulders, ribs, thoracic and cervical spine

3.7 Longitudinal stretch supine over a rolled towel

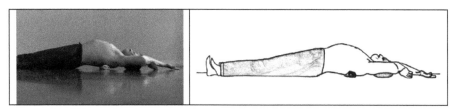

Starting position: Sitting on the floor. Place a tightly rolled up towel behind your back across the apex of your thoracic spine, where the curve is most flexed. Lie over the towel with your feet apart and your palms upwards. Bring your arms apart until your hands are above your head and your arms rest against the side of your head. Feel an increase of pressure of your body on the towel. Tuck your chin in and relax over the towel.

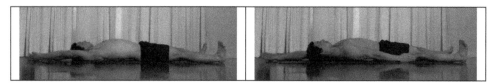

Technique: See Part A. Page 111.

Stretch one arm, both arms or combinations of arms and legs

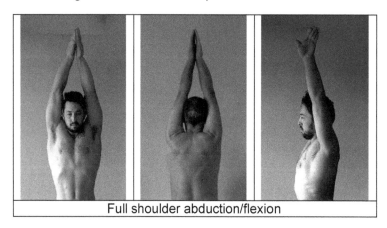

Direction and range of movement

Depending on the stretch, the main movements include shoulder abduction, elbow extension, scapula elevation or depression, scapula protraction or retraction, scapula upward or downward rotation, knee extension and ankle dorsiflexion or plantar flexion.

Other movements include scapula backward tilt, shoulder internal or external rotation, elbow supination or pronation, finger extension and abduction, thoracic extension, thoracic and lumbar spinal distraction (longitudinal stretching), cervical flexion or moving out of extension, and head flexion or moving out of extension with posterior head translation.

Full shoulder abduction/flexion

A small rolled up towel is placed under the apex of the thoracic spine. The apex of the curve is usually in the middle of the thoracic spine at about vertebra level T7, but it can be at any point between vertebra T4 and T12. The rolled up towel raises the spine and rib cage off the floor. The spine is raised to its maximum elevation off the floor at the point the towel contacts the spine. This is also the point of maximum thoracic extension

Gravity acting on the torso causes the shoulders to drop back towards the floor and the scapula to retract and acting on the head on the neck causes the cervical spine to extend.

Full shoulder abduction over a rolled up towel can be challenging for some people, but a person with normal flexibility should be able to fully abduct both shoulders, fully extend both elbows, bringing the backs of their wrists, hands and fingers together, while maintaining floor contact with their hands – a movement also requiring shoulder internal rotation and forearm pronation.

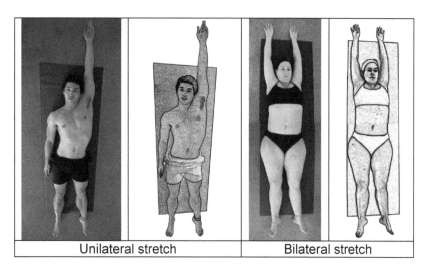

| Unilateral stretch | Bilateral stretch |

Shoulder abduction is 180 degrees, a combination or glenohumeral and scapulothoracic movement at a ratio of 2:1. Scapula tilt is between 5 and 10 degrees. Shoulder internal rotation is 90 degrees. From full supination to full pronation is 180 degrees.

Full forearm extension at the elbow means a straight arm. But in extremely flexible people, the elbow may hyperextend 10 degrees past the straight position. This may be caused by a shorter olecranon process or the result of ligament laxity, associated with congenital hypermobility.

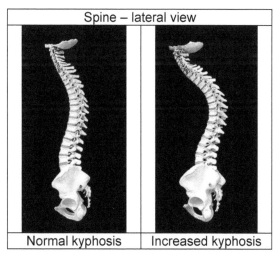

Spine – lateral view

| Normal kyphosis | Increased kyphosis |

Thoracic extension varies between different individuals and it varies in different regions of the thoracic spine. But between T1 and T12 on average there is about 25 degrees extension in the thoracic spine. Most thoracic extension occurs in individuals with a reverse kyphosis and in those with congenital hypermobility. Least thoracic extension occurs in individuals with an increase kyphosis and in those with generalised inflexibility.

This technique is most useful for people with an exaggerated kyphosis. The rolled up towel should be placed at or near to the apex of the kyphosis, which may be between T4 and T12 but is usually near T7.

Target tissue

These are a series of different stretches involving an upper limb, both upper limbs, or various combinations of upper and lower limbs and the trunk. Some are longitudinal stretches down one side of the body and others are diagonal stretches. There are five variations and each one involves different muscles.

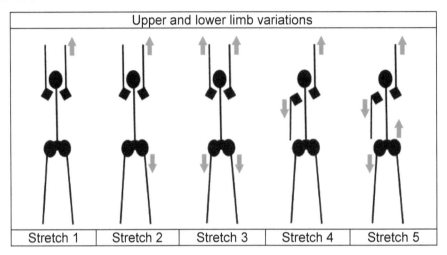

Upper and lower limb variations				
Stretch 1	Stretch 2	Stretch 3	Stretch 4	Stretch 5

Stretch 1 One upper limb abducted elevated.

This is the longitudinal movement of one upper limb and stretches the muscles of the trunk, arm, forearm and hand.

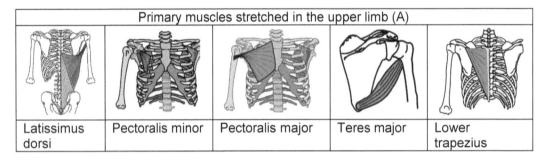

Primary muscles stretched in the upper limb (A)				
Latissimus dorsi	Pectoralis minor	Pectoralis major	Teres major	Lower trapezius

This technique primarily stretches latissimus dorsi, teres major, lower trapezius, teres minor, pectoralis minor and the lower fibres of pectoralis major. It also stretches biceps brachii, brachialis, as well as the finger flexor muscles and fascia of the anterior forearm - flexor digitorum profundus and flexor digitorum superficialis and hand – palmar interossei, flexor digiti minimi, opponens digiti minimi, lumbricales, and depending on the position of the thumb, the thenar muscles.

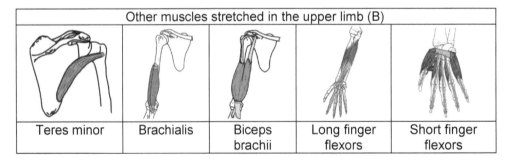

Other muscles stretched in the upper limb (B)				
Teres minor	Brachialis	Biceps brachii	Long finger flexors	Short finger flexors

In actively stretching the upper limb the following muscles are contracted: supraspinatus, middle deltoid, upper trapezius and serratus anterior. Triceps and anconeus act at the elbow to maintain extension of the forearm, and extensor digitorum, extensor indicis and extensor digiti minimi extend the fingers.

Muscles contracted in moving the upper limb (C)				
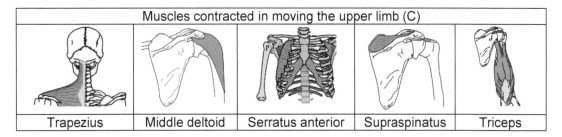				
Trapezius	Middle deltoid	Serratus anterior	Supraspinatus	Triceps

Stretch 2 Down one side of the body - upper limb, trunk, pelvis and lower limb on the same side. Upper limb up - lower limb down.

This is a longitudinal movement down one side of the body - elevating one upper limb and depressing the lower limb on the same side. It stretches the muscles of the trunk, shoulders, arm, forearm, hand, abdomen, pelvis, thigh, leg and foot, on one side of the body.

Primary muscles stretched in the trunk (D)		
Quadratus lumborum	Iliocostalis lumborum,	Abdominal muscles

This technique stretches the upper limb muscles listed above in Stretch 1 (A) and (B). In the trunk the primary muscles stretches are quadratus lumborum, iliocostalis lumborum and the lateral fibres of the abdominal muscles - the internal and external obliques. It is a weak stretch for gracilis as well as the anterior and lateral intercostal muscles. If the foot and toes are moved upwards towards your head (dorsiflexion) gastrocnemius, soleus and the toe flexor muscles are stretched, however if the foot and toes are pointed away (plantar flexion) tibialis anterior and the toe extensor muscles are stretched.

The muscles contracted to actively stretch the upper limb are listed above in Stretch 1 (C). To move the lower limb away from the upper limb on the same side and stretch one side of the body requires the contraction of erector spinae, quadratus lumborum and the lateral abdominal muscles on the opposite side.

Other muscles stretched (E)				
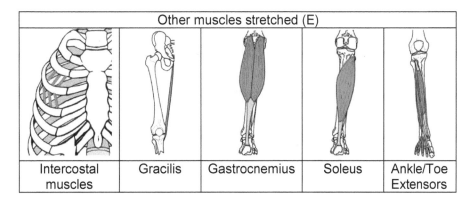				
Intercostal muscles	Gracilis	Gastrocnemius	Soleus	Ankle/Toe Extensors

In addition, the position of the heel and toes can alter which muscles being targeted. If the heel is pointed away and the foot moved upwards towards your head (ankle dorsiflexion) then tibialis anterior is contracted. If the toes are also curled upwards towards the head (toe extension) extensor hallucis longus and extensor digitorum longus are contracted. If the foot and toes are pointed away, gastrocnemius, soleus, tibialis posterior, peroneus longus, flexor hallucis longus and flexor digitorum longus are contracted.

	Variations	Muscles
Stretch 1	Unilateral upper limb	ABC
Stretch 2	Unilateral upper and lower limb	ABCDEFG
Stretch 3	Bilateral upper and lower limb	ABCDEFG
Stretch 4	Diagonal upper limb and upper thoracic spine	ABCDEHI
Stretch 5	Diagonal upper limb, lower limb, thoracic and lumbar spine	ABCDEFGHI

Stretch 3 Stretching both upper and lower limbs.

This is a longitudinal movement down both sides of the body - elevating the upper limbs and depressing the lower limbs. It stretches the muscles of the trunk, shoulders, arms, forearms, hands, abdomen, pelvis, thighs, legs and feet on both sides of the body.

Primary muscles contracted in the trunk (F)		
Quadratus lumborum	Iliocostalis lumborum	Abdominal muscles

This is mainly an active stretch for the upper limb muscles. It involves the muscles listed in Stretch 1 and 2. Other than some possible foot and ankle movement, there is very little actual lower body movement during this stretch. When the shoulder muscles on both sides of the body are contracting equally there is no sidebending of the spine or tilting of the pelvis or movement of the lower limbs. The spine remains straight, both hip bones remain level and both legs remain in a fixed position. Without movement, other than perhaps a small amount of joint play, any stretching of the lower limb muscles can only be due to a weak isometric contraction stabilising the lower body.

Tibialis anterior, extensor hallucis longus and extensor digitorum longus are responsible for moving the foot and toes upwards (dorsiflexion). Soleus and gastrocnemius are responsible for moving the foot downwards (plantarflexion) and they are assisted by tibialis posterior, peroneus longus and brevis, flexor hallucis longus and flexor digitorum longus.

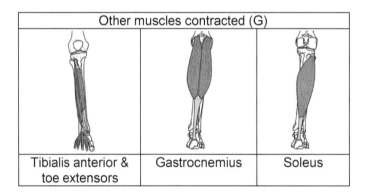

Other muscles contracted (G)		
Tibialis anterior & toe extensors	Gastrocnemius	Soleus

Stretch 4 Stretching the upper limb on one side by depressing the shoulder and the upper limb on the other side by elevating the shoulder.

The diagonal movement of the upper limbs involves the stretching of the muscles listed in Stretch 1, on the side the shoulder is elevated. However, on the side the shoulder is

364

depressed, upper trapezius, levator scapulae, rhomboid major and rhomboid minor are the muscles being stretched.

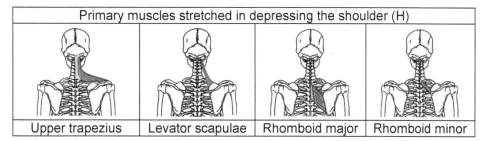

Primary muscles stretched in depressing the shoulder (H)			
Upper trapezius	Levator scapulae	Rhomboid major	Rhomboid minor

The muscles responsible for actively elevating one upper limb are listed in Stretch 1 (A). The muscles responsible for actively depressing the other upper limb include: latissimus dorsi, lower trapezius, pectoralis minor and the lower fibres of pectoralis major.

Stretch 5 Stretching by elevating the upper limb and lower limb on one side and depressing the upper limb and lower limb on the other side.

This diagonal movement involves the stretching of all the muscles listed for the upper limbs in Stretch 4, and for the lower limb the muscles listed for Stretch 2. By elevating the pelvis on one side and depressing the pelvis on the other side, the intensity of the stretch is increased.

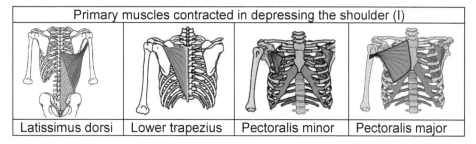

Primary muscles contracted in depressing the shoulder (I)			
Latissimus dorsi	Lower trapezius	Pectoralis minor	Pectoralis major

The muscles responsible for actively elevating one upper limb are listed in Stretch 1 and the muscles responsible for actively depressing the other upper limb are listed in Stretch 4. The muscles responsible for actively elevating one lower limb and depressing the other upper limb are the same as listed in Stretch 2 – but as both hips are involved, the force will be stronger.

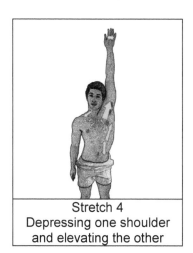

Stretch 4
Depressing one shoulder
and elevating the other

In this stretch and some of the other stretches there may also be some stretching of sternocleidomastoid, anterior scalene, teres minor, gluteus medius, gluteus minimus, sartorius, rectus femoris, tensor fasciae latae, iliopsoas, rectus abdominis, and abdominal facia as well as the anterior longitudinal ligaments in the thoracic spine. Which secondary tissues are affected depends on the posture of the individual. People with an increased kyphosis and rounded shoulders will be stretched the most.

Other tissues that may be stretched include the facia overlying the posterior leg, the Achilles tendon the plantar fascia, the pectoral fascia and ligaments of the anterior thoracic spine such as the anterior longitudinal ligaments.

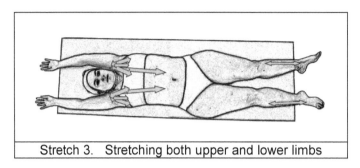

| | Stretch 3. | Stretching both upper and lower limbs |

Safety: See Rolled towel 3.6

Vulnerable areas

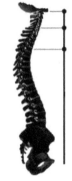

Occiput, C1 & C2

C6 & C7

T4

	Region	Level of Risk
1.	Occiput, C1 & C2	Medium
2.	Cervical spine	Low
3.	T4	Low
4.	Rotator cuff	Medium

Key:

3.7 Supine longitudinal stretches over a rolled up towel	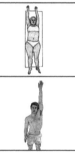

Related stretches					
1.3a, b & c Chin tuck stretches		2.3 Kneeling lateral stretch		2.4a to 2.4d Hanging stretches	
2.5a & b Upper Dog extension stretches		2.6a Half Cobra		2.7a Diagonal locust	
3.6, 3.8 & 3.9 Supine rolled towel stretches		4.0a to 4.0h Pectoralis stretches		4.6a Palms above head and supinated	
7.1h Bilateral or unilateral active calf stretch		7.2a Bilateral or unilateral active stretch for ankle dorsiflexors & toes		7.5a Squat with palms together above head	

3.8 Rolled towel - active, passive and post-isometric stretches for the shoulders, arms, forearms, wrist, hands and fingers

3.8a Bilateral anterior forearm and hand stretch supine

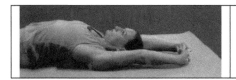

Starting position: Supine on the floor over a tightly rolled up towel and with your feet apart. The rolled towel is placed behind and across your thoracic spine at the point the curve is most flexed. Bring your arms over your head, place them on the floor, and then interlace your fingers. Pronate your forearms, placing the ulna side of your hands on the floor, while maintaining hand contact with the floor (or as near to it as possible) throughout all the stretches. Turn your hands, so your palms face away from you. Extend your elbows until both arms are completely straight. Tuck in your chin and relax over the towel.

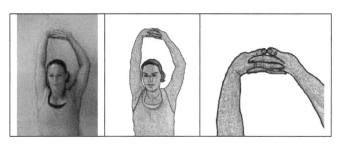

Technique: See Part A. Page 112.

3.8b Unilateral anterior forearm and hand stretch supine

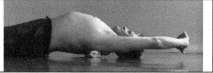

Starting position: Adopt the starting position described above in 3.8a. Flex your left elbow about 20 degrees. Press the fingertips of your left hand on the distal end of the posterior surface of the metatarsal bones of your right hand. Pull back on the fingers of your right hand with your left hand by increasing flexion at your left elbow. These push and pull levers will extend your wrist.

Technique: See Part A. Page 113.

3.8c Unilateral anterior finger and hand stretch supine

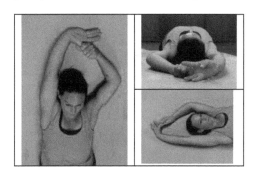

Starting position: Adopt the starting position described above in 3.8a. Grasp the index finger with your left hand and pull back on your finger. This will extend your finger at the proximal metacarpophalangeal joint and stretch tissues in your hand, wrist and forearm.

Technique: See Part A. Page 114.

3.8d Unilateral posterior forearm and hand stretch supine

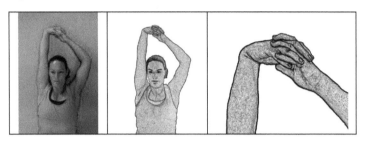

Starting position: Adopt the starting position described above in 3.8a. Interlace the fingers of both your hands but keep your forearms supinated, so that your palms face towards you. Extend your right elbow until your arm is straight. Flex your left forearm a little more at the elbow and feel a gentle pull on the back of your right hand with the fingers of your left hand.

Technique: See Part A. Page 115.

3.8e Unilateral posterior finger and hand stretch supine

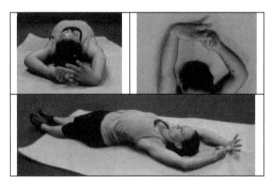

Starting position: Adopt the starting position described above in 3.8a. Grasp the index finger of your right hand with your left hand and pull on this finger to flex your finger and wrist. Keep your right arm straight and the side of your right hand in contact with the floor.

Technique: See Part A. Page 116.

Direction and range of movement

The bilateral anterior forearm and hand stretch 3.8a has active, passive, post-isometric and relaxation components. The unilateral stretches 3.8b, 3.8c, 3.8d and 3.8e have active and passive components. They are active stretches for the muscles of the shoulder and elbow, and passive stretches for the muscles and fascia of the hand and wrist.

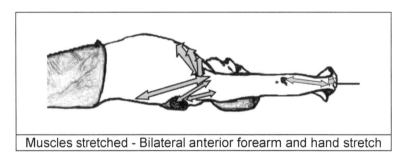

Muscles stretched - Bilateral anterior forearm and hand stretch

The spine and rib cage are raised off the floor by the rolled up towel, thus the spine is put in a position of extension. One or both arms are fully abducted, and one or both elbows are fully extended, depending on the technique. The arms should maintain contact with the floor throughout the stretch.

368

Normal joint health and a moderate level of flexibility are necessary for this stretch to be practiced as described. As a safety precaution, if there is joint degeneration and rigidity, then pillows or towels can be palace under the head or spine for support.

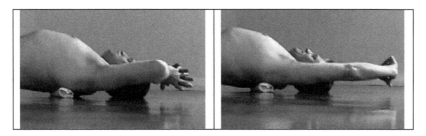

The body should allow thoracic extension, medial movement of the scapula, horizontal extension at the shoulder joints, and sufficient flexibility in the upper thoracic and lower cervical spine, to allow the head and neck to drop back safely into extension. Rotator cuff pathology may prevent comfortable shoulder abduction, in which case this stretch is probably best avoided.

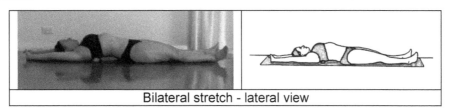
Bilateral stretch - lateral view

There is approximately 30 degrees horizontal extension at the shoulder which includes several centimetres of medial movement of the scapula on the thorax - scapula adduction or retraction.

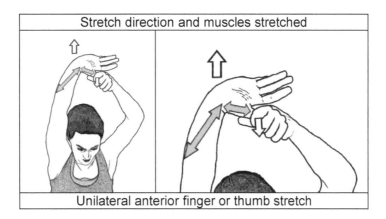
Stretch direction and muscles stretched

Unilateral anterior finger or thumb stretch

There is approximately 180 degrees shoulder abduction, 25 degrees thoracic extension, 120 degrees shoulder internal rotation, 90 degrees wrist flexion, and 90 degrees wrist extension.

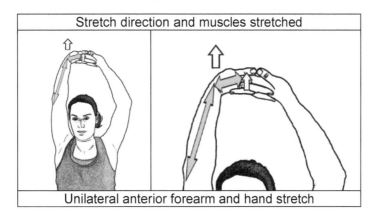
Stretch direction and muscles stretched

Unilateral anterior forearm and hand stretch

There is 90 degrees finger flexion at the metacarpophalangeal joint but finger extension can vary from zero to 20 degrees, or 90 degrees passive hyperextension in hypermobile individuals. Shoulder joint, acromioclavicular joint, sternoclavicular joint and scapulothoracic joint movement occur together simultaneously.

Target tissue

These stretches involve the abduction of one or both shoulders, including scapula protraction and upward rotation, extension of the elbow, and flexion or extension of the wrist and fingers. It stretches the muscles of the trunk, arm, forearm and hand.
In the trunk the primary muscles stretched include: latissimus dorsi, teres major, pectoralis minor, the lower fibres of pectoralis major and lower trapezius. There may be a mild stretch on brachialis with strong elbow extension, and supinator with strong forearm pronation.

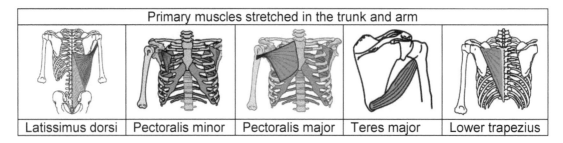

Primary muscles stretched in the trunk and arm				
Latissimus dorsi	Pectoralis minor	Pectoralis major	Teres major	Lower trapezius

In the anterior forearm and hand (3.8a, 3.8b and 3.8c) the primary muscles stretched include: forearm muscles flexing the wrist - flexor carpi radialis, flexor carpi ulnaris, palmaris longus; finger flexor muscles - flexor digitorum profundus and flexor digitorum superficialis; extrinsic thumb flexor muscle - flexor pollicis longus; intrinsic hand muscles - flexor digiti minimi, opponens digiti minimi, lumbricales and the palmar and dorsal interossei; and the intrinsic thumb flexor muscles - flexor pollicis brevis, opponens pollicis and adductor pollicis.

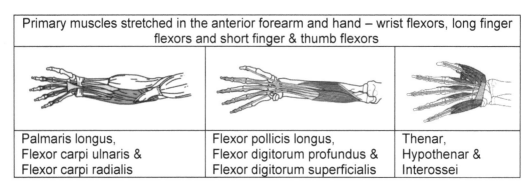

Primary muscles stretched in the anterior forearm and hand – wrist flexors, long finger flexors and short finger & thumb flexors		
Palmaris longus, Flexor carpi ulnaris & Flexor carpi radialis	Flexor pollicis longus, Flexor digitorum profundus & Flexor digitorum superficialis	Thenar, Hypothenar & Interossei

In the posterior forearm and hand (3.8d and 3.8e) the primary muscles stretched include: forearm muscles extending the wrist – extensor carpi radialis longus, extensor carpi radialis brevis and extensor carpi ulnaris; finger extensor muscles - extensor digitorum communis, extensor indicis and extensor digiti minimi; extrinsic thumb extensor muscles - extensor pollicis longus, extensor pollicis brevis and abductor pollicis longus; intrinsic hand muscles – abductor digiti minimi, lumbricales and the dorsal interossei; and the intrinsic thumb extensor muscle - abductor pollicis brevis.

Primary muscles stretched in the posterior forearm and hand	
Wrist and finger extensors	Thumb and finger extensors

In actively stretching the arm at the shoulder the following muscles are contracted: supraspinatus, middle deltoid, upper trapezius and serratus anterior. In maintaining forearm extension at the elbow triceps and anconeus are contracted. Movement at the wrist and fingers is passive, due to the force and leverage applied from the other upper limb.

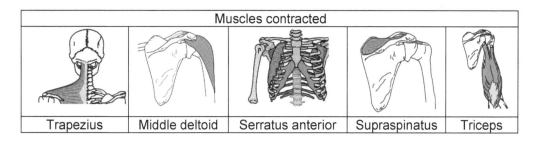

Muscles contracted				
Trapezius	Middle deltoid	Serratus anterior	Supraspinatus	Triceps

Stretching the pectoral fascia and anterior longitudinal ligaments of the thoracic spine, provides benefits for any person with an increased kyphosis and rounded shoulders.

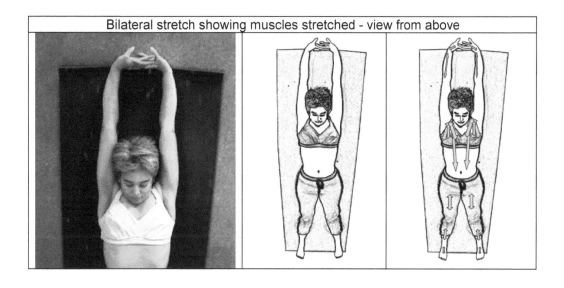

Bilateral stretch showing muscles stretched - view from above

Safety: See Rolled towel 3.6

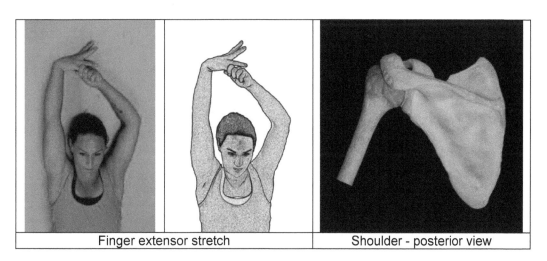

Finger extensor stretch	Shoulder - posterior view

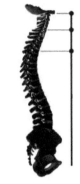

Occiput, C1 & C2

C6 & C7

T4

	Region	Level of Risk
1.	Occiput, C1 & C2	Medium
2.	Cervical spine	Low
3.	T4	Low
4.	Rotator cuff	Medium

Key:

All rolled towel stretches may be done standing, sitting or supine

3.8a Bilateral anterior forearm and hand stretch supine	
3.8b Unilateral anterior forearm and hand stretch supine	
3.8c Unilateral anterior finger and hand stretch supine	
3.8d Unilateral posterior forearm and hand stretch supine	
3.8e Unilateral posterior finger and hand stretch supine	

Related stretches					
1.3a, b & c Chin tuck stretches		2.5a & b Upper Dog extension stretches		3.6, 3.7 & 3.9 Supine rolled towel stretches	
4.0a to 4.0h Pectoralis stretches		5.3a & 5.3b Elbow flexor stretches		5.5 Supinator stretch	
5.6a Pronator stretch using a doorframe		5.7a to 5.7d Kneeling wrist extensor stretches		5.8a to 5.8e Kneeling wrist flexor stretches	

3.9 Rolled towel - active and passive stretches for shoulder, spine, ribs and hip down one side of the body

3.9a Supine hip and spine stretch over a rolled towel

Starting position: Sitting on the floor. Place a tightly rolled up towel behind your back, and then lie over the towel with your feet apart and your palms upwards. The towel should be across your spine where your thoracic curve is most flexed. Move your right arm out to the side until it is against the side of your head and your hand and forearm are above your head.

Adduct your right hip as far as possible. Bend your left hip and knee, and place your left foot on the outside of your right leg, about level with your knee to hold your leg in the adducted position. Slide your left hand down the side of your body and sidebend your spine to the left. Tuck your chin in and relax over the towel.

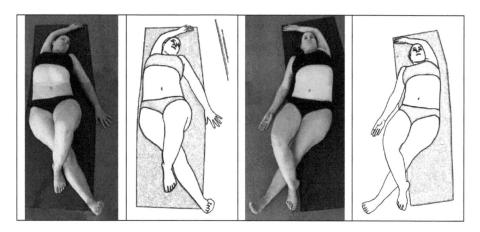

Technique: See Part A. Page 117.

3.9b Supine lumbar and thoracic spine stretch over a rolled towel

Starting position: Sitting on the floor. Place a tightly rolled up towel behind your back and then lie over the towel with your feet apart and your palms upwards. The towel should be across your spine where your thoracic curve is most flexed and at the apex of the sidebending curve. Move your right arm out to the side until it brushes against the side of your head and your hand and forearm are above your head. Slide your left hand down the side of your body and sidebend your spine to the left. Tuck your chin in and relax over the towel.

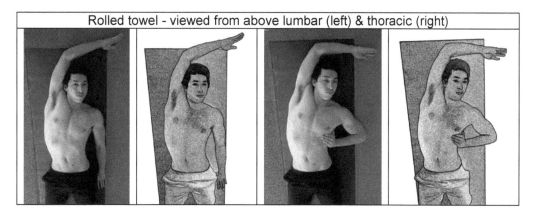

Rolled towel - viewed from above lumbar (left) & thoracic (right)

Technique: See Part A. Page 118.
Direction and range of movement

In this technique the spine and rib cage are raised above the floor by the rolled up towel, positioning the spine in extension. Also one arm is fully abducted and the spine is sidebent. In technique 3.9a one hip is adducted, while in technique 3.9b one shoulder is depressed.

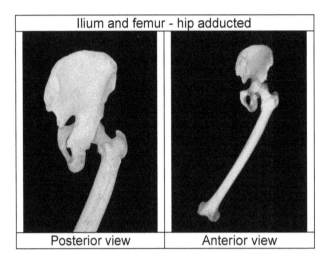

Ilium and femur - hip adducted	
Posterior view	Anterior view

There is approximately 30 degrees horizontal extension at the shoulder and this includes medial movement of the scapula on the thorax - scapula adduction or retraction. Depending on the size of the individual there is between one and three centimetres of active shoulder depression. Hip adduction is between 10 and 30 degrees. Thoracic sidebending to one side is about 20 degrees and lumbar sidebending is about 30 degrees.

Between T1 and T12 of the thoracic spine there should be about 25 degrees extension. The shape and the range of movement of the thoracic varies in different individuals. It ranges from a reverse kyphosis, to a straight 'poker' back, to a normal kyphosis, to an exaggerated kyphosis or hyperkyphosis.

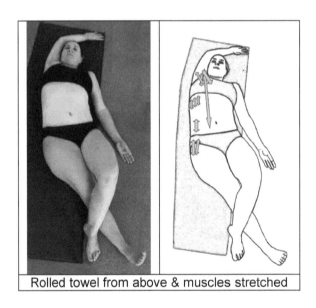

Rolled towel from above & muscles stretched

This technique is especially useful for people with an exaggerated kyphosis interacting with a scoliosis. The rolled up towel should be placed at or near to the apex of the kyphosis and the apex of the scoliosis. When these do not coincide then the rolled-up towel should be placed under the apex of the kyphosis, which may be between T4 and T12 but is usually near T7. This technique is also useful for people with round shoulders.

Target tissue

This is the longitudinal movement of one side of the body and stretches the muscles of the shoulder, lateral trunk, pelvis and thigh.

Muscles stretched in the upper limb				
Latissimus dorsi	Pectoralis minor	Pectoralis major	Teres major	Lower Trapezius

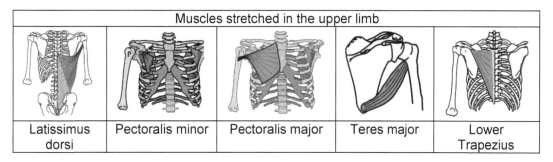

This technique primarily stretches latissimus dorsi, teres major, teres minor, pectoralis minor and the lower fibres of pectoralis major and lower trapezius. In actively stretching the upper limb the following muscles are contracted: supraspinatus, middle deltoid, upper trapezius and serratus anterior.

Muscles contracted in moving the upper limb			
Trapezius	Middle deltoid	Serratus anterior	Supraspinatus

In the trunk and hips this technique primarily stretches: the Iliocostalis fibres of Erector spinae, Quadratus lumborum, the lateral abdominal and intercostal muscles, Gluteus medius, Gluteus minimus, Tensor fasciae latae and the upper fibres of Gluteus maximus. The technique also stretches the anterior longitudinal ligaments and pectoral fascia.

Muscles stretched in the trunk and lower limb		
Erector spinae - Iliocostalis fibres	Quadratus lumborum	Lateral abdominal muscles
Lateral Intercostal muscles	Gluteus medius & Gluteus minimus	Gluteus maximus & Tensor fasciae latae

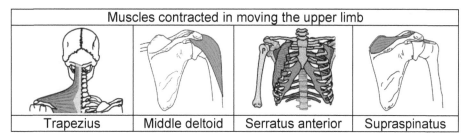

The sidebending stretch over a rolled-up towel has three features which distinguish it from the sidebending stretch standing: 1. The spine is in contact with the rolled-up towel, and the shoulders and pelvis are in contact with the floor, which provides sensory feedback to the brain about the position of the body in the frontal plane 2. Antigravity muscles are not active in maintaining a vertical posture 3. The hip is adducted, thus stretching the hip abductor muscles.

Safety: See Rolled towel 3.6

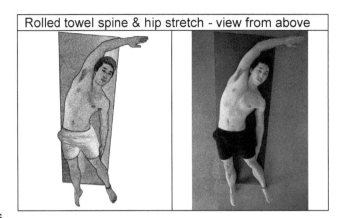

Rolled towel spine & hip stretch - view from above

Vulnerable areas

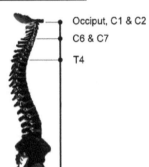

Occiput, C1 & C2

C6 & C7

T4

	Region	Level of Risk
1.	Occiput, C1 & C2	Medium
2.	Cervical spine	Low
3.	T4	Low
4.	Rotator cuff	Medium

Key:

3.9a Supine hip and spine stretch over a rolled towel	
3.9b Supine lumbar and thoracic spine stretch over a rolled towel	

Related stretches					
2.0a Standing lumbar and hip sidebending stretch		2.1a, b & c Wall supported hip & lumbar sidebend stretch		2.2a & 2.2b Thoracic and rib sidebending stretches	
2.3 Kneeling lateral stretch		2.4a to 2.4d Hanging stretches		2.5a & b Upper Dog extension stretches	
3.6, 3.7 & 3.8 Supine rolled towel stretches		5.3a & 5.3b Elbow flexor stretches		6.4a to 6.4h Unilateral hip abductor stretches	

For more detailed anatomy of the ribs, thoracic, lumbar and sacroiliac spine 2.0 – 3.9 see page 556.

4.0 Pectoralis stretches - active, passive and post-isometric stretches for pectoralis major and other anterior shoulder muscles

4.0a Easy pectoralis stretch sitting on the floor

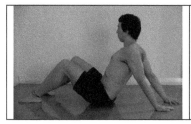

Starting position: Sitting on the floor, hips flexed and slightly abducted. Your knees may be flexed or extended. Place your hands palms down flat on the floor behind you, pointing away with fingers abducted and extended. Your wrists, elbows and shoulders are extended, and your shoulders are externally rotated. Move the top of your pelvis forward by contracting your hip flexor muscles. Allow some lumbar and sacroiliac extension but keep the rest of the spine relatively straight.

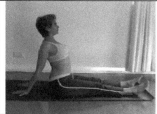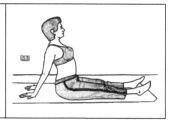

Technique: See Part A. Page 119.

In this and the following stretch, the shoulders are externally rotated and extended, while the scapula are retracted and tilted forwards.

4.0b Easy pectoralis stretch standing

Starting position: Standing straight with your feet apart, and arms abducted 20 to 30 degrees and extended 20 to 30 degrees. Your fingers are abducted, extended and spread wide apart. Externally rotate your arms and retract your scapula, so your palms point anteriorly and laterally.

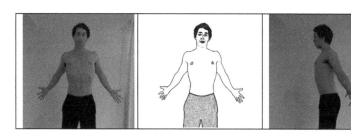

Technique: See Part A. Page 120.

4.0c Pectoralis stretch seated in a chair

Starting position: Sitting in a chair with your feet apart and planted on the floor or a block. Abduct your arms until they are level with the shoulders. Flex your elbows until your arm and forearm are at right angles. Externally rotate your arms, supinate your forearms and then horizontally extend your arms - as far as possible. Your elbows and hands move horizontally backward, parallel with the floor, while your thumbs point backwards. Sit upright.

Technique: See Part A. Page 121.

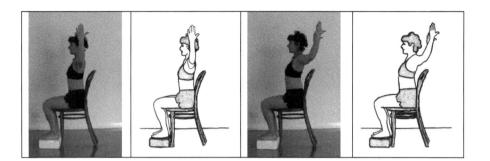

4.0d Pectoralis stretch prone

Starting position: Prone on the floor or on a carpet or mat. Abduct your arms until they are in line with your shoulders. Flex your elbows until your arm and forearm are at right angles. Your shoulders are externally rotated. Supinate your forearms so your thumbs point up towards the ceiling.

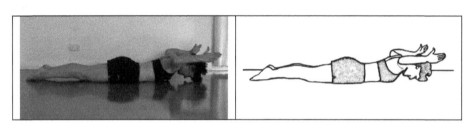

Technique: See Part A. Page 122.

4.0e Unilateral passive and post-isometric pectoralis stretch standing and wall supported

Starting position: Standing with your feet apart, the right side of your body near a wall, with your right foot about 6 cm from the wall. Raise your right arm and place your palm on the wall to the right of your head, just above shoulder height. Place the front of your right shoulder against the wall but not your right hip. Extend your right forearm until your elbow is straight. Flex your knees a little, and adjust your feet for optimum balance.

Technique: See Part A. Page 123.

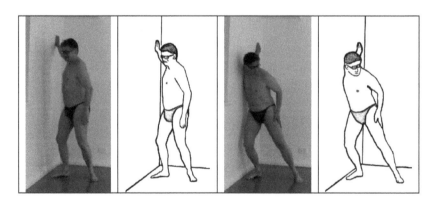

4.0f Bilateral passive and post-isometric pectoralis stretch standing and doorway supported

Starting position: Standing with your feet apart facing an open doorway or two vertical posts. Move your right foot through the doorway, placing it on the floor so that the back of your heel lines up with the doorway. Abduct your arms until your hands are level with, or just above your shoulders. Place your wrist or forearms against the side edges of the doorway. Flex your hips and knees and lunge forwards through the door. Adjust your feet for optimum balance.

Technique: See Part A. Page 124.

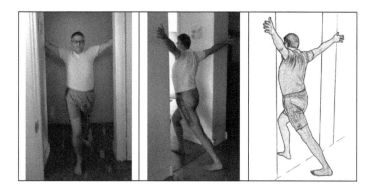

4.0g Bilateral pectoralis stretch standing walls supported

Starting position: Standing with your feet apart facing the corner of a room. Place your right foot in front of and to the right of your left foot. Abduct your arms until your hands are level with, or just above your shoulders, and place the palms of your hands on each of the walls. Extend your elbow so your arms are straight. Flex your right hip and knee, and lunge towards the corner of the room.

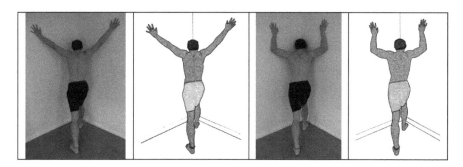

Technique: See Part A. Page 125.

4.0h Bilateral active pectoralis and latissimus dorsi stretch standing with pole or towel

Starting position: Standing with your feet apart grasping either end of a pole or towel with your hands. Raise your arms so the pole is above your head and extend your elbows so both arms are straight.

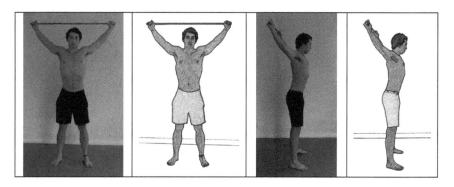

Technique: See Part A. Page 126.

Direction and range of movement

The seated and standing easy pectoralis stretches 4.0a and 4.0b are active stretches involving shoulder external rotation and extension, along with scapula retraction and forward tilting. All the remaining techniques 4.0c to 4.0h involve shoulder horizontal extension, shoulder external rotation, scapula retraction and backward tilting. Techniques 4.0c, 4.0d and 4.0h are active stretches and techniques 4.0e, 4.0f and 4.0g are passive stretches which can also be done as post-isometric stretches.

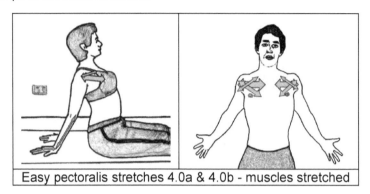

Easy pectoralis stretches 4.0a & 4.0b - muscles stretched

There is about 4 cm of scapula retraction or medial movement of the scapula along the rib cage and towards the spine. In the neutral position there is about 40 degrees external rotation of the shoulder and 50 degrees extension at the shoulder, but when the arm is abducted to 90 degrees there is about 90 degrees external rotation and 30 degrees horizontal extension at the shoulder.

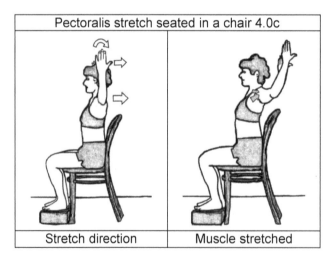

Pectoralis stretch seated in a chair 4.0c

Stretch direction	Muscle stretched

The standing unilateral wall supported pectoralis stretch 4.0e involves spinal rotation; the thoracic spine contributes about 35 degrees rotation.

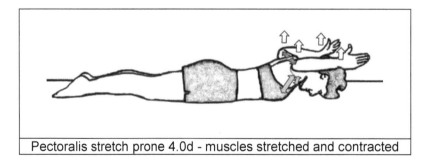

Pectoralis stretch prone 4.0d - muscles stretched and contracted

In the unilateral stretch 4.0e, muscle contraction rotates the spine, retracts both scapula and horizontally extends the shoulder being stretched. This technique works via leverage acting through the scapula to horizontally extend the shoulder and stretch the anterior shoulder

380

tissues, which is mainly the pectoralis major. In this stretch, one shoulder is fixed against the wall and acts as a pivot while the tip of the other shoulder moves away from the wall, forcing both scapulae to slide backwards around the rib cage and towards the spine.

The stretch is increased by moving the hip nearest the wall further forwards, and in a direction that is parallel with the wall, while holding the other hip in a fixed position or moving it slightly backwards. This creates another pivoting type movement, of rotation of the pelvis around an axis between the spine and the hip furthest from the wall.

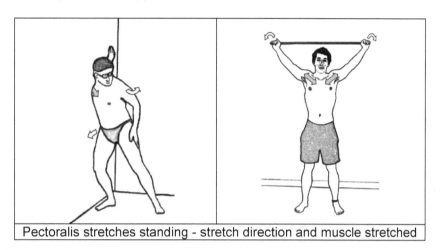
Pectoralis stretches standing - stretch direction and muscle stretched

In the bilateral passive stretches 4.0f and 4.0g, muscle contraction flexes both the knee and hip joints, which moves the body forwards. Also by contracting muscles to keep the spine rigid, both scapulae are drawn into bilateral retraction, and both shoulders into horizontally extension. Most doorways are about 80 cm wide - that is about elbow distance apart when your arms are horizontal.

In the pole or towel technique 4.0h, scapula retractor muscles and shoulder horizontal extensor muscles contract to stretch the anterior shoulder tissues, mainly pectoralis major and latissimus dorsi.

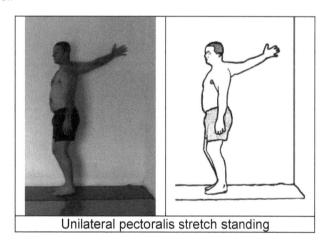
Unilateral pectoralis stretch standing

In the standing and sitting easy pectoralis stretches the arms are in extension and external rotation; this position tends to stretch the muscles responsible for shoulder flexion and internal rotation. In these stretches the scapula is tilted forwards, so stretches the muscles responsible for backward tilt.

In all the other stretches the arms are in horizontal extension, external rotation and abduction and these stretch the muscles responsible for shoulder internal rotation, horizontal flexion and adduction. In these stretches the scapula is tilted backwards so stretches the muscles responsible for forward tilt. All the techniques involve scapula retraction so stretch muscles responsible for scapula protraction.

Target tissues

These techniques mainly stretch the clavicular, sternal and abdominal parts of pectoralis major, as well as the overlying pectoral fascia.

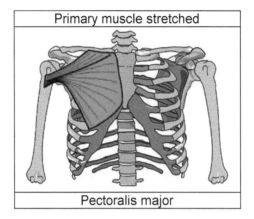

Primary muscle stretched

Pectoralis major

They also stretch the anterior deltoid, subscapularis, serratus anterior, and the joint capsule and ligaments of the anterior shoulder joints. Techniques 4.0a, b, e, f, g and h are also weak stretches for coracobrachialis and biceps brachii.

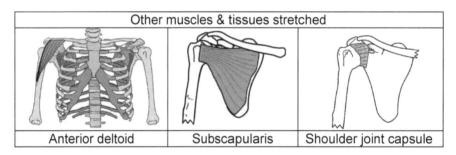

Other muscles & tissues stretched

Anterior deltoid	Subscapularis	Shoulder joint capsule

In techniques 4.0a and 4.0b shoulder abduction is less than 90 degrees, so they mainly target the upper or clavicular part of pectoralis major, whereas in techniques 4.0c to 4.0h shoulder abduction is 90 degrees or greater than 90 degrees, so they mainly target the sternal or abdominal part of pectoralis major.

In technique 4.0f and 4.0g when your arms are level with your shoulders, you will tend to localise the stretch on the upper and middle fibres of the sternal part of pectoralis major, as well as the pectoral fascia. When your arms are above your shoulders, you will tend to increase the stretch on the lower fibres of pectoralis major.

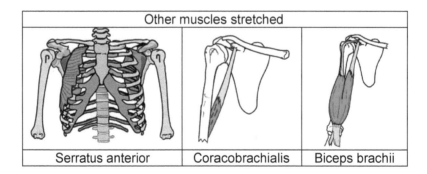

Other muscles stretched

Serratus anterior	Coracobrachialis	Biceps brachii

Between a position of 90 degrees shoulder abduction to about 135 degrees abduction, external rotation or horizontal extension of the shoulder will increases the stretch on pectoralis minor, anterior deltoid, coracobrachialis and biceps brachii, and to a lesser extent, latissimus dorsi, teres major, lower trapezius and subclavius. Shoulder abduction is only effective as a stretch for pectoralis major up to about 45 degrees above the horizontal.

With your arms horizontal and your elbows flexed 90 degrees external rotation focuses the stretch on the lower fibres of pectoralis major, and to a lesser extent pectoralis minor, anterior deltoid, coracobrachialis and latissimus dorsi.

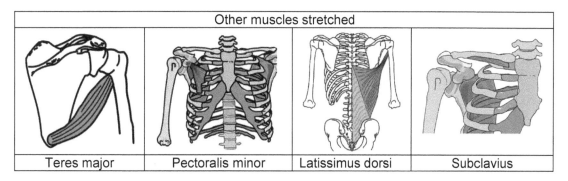

Other muscles stretched			
Teres major	Pectoralis minor	Latissimus dorsi	Subclavius

The position of the shoulders also influences which secondary muscles are stretched. Shoulder horizontal extension stretches coracobrachialis and the short head of biceps, scapular retraction stretches serratus anterior, shoulder external rotation stretches subscapularis, anterior deltoid, latissimus dorsi and teres major, scapula elevation and backward tilting stretches pectoralis minor.

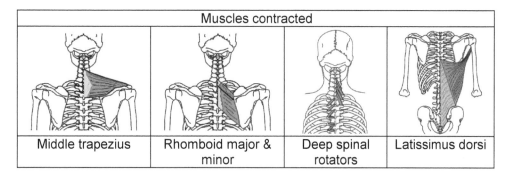

Muscles contracted			
Middle trapezius	Rhomboid major & minor	Deep spinal rotators	Latissimus dorsi

In addition to stretching pectoralis major, the prone technique has an important role in strengthening important postural muscles, thus countering the rounded shoulder posture. The technique works by actively contracting against gravity and against the resistance offered by the anteriorly located muscles.

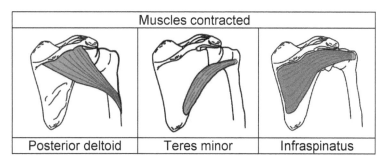

Muscles contracted		
Posterior deltoid	Teres minor	Infraspinatus

During shoulder external rotation the arms rotate around an axis passing through the elbow and down the shaft of the humerus. The active stretches technique 4.0a, b, c, d and h strengthen rhomboid major and minor, middle trapezius, infraspinatus, teres minor and posterior deltoid.

Muscles responsible for shoulder horizontal extension include posterior deltoid, latissimus dorsi, teres major, infraspinatus and teres minor. Muscles responsible for scapula retraction include rhomboid major and minor and middle trapezius. Muscles responsible for shoulder external rotation include infraspinatus, teres minor and posterior deltoid.

Stretching in 4.0e occurs as a result of muscle contraction from the deep rotator muscles of the thoracic spine, the abdominal obliques, gluteus maximums, the hip rotator muscles and shoulder retractor muscles: the rhomboids, and middle trapezius.

With the bilateral techniques there will be greater resistance from both pectoralis major muscles and their overlying fascia, as you are trying to stretch both sides of the body at the same time. The bilateral stretch may therefore be less effective than the unilateral stretch, where you are localising the stretch to one pectoralis major muscle at a time.

Muscles contracted		
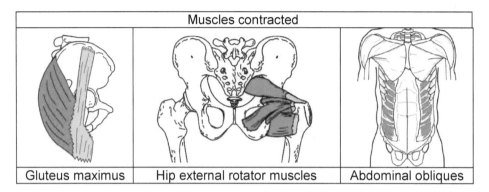		
Gluteus maximus	Hip external rotator muscles	Abdominal obliques

Safety

Do not use too much force when you pull your shoulders backwards and squeeze your shoulder blades together. Do not over-contract the shoulder retractor muscles if there is a problem in the thoracic spine or ribs; for example degenerative changes to facet joints or costovertebral joints, as well as any biomechanical dysfunction that may be present. A relatively common vulnerability in the thoracic spine occurs at or near to T4, where either a single vertebra or a group of vertebra, may be fixed in an extended position. These types of fixations are frequently sensitive and may be prone to mechanical irritation from strong muscle contraction, such as during this stretching technique. Additionally, the thoracolumbar spine may also be in an extended position and/or may be relatively hypermobile compared to the rest of the spine. With that said, this is a relatively safe technique.

In the pectoralis stretch seated in a chair 4.0 c it is important to maintain an upright sitting position to get the most optimum leverage from the shoulders, such that forces can be transmitted through the spine to the pectoralis major muscles. This can be achieved by sitting on your buttock bones (ischial tuberosites), and keeping your centre of gravity over these bony pivot points. The spine can be maintained in a neutral upright position either through active muscle contraction or by using the chair for support.

Easy pectoralis stretch	
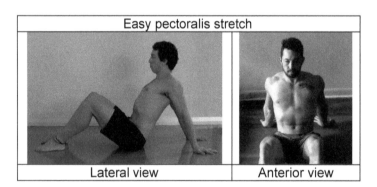	
Lateral view	Anterior view

The upper body is held in an upright position by contracting several muscles: especially the hip flexor muscles, which move the top of your pelvis forward, as well as the lower erector spinae muscles which maintain extension in the lumbar spine.

A chair with a back that is upright and congruent with the shape of your lumbar spine will help you maintain an upright position. Alternatively you can use a small pillow placed between the back of the chair and the middle of your lumbar spine, to prop you up.

With the arms straight in stretch 4.0f and 4.0g there may be some strain on the elbows. Do not use these stretches if your elbow joints are hypermobile, compromised in some way, thus vulnerable to strain and/or overstretching. Instead use alternatives such as the easy pectoralis stretches 4.0a and 4.0b, the active elbows flexed stretches 4.0c and 4.0d, or the unilateral wall supported stretch 4.0e, where the wall acts as a brace protecting your elbow against hyperextension and strain.

Shortness of pectoralis major is a contributing factor leading to rotator cuff injuries or reinjuring a previously torn rotator cuff tendon, and this muscle should be stretched regularly to prevent injury and to aid in the recovery of this problem. Other contributing factors to rotator cuff problems include hyperkyphosis and inflexibility of the thoracic spine and shoulder joints, and these are often associated with pectoralis major shortness.

To prevent shoulder injury it is important to warm up the body prior to stretching and before doing other forms of exercise involving the shoulders, with simple shoulder movements and walking. This is especially true if there is shoulder and thoracic stiffness or hyperkyphosis.

Pectoralis major is a broad fan-shaped muscle and can be divided into two main parts, clavicular fibres arising above the glenohumeral joint and the sternal and abdominal fibres arising below the glenohumeral joint. The wide separation of the origin of these fibres means the clavicular fibres are best stretched when the arm is adducted and the sternal-abdominal fibres are best stretched when the arm is abducted.

The bulk of the pectoralis major muscle is the sternal-abdominal part, and even though it needs stretching to assist in the repair of a rotator cuff strain, there is a problem: the shoulder can be very painful, and the rotator cuff can be more easily irritated or even reinjured when the shoulder is stretched in the abducted position.

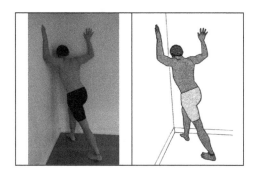

We have the paradoxical situation that the pectoralis major muscle need stretching to assist in the repair of the rotator cuff, yet the bulk of the fibres are best stretched in the abducted position where the cuff is more easily irritated.

So the safest way to stretch pectoralis major when there is an existing rotator cuff injury in the shoulder is using external rotation and extension with the shoulder in the adducted position. Initially avoid abduction by only using techniques 4.0a and 4.0b and as the rotator cuff strain show signs of improvement gradually introduce the other techniques. Treat the cuff strain and build up the structural integrity of the tendon with strengthening exercises before pursuing strong pectoralis major stretching in the abducted position.

Vulnerable areas

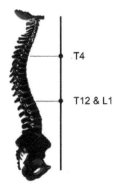

T4

T12 & L1

	Region	Level of Risk
1.	Rotator cuff	Low 4.0a & b Medium others
2.	T4	Medium
3.	Thoracolumbar	Low

Key:

4.0a Easy pectoralis stretch sitting on the floor	
4.0b Easy pectoralis stretch standing	
4.0c Pectoralis stretch seated	
4.0d Pectoralis stretch prone	
4.0e Unilateral passive and post-isometric pectoralis stretch standing and wall supported	
4.0f Bilateral passive and post-isometric pectoralis stretch standing and doorway supported	
4.0g Bilateral pectoralis stretch standing walls supported	
4.0h Bilateral active pectoralis and latissimus dorsi stretch standing with pole or towel	

Related stretches					
2.5a & b Upper Dog extension stretch kneeling		3.6, 3.7 & 3.8 Supine stretches over a rolled up towel		4.1 Unilateral subscapularis stretch	
5.2a Bilateral biceps stretches against a ledge		3.9a & b Supine hip and spine stretch over a rolled towel			

386

4.1 Subscapularis stretch - passive and post-isometric stretch for subscapularis and other anterior shoulder muscles

4.1 Unilateral passive and post-isometric subscapularis stretch

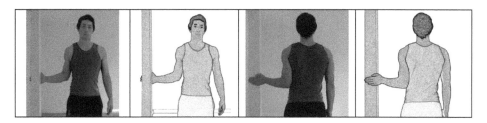

Starting position: Standing with your feet apart and with the right side of your body next to a post. Flex your right forearm, externally rotate your right arm and place the palm of your right hand on the post. Your right elbow is flexed about 90 degrees and tucked close up against the right side of your body. Rotate your pelvis to the left, until you feel the initial stages of a stretch in front of your right shoulder. You may need to reposition your feet so that your centre of gravity falls between them. Relax your shoulders and keep your spine straight.

Technique: See Part A. Page 127.

Direction and range of movement

This is a passive stretches which can also be done as post-isometric stretch. With your hand fixed against the post, hip and spinal rotation results in external rotation of the shoulder and retraction of the scapula. Thus rotation of the spine acts through the forearm, working as a lever to cause the movements and stretch the anterior shoulder muscles. The stretch can also be increased by moving the hip nearest the post forwards, while moving your other hip backwards.

External rotation of the shoulder is about 80 degrees. Rotation of the thoracic spine is about 35 degrees. There is about 4 cm retraction of the scapula along the rib cage and towards the spine.

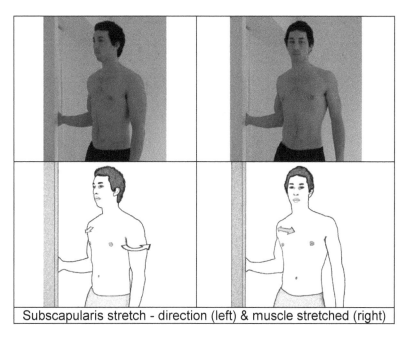

Subscapularis stretch - direction (left) & muscle stretched (right)

Target tissues

This is mainly a stretch for subscapularis. It is also a stretch for the clavicular part of pectoralis major and the upper fibres of the sternal part of pectoralis major.

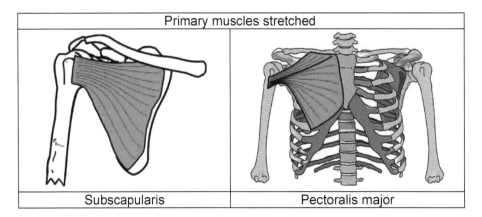

Primary muscles stretched	
Subscapularis	Pectoralis major

To a lesser extent this technique also stretches anterior deltoid, pectoralis minor, the upper part of serratus anterior and the anterior capsule and ligaments of the shoulder joint.

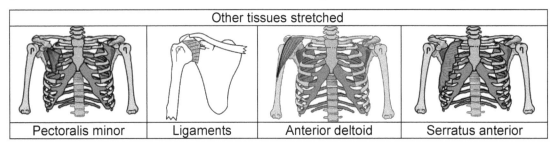

Other tissues stretched			
Pectoralis minor	Ligaments	Anterior deltoid	Serratus anterior

The stretch works due to the contraction of muscles that rotate the spine – mainly rotatores, multifidus and the oblique abdominal muscles; and muscles that retract the scapula – mainly the rhomboids and middle trapezius.

Safety

Subscapularis is an important muscle for shoulder stability. It is one of the rotator cuff group of muscles with its tendon acting as a strap supporting the anterior shoulder ligament, which acts in protecting the shoulder against injury or dislocation. Occasional stretching of this muscle will help it function more efficiently.

This is a safe technique. With the arm at the side of the body there is much less strain on the supraspinatus tendon or other vulnerable structures such as the neurovascular tissues, than in other arm positions.

Key:

4.1 Unilateral passive and post-isometric subscapularis stretch	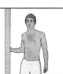

Related stretches					
4.0a Easy pectoralis stretch sitting on the floor		4.0b Easy pectoralis stretch standing		5.1b Standing winged anterior deltoid stretch	

4.2 The Shoulder Drop - passive and post-isometric stretch for the scapula depressor muscles

4.2 The Shoulder Drop

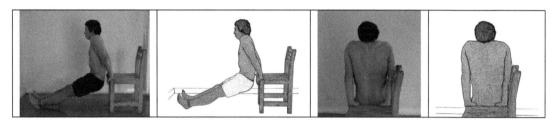

Starting position: Standing with your back facing a low table or chair. Flex your hips and knees. Place your palms on the chair with your fingers over the edge and walk your heels away from the chair until your legs are straight. Straighten your arms, relax your shoulders, and lower your pelvis and spine towards the floor. Allow your shoulders to rise but stop when you start to feel the stretch.

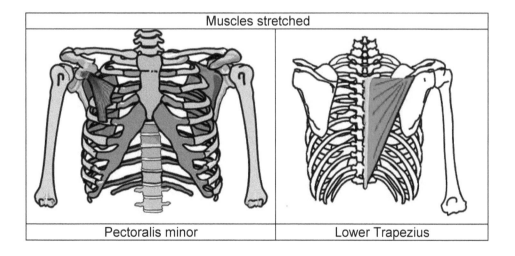

Technique: See Part A. Page 128.

Direction and range of movement

This technique involves elevation of the scapula and clavicle as well as some upwards rotation of the scapula. Total scapula elevation depression is between 10 and 12 cm. Movement occurs in the acromioclavicular, sternoclavicular, scapulothoracic and glenohumeral joints. Secondary movement occurs in the cervical and thoracic spine.

Target tissues

This is mainly a stretch for pectoralis minor and lower trapezius. It also stretches middle deltoid, supraspinatus and subclavius. This may also stretch the lowest fibres of serratus anterior and pectoralis major and the lateral pectoral fascia.

Muscles stretched	
Pectoralis minor	Lower Trapezius

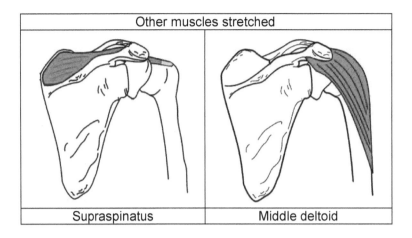

Other muscles stretched	
Supraspinatus	Middle deltoid

The passive stretch occurs as a result of gravity and body weight, causing both scapular to elevate, hence this is a stretch for the scapula depressor muscles. The post-isometric stretch occurs as a result of the contraction of the scapula depressor muscles acting on the scapula.

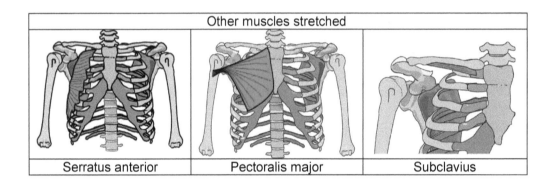

Other muscles stretched		
Serratus anterior	Pectoralis major	Subclavius

Safety

This is a safe exercise. Lower your body into the stretching position slowly. Make sure that the chair or small table is stable and strong enough to support your body weight.

Key:

4.2 The shoulder drop	

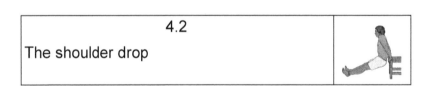

Related stretches			
1.2 The Shrug		5.1a Shoulder flexor drop	

4.3 Downward shoulder - active stretch for the muscles responsible for scapular elevation

4.3 Downward shoulder stretch

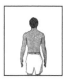

Starting position: Standing with your feet slightly apart and arms at your sides. Tuck in your chin and take your head back. Keep your head vertical and in line with your body.

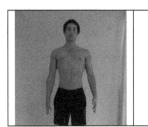 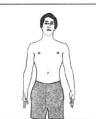 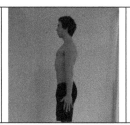 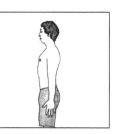

Maintain your head over your body's centre of gravity. Move your shoulders downwards but keep your arms by your side.

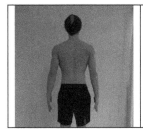 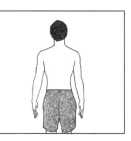

Technique: See Part A. Page 129.

Direction and range of movement

The primary movements in this technique are scapula and clavicular depression.

There is also some downward tilting of the scapula. There is only about 1 or 2 cm of scapula depression. This is because in the standing position the scapula is naturally depressed. Any further depression is as a result of the tissue compression and tension taken up during the active movement. Movement occurs in the acromioclavicular joints, sternoclavicular joints, scapulothoracic joints and glenohumeral joints. Secondary movement occurs in the cervical and thoracic spine.

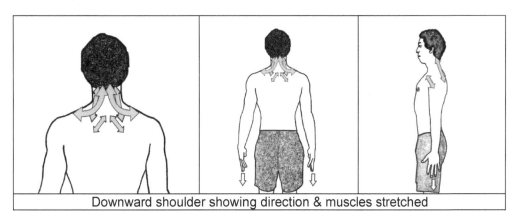

Downward shoulder showing direction & muscles stretched

Target tissues

This is an active stretch involving the contraction of scapula and clavicular depressor muscles to stretch scapula and clavicular elevator muscles

The primary muscles stretched are upper trapezius, levator scapulae, rhomboid major and minor, and the clavicular part of pectoralis major. These muscles attach on the occiput, scapula and clavicle, and cervical and upper thoracic spine.

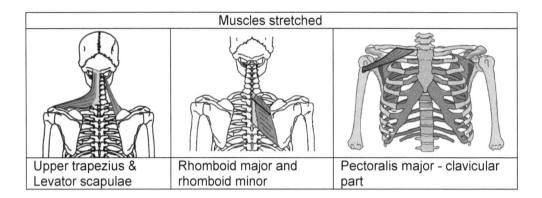

Muscles stretched		
Upper trapezius & Levator scapulae	Rhomboid major and rhomboid minor	Pectoralis major - clavicular part

The active stretch involves the contraction of latissimus dorsi, lower trapezius, subclavius, pectoralis minor and the lower or sternal part of pectoralis major.

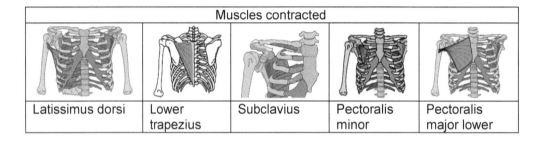

Muscles contracted				
Latissimus dorsi	Lower trapezius	Subclavius	Pectoralis minor	Pectoralis major lower

Key:

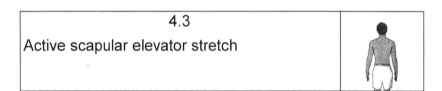

4.3 Active scapular elevator stretch	

Related stretches			
1.1a, b & c Lion stretches		4.5 Shoulder abductor stretch behind	

4.4 Shoulder abductor front stretch - a passive and post-isometric stretch for the muscles responsible for shoulder abduction and scapula retraction

4.4 Shoulder abductor front stretch

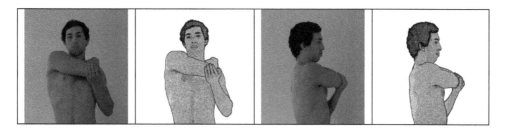

Starting position: Standing with your feet apart and arms at your sides. Flex your right elbow, and then take your right hand across the front of your body, as far as you can comfortably go to the left. Grasp your right arm, just above your elbow with your left hand.

Depending on your flexibility and the angle you wish to apply the stretch you can cradle your right forearm in your left forearm with your hand and wrist resting in the crease of your elbow, alternatively you can rest your right hand and wrist on the top of your shoulder. Pull your arm across the front of your body until you feel the initial stage of resistance from the shoulder muscles and ligaments, then stop. Stand up straight and relax your shoulders.

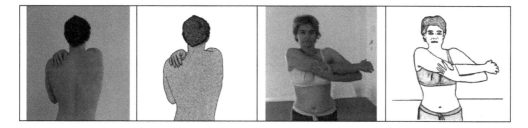

Technique: See Part A. Page 130.

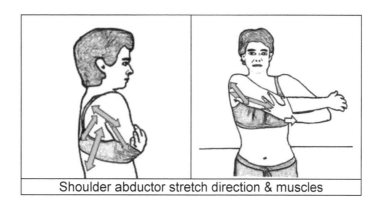

Direction and range of movement

The range of movement and which muscles are stretched depends on how this technique is done. If it is done with the arm close to the body, the stretch involves full shoulder adduction, partial shoulder internal rotation, partial shoulder flexion and a combination of scapular protraction and downwards rotation.

Shoulder abductor stretch direction & muscles

393

If it is done with the arm away from the body, the stretch involves full shoulder adduction and full shoulder internal rotation and a combination of scapular protraction, upwards rotation and lateral tilt. This position is part way between 2 planes of movement, i.e. sagittal and coronal, and may be described as horizontal shoulder flexion

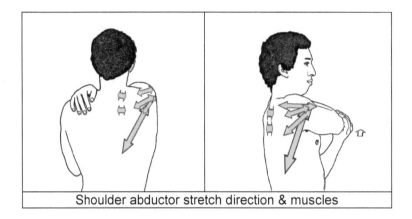

| Shoulder abductor stretch direction & muscles |

Adduction of the arm in front of the body (in flexion) is greater than behind the body (in extension), due to the shoulder having greater clearance. Adduction in front of the body varies between individuals and usually ranges from 30 degrees to 45 degrees.

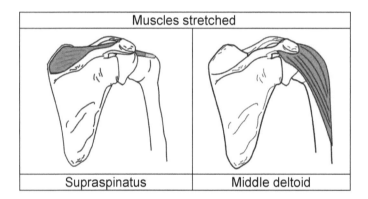

Muscles stretched	
Supraspinatus	Middle deltoid

In hypermobile individuals where the shoulder capsule and ligaments are extremely lax, shoulder adduction can exceed 70 degrees. During adduction there is about 10 cm protraction or lateral movement of the scapula along the rib cage, away from the spine. Shoulder internal rotation is about 95 degrees.

Target tissues

Primarily this is a stretch for the shoulder abductors muscles - supraspinatus and middle deltoid. It will be a mild to moderate stretch for latissimus dorsi, teres major, teres minor, infraspinatus and posterior deltoid. It may also stretch levator scapulae and the long head of triceps brachii.

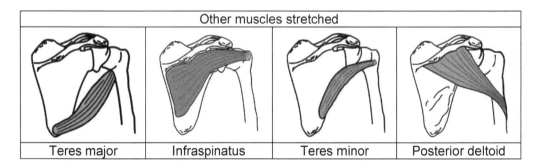

Other muscles stretched			
Teres major	Infraspinatus	Teres minor	Posterior deltoid

Variations

When the arm is adducted and close to the body, this increases the stretch in supraspinatus and middle trapezius. When the arm is adducted and is away from to the body, this increases the stretch in all the other muscles listed.

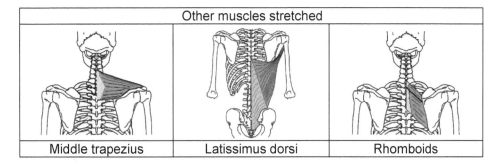

Other muscles stretched		
Middle trapezius	Latissimus dorsi	Rhomboids

Safety

If the general safety protocol is in place, for example moving slowly and with an exhalation, then this is a safe stretch and is unlikely to cause problems.

Shortness in supraspinatus is a contributing factor leading to rotator cuff strain, thus stretching the muscle may prevent injury. Strengthening should also be combined with stretching because the muscle may also be weak. Supraspinatus is one of four rotator cuff muscles working with ligaments to support the shoulder joint, helping to maintain stability in a very mobile joint. Of the four rotator cuff muscles, supraspinatus is the one most commonly torn. The stretch may be useful if there is a frozen shoulder.

Key:

4.4 Shoulder abductor front stretch	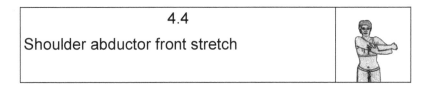

Related stretches					
4.0a & 4.0b Easy pectoralis stretches sitting or standing		4.5 Shoulder abductor stretch behind		4.8 Multi shoulder stretch	
4.9d Scapula wrap stretch standing		5.0b Active scapular retractor & stretch			

4.5 Shoulder abductor behind stretch - passive and post-isometric stretch for the shoulder abductors

4.5 Shoulder abductor behind stretch

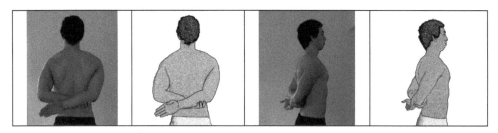

Starting position: Standing with your feet apart. Flex your right forearm and then place your right hand behind your back. Reach as far as you can across your back and to the left of your spine. Flex your left forearm and place your left hand behind your back. Reach as far as you can across your back to the right of your spine, and depending on your flexibility, grasp your right forearm as near to your elbow as you can. Pull your right arm and forearm further across your back with your left hand until you feel the initial stage of resistance from your shoulders.

Technique: See Part A. Page 131.

Direction and range of movement

This technique involves full shoulder adduction, full shoulder internal rotation, partial shoulder extension, partial scapular retraction and downwards rotation. Adduction of the arm behind the back is about 10 degrees but varies between individuals; ranging from 5 to 25 degrees.

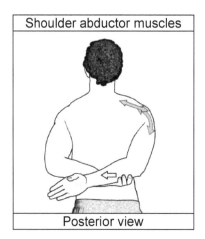

Shoulder abductor muscles

Posterior view

During adduction there is about there is about 4 cm retraction or medial movement of the scapula along the rib cage and towards the spine. Shoulder internal rotation is about 95 degrees, while shoulder extension is about 50 degrees.

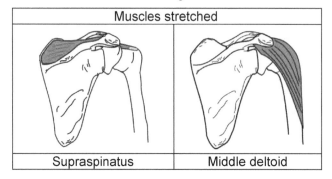

Muscles stretched	
Supraspinatus	Middle deltoid

Target tissues

This is primarily a stretch for the shoulder abductors supraspinatus and middle deltoid. Other muscles that may be stretched include serratus anterior, teres minor and the long head of triceps brachii.

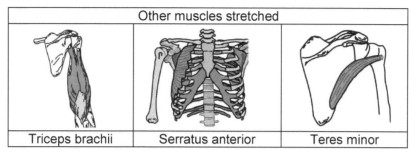

Other muscles stretched		
Triceps brachii	Serratus anterior	Teres minor

Variations

Cervical sidebending can be introduced into the technique to stretch upper trapezius, anterior, middle and posterior scalene, sternocleidomastoid and levator scapulae.

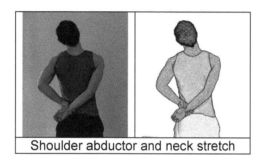

Shoulder abductor and neck stretch

Grasp your wrist with the other hand and pull your arm down and across your back to depress the shoulder, then actively sidebend your head and cervical spine away from the side of the depressed shoulder.

Safety

This is a safe stretch that is unlikely to cause problems. This is an especially good stretch for lengthening supraspinatus, which is the muscle most commonly torn in rotator cuff injuries. By stretching supraspinatus and middle deltoid regularly this will reduce the probability of a rotator cuff strain. This is also a mild stretch for the upper part of the shoulder joint capsule and ligaments, hence may be used when there is a frozen shoulder.

Key:

4.5 Shoulder abductor behind back stretch	

Related stretches					
3.1b & 3.2b Active spinal twists seated or standing		4.0a & 4.0b Easy pectoralis stretch sitting or standing		4.4 Shoulder abductor front stretch	
4.7 Palms together behind back		4.8 Multi shoulder stretch		5.1b Standing winged stretch	

4.6 Palms together above head - active stretch for shoulder muscles and strengthening technique for muscles of the spine, thighs and legs

4.6a & 4.6b Palms together above head

Starting position: Standing with your feet together or apart, and your arms at your sides. Abduct your arms until your hands are above your head and then bring your palms together. Your arms are externally rotated, and your forearms are supinated and fully extended.

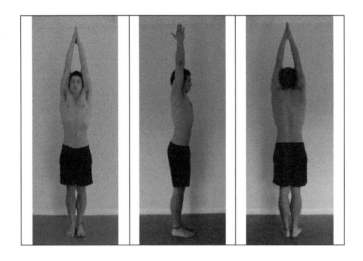

Technique: See Part A. Page 132.

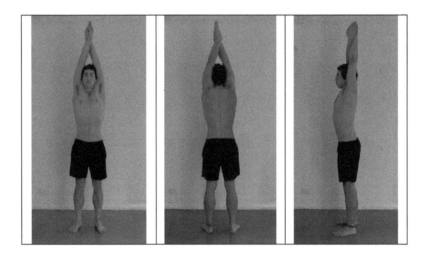

Technique: See Part A. Page 133.

Direction and range of movement

These techniques mainly involve full shoulder abduction and elbow extension. Technique 4.6a involves shoulder external rotation and elbow supination, while technique 4.6b involves shoulder internal rotation and elbow pronation.

Shoulder abduction is 180 degrees, a combination of sternoclavicular, acromioclavicular, glenohumeral and scapulothoracic joint movement.

Target tissues

This is an active stretch which also strengthens muscles important for the maintenance of good posture. This longitudinal technique affects the upper limbs and trunk bilaterally, stretching the muscles of the spine, ribs, abdomen, shoulders, arms, forearms and hands.

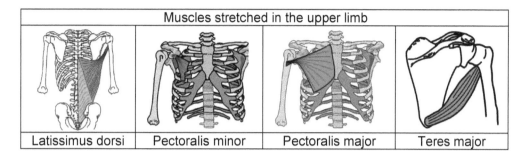

Muscles stretched in the upper limb			
Latissimus dorsi	Pectoralis minor	Pectoralis major	Teres major

This technique primarily stretches trunk muscles: latissimus dorsi, teres major, teres minor, pectoralis minor and the lower fibres of pectoralis major.

It also stretches muscles of the upper limb: biceps brachii, brachialis, coracobrachialis; finger flexor muscles of the anterior forearm: flexor digitorum profundus and flexor digitorum superficialis, and hand muscles: palmar interossei, flexor digiti minimi, opponens digiti minimi, lumbricales, as well as any associated fascia of the upper limb. There may be secondary stretching of the intercostal muscles and lumbodorsal fascia.

Technique 4.6a is a better stretch for latissimus dorsi, teres major, pectoralis major and pronator teres. Technique 4.6b is a better stretch for teres minor and biceps brachii, and may also stretch brachioradialis and supinator.

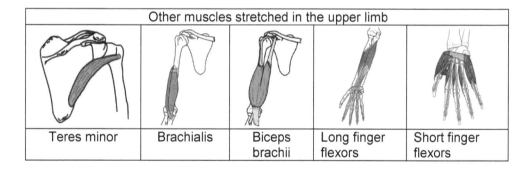

Other muscles stretched in the upper limb				
Teres minor	Brachialis	Biceps brachii	Long finger flexors	Short finger flexors

In actively stretching the upper limb the following muscles are contracted: supraspinatus, middle deltoid, serratus anterior, and upper and lower trapezius. Triceps extends the forearm, while extensor digitorum, extensor indicis and extensor digiti minimi extend the fingers.

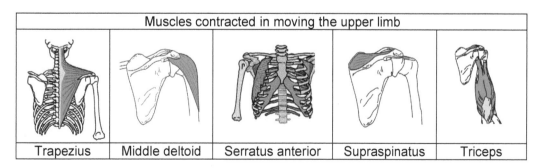

Muscles contracted in moving the upper limb				
Trapezius	Middle deltoid	Serratus anterior	Supraspinatus	Triceps

Variations

As an alternative to the stretch the forearms can be pronate, with your fingers interlaced and wrists turned outwards, so your palms face towards the ceiling.

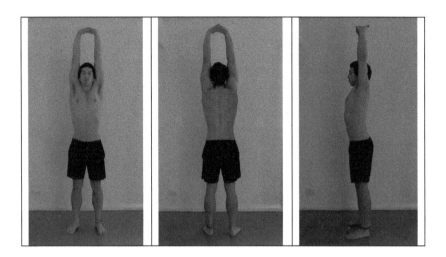

Safety

This is a relatively safe stretch. Existing rotator cuff injuries may be a problem.

Key:

4.6a Palms together above head with forearms supinated	
4.6b Palms together above head with forearms pronated	

Related stretches					
2.0a Standing lumbar and hip sidebending stretch		2.3 Kneeling lateral side stretch		2.4a to 2.4d Hanging stretches	
2.5a & 2.5b Upper Dog extension stretches		2.7b Diagonal locust		3.7, 3.8 & 3.9 Supine rolled up towel stretches	
7.5a Squat with palms together above head					

4.7 Palms together behind back - an active stretch for pectoralis minor, and a passive stretch for the flexor carpi ulnaris and other anterior forearm muscles, and wrist and finger flexor muscles and fascia of the hand

4.7 Palms together behind back

Starting position: Standing with your feet apart and arms by your sides. Flex your elbows, then abduct and internally rotate your shoulders. Your hands should now rest on your iliac crests and lateral lumbar spine.

Slide your hands behind your back, and bring your palms together. If this is difficult then start with the index finger and forefinger of each hand touching, gradually working your way into a full contact of both palms with the little fingers of both hands touching your back.

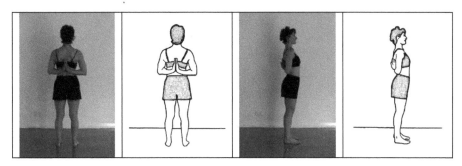

Technique: See Part A. Page 134.

Direction and range of movement

This technique involves a combination of scapula retraction, also known as adduction and shoulder external rotation.

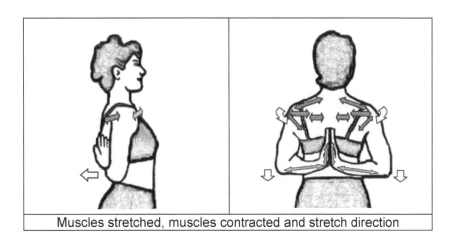

Muscles stretched, muscles contracted and stretch direction

To get to the starting position you must flex your elbows 90 degrees, then abduct your arm about 45 degrees and then internally rotate your arms as far as possible, so that your hands rest on the your iliac crests, just lateral to your lumbar spine. You then must adduct your arms and slide your hands behind your back, and press the palms of your hands together.

If getting to the starting position is difficult then start with the index and forefinger of each hand touching and gradually work your way into a full contact of both palms.
There is about 4 cm of scapula adduction or medial movement of the scapula along the rib cage and towards the spine. There is about 40 degrees external rotation at the shoulder.

Target tissues

This technique mainly stretches the pectoralis minor. It also stretches serratus anterior, the wrist flexor muscles in the anterior forearm, and the finger flexor muscles in the hand and forearm.

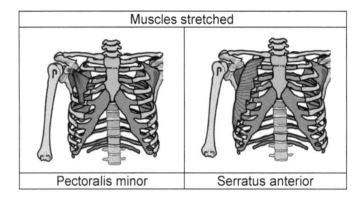

Muscles stretched	
Pectoralis minor	Serratus anterior

This is a passive stretch for the wrist and finger flexor muscles. In the forearm it stretches the wrist flexor muscles flexor carpi ulnaris, flexor carpi radialis and palmaris longus and the finger flexor muscles flexor digitorum profundus and flexor digitorum superficialis.

In the hand it stretches the finger flexor muscles flexor digiti minimi, opponens digiti minimi, lumbricales, the palmar and dorsal interossei, and the palmar aponeurosis. With the arms internally rotated pectoralis major and superficial pectoral fascia are in a shortened state. Other muscles attaching anteriorly or laterally on the humerus such as anterior deltoid, subscapularis, latissimus dorsi and teres major are also shorter.

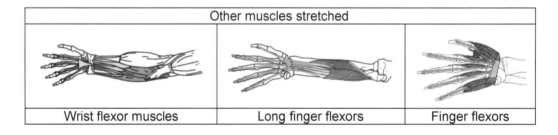

Other muscles stretched		
Wrist flexor muscles	Long finger flexors	Finger flexors

In contrast pectoralis minor, which is attached on the coracoid process of the scapula, is not affected by rotation of the humerus. With less pull on the shortened shoulder muscles more emphasis can be placed on stretching pectoralis minor. Anterior deltoid may be mildly stretched by the extension.

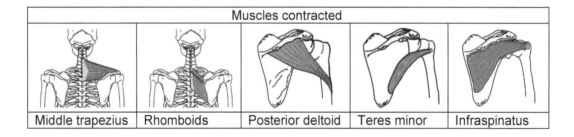

Muscles contracted				
Middle trapezius	Rhomboids	Posterior deltoid	Teres minor	Infraspinatus

402

This is also an active stretch which utilises the contraction of scapular retractor muscles as well as the external rotator muscles of the arm. This technique helps strengthen rhomboid major, rhomboid minor, middle trapezius, infraspinatus, teres minor and posterior deltoid.

Safety

This is a safe stretch, good for strengthening posterior postural muscles.

Key:

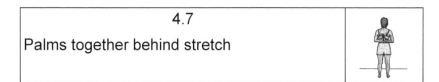

4.7 Palms together behind stretch	

Related stretches					
4.0a & 4.0b Easy pectoralis stretch sitting or standing		4.5 Shoulder abductor stretch behind		4.8 Multi shoulder stretch	
5.0a Shoulder external rotator stretch		5.1b Standing winged stretch		5.2a, b & c Biceps stretch against a ledge	

4.8 Multiple shoulder muscle stretch - active and passive stretch for many shoulder muscles

4.8 Multiple shoulder muscle stretch

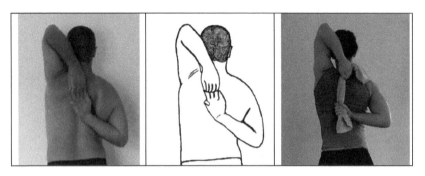

Starting position: Standing with your feet apart. Bend your left elbow to the fully flexed position and lift your left arm to the fully abducted position. Your arm and forearm are near your ear, and your hand is on your upper thoracic spine. Internally rotate your right arm, placing your right hand behind your back. Clasp the fingers of both hands together behind your back. If you are unable to clasp your hands together, then grasp as close as possible on a towel. Keep your head and spine straight, while relaxing your shoulders.

Technique: See Part A. Page 135.

Direction and range of movement

The clasped hands are fixed points around which movement of the scapula and arm can occur. The scapula can glide over the ribs in several directions - superior-inferior, medial-lateral, forwards-backwards tilt and upward-downwards rotation: these movements act in combination.

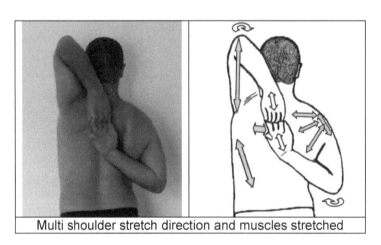

Multi shoulder stretch direction and muscles stretched

This is both an active and a passive stretch. In the active part agonists stretch their antagonists. In the passive part the agonists act through levers to stretch muscles in other parts of the body. The stretch uses multiple joint movements. As in the technique described above, I will describe the right shoulder as the extended low side and the left shoulder as the abducted high side.

In the starting position the right shoulder is positioned in internal rotation and extension, while the right scapula is positioned in combined forward tilt, downward rotation, depression and

404

retraction. The left shoulder is positioned in external rotation and abduction, while the left scapula is positioned in combined upward rotation, elevation and protraction.

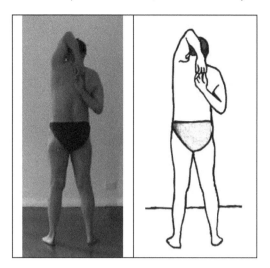

When the point of the right elbow moves backwards this increases extension at the shoulder and forward tilt of the scapula.

When the point of the right elbow moves right or outwards away from the spine this increases abduction at the shoulder, as well as upward rotation, protraction and elevation of the scapula.

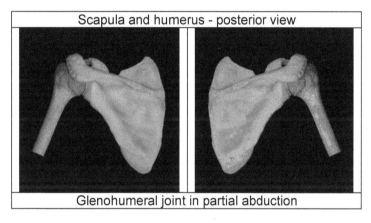

When the point of the right elbow moves left or inwards towards the spine this increases adduction at the shoulder, as well as increasing downward rotation, retraction and depression of the scapula.

When the point of the left elbow moves backwards this increases flexion at the shoulder, as well as backward tilt and upward rotation of the scapula. When the point of the left elbow moves right or behind the head, this increases abduction at the shoulder, as well as upward rotation, protraction and elevation of the scapula.

When the point of the left elbow moves left or away from the head this decreases the abduction at the shoulder, and decreases the upward rotation, protraction and elevation position of the scapula.

This technique involves multiple planes of movement in both shoulders, with each shoulder generally doing the opposite motion - on the right side there is full extension and internal rotation at the shoulder, plus a combination of scapula movements, while on the left side there is full flexion, abduction and external rotation at the shoulder, plus a combination of the opposite scapula movements.

The active shoulder technique is a combined movement of the clavicle, scapula and humerus at the glenohumeral, acromioclavicular, sternoclavicular and scapulothoracic joints.
Full shoulder abduction is about 180 degrees. In the anatomical position there is about 60 degrees external rotation of the shoulder. At full abduction there is about 35 degrees external rotation.

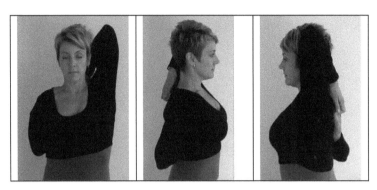

Active hyperextension of the shoulder is about 50 degrees, while passive hyperextension of the shoulder is about 80 degrees. About 10 cm scapula abduction and 4 cm scapula adduction is possible; each scapulae can translate about 14 cm in total across the rib cage.

Target tissues

Different muscles are stretched on the left and right sides of the body because there is a completely different combination of shoulder and scapula movements. Also by varying the direction and distance you are moving the right or left elbow you can place greater emphasis on stretching some muscles and less on others.

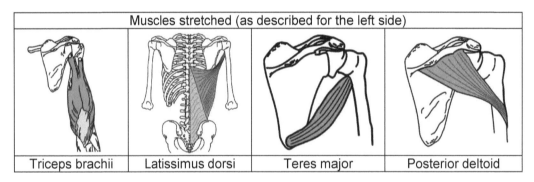

Muscles stretched (as described for the left side)			
Triceps brachii	Latissimus dorsi	Teres major	Posterior deltoid

On the left side of the body this is primarily a stretch for triceps brachii, latissimus dorsi, teres major and the lower fibres of posterior deltoid. To a lesser extent on the left side this is also a stretch for the middle to lower fibres of trapezius and the lower fibres of pectoralis major.

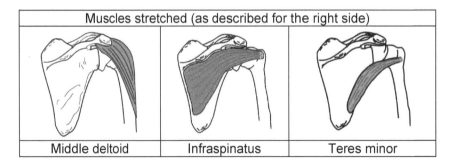

Muscles stretched (as described for the right side)		
Middle deltoid	Infraspinatus	Teres minor

On the right side of the body this is primarily a stretch for middle deltoid, infraspinatus and teres minor. When the right elbow points backwards it increases the stretch on coracobrachialis, anterior deltoid and the lower fibres of serratus anterior. When the right elbow points towards the spine it increases the stretch on supraspinatus, middle deltoid and

406

the upper fibres of serratus anterior. This is also a stretch for anterior shoulder capsule, ligaments and fascia.

Other muscles stretched			
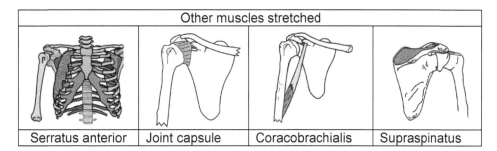			
Serratus anterior	Joint capsule	Coracobrachialis	Supraspinatus

Flexion of the forearm at the elbow stretches the two heads of the triceps which attach on the humerus. When the point of the elbow moves right and behind the head this increases the stretch on the long head of the triceps which attaches on the scapula.

Variations

This stretch may be done seated on a stool, which fixes the pelvis and helps maintain stability of the spine and ribs for better control over the stretch. The technique may also be done as a post-isometric stretch, provided both hands are clasped together or grasp a towel. Then the muscles attaching the scapula to the torso and the humerus can be contracted isometrically, then relaxed and the shoulder can be moved to a new position. The contractions can involve pulling, pushing or moving the arms in a variety of directions.

Safety

If there is a pre-existing rotator cuff strain then this technique may cause irritation to the tendon. If you have a history of shoulder dislocation or you are congenitally hypermobile, then this technique should be done with caution.

Key:

4.8 Multi shoulder stretch	
Multi shoulder stretch	

Related stretches					
2.4a to 2.4d Hanging by the arm		4.5 Shoulder abductor stretch behind		4.7 Palms together behind back	
5.0a Shoulder external rotator stretch		5.1b Standing winged stretch		5.4 Passive triceps stretch	

407

4.9 Scapula retractor stretches - active, passive and post-isometric stretches for the shoulder, spine and scapula retractor muscles

4.9a Scapula retractor stretch standing

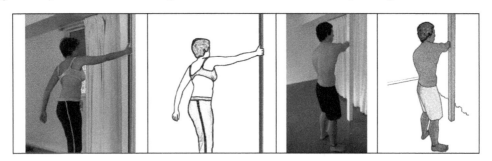

Starting position: Standing with your feet apart. Raise your right arm and grasp a strong vertical pole with your right hand. Grasp the pole at a height level with your shoulders, so that when your arm is straight it is horizontal with the floor. Bend your hips and knees, allowing your body to drop towards the floor. Lean backwards until your right arm is straight and you feel the initial stages of tension down the side of your right arm and shoulder.

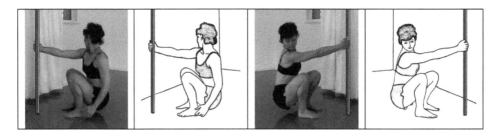

Technique: See Part A. Page 136.

4.9b Scapula retractor stretch squatting unilateral

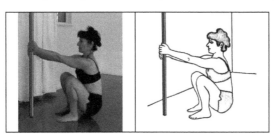

Starting position: Squatting in front of a strong vertical wooden or metal pole. Grasp the pole with your right hand, at a height that is level with or slightly above your shoulders. Lean back until your right arm is straight. If you are unable to squat easily then grasp the pole first, then bend your hips and knees to move into the squatting position.

Technique: See Part A. Page 137.

4.9c Scapula retractor stretch squatting bilateral

Starting position: Squatting in front of a strong vertical wooden or metal pole. Grasp the pole with both your hands at a height that is slightly above your shoulders. Lean backward until your arms are straight. If you are unable to squat easily then grasp the pole first, then bend your hips and knees, to move into the squatting position.

Technique: See Part A. Page 138.

4.9d Scapula wrap stretch standing

Starting position: Standing straight. Lift your right arm, then reach forward and take it around the left side of your rib cage. Grasp your ribs and the lateral border of your left scapula with your right hand. Repeat the process with your left arm, grasping your ribs and the lateral border of your right scapula with your left hand. Make sure your arms and forearm fit comfortably together and wrap around your rib cage.

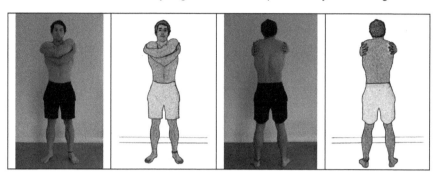

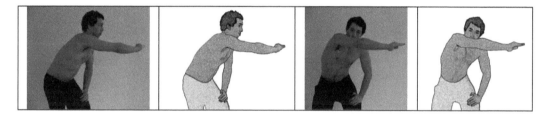

Technique: See Part A. Page 139.

4.9e Scapula active retractor stretch standing

Starting position: Standing with flexed hips and knees. Place the palm of your left hand on top of your left thigh and flex your left elbow to about 20 degrees. Use your left arm to help keep a fixed posture and to steady your body during the stretch. Raise your right arm and reach forward, down and away with your hand. Your spine is straight and angled slightly forward on your hips. Your right arm should be straight and angled down towards the floor. The angle of your right arm relative to your spine, will determine which muscles are stretched but should average at about 90 degrees.

Technique: See Part A. Page 140.

Direction and range of movement

All these techniques involve scapular protraction or lateral movement of the scapula along the rib cage and away from the spine as the primary movements. Techniques 4.9a, 4.9b, 4.9c and 4.9e also involve lateral tilt and upward rotation of the scapula. In technique 4.9d there is a small amount of downward rotation of the scapula.

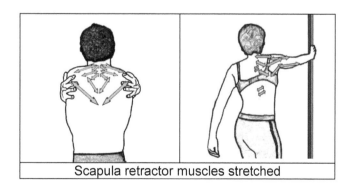

Scapula retractor muscles stretched

There is some horizontal flexion of the shoulder joint in all the techniques. In technique 4.9d this is combined with internal rotation and adduction. Techniques 4.9a, 4.9b and 4.9e involve some thoracic rotation. Techniques 4.9b and 4.9c are done squatting, which involves full hip and knee flexion.

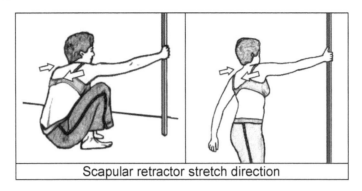

Scapular retractor stretch direction

The scapula has approximately 10 cm of protraction. Taken from the coronal plane and with the arm in 90 degrees abduction there is about 140 degrees horizontal flexion at the shoulder - a combination of scapulothoracic and glenohumeral joint movement. In the thoracic spine there is a total of about 35 degrees rotation, however only part of this range of movement is taken up during this stretch.

Target tissues

These techniques mainly stretch muscles connecting the scapula to the lower cervical and upper thoracic spine. These are rhomboid major and minor and middle trapezius (part III), which are the trapezius fibres attaching on the spine of the scapula.

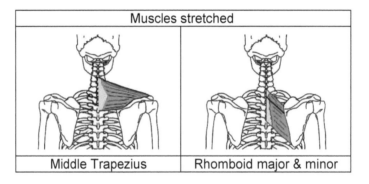

Muscles stretched	
Middle Trapezius	Rhomboid major & minor

To a lesser extent these techniques also stretch muscles attaching on the humerus, ribs and lumbar spine. Secondary muscles stretched include posterior deltoid, infraspinatus, teres minor, middle trapezius (part II), which are the trapezius fibres attaching on the acromion process, lower trapezius (part IV), teres major, upper fibres of latissimus dorsi, serratus posterior inferior, the deep posterior muscles of the thoracic spine - the rotatores.

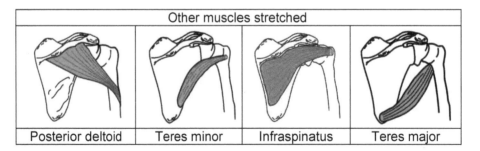

Other muscles stretched			
Posterior deltoid	Teres minor	Infraspinatus	Teres major

Techniques 4.9a to 4.9c are passive stretches that use the weight of the body plus contraction of muscles in the spine. In the post-isometric component of technique 4.9a muscles of the spine, pelvis and legs stabilise the body during shoulder retraction.

410

Technique 4.9d is an isometric contraction followed by an active stretch. Isometric scapula retractor muscles contraction is followed by scapula protractor muscles contraction and a repositioning of the hands around the rib cage. Technique 4.9e is an active stretch that uses protractor muscles to stretch retractor muscles.

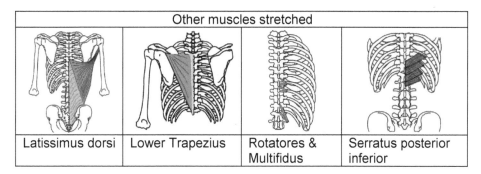

Other muscles stretched			
Latissimus dorsi	Lower Trapezius	Rotatores & Multifidus	Serratus posterior inferior

Although these are primarily techniques for stretching scapula retractor muscles, technique 4.9a, 4.9b and 4.9e will also stretch muscles in the shoulder and spine, 4.9c and 4.9d will also stretch muscles around the shoulder joint. Techniques 4.9b and 4.9c involve squatting, requiring lumbar, hip and knee flexion, and sacroiliac extension.

Lumbar flexion will stretch the thoracolumbar fascia and the posterior fibres of the lumbar erector spinae; hip flexion will stretch gluteus maximus and the lowest fibres of adductor magnus; and knee flexion will stretch vastus medialis, lateralis and intermedius.

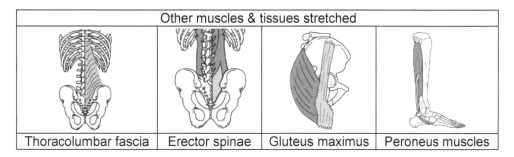

Other muscles & tissues stretched			
Thoracolumbar fascia	Erector spinae	Gluteus maximus	Peroneus muscles

Depending on ankle flexibility and how the squat is done, this may also stretch soleus, tibialis posterior and the peroneus longus and brevis muscles.

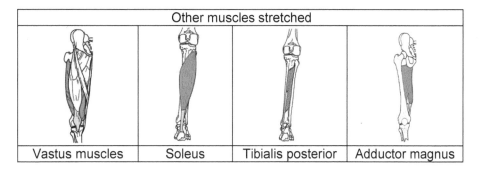

Other muscles stretched			
Vastus muscles	Soleus	Tibialis posterior	Adductor magnus

Safety

In techniques 4.9a, 4.9b and 4.9c make sure that the pole is made from metal or a strong wood that is firmly attached to the floor and ceiling, thus will support your body weight when you pull on it or lean back on it.

Avoid moving into any of the stretches too quickly. Two possible problems may arise from overzealous stretching. Firstly, the supraspinatus tendon may become trapped between the head of the humerus and the acromion process, possibly creating a tear; Secondly, thoracic ligaments or muscles attaching on the thoracic spine may be strained, resulting in muscle spasm and vertebral joint dysfunction. The most vulnerable area of the spine is a single or group of extended vertebrae at or near T4.

An intervertebral disc may be prolapsed or herniated. This is more likely to occur in technique 4.9d, especially if excessive force is used and if the breath is held in during the stretch. The combination of force and intrathoracic pressure could result in a vulnerable disc being pushed beyond its loading capacity.

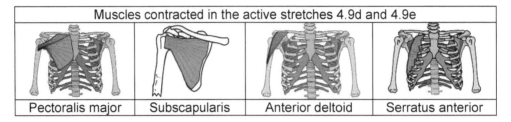

Muscles contracted in the active stretches 4.9d and 4.9e			
Pectoralis major	Subscapularis	Anterior deltoid	Serratus anterior

If there is a knee problem which prevents full knee flexion, then techniques 4.9b and 4.9c should be avoided. Knee cartilage or ligament tears or degenerative changes to the knee joint are the most likely causes of knee restriction.

All of the stretches should be done with a straight spine and with the head in line with the spine. A common error is to point the chin forward, taking the occiput into an anterior position. This reinforces the common bad head forward posture, which may result in suboccipital muscle strain, neck pain and headaches.

Typically the thoracic spine is in a flexed forward position or kyphosis. In some people years of slouching may result in this kyphosis becoming exaggerated. Genetics may also play a role in increasing the kyphosis with one or several vertebrae being involved.

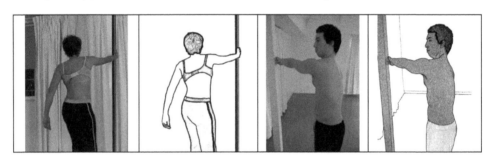

Gravity always acts on the body but when there is an increased kyphosis the body's centre of gravity shifts forwards, meaning gravity has greater effect. The result is that it pushes the flexed spine into even greater flexion, while it also pushes the scapula forwards and around the sides of the rib cage, into a protracted position and creating the characteristic round shoulder stooping posture. In this posture the erector spinae muscles and the scapula retractor muscles must work harder to hold the body erect, and over time straightening the spine and shoulders becomes very difficult. Under these conditions prolonged standing or sitting can result in muscle fatigue and pain.

Although stretching can relieve these tired and achy muscles, these muscles are not short, hence should not be stretched too far. If the retractor muscles are stretched too hard or too frequently, this may make a bad posture worse. Stretching the retractor muscles should only be done gently and only to relieve the pain from postural fatigue.

An exaggerated thoracic kyphosis is associated with shortness through the front of the trunk, in the pectoral fascia and muscles. Stretching pectoralis major and minor muscles, and doing spinal extension exercises such as the upper dog stretch, is far more important for the correction of an exaggerated kyphosis. In combination with these stretches the scapula retractor muscles should be strengthened. The pectoralis stretches 4.0a to 4.0d are good examples of active stretches that combines stretching the pectoralis muscles with strengthening the scapula retractors muscles.

Vulnerable areas

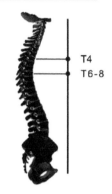

T4

T6-8

	Region	Level of Risk
1.	T4	Medium
2.	T6-8	Low

Key:

4.9a Scapula retractor stretch standing	
4.9b Scapula retractor stretch squatting unilateral	
4.9c Scapula retractor stretch squatting bilateral	
4.9d Scapula wrap stretch standing	
4.9e Scapula active retractor stretch standing	

Related stretches					
2.9a & 2.9b Flexed cat stretches		3.4 Active spinal twist kneeling		4.4 Shoulder abductor front stretch	
5.0a & 5.0b Shoulder external rotator stretches		7.5b Squat with arms in front of body			

413

5.0 Shoulder external rotator stretches - passive, post-isometric and active stretches for muscles responsible for shoulder external rotation and scapular retraction

5.0a Shoulder external rotator stretch

Starting position: Standing with your feet slightly apart and arms at your sides. Flex your right elbow, abduct and internally rotate your right shoulder, placing the back of your right hand against the right side of your lower back. Your right wrist rests on the right iliac crest on the side of your pelvis.

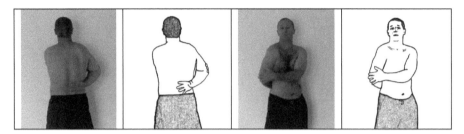

Internally rotate your arm more, by moving your right elbow forwards. Reach forwards and to your right with your left arm, and grasp your right elbow with your left hand. If you can't reach your elbow grasp it as near to your elbow as possible. Relax your right shoulder.

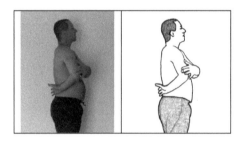

Technique: See Part A. Page 141.

5.0b Active shoulder external rotator stretch

Starting position: Standing with your feet apart and arms at your sides. Internally rotate and flex your arms forwards, thereby bringing the backs of your wrists, hands and fingers together in front of you. Keep both your arms and your spine straight.

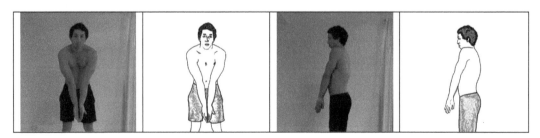

Technique: See Part A. Page 142.

Direction and range of movement

These techniques involve a combination of scapula protraction and shoulder internal rotation. Movement occurs at the acromioclavicular, sternoclavicular, glenohumeral and scapulothoracic joints. In technique 5.0b, pronation occurs in both the radioulnar and radiohumeral joints of the elbow.

414

There is about 10 cm of scapula protraction or lateral movement of the scapula along the rib cage and away from the spine. There is about 100 degrees of internal rotation at the shoulder.

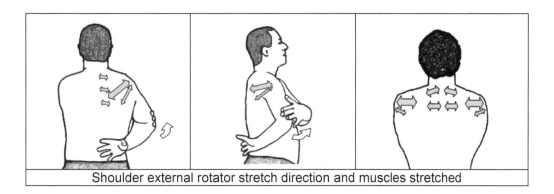

Shoulder external rotator stretch direction and muscles stretched

Target tissues

These techniques stretch posterior shoulder muscles responsible for external rotation – infraspinatus, teres minor and posterior deltoid; and scapulothoracic muscles responsible for scapula retraction – rhomboid major, rhomboid minor and middle trapezius. Technique 5.0a may also be a mild stretch for the long head of triceps brachii.

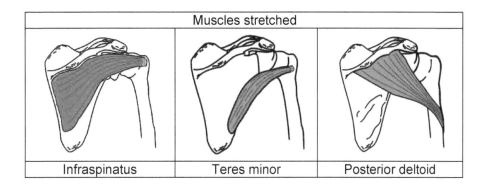

Muscles stretched		
Infraspinatus	Teres minor	Posterior deltoid

The passive stretch 5.0a uses the muscles of one upper limb to pull on the forearm of the other upper limb, creating leverage to localise a strong stretch to the posterior shoulder region. The active stretch 5.0b mainly involves the contraction of pectoralis major and serratus anterior, supported by anterior deltoid, subscapularis, latissimus dorsi and teres major. Pronator teres is also involved in pronating the forearm.

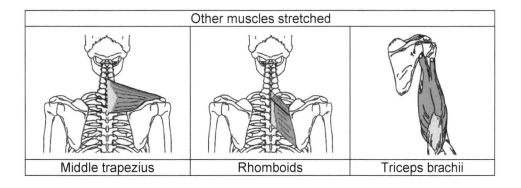

Other muscles stretched		
Middle trapezius	Rhomboids	Triceps brachii

Safety

These are relatively safe techniques. They help relieve tension in antigravity muscles such as the middle trapezius and rhomboids, affected by postural stresses. These muscles have a stabilising role, so as well as stretching them, they should also be strengthened. Also infraspinatus and teres minor, which stabilise the shoulder via the rotator cuff, should be strong as well as flexible.

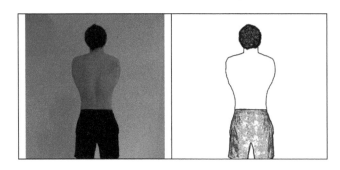

Avoid overstretching middle trapezius and the rhomboids, which may already be in a stretched state due to an existing kyphosis, round shoulders posture and postural distortions from prolonged sitting. Stretching frequency and force should be based on the unique posture of the individual and the situation. The stretch may only need to be done infrequently with a mild to moderate force for tension, but individuals with lost movement, for example a frozen shoulder, may need to stretch daily and with a stronger force. Aim to localise the stretch on the glenohumeral joint, scapulothoracic joint or both, depending on need.

Key:

5.0a Shoulder external rotator stretch	
5.0b Active scapular retractor & shoulder external rotator stretch	

Related stretches			
4.7 Palms together behind back		4.8 Multi shoulder stretch	

416

5.1 Shoulder flexor stretches - passive and post-isometric stretches for the shoulder flexor muscles

5.1a Shoulder flexor drop

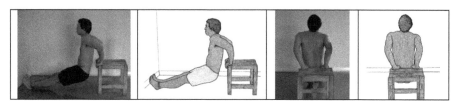

Starting position: Standing with your back facing a low table or chair. Flex your hips and knees. Place your palms on the chair, shoulder width apart and with your fingers curled over the edge of the chair. Walk your heels away from the chair until your legs are straight. Flex your forearms and extend your arms, slowly lowering your body towards the floor. Move your elbows backwards and towards each other. Relax your shoulders but stop the decent to the floor when you start to feel the initial stage of a stretch.

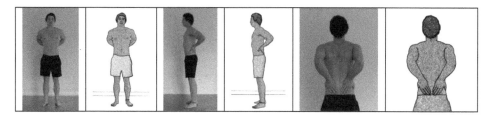

Technique: See Part A. Page 143.

5.1b Winged anterior deltoid stretch standing

Starting position: Standing with your feet apart. Place your hands behind your back, palms down and with your fingers pointing down towards the floor. Point your elbows backwards and stand up straight.

Technique: See Part A. Page 144.

Direction and range of movement

Both techniques involve extension of the shoulders and retraction of the scapulae. Technique 5.1a also involves partial elevation of the scapula and clavicle, and some forwards tilting of the scapula. Shoulder extension is about 50 degrees. Scapula forward tilt is integrated with shoulder extension and is about 15 degrees. Scapula elevation is between 10 and 12 cm. Total scapula forward-backward tilt is between 20 and 30 degrees.

Movement occurs in the acromioclavicular joints, sternoclavicular joints, scapulothoracic joints and glenohumeral joints. Secondary movements occur in the upper spine, hips and elbows.

Target tissues

These are mainly stretches for anterior deltoid and serratus anterior. They are also stretches for coracobrachialis, the clavicular part of pectoralis major and the joint capsule and ligaments overlaying the anterior glenohumeral joints.

Technique 5.0a has a scapula elevation component so will also stretch subclavius and lower trapezius. With both forearms pronated the biceps brachii may be stretched. This may also be a mild stretch for pectoralis minor. How much pectoralis minor stretches will depend on the tightness of other muscles and whether during the stretch, the scapula tilts forward rather than elevates. Elevation and backward tilting movements stretch the muscle, and forward tilting would keep pectoralis minor short.

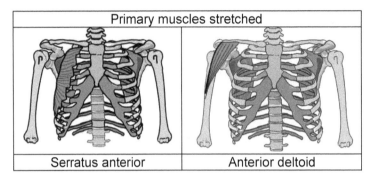

Primary muscles stretched	
Serratus anterior	Anterior deltoid

The passive stretch in technique 5.1a occurs as a result of gravity and body weight, causing the glenohumeral joint to move into extension, thereby stretching the shoulder flexor muscles, as well as causing the scapula to move into retraction, elevation and forward tilt, thereby stretching the scapular protractor and depressor muscles.

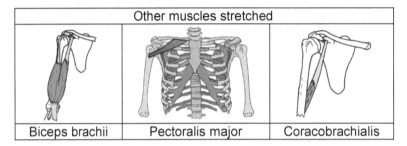

Other muscles stretched		
Biceps brachii	Pectoralis major	Coracobrachialis

The post-isometric stretch occurs as a result of the contraction of the shoulder flexor muscles and scapula protractor muscles.

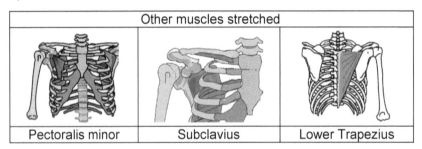

Other muscles stretched		
Pectoralis minor	Subclavius	Lower Trapezius

Safety

This is a safe exercise. Lower your body into the stretching position slowly. Make sure that the chair or small table is stable and strong enough to support your body weight.

Key:

5.1a Shoulder flexor drop	
5.1b Winged anterior deltoid stretch standing	

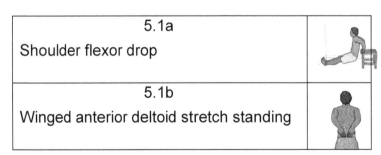

Related stretches	
5.2a, b & c Biceps stretches against a ledge	

5.2 Ledge squat stretches - passive and post-isometric stretches for the anterior shoulder muscles and fascia

5.2a Bilateral passive stretch against a ledge

Starting position: Standing with your feet slightly apart and your back towards a ledge or shelf. The ledge shoulder is about level with your lower lumbar spine. Flex your elbows, extend your shoulders and interlace the fingers of both hands behind your back. Place your interlaced hands on the ledge. Your index fingers and thumbs are in contact with the ledge. Extend your forearms until your elbows are straight. Flex your knees until you feel a stretch across the front of your shoulders and down the front of your arms.

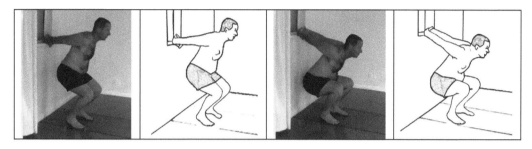

Technique: See Part A. Page 145.

5.2b Bilateral post-isometric stretch against a ledge

Starting position: The same as for technique 5.2a described above.

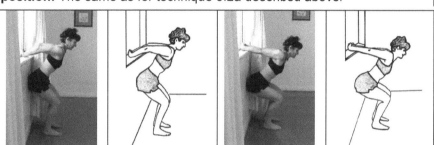

Technique: See Part A. Page 146.

5.2c Unilateral passive and post-isometric stretch against a ledge

Starting position: Standing with your feet apart and your back towards a ledge or shelf. The ledge shoulder is about level with your lower back. Extend your right arm and place the palm of your right hand on the ledge. Do not allow your arm to abduct. Rotating your thoracic spine to the left will help put your arm into extension. Your right hand should be behind your shoulder and your elbow straight. Flex your hips and knees until you feel a stretch across the front of your shoulder and down the front of your arm.

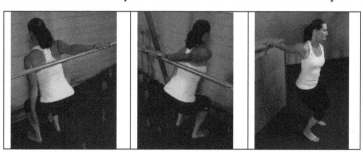

Technique: See Part A. Page 147.

Direction and range of movement

Active extension of the shoulder is about 45 degrees but passive extension is about 90 degrees. Movement is a combination of extension of the glenohumeral joint and forward tilting of the scapula on the ribs.

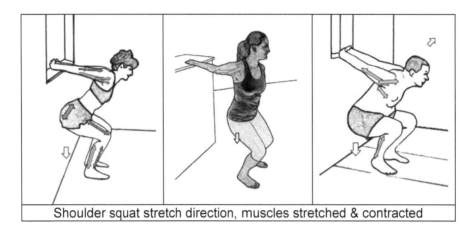

Shoulder squat stretch direction, muscles stretched & contracted

In addition there is forward rotation of the clavicle at the sternoclavicular and acromioclavicular joints, full elbow extension, partial hip and knee flexion and between 20 and 30 degrees dorsiflexion of the ankle. A small amount of movement also occurs within the tarsal joints of the foot. In the unilateral stretch the arm is externally rotated and in the bilateral stretch the arm is more internally rotated.

Target tissues

These techniques mainly stretch biceps brachii and anterior deltoid. They also stretch coracobrachialis, the lower fibres of serratus anterior, the clavicular part of pectoralis major and overlying pectoral fascia.

As the squat becomes deeper other muscles may be stretched including: brachialis, brachioradialis, the wrist extensor muscles, as well as the anterior ligaments and capsule of the shoulder joint. There may be a small stretch on subscapularis when the arm is externally rotated in unilateral stretch 5.2c.

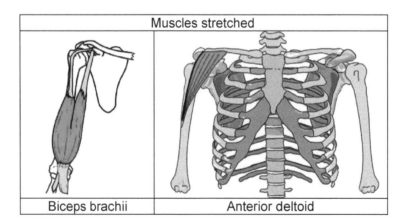

Muscles stretched	
Biceps brachii	Anterior deltoid

In the unilateral stretch the arm is in greater external rotation, increasing the stretch on anterior deltoid, coracobrachialis, the upper fibres of pectoralis major, and the short head of biceps brachii. Rotating the thoracic spine away from the side being stretched increases horizontal extension at the shoulder, further increasing the stretch on these muscles and initiating a stretch of middle deltoid and supraspinatus.

To include soleus and other deep calf muscles in the stretch you must keep your heels on the ground. In the bilateral techniques 5.2a and 5.2b, the fingers are interlaced, internally rotating the shoulders, which results in a more general stretch of all the muscles.

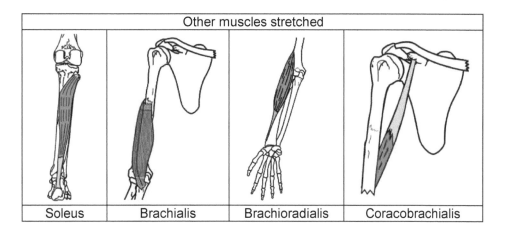

Other muscles stretched			
Soleus	Brachialis	Brachioradialis	Coracobrachialis

Stretching occurs mainly as a result of muscle contraction of the quadriceps and gluteus maximus lowering the body into a squatting position. These muscles act as brakes against gravity pulling the body towards the ground. The deeper the squat the greater the leverage exerted on the anterior shoulders.

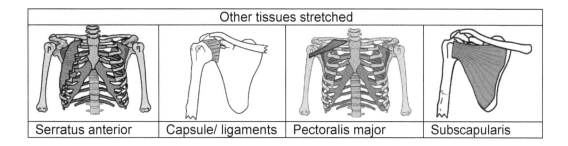

Other tissues stretched			
Serratus anterior	Capsule/ ligaments	Pectoralis major	Subscapularis

During the unilateral stretch 5.2c the elbows are held in extension by the force of the ledge pushing up against the wrist, and by contraction of the triceps.

During the bilateral stretches 5.2a and 5.2b the interlocking fingers, clasped hands, and locked extended elbows, turn the upper limbs into a single long rectangular lever which acts on the glenohumeral, acromioclavicular, sternoclavicular and scapulothoracic joints.

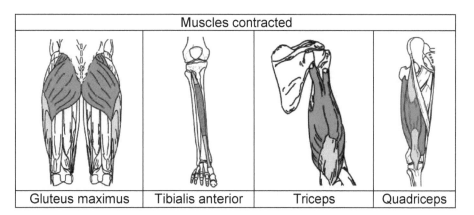

Muscles contracted			
Gluteus maximus	Tibialis anterior	Triceps	Quadriceps

During all the stretches the hands are held back by the ledge as the body descends. The ledge is a fulcrum about which the wrist pivots, creating leverage through the arm to increase shoulder extension and forward tilt of the scapula.

This technique strengthens triceps brachii, tibialis anterior, gluteus maximus and the quadriceps group of muscles.

In the post-isometric stretch pectoralis major, anterior deltoid and biceps muscles are contracted and then allowed to relax, thereby facilitating muscle lengthening during the relaxation stage.

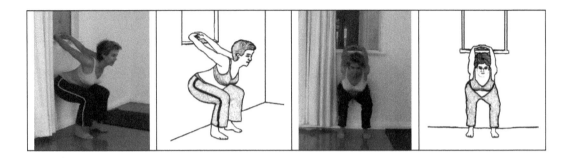

Safety

Biceps brachii can become short particularly after repetitive activities such as digging in the garden or lifting things; if this is the case it may prevent an injury or tear in the muscle or tendon. If the biceps or any of its tendons have been strained or ruptured then scar tissue may be present which will result in weakness.

Do not do this technique if you have damage to your articular capsule, glenoid labrum, transverse humeral ligaments, biceps tendon, or if you have a congenitally shallow bicipital groove. Although it is good to stretch the biceps, seek advice on whether this exercise is appropriate or should be modified to suit your unique needs or to take into account any damaged area

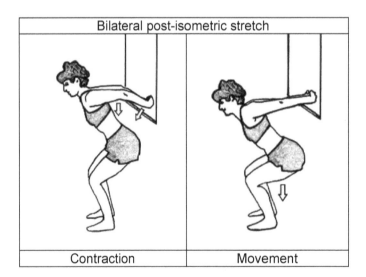

Capsule and ligament laxity as well as a congenitally hypermobile shoulder joint can result in dislocation. If there is a history of shoulder dislocation then caution should be taken when doing this stretch.

The biceps tendon can rupture if weakened by trauma, rheumatoid arthritis or other degenerative processes. This stretch may irritate a pre-existing rotator cuff tear. Warm up the shoulder with simple movements and walking before stretching.

	Region	Level of Risk
1.	Biceps tendon changes & weakness	Medium
2.	Rotator cuff strain	Medium
3.	Shoulder capsule or ligament laxity	Medium

Key:

5.2a Bilateral passive or post-isometric biceps stretch squatting	
5.2b Unilateral passive and post-isometric biceps stretch against a ledge	

Related stretches					
4.0a & 4.0b Easy pectoralis stretches		4.5 Shoulder abductor stretch behind		5.1a Shoulder flexor drop	
5.1b Standing winged anterior deltoid stretch					

For more detailed anatomy of the shoulder - scapula, clavicle and humerus 4.0 - 5.2 see page 571.

5.3 Elbow flexor stretches - passive and post-isometric stretches for muscles responsible for forearm flexion

5.3a & 5.3b Passive and post-isometric elbow flexor stretches

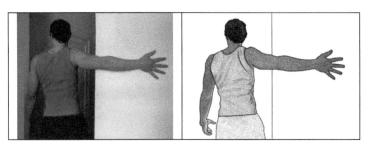

Starting position: Standing with your feet apart, under a doorframe or near the corner of a room with your right side facing the doorframe/corner. Place your right foot through the doorway but leave your left foot outside the doorway behind you. Extend your right arm until it is horizontal and level with your shoulder; hence at right angles to the doorframe. The doorframe should cross your arm about a third of the way from your elbow to your shoulder. Keep your right elbow straight and your fingers, palm, wrist, forearm, elbow as well as part of your arm in contact with the wall.

Technique: See Part A. Page 148 and 149.

In the post-isometric stretch combine flexion of the elbow with: supination and shoulder horizontal flexion for biceps; forearm pronation for brachialis and brachioradialis; wrist and finger flexion for the anterior forearm muscles. Then relax and increase elbow extension to target the elbow flexors; increase elbow supination to target brachialis and brachioradialis; increase wrist and finger extension to target the anterior forearm muscles.

Direction and range of movement

In this technique, the thoracic spine is rotated away from the arm, both scapula are retracted, and on one side of the body, a shoulder is horizontally extended, and an elbow is extended.

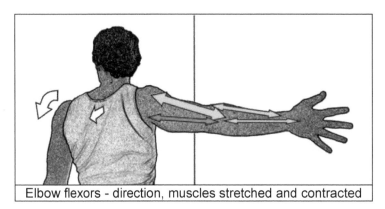

Elbow flexors - direction, muscles stretched and contracted

In the thoracic (T1 to T12) there is about 35 degrees rotation and about 4 cm of medial movement of the scapula along the ribs. During the stretch the scapula move towards the spine, a movement known as retraction or adduction. Horizontal extension of the shoulder is about 30 degrees. Pronation of the elbow is 85 degrees and supination is 90 degrees.

Full elbow extension is 0 degrees, by convention this is the start of the range of elbow movement; it is also the default anatomical position. Bone against bone contact prevents any movement past the straight, extended arm position, except in hypermobile individuals who may have up to 15 degrees hyperextension at the elbow.

Target tissues

This technique can be done as an active, passive or post-isometric stretch. It uses leverage from the contraction of muscles in the shoulder and spine. It is primarily a stretch for biceps brachii, brachialis and brachioradialis.

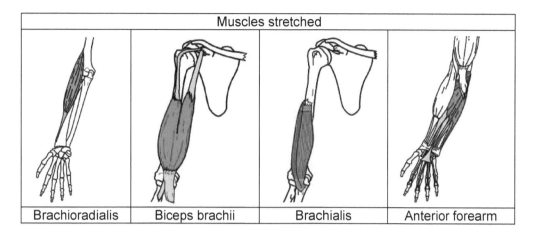

Muscles stretched			
Brachioradialis	Biceps brachii	Brachialis	Anterior forearm

The elbow flexor stretch is also a stretch for anterior deltoid, serratus anterior, the middle fibres of pectoralis major, and in the forearm, flexor carpi ulnaris, flexor carpi radialis, palmaris longus and pronator teres.

All the muscles contracted in the post-isometric stretch are the same as the muscles that are stretched. Triceps brachii is contracted in the active stretch. During the passive stretch middle trapezius, rhomboid major and minor, multifidus, rotatores, erector spinae, infraspinatus, teres minor and posterior deltoid play an indirect role in rotating the trunk and stabilise the body.

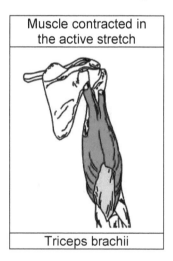

Muscle contracted in the active stretch
Triceps brachii

Safety

If you have an exaggerated thoracic kyphosis, an inflexible thoracic spine or rounded shoulders, then the rotator cuff tendon in your shoulder is vulnerable to injury with this technique.

Make sure you have warmed up your body, in particular your shoulder muscles prior to doing this stretch. Simple circles of the shoulders, other shoulder movements or even brisk walking for about ten minutes are usually adequate.

If you are congenitally hypermobile, or have localised elbow hypermobility as a result of injury or overstretching, your elbow may hyperextend past the neutral straight position by as much as 15 to 20 degrees. If this applies to you then this technique must be done with caution. Do not take a hyperextended elbow further into extension and stretch lax elbow ligaments. If it is absolutely necessary to stretch the elbow flexor muscles, then the elbow joint should be protected during the stretch either with a firm brace or by taking advantage of the rigidity of the wall to protect the elbow. Do not use force and leverage to extend the elbow past the straight position.

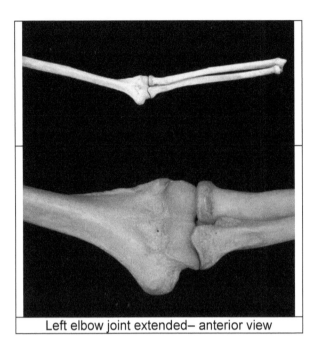

| | Left elbow joint extended– anterior view |

<u>Vulnerable areas</u>

	Region	Level of Risk
1.	Rotator cuff	Medium
2.	Hypermobile elbow	High

Key:

5.3a & 5.3b	
Passive and post-isometric elbow flexor stretches	

Related stretches					
2.0a Standing sidebending stretch		2.4a, b & c Hanging stretches		2.5a & 2.5b Upper Dog extension stretches	
3.6, 3.7 & 3.8 Supine pectoralis stretch over a rolled up towel		4.0a, b & c Pectoralis stretches		5.7 & 5.8 Kneeling wrist stretches	
Many more elbow extension stretches are listed in the appendix section					

5.4 Triceps stretch - passive stretch for the triceps and muscles responsible for shoulder adduction

5.4 Triceps stretch

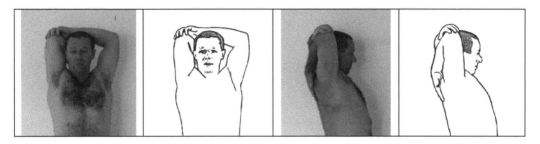

Starting position: Standing with your feet apart and arms at your sides. Flex your right forearm until it is fully flexed. Abduct your right arm to the fully abducted position. Your right elbow should now be near your right ear and the palm of your right hand should rest on your upper thoracic spine.

Abduct your left arm and grasp your right elbow with your left hand. Keep both your arms and forearms back, and slightly behind your head. Keep a straight spine, maintaining spine and head alignment. Don't let your forearms push your head forward into a flexed position. Relax your shoulders.

Technique: See Part A. Page 150.

Direction and range of movement

This technique involves full shoulder abduction combined with partial scapula protraction and upward rotation. The elbow is in full flexion.

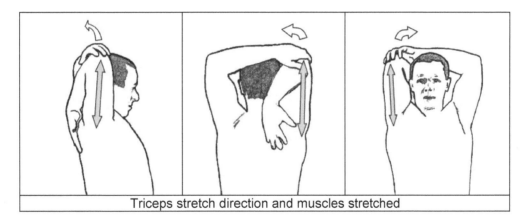

Triceps stretch direction and muscles stretched

Full shoulder abduction is 180 degrees. At full abduction there is about 35 degrees upward rotation and about 8 cm of lateral movement of the scapula.

Target tissues

This technique primarily stretches triceps brachii and overlying fascia.

The fully flexed elbow places the two shorter heads of triceps, the medial and lateral humeral heads, into a lengthened position and thus stretches them.

The fully abducted shoulder combined with the flexed elbow, places the third, or long head of triceps into a lengthened position and stretches it. As the long head is anchored on the scapula, any additional abduction or flexion of the arm will stretch that head further.

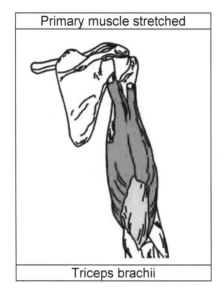

Primary muscle stretched
Triceps brachii

Other muscles stretched include latissimus dorsi, teres major and the lower fibre of pectoralis major. This may be a mild stretch for the lower fibres of anterior deltoid and posterior deltoid.

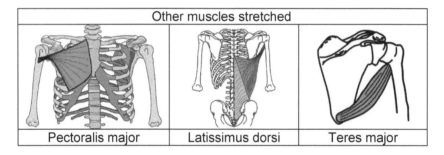

Other muscles stretched		
Pectoralis major	Latissimus dorsi	Teres major

Directing the stretch by pulling the elbow upwards or towards the ceiling (shoulder elevation), increases the stretch on the latissimus dorsi.

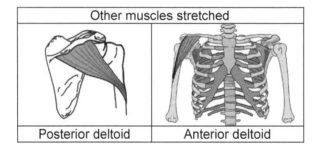

Other muscles stretched	
Posterior deltoid	Anterior deltoid

Variations

This stretch may also be done seated. This variation fixes the ischial bones of the pelvis on the seat, which helps you to hold the spine still for better control over the stretch. This can easily be converted to a post-isometric stretch by resisting shoulder adduction with the hand holding the elbow, and then stretching the triceps as described above for the passive stretch. If this stretch is done with the forearm extended there is less stretch on the triceps and a greater emphasis placed on stretching the other muscles.

Safety

If this stretch is done correctly, it is unlikely to cause any problems. You need to be able to flex your shoulder sufficiently, such that you can take your arm behind your head. What you should not do is let your arm push your head and cervical spine forwards into flexion. This will put strain on cervical ligaments, muscles and intervertebral discs which if repeated may cause unwanted postural changes and degenerative changes. When you do this stretch ensure your arms and forearms are brought as far backwards behind your head as possible so your spine stays straight and in line with your head.

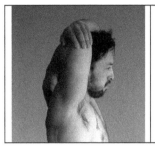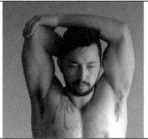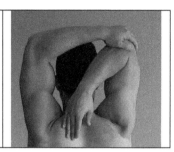

If there is an existing rotator cuff strain then this technique may compress the tendon or bursa and may cause irritation. Discontinue the movement if there is shoulder pain during the stretch; if it persists seek advice about the cause. If the shoulder is hypermobile do not overstretch it - or any hypermobile joint.

Triceps stretch with forearms partially extended
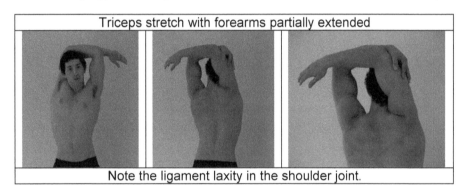
Note the ligament laxity in the shoulder joint.

Key:

5.4 Passive triceps stretch	

Related stretches			
1.2 The Shrug standing	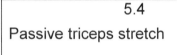	4.8 Multi shoulder stretch	

5.5 Supinator stretch - active and post-isometric stretch for the muscles responsible for forearm supination

5.5 Supinator stretch

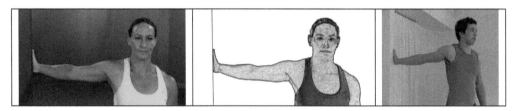

Starting position: Standing with your feet apart and with your right side opposite a doorframe or firmly anchored vertical pole. Partially abduct and flex your right arm, and grasp the doorframe with your right hand at point just below the level of your shoulder. Your thumb should point upwards towards the ceiling, your forearm should be extended and your arm should be relaxed.

Technique: See Part A. Page 151.

Direction and range of movement

Supination is about 90 degrees. It is measured from the mid or neutral position, with the elbow flexed at 90 degrees. This stretch involves full elbow extension and forearm supination. Partial shoulder flexion, abduction and external rotation places the arm in a good starting position, with the arm muscles maximally relaxed.

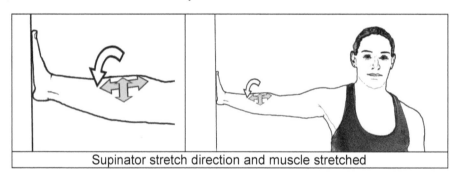

Supinator stretch direction and muscle stretched

The supinator stretch can be done either as an active stretch or as an active stretch combined with a post-isometric contraction. During the active stretch the forearm is pronated at the elbow. The hand and arm are in fixed positions with the hand grasping the doorframe while the shoulder muscles hold the arm steady. With the shoulder and hand fixed, and the elbow fully extended, movement at the forearm is limited to either supination or pronation, as the radius is free to rotate relative to the humerus and the ulna.

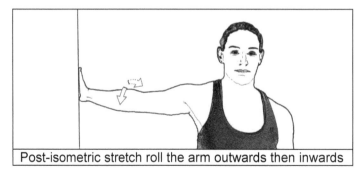

Post-isometric stretch roll the arm outwards then inwards

During the active stretch the forearm is pronated at the elbow due to contraction of the pronator teres and pronator quadratus muscles, which thereby stretches the supinator

430

muscle. During the post-isometric stretch, the supinator is contracted but as the hand and shoulder are fixed, there is muscle contraction but no actual movement.

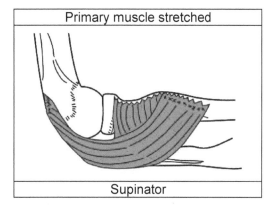

Primary muscle stretched
Supinator

After the isometric contraction the techniques switches to an active stretch, where as above, the pronator muscles contract to stretch the supinator muscle. As with all active stretches, reciprocal inhibition assists in lengthening supinator.

Target tissues

This mainly stretches supinator. To a lesser extent it also stretches biceps brachii, brachialis and brachioradialis.

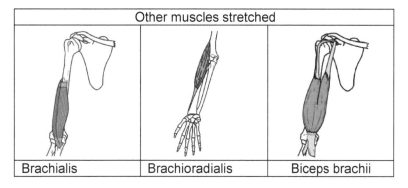

Other muscles stretched		
Brachialis	Brachioradialis	Biceps brachii

Forearm extension is maintained by triceps brachii. Shoulder stability is maintained by the contraction of pectoralis major, deltoid, serratus anterior, latissimus dorsi, supraspinatus, trapezius, subscapularis, infraspinatus, teres major and minor, rhomboid major and minor.

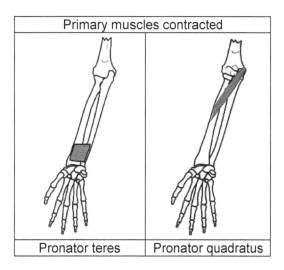

Primary muscles contracted	
Pronator teres	Pronator quadratus

The fixed hand position is maintained by the contraction of short and long finger flexors. Forearm pronation is produced by the contraction of pronator teres and pronator quadratus.

Safety

This is a safe stretch that is unlikely to cause problems. The stretch may be useful for assisting in the recovery of a tennis elbow or overuse problem in the forearm.

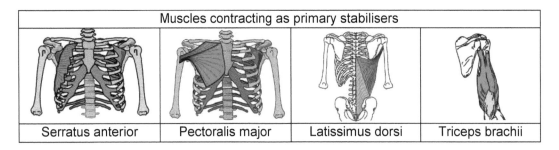

Muscles contracting as primary stabilisers			
Serratus anterior	Pectoralis major	Latissimus dorsi	Triceps brachii

Other muscles contracting as stabilisers			
Teres minor	Rhomboids	Teres major	Infraspinatus
Subscapularis	Middle trapezius	Deltoid	Supraspinatus

Key:

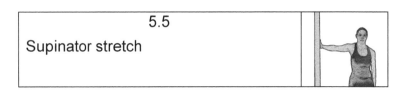

5.5	
Supinator stretch	

Related stretches					
2.5b & 2.5c Upper Dog extension stretches		3.8 & 3.9 Supine hand & forearm stretches		4.0a, b, e & f Pectoralis stretches	
4.6b Palms together above head forearms pronated		5.3a & 5.3b Elbow flexor stretches		5.7c Kneeling wrist extensor stretch	
5.8d & 5.8e Wrist flexor stretches					

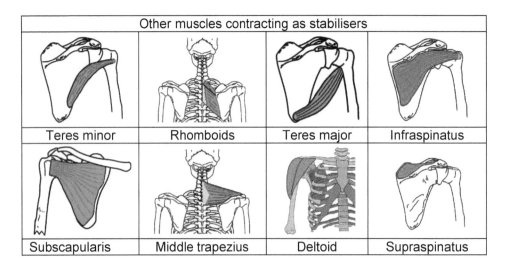

5.6 Pronator stretches - active, passive and post-isometric stretches for pronator teres and pronator quadratus

5.6a Pronator stretch using a doorframe

Starting position: Standing with your feet apart and your right side near to a doorframe or pole. Grasp the doorframe with your right hand - just below shoulder level. Keep your arm straight and have your thumb pointing downwards. Place your right arm about midway between abduction and extension and grasp the doorframe at a height where shoulder muscle tension is minimal and the stretch is easy to execute.

Technique: See Part A. Page 152.

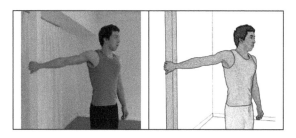

5.6b Passive pronator stretch assisted by the other hand

Starting position: Standing with your feet apart. Flex your right elbow to 90 degrees. Supinate your right forearm by rotating it outwards as far as possible. Grasp your right wrist with a firm hold of your left hand.

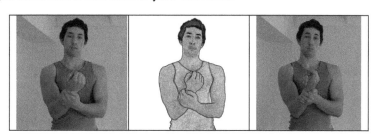

Technique: See Part A. Page 153.

Direction and range of movement

Pronation is about 90 degrees. It is measured from the mid or neutral position, with the elbow flexed at 90 degrees. Pronation may be slightly less than 90 degrees in some people.

Technique 5.6a involves full elbow extension and forearm pronation. There is partial shoulder extension, abduction and internal rotation to place the arm in a good starting position and put the arm muscles in a maximally relaxed state. The stretch can be done either as an active stretch or as a post-isometric technique.

During the active stretch, the forearm is supinated at the elbow due to contraction of the supinator muscle, which thereby stretches pronator teres and pronator quadratus. The hand and arm are in fixed positions with the hand grasping the doorframe, while the shoulder muscles hold the arm steady. With the shoulder and hand fixed, and the elbow fully extended, movement at the forearm is limited to either supination or pronation, as the radius is free to rotate relative to the humerus and the ulna.

During the post-isometric stretch, the pronator muscles are contracted but as the hand and shoulder are fixed, there is muscle contraction but no actual movement. Isometric pronation involves pushing your thumb and the radial side of your hand against the side of the doorframe, while attempting to rotate your forearm inwards and downwards.

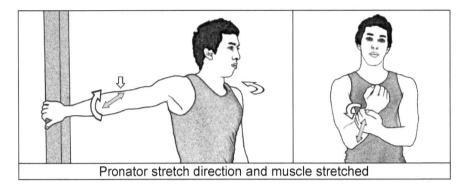

Pronator stretch direction and muscle stretched

As pronator teres is also a weak forearm flexor, isometric pronation can be combined with forearm flexion; this flexion action involves pushing your hand downward against the doorframe. After the isometric contraction the techniques becomes an active stretch, where as above, supinator contraction stretches the pronator muscles. As with all active stretches, reciprocal inhibition aids in lengthening the pronators.

Technique 5.6b involves full forearm supination with the elbow flexed 90 degrees. During the passive stretch the forearm is supinated by the hand of the opposite upper limb. During the post-isometric stretch the pronator muscles are contracted but the forearm is held in a fixed position by the hand of the opposite limb, and no actual movement occurs. The action involves pushing your wrist against the pads of your fingers for about five seconds.

Primary muscle stretched

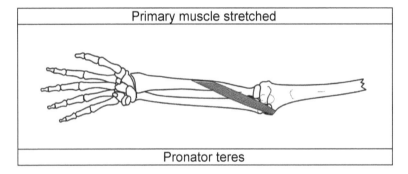

Pronator teres

Target tissues

These techniques stretch pronator teres and pronator quadratus. Technique 5.6a is a mild stretch for brachialis, brachioradialis and biceps. If the shoulder is extended, there may be an unintended stretch for anterior deltoid, coracobrachialis, subscapularis and pectoralis major.

Other muscles stretched

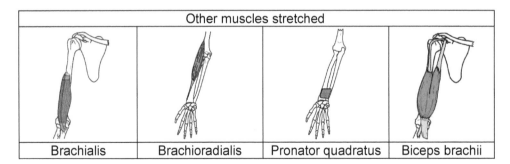

Brachialis	Brachioradialis	Pronator quadratus	Biceps brachii

For successful stretching of pronator teres it is important to find the right combination of shoulder abduction and extension to create minimum muscle tension. In addition for a good pronator teres stretch, it is important to grasp the doorframe at a height where it is easy to roll the forearm outwards.

In the active part of technique 5.6a, supinator stretches pronator teres by supinating the forearm at the elbow. The movement produces supination at the elbow because the hand and wrist are fixed at the doorframe, while the shoulder is relatively fixed by the action of shoulder stabiliser muscles. Actively contracting triceps results in reciprocal inhibition of the forearm flexor muscles including pronator teres, further assisting the stretching process. In technique 5.6b the pronators are passively stretched using force generated by upper limb muscles on the opposite side of the body, mainly finger flexor muscles and wrist extensor muscles.

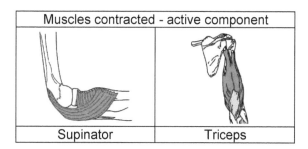

Muscles contracted - active component	
Supinator	Triceps

Safety

If you have a hyperextended elbow, either as a result of generalised congenital hypermobility or localised hypermobility caused by trauma, then modifications may be necessary if you are to prevent ligament strain and overstretching of the elbow. The elbow joint can be protected with a firm brace or by using the forearm flexor muscles as stabilisers, countering the contraction of triceps brachii.

Vulnerable areas

Key:

	Region	Level of Risk
1.	Hypermobile elbow	Medium

5.6a Pronator stretch using a doorframe	
5.6b Pronator stretch assisted by the hand of the other limb	

Related stretches					
3.8d Supine rolled towel posterior forearm stretch		4.0a & 4.0b Easy pectoralis stretches		4.0e Pectoralis stretch against wall standing	
5.0b Active shoulder retractor & rotator stretch		5.3a & 5.3b Elbow flexor stretches		5.7d Kneeling wrist extensor stretch	
5.8b Wrist flexor stretches					

For more detailed anatomy of the elbow and forearm - humerus, radius and ulna 5.3 - 5.6 see page 585.

5.7 Wrist extensor stretches - passive and post-isometric stretches for the extensor muscles of the wrist and hand

5.7a Kneeling unilateral wrist extensor stretch

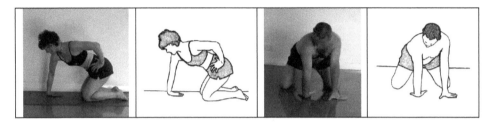

Starting position: Kneeling on the floor, preferably on a carpet or on a mat. Bend forwards at the hips and place the palm of your left hand on the floor in front of you. Flex your right arm, forearm and hand and place the back of your right hand on the floor so your palm faces upwards. Your arms are straight and vertical, with your hands directly below your shoulders. Keep your knees and feet apart for easier balance. Your spine should be in a neutral position, neither flexed nor extended.

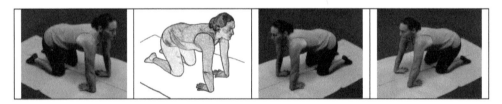

Technique: See Part A. Page 154.

5.7b Kneeling bilateral wrist extensor stretch

Starting position: Kneeling on the floor, preferably on a carpet or on a mat. Bend forwards at the hips, flex your elbows and wrists, and place the backs of both hands on the floor with your fingers pointing towards your knees. Extend your elbows so your arms are straight and vertical and your hands are directly under your shoulders. Keep your knees and feet apart for easier balance. Your spine should be in a neutral position - neither flexed nor extended. Do not take the weight of your upper body through your wrists.

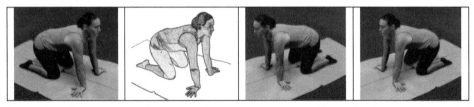

Technique: See Part A. Page 155.

5.7c Kneeling wrist extensor and ulna deviator stretch

Starting position: Kneeling on the floor, preferably on a carpet or on a mat. Bend forwards at the hips, flex your elbows and wrists, fully internally rotate your arms, and place your backs of your hands on the floor with your fingers pointing outwards, laterally and away from your body. In all other respects the starting position is the same as in technique 5.7b.

Technique: See Part A. Technique 1.4c Page 59. By combining wrist flexion with radial deviation and forearm pronation, this becomes a localised stretch for extensor carpi ulnaris.

5.7d Kneeling wrist extensor and radial deviator stretch

Starting position: Kneeling on the floor. Bend forwards at the hips, flex your elbows and wrists and place the backs of your hands on the floor with your fingers pointing inwards, medially and towards each other. In all other respects the starting position is the same as in technique 5.7b.

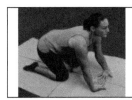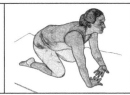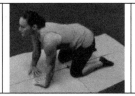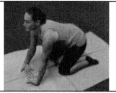

Technique: See Part A. Page 157. By combining wrist flexion with ulna deviation and forearm supination, this becomes a localised stretch for extensor carpi radialis longus and brevis.

Direction and range of movement

This technique involves full elbow extension and full wrist flexion. Radial deviation and ulna deviation may be combined with wrist flexion.

Full elbow extension is a straight arm set at 0 degrees, but in a hypermobile person the elbow may extend up to15 degrees beyond neutral. Wrist flexion occurs between the radius and the proximal row of carpal bones - the radiocarpal joint, and between the proximal and the distal row of carpal bones - the midcarpal joint. There is about 80 to 90 degrees of flexion at the wrist, 50 degrees at the radiocarpal joint and 35 degrees at the midcarpal joint.

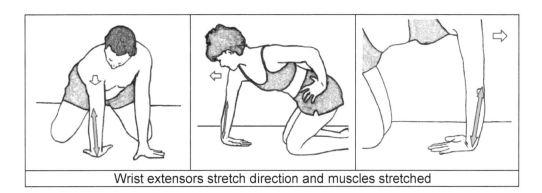

Wrist extensors stretch direction and muscles stretched

Target tissues

These are passive stretches primarily for the extensor muscles of the wrist and hand. They also stretch the finger extensor muscles, fascia in the posterior forearm and ligaments in the posterior wrist. The extensor muscles are part of the posterior compartment of the forearm, most of them arising from the lateral epicondyle at the distal end of the humerus.

The muscles stretched the most are the wrist extensor muscles: extensor carpi ulnaris, extensor carpi radialis longus and extensor carpi radialis brevis.

The finger extensor muscles, extensor digitorum, extensor digiti minimi and extensor indicis are stretched less than the wrist extensors, but active finger flexion can be used to increase the stretch on these muscles. Also a passive stretch may be possible in the unilateral techniques if you use your free hand.

The kneeling unilateral and bilateral wrist extensor stretches 5.7a and 5.7b are general stretches for the wrist extensors: extensor carpi ulnaris, extensor carpi radialis longus and extensor carpi radialis brevis. They may also stretch brachioradialis, supinator, brachialis, biceps brachii and extensor digitorum.

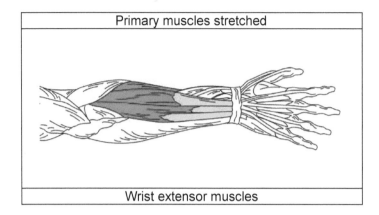

The kneeling wrist extensor and ulna deviator stretch 5.7c is mainly for extensor carpi ulnaris. It may also stretch extensor digitorum communis, supinator, brachioradialis and biceps brachii. To a lesser extent it may also stretch brachialis, and extensor carpi radialis longus and brevis.

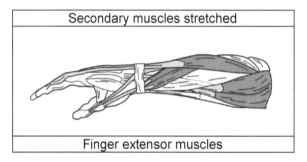

Kneeling wrist extensor and radial deviator stretch 5.7d is mainly for extensor carpi radialis longus and extensor carpi radialis brevis. It may also stretch extensor digitorum communis, abductor pollicis longus and extensor pollicis longus and brevis. To a lesser extent it may stretch, brachioradialis, brachialis and extensor carpi ulnaris.

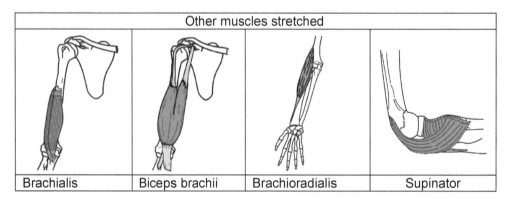

Variations

These stretches may be done standing with the back of your hand on a table or against a wall. They can be done as passive or post-isometric stretches.

In technique 5.7a the back of your hand on the floor with your fingers pointing backwards, which pronates your forearm, stretching most of the extensor muscles. If however your fingers are pointing forwards, this will supinate your forearm, slightly increasing the stretch on extensor carpi ulnaris and extensor digiti minimi but decreasing the stretch on all the other muscles.

438

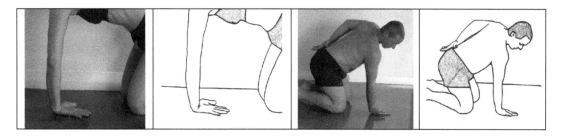

Safety

Do not put the weight of the body through the wrist when you do this stretch; use just enough pressure on the wrist to keep the hand in flexion.

If there is a pre-existing wrist strain or a history of osteoarthritis, rheumatoid arthritis or tendonitis involving the wrist, then there may be joint hypermobility or restriction, which may create wrist pain during the stretch. If this is the case, then this technique may be contraindicated, and professional advice should be sought before doing the stretch.

Key:

5.7a Kneeling unilateral wrist extensor stretch	
5.7b Kneeling bilateral wrist extensor stretch	
5.7c Kneeling wrist extensor and ulna deviator stretch	
5.7d Kneeling wrist extensor and radial deviator stretch	

Related stretches			
3.8d & 3.8e Supine forearm stretches over a rolled up towel		5.2a & 5.2b Bilateral biceps stretch against a ledge	

5.8 Wrist flexor stretch - passive and post-isometric stretches for the flexor muscles of the wrist and hand

5.8a Kneeling unilateral wrist flexor stretch

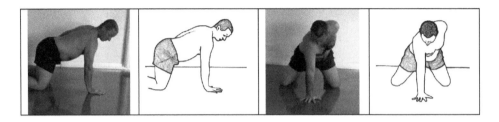

Starting position: Kneeling on the floor, preferably on a carpet or on a mat. Bend forwards at the hips, flex your right arm and forearm and place the palm of your right hand on the floor in front of you. Fully extend your right elbow, so that your arm is straight. Your arm should be vertical, your wrist below your shoulder and your knees and feet apart for balance. Your spine should be in a neutral position, neither flexed nor extended.

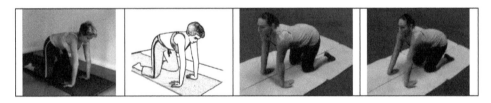

Technique: See Part A. Page 158.

5.8b Kneeling bilateral wrist flexor stretch

Starting position: Kneeling on the floor, preferably on a carpet or on a mat. Bend forwards at the hips, externally rotate your arms, and then place your palms on the floor with your fingers pointing backwards towards your knees. Extend your elbows so your arms are straight and vertical. For optimal balance place your hands directly in line with and below your shoulders, and have your knees and feet apart. Your spine should be in a neutral position, neither flexed nor extended.

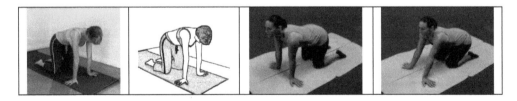

Technique: See Part A. Page 159.

5.8c Kneeling wrist flexor and radial deviator stretch

Starting position: Kneeling on the floor, preferably on a carpet or on a mat. Bend forwards at the hips, externally rotate your arms and place your palms on the floor with your fingers pointing outwards, laterally and away from your body. In other respects the starting position is the same as in technique 5.8b.

Technique: Technique: See Part A. Page 160. This is a localised stretch for flexor carpi radialis, combining wrist extension with ulna deviation and forearm supination.

5.8d Kneeling wrist flexor and ulna deviator stretch

Starting position: Kneeling on the floor, preferably on a carpet or on a mat. Bend forwards at the hips, internally rotate your arms and place your palms on the floor with your fingers pointing inwards, medially and towards each other. In all other respects the starting position is the same as in technique 5.8b.

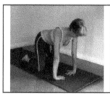
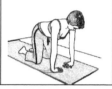
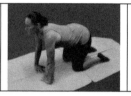
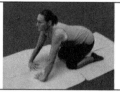

Technique: See Part A. Page 161. This is a localised stretch for flexor carpi ulnaris, combining wrist extension with radial deviation and forearm pronation.

5.8e Standing unilateral wrist flexor stretch

Starting position: Standing next to a table, with your feet apart. Place the palm of your right hand on the table in front of you. Place the palm of your left hand over the back of your right hand, perpendicular to it and covering the whole hand up to the wrist. Fully extend your elbows, so that your arms are straight. Flex your hips and knees, so that your spine remains straight.

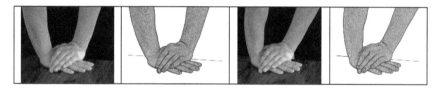

Technique: See Part A. Page 162.

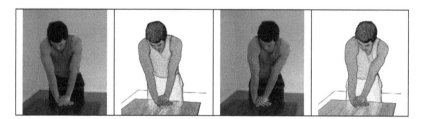

Direction and range of movement

There is between 75 and 85 degrees of extension at the wrist, about 35 degrees at the radiocarpal joint and 50 degrees at the midcarpal joint.

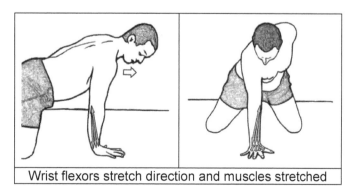
Wrist flexors stretch direction and muscles stretched

This technique involves full elbow extension and full wrist extension. Radial deviation and ulna deviation may be combined with wrist flexion.

441

Full elbow extension is a straight arm set at 0 degrees, but in hypermobile people the elbow may extend up to 15 degrees beyond neutral. Wrist extension occurs between the radius and the proximal row of carpal bones - the radiocarpal joint and between the proximal and the distal row of carpal bones - the midcarpal joint.

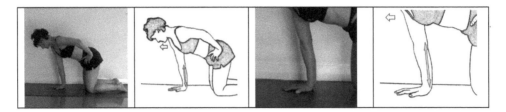

Target tissues

These are passive stretches primarily stretching the flexor muscles of the wrist and hand. They also stretch the finger flexor muscles, fascia in the anterior forearm and anterior ligaments in the wrist. The flexor muscles are part of the anterior compartment of the forearm, most arising from the medial epicondyle at the distal end of the humerus.

The muscles stretched the most are the wrist flexor muscles: flexor carpi ulnaris, flexor carpi radialis and palmaris longus.

Primary muscles stretched
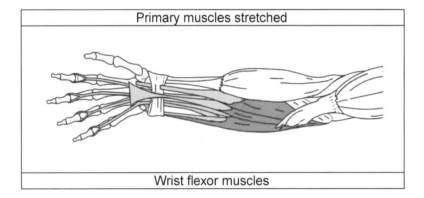
Wrist flexor muscles

The finger flexor muscles are also stretched: flexor digitorum profundus, flexor digitorum superficialis and flexor pollicis longus. This is also a stretch for pronator teres, biceps brachii, brachialis and brachioradialis.

The unilateral wrist flexor stretches 5.8a and 5.8e are general stretches for the wrist flexors: flexor carpi ulnaris, flexor carpi radialis and palmaris longus. The kneeling bilateral wrist flexor stretch 5.8b is also a good stretch for brachioradialis and the finger flexor muscles, as well as being a mild stretch for pronator teres, biceps brachii and brachialis.

Secondary muscles stretched	
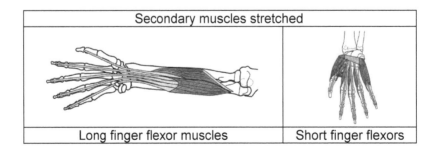	
Long finger flexor muscles	Short finger flexors

The kneeling wrist flexor and radial deviator stretch 5.8c is mainly for flexor carpi radialis. It may also stretch flexor digitorum profundus, flexor digitorum superficialis and palmaris longus. To a lesser extent in may stretch flexor carpi ulnaris and flexor pollicis longus.

The kneeling wrist flexor and ulnar deviator stretch 5.8d is mainly for flexor carpi ulnaris. It may also stretch flexor digitorum profundus, flexor digitorum superficialis and palmaris longus. To a lesser extent in may stretch flexor carpi radialis and flexor pollicis longus.

These can be done as passive or post-isometric stretches. If the fingers are extended there will be greater stretch on the finger extension muscles.

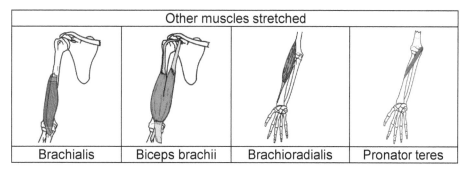

Other muscles stretched			
Brachialis	Biceps brachii	Brachioradialis	Pronator teres

Safety

If there is a pre-existing strain, osteoarthritis, rheumatoid arthritis or tendonitis of the wrist with pain and restriction, this technique may be contraindicated; professional advice should be sought before doing this stretch.

Key:

5.8a Kneeling unilateral wrist flexor stretch	
5.8b Kneeling bilateral wrist flexor stretch	
5.8c Kneeling wrist flexor and radial deviator stretch	
5.8d Kneeling wrist flexor and ulna deviator stretch	
5.8e Standing unilateral wrist flexor stretch	

Related stretches			
3.8a, b & c Supine stretches over a rolled up towel		4.7 Palms together behind back	

5.9 Finger flexor stretch - post-isometric and passive stretch for the forearm, wrist, hand and fingers

5.9 Standing finger flexor muscle stretch on a table

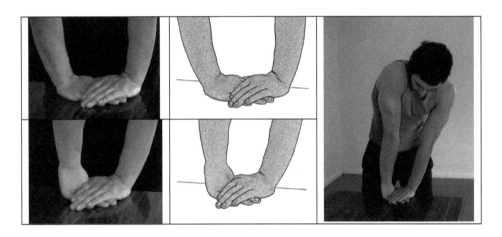

Starting position: Standing with the palm of your right hand on the top of a table. Place your left hand across the back of your right hand perpendicular to your hand and just distal to your metacarpophalangeal joints. Your shoulders sit directly above your wrists and your elbows are straight.

Sideshift your shoulders and upper spine to your left and allow your fingers to extend at the metacarpophalangeal joints. Stop when you feel the initial stages of a stretch in your fingers or forearm.

Technique: See Part A. Page 163.

Direction and range of movement

Movement is localised to the metacarpophalangeal joints or interphalangeal joint of the hand. The technique uses the contraction of shoulder and spinal muscles, to move the upper body to one side, and shift the weight of the body over the fingers.

Target tissue

This is a passive stretch for the finger flexor muscles in the anterior forearm and hand.

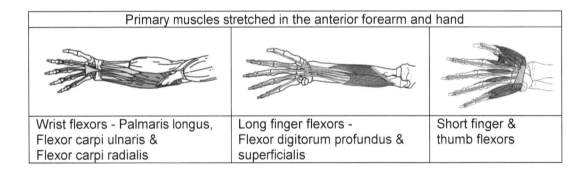

Primary muscles stretched in the anterior forearm and hand		
Wrist flexors - Palmaris longus, Flexor carpi ulnaris & Flexor carpi radialis	Long finger flexors - Flexor digitorum profundus & superficialis	Short finger & thumb flexors

The technique primarily stretches the extrinsic finger muscles in the forearm including flexor digitorum profundus and flexor digitorum superficialis, and the intrinsic finger muscles including flexor digiti minimi, opponens digiti minimi, lumbricales and the palmar and dorsal interossei.

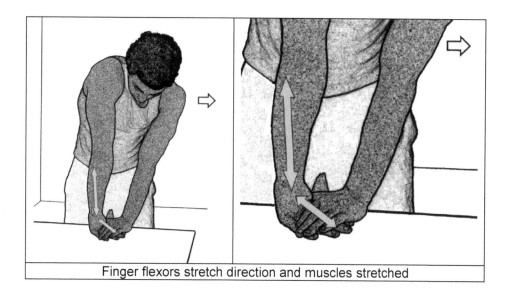

| Finger flexors stretch direction and muscles stretched |

Other muscles stretched include the forearm muscles flexing the wrist - flexor, flexor carpi ulnaris, palmaris longus and flexor carpi radialis longus and brevis. The palmar aponeurosis and fascia of the forearm are also stretched.

Safety

This is a safe stretch if done correctly. The technique uses leverage created by the length of the upper limb and relatively powerful shoulder muscles, plus the weight of the upper body, to extend the finger joints. As a consequence there is always the danger with this type of passive stretch of overstretching the finger joints. It is important therefore that you do not go beyond the anatomical limits of the joint, thereby straining the ligaments. Stretch the finger muscles but do not overwhelm the ligaments supporting the joints.

Key:

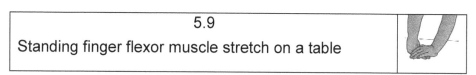

| 5.9 |
| Standing finger flexor muscle stretch on a table |

Related stretches			
3.8a, b, c & d Supine anterior forearm and hand stretches over a rolled up towel		5.8b Kneeling bilateral wrist flexor stretch	

For more detailed anatomy of the wrist and hand - radius, ulna, carpal, metacarpal & phalanges 5.7 – 5.9 see page 594.

6.0 Iliopsoas stretches - passive and post-isometric stretches for iliacus, psoas and other hip flexor muscles

6.0a The Lunge

Starting position: Kneeling on the floor with a chair at your left side to help maintain balance. Place a small pillow under your right knee. Flex your left hip and place the sole of your left foot on the floor about 50 cm in front of your body. Grasp the chair with your left hand. Take your left knee forwards and allow your body to descend. Reposition your left foot so your left thigh and leg form a right angle, and your knee is directly over your foot. Your spine should be straight and vertical.

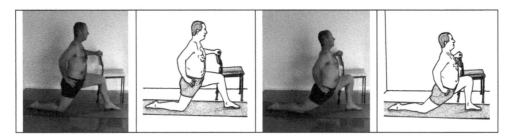

Technique: See Part A. Page 164.

6.0b The forwards splits

Starting position: Kneeling on the floor with a chair at your left side to help maintain balance. Place a small pillow under your right knee or use a mat. Flex your left hip and place the heel of your left foot on the mat about 1 m in front of your body, and your left knee on a foam roll. You will not need the roll or chair if you can do this stretch easily. Slide your left heel forwards to extend your right hip and extend your left knee. Allow your body to descend but stop as soon as you feel the initial stages of a stretch in front of your right hip or behind your left knee. Your spine should be straight and vertical.

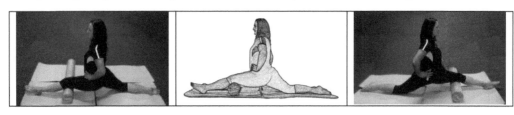

Technique: See Part A. Page 165.

6.0c The hanging hip stretch

Starting position: Laying on your back on a strong and stable table with the right side of your pelvis near to the edge of the table. Flex your left hip and knee, grasp your knee with both hands, pull it towards your body and hold your thigh against your chest. Lower your right leg over the side of the table.

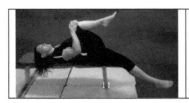
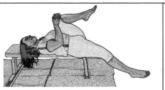
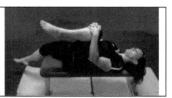

Technique: See Part A. Page 166.

446

Direction and Range of Movement

Technique 6.0a and 6.0b involve partial knee flexion on both sides, full hip extension on one side and full hip flexion on the other side. In technique 6.0b hip flexion and knee extension on one side will depend on the flexibility of the hamstrings, and hip extension and knee flexion on the other side will depend on the flexibility of the hip flexors and knee extensors.

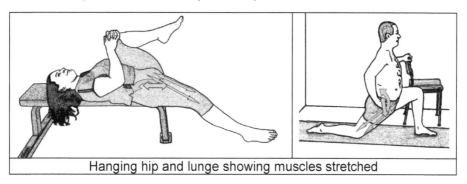

Hanging hip and lunge showing muscles stretched

Technique 6.0c involves partial knee flexion on one side and full knee flexion on the other side, and full hip flexion on one side and full hip extension on the other side. The amount of hip extension and knee flexion on the side being stretched will depend on the flexibility of the hip flexors and knee extensors.

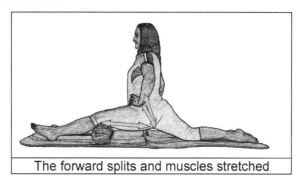

The forward splits and muscles stretched

Passive hip extension is 30 degrees and active hip extension is 20 degrees. Hip extension is reduced when the knee is flexed due to tension of rectus femoris.

Target tissues

This is primarily a stretch for the flexor muscles of the hips, the iliacus and psoas major. These techniques stretch rectus femoris, tensor fasciae latae and sartorius if they are short. Technique 6.0b also stretches the hamstrings.

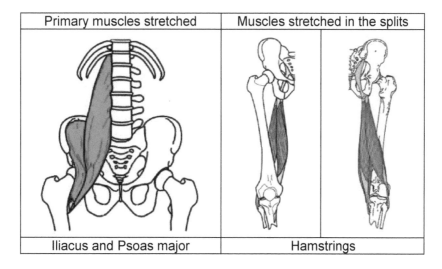

Primary muscles stretched	Muscles stretched in the splits
Iliacus and Psoas major	Hamstrings

447

Full hip flexion stretches adductor magnus, whereas full hip extension stretches adductor longus and brevis and gracilis.

Other muscles stretched			
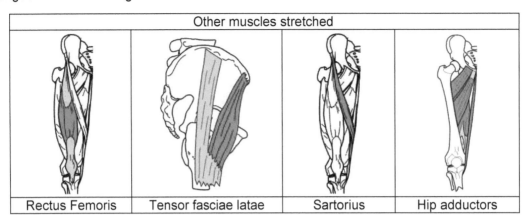			
Rectus Femoris	Tensor fasciae latae	Sartorius	Hip adductors

Safety

If there is a pre-existing groin strain, either in the inguinal ligament or one of the abdominal muscles, then there will be pain and restriction. If this is the case then these techniques may be contraindicated and professional advice should be sought before doing them.

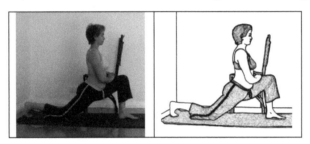

After muscle tightness has been excluded, hip extension is constrained by strong iliofemoral ligaments. Regular, intense stretching of these ligaments with the forward splits will produce greater flexibility, but that flexibility will be obtained at the expense of stability, the role of which will fall increasingly to muscles. Do not attempt the splits if there is a history of hip bursitis, tendinitis, osteoarthritis, sciatica ligament strain, inguinal hernia or muscle strain.

Key:

6.0a The lunge	
6.0b The forwards splits	
6.0c The hanging hip stretch	

Related stretches					
2.6a, b, c & d The Cobra stretches		2.7a, b & c The locust stretches		6.6a, b & c Standing quadriceps stretches	

6.1 Mixed Gluteus stretches - passive and post-isometric stretches for piriformis and gluteus minimus, medius and maximus in hip flexion and external rotation

6.1a & 6.1b Passive and post-isometric stretches for hip extensors and rotators

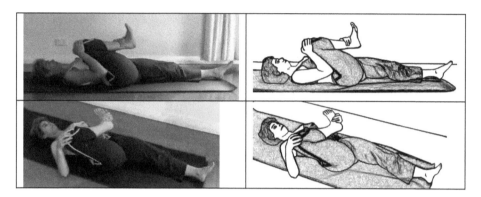

Starting position: Supine on a mat or carpet. Flex your right hip and knee. Grasp your right knee with your right hand and grasp your right foot with your left hand. Pull your right knee towards your right shoulder and flex your hip further. Pull your right foot towards your left shoulder to externally rotate your hip. Move your right knee across your chest and towards your left shoulder to adduct your hip but without losing the flexion and rotation.

Technique: See Part A. Pages 167 and 168.

Hip flexion and external rotation may be combined, and hip adduction and external rotation may be combined. Each variation will place a stretch on a different muscle or muscle group.

6.1c & 6.1d Passive and post-isometric cross leg stretches for hip extensors and rotators

Starting position: Supine on a mat or carpet with your hips and knees partially flexed. Fully flex your right hip, then externally rotate it and place your right foot on your left thigh just above your knee. Reach through the space between your thighs and right leg with your right hand, and grasp your left thigh and leg just below your knee. Reach around the outside of your left thigh with your left hand, and grasp your left thigh and leg just below your knee. Interlace the fingers of both hands around your left knee. Pull your left knee towards your chest. This flexes and externally rotates your right hip.

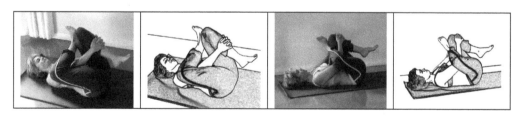

Technique: See Part A. Pages 169 and 170.

6.1e Passive and post-isometric stretch for hip extensors and rotators on a table

Starting position: Standing facing a table. Place the outside of your right foot and ankle on the table in front of your left hip. Your right hip is flexed, externally rotated and abducted. Flex your trunk by leaning forwards and taking your body weight over your right foot.

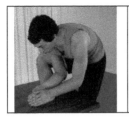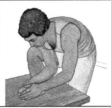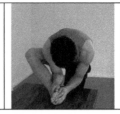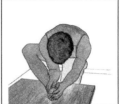

Technique: See Part A. Page 171.

6.1f Passive and post-isometric stretch for hip extensors, rotators and abductors on a table

Starting position: Standing facing a table. Place the outside of your right thigh, knee, leg and ankle on the table in front of you. Your right hip is flexed, externally rotated and adducted. Grasp your right knee with both hands. Straighten your body by extending your spine and by pushing your hands against your knee and extending your elbows. Rotate your spine and pelvis to the right.

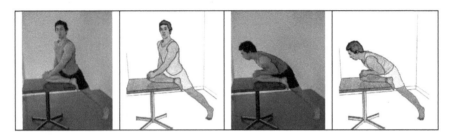

Technique: See Part A. Page 172.

6.1g Post-isometric stretch for gluteus minimus with your hips in flexion seated on a chair

Starting position: Sitting on a chair with your back straight, your feet apart and firmly planted on the floor. Flex your right hip and knee, and place the outside of your right ankle on your left thigh just above your knee. Allow your right knee to drop until you feel a mild stretch in your groin. Place your right hand on you right thigh just above your knee.

Technique: See Part A. Page 173.

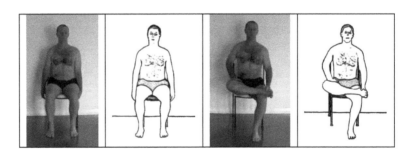

Direction and range of movement

These techniques mainly involve hip flexion, external rotation and abduction. Passive hip flexion with the knee flexed, as in these stretching techniques, is about 150 degrees. This can be 170 degrees or more in people with hypermobile hip joints.

Active hip external rotation is about 45 degrees. Active hip abduction is about 45 degrees. For passive external rotation or abduction add about 20 or 30 degrees more. When hip flexion, external rotation and abduction are combined there will be less range available for these movements individually.

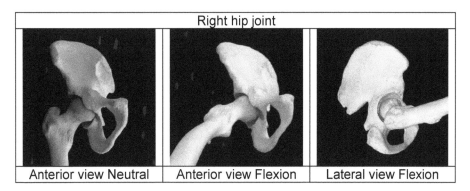

Right hip joint		
Anterior view Neutral	Anterior view Flexion	Lateral view Flexion

Target tissues

These techniques mainly stretch piriformis, gluteus minimus, the anterior fibres of gluteus medius and the upper fibres of gluteus maximus. Which muscles or muscle fibres are stretched and the extent of their stretch, depends on the amount and combination of hip flexion, external rotation and abduction/adduction used.

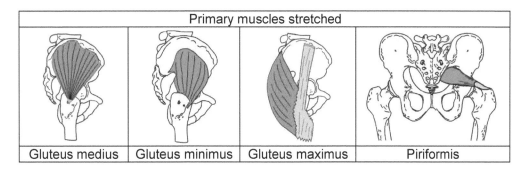

Primary muscles stretched			
Gluteus medius	Gluteus minimus	Gluteus maximus	Piriformis

The piriformis is an external rotator of the hip when the hip is in a neutral position. Above 60 degrees hip flexion the piriformis becomes an internal rotator and a horizontal abductor of the hip. In order to effectively stretch the piriformis the hip must be put into flexion, external rotation and adduction.

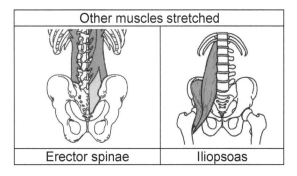

Other muscles stretched	
Erector spinae	Iliopsoas

The upper fibres of gluteus maximus, attaching on the ilium, are stretched the most in hip flexion and adduction, such as in technique 6.1a, b, c and f. The lower fibres of gluteus maximus, mainly attach on the sacrum, and are stretched the most in hip flexion and internal rotation. Most of the techniques in this chapter involve external rotation; which shortens the lower fibres of gluteus maximus, which results in a slightly reduced intensity in the stretch.

When the hip is in extension (i.e. the neutral standing position), gluteus minimus and most of the gluteus medius fibres are hip internal rotators and abductors, and so are stretched most when hip external rotation is combined with hip adduction. In both muscles, the anterior fibres are stretched most with external rotation, and the posterior fibres are stretched most with adduction.

In hyperextension the posterior fibres of gluteus medius become weak hip external rotators, and are therefore stretched with internal rotation. When the hip is in flexion, gluteus medius and gluteus minimus abduct the hip towards the coronal plane. Both muscles are important hip stabilisers.

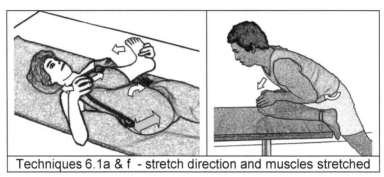

Techniques 6.1a & f - stretch direction and muscles stretched

Techniques 6.1a to 6.1f involve lumbar flexion and will stretch erector spinae. All the techniques involves hip flexion and external rotation and so will stretch the lower (condyloid) part of adductor magnus. Techniques 6.1a and 6.1b will also stretch a short iliopsoas, but on the opposite side to the primary hip muscles being stretched.

In the unilateral passive and post-isometric stretch 6.1a and 6.1b pure hip flexion stretches all fibres of gluteus maximus, but if hip flexion is combined with external rotation this reduces the stretch on the lower part of gluteus maximus; hip flexion combined with horizontal hip adduction stretches gluteus medius and piriformis and increases the stretch on the upper fibres of gluteus maximus; hip flexion combined with hip external rotation stretches gluteus minimus and the anterior fibres of gluteus medius.

Piriformis is a weak hip abductor and the best way to stretch piriformis is to keep hip abduction to a minimum. In techniques 6.1a, 6.1b, 6.1e and 6.1g you can control the amount of hip adduction and abduction. In 6.1a and 6.1b this is done by moving your leg across your body with both hands. In 6.1e this is done by positioning your foot as far across the table and to the side of your body as possible. In 6.1g this is done by resting your leg on your thigh so that your knee stays as close as possible to the midline of your body.

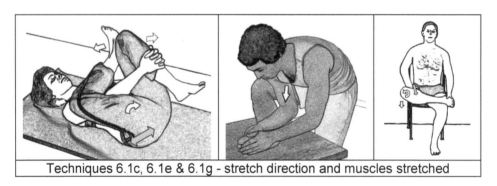

Techniques 6.1c, 6.1e & 6.1g - stretch direction and muscles stretched

In techniques 6.1c and 6.1d the hip is in flexion, external rotation and abduction. This is not a good stretch for piriformis because you cannot prevent your knee from dropping out to the side and further into abduction. It is however a good stretch for gluteus minimus, the anterior fibres of gluteus medius and gluteus maximus, especially the upper fibres. In techniques 6.1f the hip is in flexion, external rotation and adduction. This is a good stretch for piriformis, gluteus minimus, gluteus medius and gluteus maximus.

Safety

If there is a pre-existing problem in the knee then these stretches may be contraindicated. Collateral ligaments strains, tears in one of the menisci, joint hypermobility and/or osteoarthritis of the knee, are the most common pathologies which may be aggravated with this stretch.

452

In technique 6.1e avoid extreme flexion of the lumbar spine as this may strain the lumbar muscles or ligaments, or sacroiliac ligaments or overload the intervertebral discs. A major part of the flexion created in the stretch should be in the hip joint.

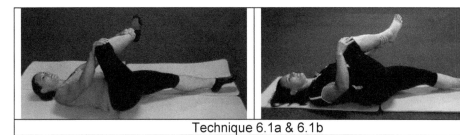

Technique 6.1a & 6.1b

Vulnerable areas

	Region	Level of Risk
1.	Knee	Low
2.	Lumbar or sacroiliac	Low

Key:

6.1a & 6.1b Passive and post-isometric stretches for hip extensors and rotators	
6.1c & 6.1d Passive and post-isometric cross leg stretch for hip extensors and rotators	
6.1e Passive and post-isometric stretch for hip extensors and rotators on a table	
6.1f Passive and post-isometric stretch for hip extensors, rotators and abductors on a table	
6.1g Post-isometric stretch for gluteus minimus with your hips in flexion seated on a chair	

Related stretches					
3.0a Passive back stretch - knees to chest supine		3.0e Unilateral stretch for the lumbar & gluteus maximus		6.3a, b & c Unilateral stretches for gluteus minimus	
6.5a, b & g Bilateral stretches for hip adductors & internal rotators					

6.2 Hip external rotator stretches - passive and post-isometric stretches for the hip external rotators and abductors

6.2a Hip external rotator stretch supine

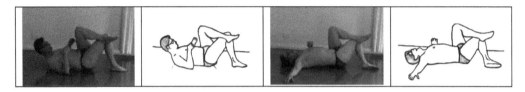

Starting position: Supine, hips and knees flexed, with feet planted on the floor slightly apart. Lift your left leg over the top of your right knee and hook it around your right thigh in a cross legged position. Pull your right knee to the left with your left leg and internally rotate and adduct your hip but stop when you feel the initial stages of hip tension. Keep your head, shoulders, arms, spine, pelvis and right foot on the floor.

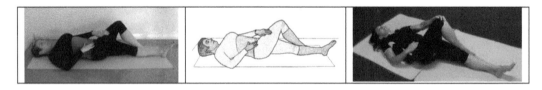

Technique: See Part A. Page 174. In this technique and the piriformis stretch following, the passive stretch involves hip horizontal adduction and internal rotation and the post-isometric component involves attempting hip horizontal abduction and externally rotation.

6.2b Piriformis stretch supine

Starting position: Supine with the right hip and knee flexed and the sole of your right foot placed on the floor on the outside of your left leg just below your knee. Place the fingers of your left hand on the lateral side of your right knee. Place the fingers of your right hand on the right anterior superior iliac spine. Push your right knee to the left with your left hand while holding your pelvis firmly down on the floor with your right hand.

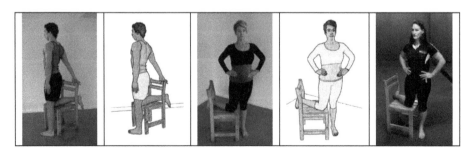

Technique: See Part A. Page 175.

6.2c Hip external rotator stretch standing using a chair

Starting position: Standing at the front of a chair. Face the right side of the chair with the outside of your right leg touching the front of the chair. Flex your right knee, internally rotate your right hip, and place your right knee and leg on the seat of chair with your foot overhanging the back of the chair. Your leg is on the seat and the inside of your right ankle rests against the inside of back of the chair on the left side.

Technique: See Part A. Page 176.

Direction and range of movement

These techniques all involve hip internal rotation. Techniques 6.2a and 6.2b also involve hip adduction and hip flexion whereas technique 6.2c is pure hip internal rotation and the stretch is done in a neutral hip position.

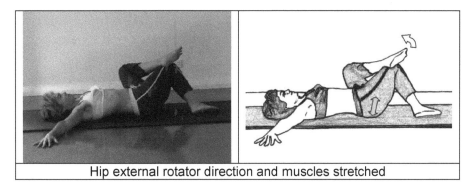

Hip external rotator direction and muscles stretched

Hip adduction without any movement of the pelvis is between 10 and 30 degrees. Hip adduction varies considerably and can be as high as 45 degrees in some individuals. Hip internal rotation when the hip is in flexion is about 35 degrees. When the hip is in neutral, internal rotation is about 35 degrees.

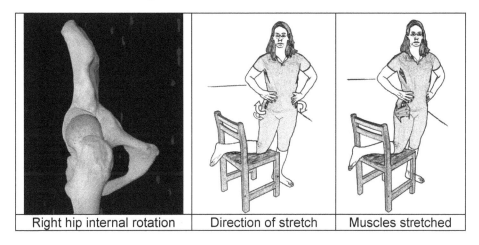

Right hip internal rotation	Direction of stretch	Muscles stretched

Target tissues

These are stretches for gamellus superior and inferior, obturator internus and externus, quadratus femoris, piriformis and the lower part of gluteus maximus. They may act as a weak stretch for the posterior fibres of gluteus medius.

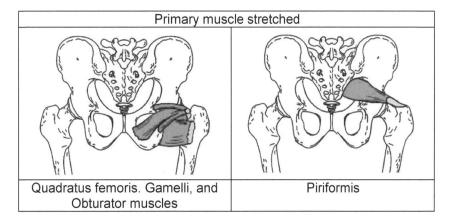

Primary muscle stretched	
Quadratus femoris. Gamelli, and Obturator muscles	Piriformis

In the neutral hip position, piriformis is a hip external rotator and is stretched with internal rotation. With increasing levels of hip flexion there is diminishing return using internal rotation to stretch piriformis and by 60 degrees hip flexion the stretch on piriformis using internal rotation is negligible.

In partial hip flexion, piriformis becomes a hip abductor and is stretched with adduction. In extreme hip flexion, piriformis becomes a weak hip internal rotator and is stretched with external rotation. Increased the stretch by combining the external rotation with adduction.

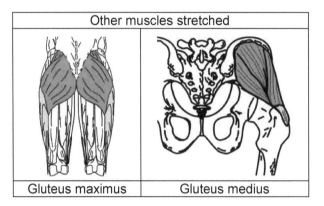

Other muscles stretched	
Gluteus maximus	Gluteus medius

In technique 6.2a the foot that is fixed on the floor can be positioned medially to make this more of an adduction stretch for piriformis or laterally to make this more of an internal rotation stretch for the hip external rotator muscles. With the hip in flexion, techniques 6.2b uses adduction to stretch piriformis. In techniques 6.2c the hip is in the neutral extended position and uses internal rotation to stretch both piriformis and the other hip external rotator muscles.

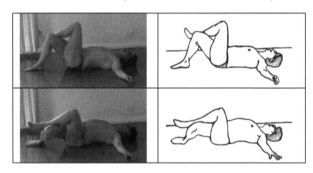

Key:

6.2a Hip external rotators stretch supine	
6.2b Piriformis stretch supine	
6.2c Hip external rotator stretch standing using a chair	

Related stretches					
3.1c Spinal twist sitting on the floor		6.4d Unilateral hip abductor stretch supine		7.4b Unilateral stretch for hip abductors and rotators and lumber	

6.3 Hip internal rotator stretch - active, passive and post-isometric stretches for gluteus minimus and anterior fibres of gluteus medius

6.3a Gluteus minimus stretch supine

Starting position: Supine on a mat or carpet. Flex your right hip and knee. Place the outside of your right foot on your left leg just above your ankle. Bring your right knee towards the mat and externally rotate your right hip.

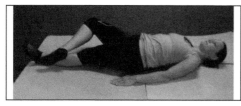
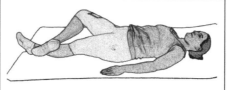

Technique: See Part A. Page 177.

6.3b Active and post-isometric stretches for gluteus minimus sidelying

Starting position: Sidelying on your left side on a mat or carpet. Flex your right hip and knee. Place your right foot in front of your left knee. Lift your right knee and point it towards the ceiling but keep the sole of you right foot firmly planted on the mat - externally rotate your right hip.

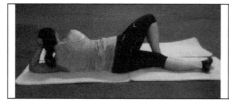
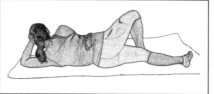

Technique: See Part A. Page 178.

6.3c Post-isometric stretch for gluteus minimus prone

Starting position: Prone on a mat or carpet. Flex your knee and abduct and externally rotate your right hip. Place the inside your right knee, leg and foot flat on the mat. Slide your right foot under your left leg at a point just above your ankle. The weight of your pelvis and right leg puts your hip into external rotation.

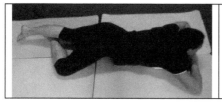
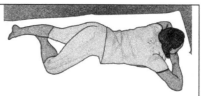

Technique: See Part A. Page 179.

6.3d Gluteus minimus stretch standing using a chair

Starting position: Standing on the right side of a chair, near its back leg. Face the rear of the chair, with your body parallel to the back of the chair and the outside of your right leg touching the side of the chair. Grasp the back of the chair and stand up straight. Flex your right knee and then flex and externally rotate your right hip. Place your right leg on the seat of chair so the inside of your knee is against the back of the chair, the outside of your ankle is against the front of your left leg and your leg is supported by the seat.

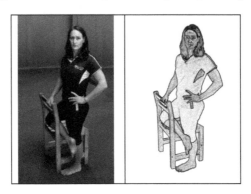

Technique: See Part A. Page 180.

Direction and range of movement

These techniques mainly involve hip external rotation. Hip flexion is unwanted and should be zero or kept to a minimum. It may be necessary to have hip abduction to complete the stretches or varying degrees hip abduction may be deliberately introduced. Hip external rotation in the neutral position (i.e. without other movements) about 45 degrees.

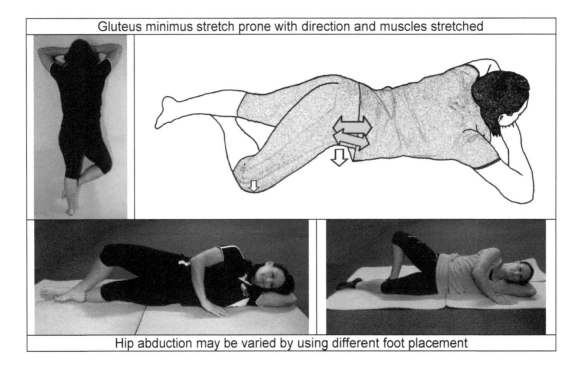

Gluteus minimus stretch prone with direction and muscles stretched

Hip abduction may be varied by using different foot placement

Technique 6.3a may be done as an active stretch by contracting the hip external rotator muscles and the rotator fibres of gluteus maximus, or as a passive stretch using the weight of the thigh and leg, or as a post-isometric stretch by resisting the upward movement of the knee with one hand. Technique 6.3b may be done as an active or post-isometric stretch.

Technique 6.3c may be done as an active stretch by contracting the hip external rotator muscles and gluteus maximus or as a passive stretch using the weight of the pelvis or as a post-isometric stretch by pushing the knee into the floor. Technique 6.3d may be done as a passive stretch by moving the groin forward and using leverage of the thigh and leg or as a post-isometric stretch by pushing the knee against the back of the chair.

458

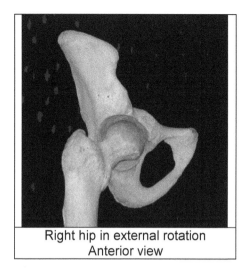

Right hip in external rotation
Anterior view

Target tissues

These are localised stretches for gluteus minimus and the anterior fibres of gluteus medius and involve full external rotation of the hip. They may be a weak stretch for tensor fasciae latae. By increasing the amount of hip abduction more stretch is placed on gluteus minimus relative to gluteus medius and tensor fasciae latae. In technique 6.3c and 6.3d there may be a moderate stretch in the hip adductor muscles. Also technique 6.3d may stretch the hip joint capsule and tensor fasciae latae in the opposite hip.

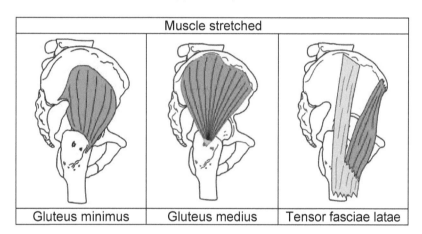

Muscle stretched		
Gluteus minimus	Gluteus medius	Tensor fasciae latae

The active stretches involve the contraction of gluteus maximus and the hip external rotator muscles. Of the post-isometric stretches, 6.3a involves the contraction of the abdominal muscles to flex the torso, and 6.3a, and 6.3b involve the unilateral contraction of pectoralis major, latissimus dorsi, triceps brachii and shoulder stabiliser muscles to resist the isometric contraction.

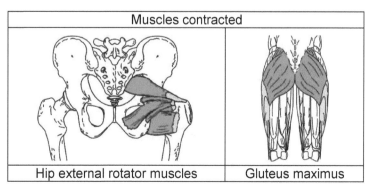

Muscles contracted	
Hip external rotator muscles	Gluteus maximus

Techniques 6.3c involve the unilateral contraction of quadriceps femoris and iliopsoas to resist the isometric contraction of gluteus minimus and medius in the opposite hip. In addition to the isometric contraction of gluteus minimus and medius there is the contraction of the adductors and tensor fascia latae.

Safety

These are relatively safe techniques provided there is no joint hypermobility or degeneration in the hip or knee.

Vulnerable areas

	Region	Level of Risk
1.	Knee	Low

Key:

6.3a Unilateral gluteus minimus stretch supine	
6.3b Unilateral active and post-isometric stretches for gluteus minimus sidelying	
6.3c Unilateral post isometric stretch for gluteus minimus prone	
6.3d Unilateral gluteus minimus stretch standing using a chair	

Related stretches					
6.1e Unilateral stretch for hip extensors and rotators		6.1g Unilateral gluteus minimus stretch seated		6.5a Bilateral stretch for hip adductors & rotators sitting	
6.5g Bilateral stretch hip adductors & rotators on wall		6.5j Bilateral stretch for hip adductors and rotators supine		7.0a, b & c Forward bends sitting	

6.4 Hip abductor stretches - passive and post-isometric stretches for tensor fasciae latae, gluteus medius, minimus and the upper fibres of gluteus maximus

6.4a Passive stretch for tensor fasciae latae standing

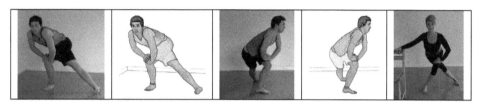

Starting position: Standing with your feet apart. Flex your hips and knees about 45 degrees. Extend and adduct your right hip, and move your right leg behind your left leg and to your left. Flex your left knee to about 90 degrees and grasp it with both hands. Grasp a chair or use your knee to support your upper body. Adjust the position of your right foot for optimum balance. Most of your body weight should be over your left knee and foot.

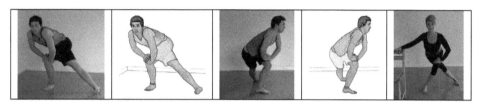

Technique: See Part A. Page 181.

6.4b Passive stretch for gluteus maximus and medius kneeling

Starting position: Kneeling on a small pillow or mat beside a chair or stool. Flex your left hip and place the outside of your left foot on the floor in front of you and to your right. Place your right hand on the chair for support. Slide your left foot diagonally forwards and away from your body, and as you do so extend your right hip by moving your pelvis forwards. Slide your left foot as far as possible to your right, and as you do so, sideshift your pelvis to the right, and adduct your right hip.

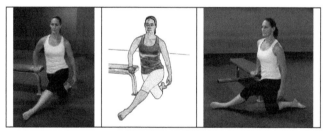

Technique: See Part A. Page 182.

6.4c Passive stretch for tensor fasciae latae standing

Starting position: Standing with your feet together and the right side of your body, arm length away from a wall or post. Abduct your right arm until it is level with your shoulder and place the palm of your hand on the wall. Extend your right hip and then adduct your hip and place your right foot on the floor behind and to the side of your left foot. Place your left hand on the left side of your pelvis. Sideshift your pelvis to the right and towards the wall. Make sure both your knees and your spine is straight.

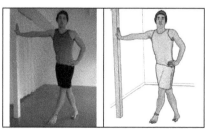

Technique: See Part A. Page 183.

6.4d Passive or post-isometric hip abductor stretch supine

Starting position: Supine on a mat. Flex your left hip and knee and lift your left foot off the ground. Adduct your right leg to the left until you feel the initial stages of resistance from the muscles and fascia of the lateral thigh, then place it on the mat. Place your left foot down on the mat against the outside of your right knee to pin down the right leg in adduction. Flex your right hip and knee, until the top of your right thigh presses against the bottom of the calf muscle of your left leg.

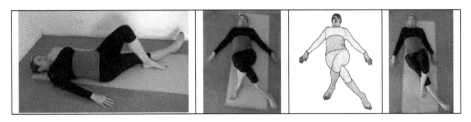

Technique: See Part A. Page 184.

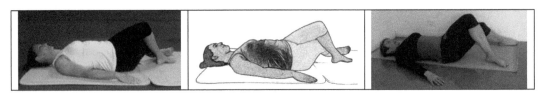

6.4e Passive stretch for quadratus lumborum, tensor fasciae latae and gluteus maximus sidelying on a table

Starting position: Sidelying on your left side, diagonally across a table or couch with a small pillow for your head. Flex your left hip and knee to 90 degrees.
Extend your right hip and drop your right lower limb over the side of the table and lower it towards the floor. Rest the inside of your right knee on the edge of the table or if the table is too hard, on a small pillow on the table on the soft part of your left foot.

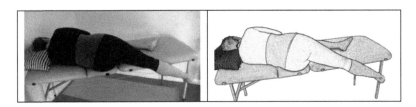

Technique: See Part A. Page 185.

6.4f Post-isometric stretch for quadratus lumborum, tensor fasciae latae and gluteus maximus sidelying on a table

Starting position: Sidelying on your left side on a table or couch with a small pillow for your head. Then follow the instructions for the sidelying stretch 6.4e. Hook your right foot under the table or hook your right knee under your left foot.

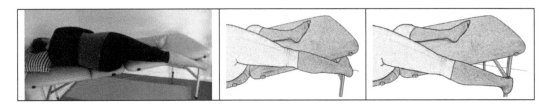

Technique: See Part A. Page 186.

6.4g Passive and post-isometric stretch for tensor fasciae latae and gluteus maximus sidelying with the knee straight

Starting position: Sidelying on your right side with your legs straight and arms in front. Place your palms flat on the floor shoulder width apart. Push your hands into the floor and raise your upper body off the floor. Your shoulders are horizontal and level. Your head, cervical and upper thoracic spine are vertical. Most of the sidebending is in your hips but with some in the lumbar spine.

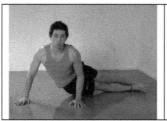 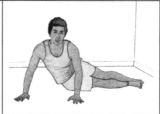

Technique: See Part A. Page 187.

6.4h Passive and post-isometric stretch for gluteus medius and gluteus minimus sidelying with the knee bent

Starting position: Sidelying on your right side with your legs flexed and arms in front. Place your palms flat on the floor, shoulder width apart. Push your hands into the floor and raise your upper body off the floor. Your shoulders are horizontal and level. Your head, cervical and upper thoracic spine are vertical. Most of the sidebending is in your hips but with some in the lumbar spine.

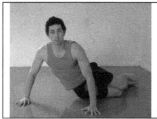 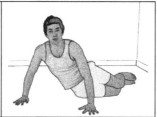

Technique: See Part A.Page 188.

Direction and range of movement

All these techniques involve hip adduction with either knee flexion or knee extension. In addition technique 6.4a also involves hip flexion and a small amount of lumbar flexion, technique 6.4d involves a small amount of hip flexion and techniques 6.4e, 6.4f, 6.4g and 6.4h involve a small amount of lumbar sidebending.

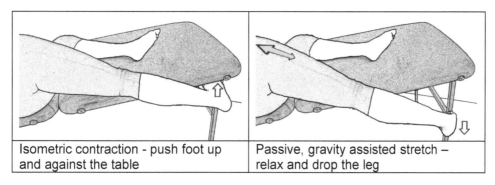

| Isometric contraction - push foot up and against the table | Passive, gravity assisted stretch – relax and drop the leg |

Technique 6.4b can be modified by introducing hip internal or external rotation or different amounts of hip extension with the adduction. Tensor fasciae latae and the most anterior fibres

of gluteus minimus and medius are best stretched with the hip adducted, extended and externally rotated.

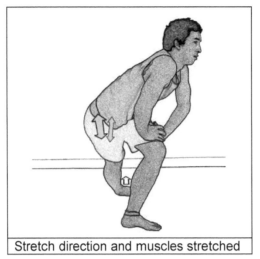

Stretch direction and muscles stretched

In technique 6.4b secondary stretches may be got in muscles of the lower limb on the opposite side to the primary one being stretched. If the hip is flexed and abducted so the foot is inverted, then lateral leg muscles, peroneus longus and brevis can be stretched; and if the hip is extended and adducted, then lateral thigh muscles can be stretched. Care should be taken not to strain the knee. This is primarily a stretch for the other hip.

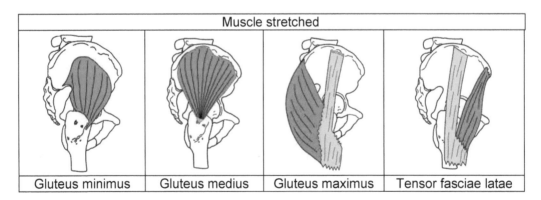

Stretch direction and muscles stretched

Target tissues

These are primarily stretches for tensor fasciae latae, gluteus medius, the posterior fibres of gluteus minimus and the upper fibres of gluteus maximus.

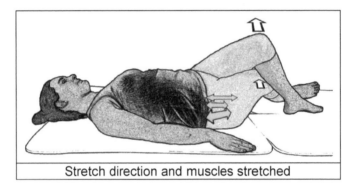

Muscle stretched			
Gluteus minimus	Gluteus medius	Gluteus maximus	Tensor fasciae latae

Hip adduction stretches all these muscles. Between full knee extension and 30 degrees flexion the iliotibial band is taught and it is a stretch for tensor fasciae latae and the upper fibres of gluteus maximus. With knee flexion greater than 30 degree iliotibial band tension

464

decreases and it is a stretch for gluteus medius and minimus. Stretches 6.4d, 6.4e, 6.4f, 6.4g and 6.4h are also stretches for quadratus lumborum and the abdominal oblique muscles.

In techniques 6.4d, 6.4e and 6.4f when the arm on the side being stretched is fully abducted this stretches latissimus dorsi and increases tension on the lumbodorsal fascia, which fixes the pelvis, reduces lumbar sidebending and increases the stretch in the hip. When the arm remains at the side of the body there is no stretch on latissimus dorsi, which reduced tension on the lumbodorsal fascia and allows for a greater stretch on quadratus lumborum.

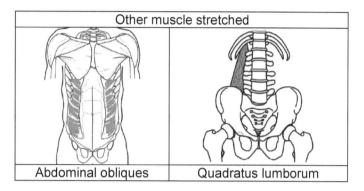

Other muscle stretched	
Abdominal obliques	Quadratus lumborum

In technique 6.4e, if you turn your leg so your toes point towards the floor you internally rotate your hip joint, and this focuses the stretch on the upper fibres of gluteus maximus and the posterior fibres of gluteus medius. If you turn your leg so your toes point towards the ceiling you externally rotate your hip joint and this focuses the stretch on tensor fasciae latae and the anterior fibres of gluteus minimus.

Safety

These are relatively safe techniques. However with extreme hip adduction there is concern that some of the force may be carried through to the lower lumbar spine and sacroiliac joints.

Techniques 6.4a, 6.4e, 6.4f, 6.4g and 6.4h are most problematic with respect to the lower back; care should be taken not to place strain on lumbar ligaments and intervertebral discs. An option for technique 6.4e is to abduct your right arm and grasp the end of the table with your right hand, to stretch latissimus dorsi and use the lumbodorsal fascia to stabilise the pelvis.

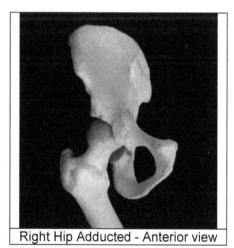

Right Hip Adducted - Anterior view

Care should be taken in technique 6.4a not to put excessive load on the flexed weight-bearing knee, and especially avoid twisting forces which can damage menisci (cartilages) and strain ligaments. If there is potential weakness, instability or hypermobility in the knee or a history of knee pathology or injury then do not do this technique or approach it cautiously using a chair or table for support. Similarly in technique 6.4b avoid putting excessive load on the knee and straining the lateral collateral ligament or meniscus.

465

Key:

6.4a Unilateral passive stretch for tensor fasciae latae standing	
6.4b Unilateral passive stretch for gluteus maximus and medius kneeling	
6.4c Unilateral passive stretch for tensor fasciae latae standing	
6.4d Unilateral passive or post-isometric hip abductor stretch	
6.4e Unilateral passive stretch for quadratus lumborum, tensor fasciae latae and gluteus maximus sidelying on a table	
6.4f Unilateral post-isometric stretch for quadratus lumborum, tensor fasciae latae & gluteus maximus sidelying on a table	
6.4g Unilateral passive and post-isometric stretch for tensor fasciae latae & gluteus maximus sidelying with knee straight	
6.4h Unilateral passive and post-isometric stretch for gluteus medius and gluteus minimus sidelying with the knee bent	

Related stretches					
2.0a Standing lumbar and hip sidebending stretch		2.1a, b & c Wall lumbar & hip sidebend stretches		2.4a & 2.4d Hanging sidebending stretches	
3.9a Supine hip and spine stretch over a rolled towel		6.2a & 6.2b Unilateral stretches for hip rotators		7.4b Unilateral stretch for hip abductors rotators	

6.5 Passive, active and post-isometric stretches for the hip adductors

6.5a & 6.5b Bilateral passive and post-isometric stretches for the hip adductors and internal rotators sitting

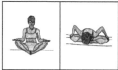

Starting position: Sitting on the floor with your pelvis and back against a wall. Flex your hips and knees, and bring your heels to your groins. Allow your knees to drop towards the floor and bring the soles of your feet together. Place your hands on your thighs just above your knees and gently press down.

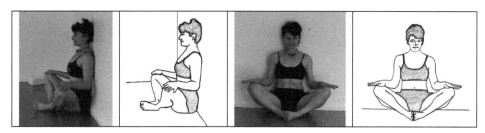

Technique: See Part A. Pages 189.

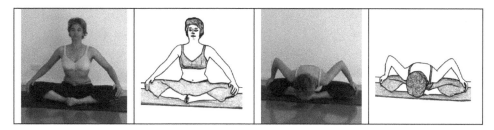

Technique: See Part A. Page 190.

6.5c & 6.5d Bilateral active, passive and post-isometric stretch for the hip adductors and extensors sitting

Starting position: Sitting on the floor with your pelvis and back against a wall. Push your ischial tuberosities back into the corner of the room. Grasp your knees and move your legs apart, but stop when you feel a stretch down the inside of one or both of your thighs. Keep your legs an equal distance apart and your pelvis in contact with the wall. Lean forwards and walk your fingers across the floor until you feel a stretch in your groins and inside thighs. Depending on your flexibility grasp the inside of your knees, legs, or toes. Flex at the hips and tilt your pelvis forwards. Stretch while maintaining a firm hold with both hands.

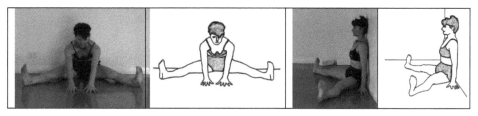

Technique: See Part A. Technique 6.5c on page 191 and 6.5d on page 192.

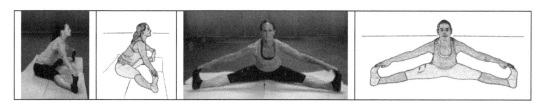

6.5e, 6.5f & 6.5g Bilateral active and passive stretch facilitated by gravity for the hip adductors, supine and with legs against a wall

Starting position: Sitting on the floor facing a wall. Move your body so the bottom of your pelvis is in contact with the wall. Lean backwards and lay your upper body on the floor. Straighten your knees and place the back of your legs against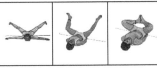
the wall. Move your legs apart but stop when you feel the initial stages of a stretch down the inside of one or both of your thighs or groins. Your legs are an equal distance apart.

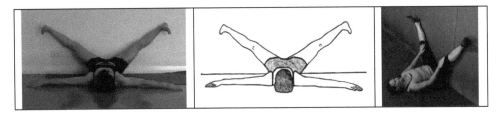

Technique: See Part A. Pages 193, 194 and 195.

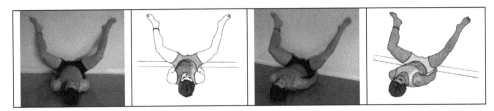

In technique 6.5f flex your hips and knees so only your heels are in contact with the wall, which become a pivot for hip movement. In technique 6.5g flex your knees and bring your heels towards your groins.

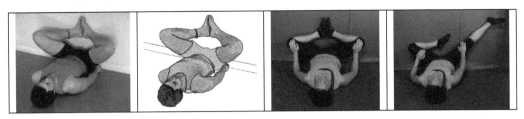

6.5h Bilateral stretch for the hip adductors standing

Starting position: Standing with your feet wide apart facing a chair. Bend forwards and place the palms of your hands on a chair. If you have good flexibility and can keep your knees and spine straight, place your hands on the floor. Feel the initial stages of a stretch down the inside your thighs.

Technique: See Part A. Page 196.

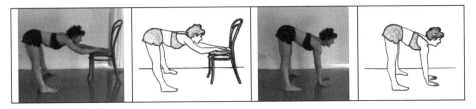

6.5i Unilateral passive stretch for the hip adductors standing

Starting position: Standing with your feet wide apart. Flex your left hip and knee but keep your right leg straight. Bend forwards and place the palms of your hands on the floor, or if you are unable to reach the floor then grasp the edge of a table.

468

Continue flexing your left hip and knee until you feel the initial stages of a stretch in your groin or down the inside your right thigh.

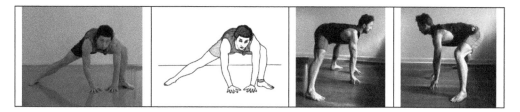

Technique: See Part A. Page 197.

6.5j Bilateral stretch for the hip adductors and internal rotators supine

Starting position: Supine on a mat on the floor. Flex your hips and knees so your feet are on the floor near your groins. Drop your knees out to the side and bring the soles of your feet together. Feel the initial stages of a stretch down the inside of your thighs. Use pillows under your thighs if your hips are stiff or for your head.

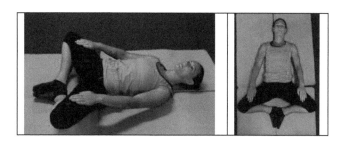

Technique: See Part A. Page 198.

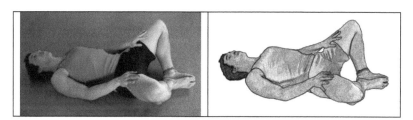

6.5k Bilateral stretch for the hip adductors kneeling and with knees flexed and hips externally rotated

Starting position: Kneeling on a mat on the floor with your hands palms down on the floor in front of you about shoulder distance apart. Two mats may be used under your knees, which slide across the floor during the stretch. Move your knees apart and then move your feet apart. Your spine should be straight.

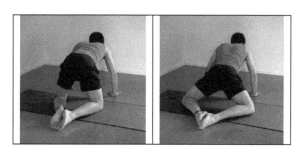

Technique: See Part A. Page 199.

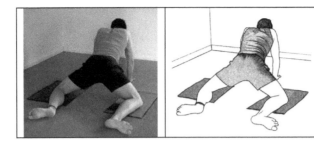

6.5l Bilateral stretch for the hip adductors kneeling with the hips extended and knees flexed

Starting position: Kneeling on a mat on the floor and grasp the back of a chair. Two mats may be used under your knees, which slide across the floor during the stretch. Move your knees apart and then move your feet apart. Your toes are pointing backwards and your spine should be straight, vertical and in a neutral position.

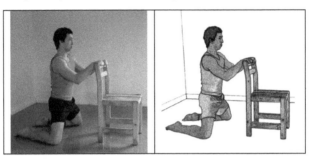

Technique: See Part A. Page 200.

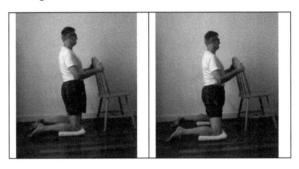

6.5m Bilateral stretch for the hip adductors standing with hips and knees extended

Starting position: Standing with your feet wide apart and grasp the back of a chair. Your arms are extended at your sides and your elbows are partly flexed. Move your feet further apart but keep your toes pointing forward. If your feet do not slide on the floor easily then wear a pair of socks. Your spine should be straight, vertical and in a neutral position.

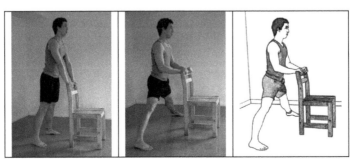

Technique: See Part A. Page 201.

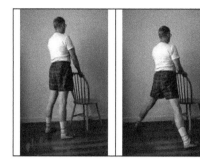

6.5n Unilateral stretch for the hip adductors sidelying with your back against a wall, and your hips and knees extended

Starting position: Sidelying on your left side with your back against a wall. Flex your left hip and knee, and find a comfortable stable position. Flex your left elbow and shoulder, and support your head with your hand. Flex your right elbow and shoulder, and place your palm flat on the floor. Lift your right leg as high up the wall as possible and fix it on the wall.

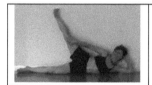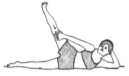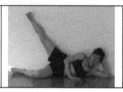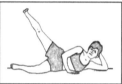

Technique: See Part A. Page 202.

Direction and range of movement

These techniques are primarily for increasing hip abduction, hence stretching the hip adductor muscles. Hip abduction may be combined with hip external rotation, and hip abduction may be done either in hip extension or hip flexion.
Ideally the techniques should be done with the lumbar spine in neutral or a small amount of extension. But posture and flexibility vary and some people may have to do this stretch in a slightly flexed position. But the stretch direction should always be towards extension.

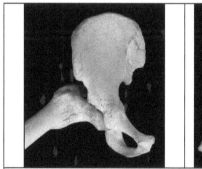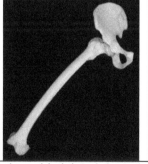

Right ilium and femur - anterior view - hip joint abducted

Active hip abduction is about 45 degrees, active hip external rotation is about 45 degrees and active hip flexion with the knee flexed is about 125 degrees.

Target tissues

These techniques mainly stretch the hip adductors including adductor magnus, adductor longus, adductor brevis and gracilis. Some techniques also stretch hip internal rotator muscles such as gluteus minimus and the anterior fibres of gluteus medius, hip flexors such as pectineus, and hip extensor muscles such as the hamstrings and the lower part of gluteus maximus.

The starting position of each stretch and the direction of movement determine which muscles are stretched the most, as well as the combination of muscles stretched.

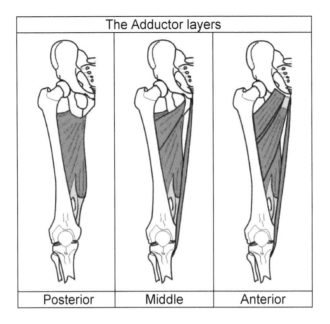

Hip abduction is a constant movement present in all the techniques. Hip external rotation is present in many of the techniques, but in varying amounts. Hip flexion is present in techniques 6.5a to 6.5k, which is about 80% of the techniques. Hip extension is present in the last three techniques 6.5l, 6.5m and 6.5n, which is about 20% of the techniques.

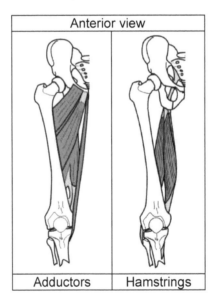

Hip abduction combined with hip flexion increases the stretch on adductor magnus, especially the part attached to the ischial tuberosity, and reduces the stretch on the other hip adductor muscles. In contrast, hip abduction combined with hip extension increases the stretch on adductor longus, adductor brevis, gracilis and pectineus and reduces the stretch on adductor magnus.

When hip abduction with flexion or extension is combined with knee flexion, the knee flexion reduces the stretch on the hamstrings and gracilis, allowing an increased stretch on other

472

muscles. Techniques 6.5a, 6.5b, 6.5f, 6.5g, 6.5j and 6.5k, and 6.5i on one side, involve knee flexion and hip flexion. Only techniques 6.5l is in knee flexion and hip extension.

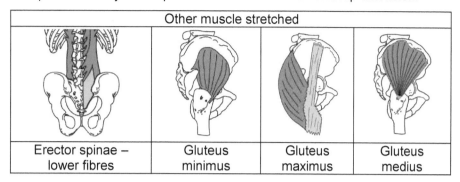

Other muscle stretched			
Erector spinae – lower fibres	Gluteus minimus	Gluteus maximus	Gluteus medius

Hip abduction combined with knee extension increase the stretch on gracilis Techniques 6.5c, 6.5d, 6.5e, 6.5h, 6.5m, 6.5n and 6.5i on one side, are in knee extension. Technique 6.5m and n are in knee extension and hip extension and stretch gracilis most. Hip abduction combined with knee extension and hip flexion also stretch the hamstrings. Techniques 6.5c, 6.5d, 6.5e, 6.5h and 6.5i on one side, are in knee extension and hip flexion.

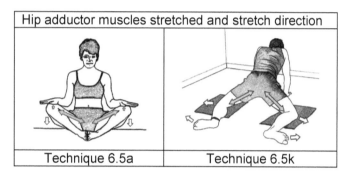

Hip adductor muscles stretched and stretch direction	
Technique 6.5a	Technique 6.5k

Hip abduction combined with hip external rotation increases the stretch on the condyloid portion of adductor magnus, especially if the hip is also in flexion. Techniques 6.5a, 6.5b, 6.5c, 6.5d, 6.5e, 6.5f, 6.5g, 6.5j and 6.5k are in hip external rotation and hip flexion.
If hip abduction is kept to a minimum, and hip external rotation is emphasised, some of these techniques may also stretch some of the fibres of gluteus minimus and medius - especially 6.5b, 6.5f, 6.5g and 6.5j.

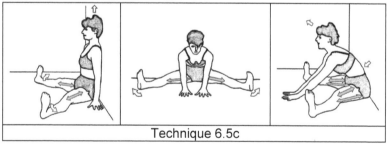

Technique 6.5c		

Hip abduction combined with hip internal rotation and hip flexion may stretch some of the fibres of gluteus maximus and some of the external rotator muscles. Techniques 6.5k can be done in hip flexion and internal rotation.

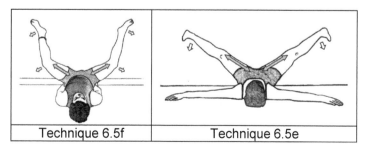

Technique 6.5f	Technique 6.5e

473

Techniques 6.5b, 6.5c, 6.5d, 6.5h and 6.5i involve some lumbar and thoracolumbar flexion and stretch the lumbar extensors, especially erector spinae.

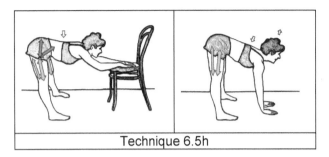

Technique 6.5h

Safety

With time and effort the good levels of adductor flexibility can be achieved by people with low flexibility. An optimum level of adductor flexibility should be the goal of a good exercise program.

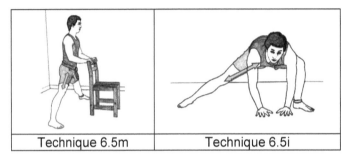

| Technique 6.5m | Technique 6.5i |

The adductor muscle stretches, as described, are safer when done slowly and with controlled breathing. Techniques 6.5a, 6.5b, 6.5f, 6.5g and 6.5j, if forced can overstretch the lateral collateral ligament supporting the knee joints. If too much flexion and force is used in techniques 6.5b, 6.5c, 6.5d and 6.5h this can overstretch ligaments supporting the sacroiliac and lumbar spine.

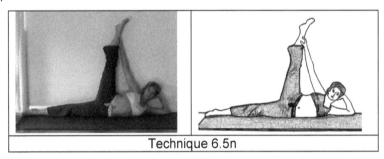

Technique 6.5n

Individuals with congenital hypermobility may have exceedingly high levels of hip flexibility and will be able to do these technique with ease. High levels of adductor flexibility may be useful for dancers or gymnasts, but under most circumstances extreme adductor flexibility is unnecessary and may cause problems such as hip joint instability or hypomobility in other areas. Hypermobile people should do isometric strengthening exercises, such as the isokinetic techniques using a rubber band to increase tone in the adductors.

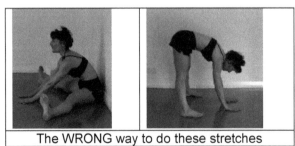

The WRONG way to do these stretches

474

If this is your first time attempting these stretches support the body using strong, stable and appropriately placed furniture. Furniture can be especially useful if you are wearing socks to slide into positions of increased hip abduction. If you are wearing socks take care to select a floor that offers some friction resistance to movement and is not too slippery.

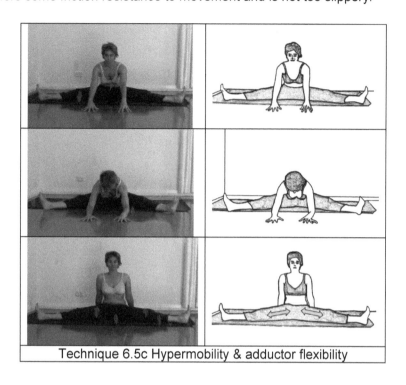

Technique 6.5c Hypermobility & adductor flexibility

Key:

6.5a Bilateral stretch for the hip adductors and internal rotators sitting	
6.5b Bilateral active stretch for the hip adductors, extensors and internal rotators sitting	
6.5c Bilateral passive stretch for the hip adductors and extensors sitting	
6.5d Bilateral post-isometric stretch for the hip adductors and extensors sitting	
6.5e Bilateral stretch for the hip adductors supine and with legs against a wall	
6.5f Bilateral stretch for the hip adductors and internal rotators supine and with knees flexed and heels against a wall	

6.5g Bilateral stretch for the hip adductors and internal rotators supine and with knees flexed and feet against a wall	
6.5h Bilateral stretch for the hip adductors standing	
6.5i Unilateral stretch for the hip adductors standing	
6.5j Bilateral stretch for the hip adductors and internal rotators supine	
6.5k Bilateral stretch for the hip adductors kneeling with knees flexed and hips externally rotated	
6.5l Bilateral stretch for the hip adductors kneeling with hips extended and knees flexed	
6.5m Bilateral stretch for the hip adductors standing and with hips and knees extended	
6.5n Unilateral stretch for the hip adductors sidelying with your back against a wall, and your hips and knees extended	

Related stretches					
6.1e Unilateral stretch for hip over a table		6.1g Unilateral gluteus minimus stretch seated		6.3a, b & c Unilateral gluteus minimus stretches	
7.0abc Forward bend sitting					

6.6 Quadriceps stretch - active and passive stretches for the quadriceps, tibialis anterior and the toe extensor muscles

6.6a Quadriceps stretch standing

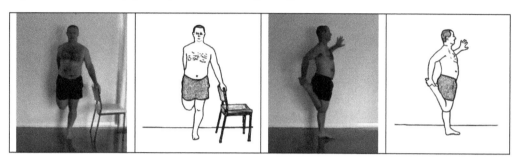

Starting position: Standing beside a chair or wall and grasp the back of the chair with your left hand. Flex your right hip and knee, and grasp the front of your right ankle with your right hand. Extend your right hip but keep your right knee in full flexion. Hold your foot and keep your spine and left leg straight and vertical.

Technique: See Part A. Page 203.

6.6b & 6.6c Passive and post-isometric knee, ankle and toe stretch standing

Starting position: Adopt the same standing position as in 6.6a except grasp the front of your right foot and toes with your right hand.

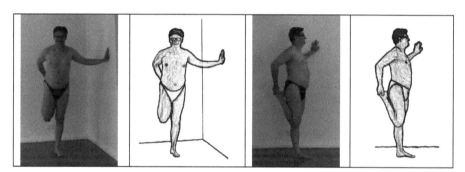

Technique: See Part A. Page 204 and 205.

Quadriceps stretch semi-supine 6.6d

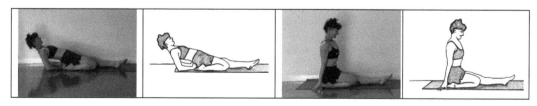

Starting position: Sitting on a mat with your legs straight and in front of you. Flex your right hip and knee. Grasp your right ankle with your right hand, lean to the left and take your foot under your thigh, and place it to the side of your right hip and pelvis. You are now in a half kneeling position. Extend your shoulders and flex your elbows. Lean backwards and support your upper body on your bent elbows. Your right knee is in full flexion and your right foot is beside your right hip. Keep your spine and left leg straight.

Technique: See Part A. Page 206.

6.6e Passive and post-isometric quadriceps stretch prone

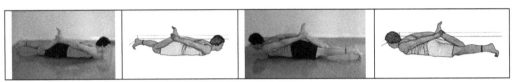

Starting position: Prone on a mat with your legs straight. Flex your right knee and bring your foot towards your buttocks. Lean backwards and grasp your right foot behind your right ankle with your right hand or both hands. Pull your right foot nearer to your buttocks. Your right knee is in full flexion and your left knee is in extension.

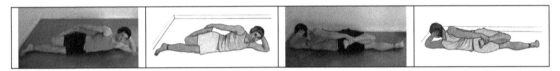

Technique: See Part A. Page 207.

6.6f Quadriceps stretch sidelying

Starting position: Sidelying on your left side on a mat on the floor. Flex your right hip and knee, and grasp your right ankle or foot with your right hand. Extend your right hip but keep your knee flexed. Flex your left shoulder and elbow, and rest the left side of your head in the palm of your left hand. Straighten your spine and left leg. Pull your right foot towards your body and into your right buttock.

Technique: See Part A. Page 208.

Direction and range of movement

In hip flexion the knee joint has a passive range of movement of about 160 degrees and an active range of movement of about 150 degrees. In hip extension or hyperextension rectus femoris tension reduces the range of movement.

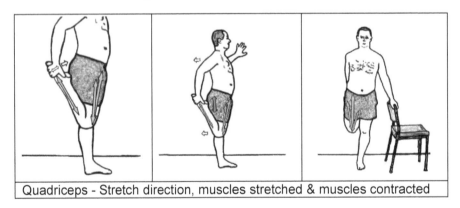

Quadriceps - Stretch direction, muscles stretched & muscles contracted

Foot mobility varies a lot between individuals and depends on the shape of the bones and the level of ligament laxity. Plantarflexion is between 30 and 50 degrees, and dorsiflexion is between 20 and 30 degrees. Most dorsiflexion and plantarflexion movement is at the ankle joint, and some is in the tarsal joints. Dorsiflexion is greater by about 10 degrees when the knee is flexed due to tension of gastrocnemius.

Target tissues

These are primarily techniques for stretching the quadriceps group of muscles, rectus femoris, vastus intermedius, vastus lateralis and vastus medius. All of these muscles extend the knee and pass over the knee joint via the patella, but only rectus femoris passes over both the hip and knee joint. Consequentially it is the only quadriceps muscle stretched by hip extension. Compared with iliopsoas, rectus femoris is a relatively weak hip flexor, accounting for about 1/3 of the flexion force.

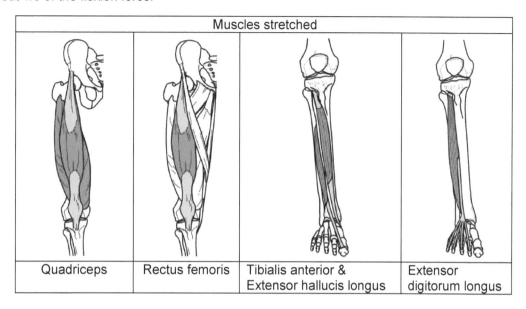

Muscles stretched			
Quadriceps	Rectus femoris	Tibialis anterior & Extensor hallucis longus	Extensor digitorum longus

This is also a stretch for the muscles of anterior compartment of the leg, tibialis anterior, extensor digitorum longus and extensor hallucis longus.

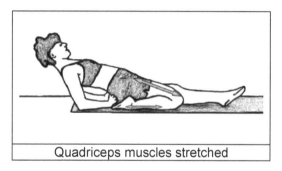

Quadriceps muscles stretched

Safety

Care should be taken not to overextend the spine by arching your back. It is most vulnerable in the thoracolumbar, lumbosacral or sacroiliac regions and injury is most likely to occur if there is limited hip, knee or ankle flexibility. Care should be taken if there are osteoarthritic changes in any of these areas or in the spine.

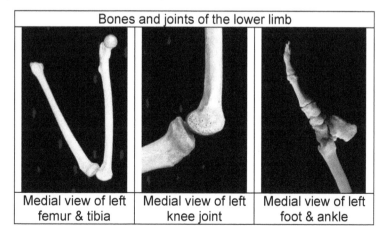

Bones and joints of the lower limb		
Medial view of left femur & tibia	Medial view of left knee joint	Medial view of left foot & ankle

The semi-supine quadriceps stretch 6.6d is the technique most likely to cause spinal hyperextension because of the weight of the pelvis and having less control over the pelvis in this position. A short psoas can pull the lumbar spine into extension, and a short iliacus can tilt the pelvis anteriorly. If this is the case then it is would be wise to stretch iliopsoas for several weeks prior to attempting the quadriceps stretches and especially techniques 6.6d. Unless they are lengthened sufficiently, the quadriceps stretches can put intervertebral discs, lumbar and sacroiliac ligaments and vulnerable tissues in the knees under dangerous stress.

This stretch should not be attempted if there is knee damage such as a meniscus tear or thinning, ligament strain or any osteoarthritis in the knee. As is true for all standing stretches, avoid the poor head forward posture when doing the standing quadriceps stretch (see Chin tuck 1.3). Keep the spine straight and the head in line with the centre of gravity.

Vulnerable areas

	Region	Level of Risk
1.	Knee	Medium
2.	Thoracolumbar spine	Low
3.	Lumbosacral spine	Low
4.	Sacroiliac joint	Low

Key:

6.6a Standing quadriceps stretch	
6.6b Standing passive knee, ankle & toe stretch	
6.6c Standing post-isometric knee, ankle and toes stretch	
6.6d Supine quadriceps stretch	
6.6e Prone passive and post-isometric quadriceps stretch	
6.6f Sidelying quadriceps stretch	

Related stretches					
1.1a Lion stretch kneeling		2.2b Thoracic and rib sidebending stretch kneeling		3.0a, b & e Knees to chest stretch supine	
4.9b & 4.9c Scapula retractor stretch squatting					

480

6.7 Hamstring stretches – active, passive and post-isometric stretches for semitendinosus, semimembranosus and biceps femoris

6.7a Active and passive stretch for the hamstrings standing

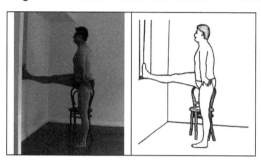

Starting position: Standing facing a table or window ledge. Flex your right hip and knee and place the heel of your right foot on the table or ledge. Extend your right knee until your leg is straight. Hold the back of a chair for support or hold your hips if you have good balance. The height of the table should be sufficient to challenge the hamstrings.

Technique: See Part A. Page 209.

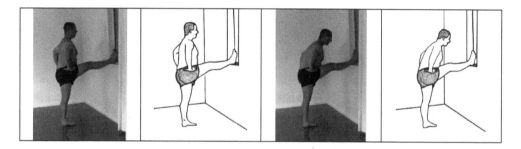

6.7b Combined active and passive stretch for the hamstrings standing

Starting position: See previous technique 6.7a. Reach forwards and grasp a suitable point down your right leg with your right hand. Grasp your knee or ankle if you have below average hamstring flexibility, or grasp your foot and toes if you have above average hamstring flexibility. Keep your right arm in a fixed position. Depending on your flexibility it can either be straight or flexed at the elbow. Keep your spine and both legs straight throughout the stretch.

Technique: See Part A. Page 210.

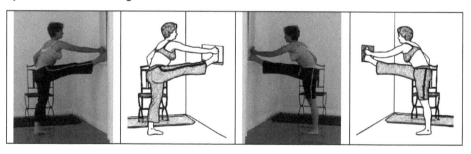

The passive stretch involves the contraction of elbow flexors, shoulder extensors and scapula retractors, to pull the trunk forwards, and the active stretch involves the hip flexors tilting the pelvis forward at the hip joint. The diagonal hold is a greater challenge than the same side hold because there is a greater distance to reach.

Different starting positions can be used to target individual muscles of the lower limb. Rotation of the hip inwards increase the stretch on the lateral hamstring muscle, biceps femoris; rotation of the hip outwards stretches the medial hamstring muscle, semitendinosus; pointing the heel away stretches the gastrocnemius; rotation of the pelvis outwards combined with turning the weight bearing foot outwards increases the stretch on adductor magnus.

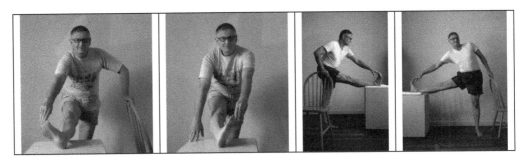

6.7c & 6.7d Passive and post-isometric stretch for the hamstrings supine

Starting position: Supine on a carpet or mat. Flex your hips and knees, and place your feet on the mat. Flex your right hip more, lift your right foot off the mat and move it towards your head. Flex your head and upper spine, and grasp your right foot behind your ankle with both hands. If you cannot reach your foot, flex your left hip and knee more. Pull your right foot up and over your head until you feel tension.

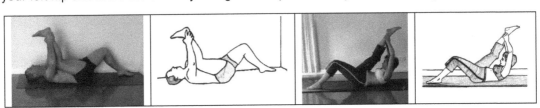

Technique: See Part A. Page 211 and 212.

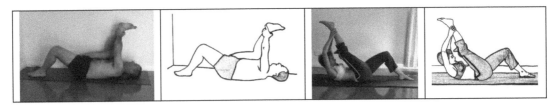

6.7e Active and post-isometric stretch for the hamstrings supine with your leg vertical and against a post or wall

Starting position: Supine on a carpet or mat. Position the inside your left thigh beside a vertical post or the outside corner of a wall. Flex your right hip and place the back of your heel against the post. Your left hip is extended. Straighten your left leg and feel the initial stages of tension in the back of your right thigh or behind your right knee.

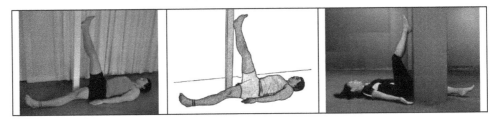

Technique: See Part A. Page 213.

6.7f Passive and post-isometric stretch for the hamstrings standing with hips flexed

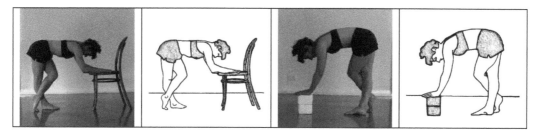

Starting position: Standing with your feet apart and facing a chair, blocks or the empty floor. Use a chair if your hamstrings are short, blocks if they are moderately flexible or the floor if they are very flexible. As your flexibility increases progress from fingertips to palms, and from a chair to two blocks, to one block and finally to the floor.

Bend forwards at the hips and place your hands on a chair, blocks or floor.
Flex your left hip and knee, then adduct your hip, then extend it and place the toes and balls of your left foot on the floor outside and just behind your right foot. Your left thigh and leg, wrap around your right thigh and leg.

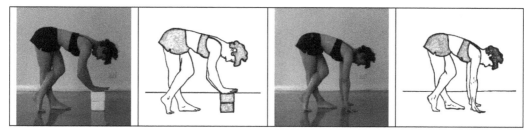

Move your left foot backwards, sliding your toes along the floor until your left calf presses against the front of your right leg. Flex your elbows and lower your body towards the floor - bend at the hips. Stop when you feel the start of a stretch behind your thigh and knee.

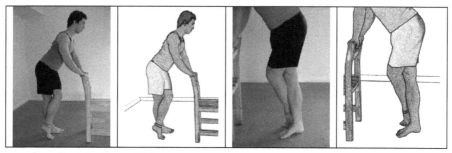

Technique: See Part A. Page 214.

6.7g Active and passive stretch for the short head of biceps femoris standing with legs vertical

Starting position: Adopt the starting position in technique 6.7f. In this technique there is no need to bend forwards at the hips because hip flexion does not influence the short head of biceps femoris which only passes over the knee joint. So a chair is only used for support.

Internally rotate your right hip and place your right foot on the floor turned inwards about 45 degrees. Push your left knee backwards against your right leg, and extend your right knee by contracting the quadriceps in your left thigh. Keep most of your weight on the right leg but do not let your left foot slide on the floor.

Technique: See Part A. Page 215.

Direction and range of movement

These techniques are primarily for increasing hip flexion and knee extension, and stretching the hamstring muscles. Hip flexion and knee extension may be combined with other movements to localise the stretch on individual hamstring muscles or to include other lower limb muscles in the stretch (see 6.7b).

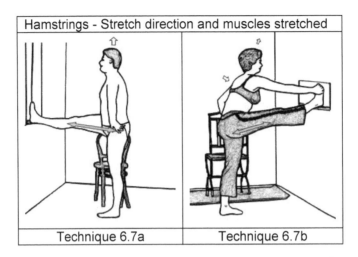

Hamstrings - Stretch direction and muscles stretched	
Technique 6.7a	Technique 6.7b

When the hip is flexed and knee extended, these movements will target: Biceps femoris (long head) if the hip is internally rotated; Semitendinosus if the hip is externally rotated; Gastrocnemius if the foot is dorsiflexed; Adductor magnus if the hip is abducted horizontally.

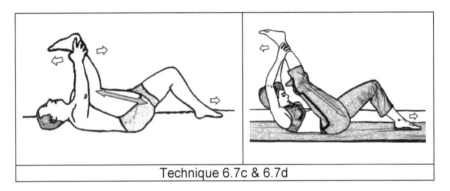

Technique 6.7c & 6.7d

All the techniques involve some hip flexion. Hip flexion stretches all the hamstrings except the short head of biceps femoris, covered in technique 6.7g. Hip flexion is combined with full knee extension in techniques 6.7a, 6.7b, 6.7e, 6.7f and 6.7g. Hip flexion is combined with partial knee flexion in techniques 6.7c and 6.7d. Full knee flexion shortens the hamstrings and prevents hamstring stretch, even in full hip flexion.

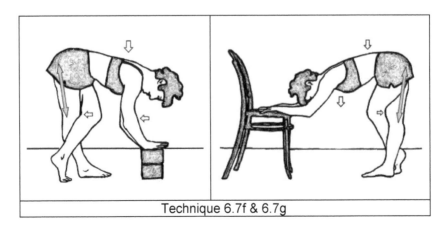

Technique 6.7f & 6.7g

Partial hip flexion combined with full knee extension, focuses the stretch on the lower part of the hamstrings just above the knee. Partial hip flexion combined with partial knee extension is a better stretch for the hamstrings because it focuses the stretch on the middle part of the hamstrings, thus stretching more of the muscle fibres. It uses both the knee and the hip as levers to localise the stretch in the belly of the muscles.

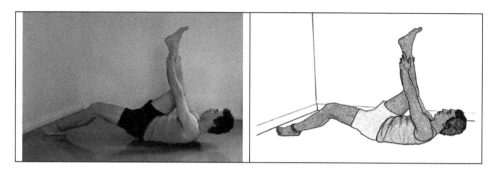

The partial knee extension stretch is an excellent technique when done with a partner, but it is hard for an individual to pull against the hamstrings in this position. This technique cannot generate as great a force as the other hamstrings stretches which use levers and body weight. It works if you have good upper limb strength, can be used to develop upper limb strength, and is a useful stretch for iliopsoas and other hip flexors of the opposite lower limb.

Target tissues

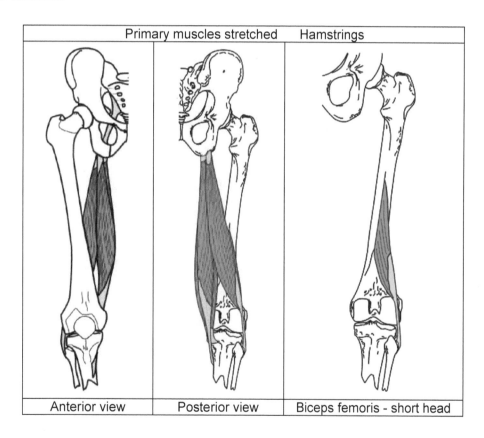

Primary muscles stretched		Hamstrings
Anterior view	Posterior view	Biceps femoris - short head

These are stretches for the hamstrings: semimembranosus, semitendinosus and the long head and the short head of biceps femoris. To a lesser extent this is also a stretch for adductor magnus, especially when the hip is abducted. With the foot is dorsiflexed this is also a stretch for gastrocnemius.

Secondary muscles stretched	
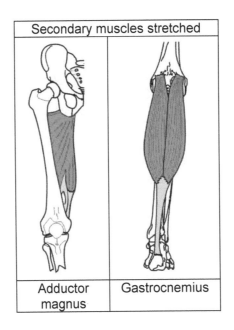	
Adductor magnus	Gastrocnemius

Safety

The techniques should be done with the spine in neutral or slight extension. Avoid excessive spinal flexion, which can place dangerous loads on intervertebral discs, and posterior spinal muscles and ligaments. Lumbar supraspinous and erector spinae muscles and sacroiliac ligaments are most vulnerable to strain.

If there is a pre-existing intervertebral disc problem in the lumbar spine, then technique 6.7a, 6.7b and 6.7f may be contraindicated. Very tight hamstrings can result in significant spinal flexion if care is not taken to maintain a straight spine during these stretches.

Pelvis, femur & proximal tibia & fibula		
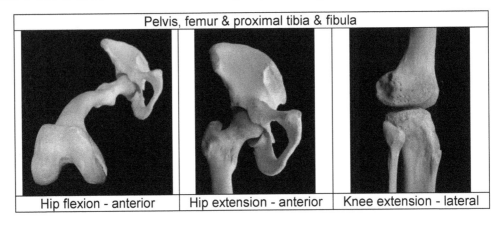		
Hip flexion - anterior	Hip extension - anterior	Knee extension - lateral

People with congenital hypermobility may have genu recurvatum, a deformity where the knee joint bends backwards beyond the straight position. Knee hyperextension is more common in women and may be between 5 and 20 degrees. It may also be caused by trauma resulting in cruciate ligament laxity. If genu recurvatum is present then technique 6.7a, 6.7b, 6.7e, 6.7f and 6.7g may be contraindicated and strengthening exercise may be more appropriate.

Vulnerable areas

	Region	Level of Risk
1.	Lumbar	Medium
2.	Knee	Low

Key:

6.7a Unilateral active and passive stretch for the hamstrings standing with one leg horizontal	
6.7b Unilateral combination active and passive stretch for the hamstrings standing with one leg horizontal	
6.7c Unilateral passive stretch for the hamstrings supine	
6.7d Unilateral post-isometric stretch for the hamstrings supine	
6.7e Unilateral active and post-isometric stretch for the hamstrings supine with your leg vertical and against a post or wall	
6.7f Unilateral passive stretch for the hamstrings standing with legs vertical	
6.7g Unilateral active and passive stretch for the short head of biceps femoris standing with legs vertical	

Related stretches					
6.0b Forwards splits		6.5c & 6.5d Bilateral stretches for hip adductors		6.5e Bilateral stretch for the hip adductors against a wall	
6.5h Bilateral stretch for the hip adductors standing		6.5n Unilateral stretch for the hip adductors sidelying		6.9a, b & c Stretches for hamstrings and calf	
7.0a, b, c & d Seated forward bend for the hips		7.4 Unilateral straight leg stretch for the hamstrings			

6.8 Popliteus stretch - active, passive, and post-isometric stretches for popliteus

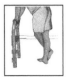

6.8a & 6.8b Active, passive and post-isometric stretches for popliteus standing with legs vertical

Starting position: Standing with your feet apart facing the back of a chair. Externally rotate your right hip and place your right foot on the floor pointing outwards about 45 degrees.

Grasp the back of the chair. Wrap your left leg around your right leg, and place the toes and balls of your left foot on the floor on the outside of your right foot. Press the back of your left leg against the front of your right leg. Extend both knees but stop when your feel the initial stages of a stretch behind your right knee.

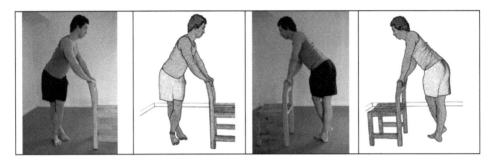

Technique: See Part A. Pages 216 and 217.

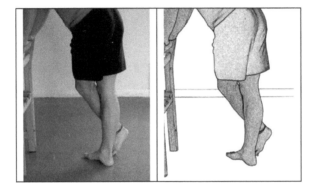

Direction and range of movement

This technique is for increasing knee extension and external rotation of the leg (as opposed to the hip and thigh). It is an active stretch combined with a passive stretch.

The active stretch involves the quadriceps muscles of the target leg, contracting and extending that knee. The passive stretch is caused by the contraction of the quadriceps muscles of the other thigh, further extending the knee being stretched by pushing back against the target knee.

488

Target tissues

These are active, passive and post isometric stretches for popliteus.

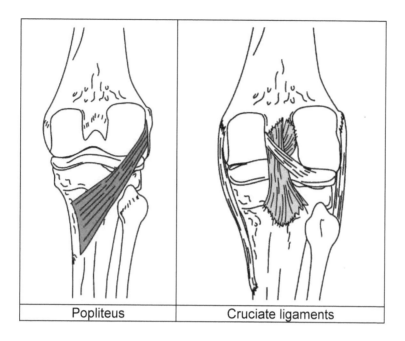

| Popliteus | Cruciate ligaments |

Safety

Genu recurvatum, a deformity where the knee joint extends beyond the straight position, may exist in people with congenital hypermobility or may be the result of trauma to cruciate ligaments. It is more common in women and may be between 5 and 20 degrees. If genu recurvatum is present then this technique should be modified to avoid increasing knee hyperextension, or it may be contraindicated and strengthening exercise adopted instead.

Vulnerable areas

	Region	Level of Risk
1.	Knee	Low

Key:

6.8a & 6.8b	
Unilateral active, passive and post-isometric stretch for popliteus standing with legs vertical	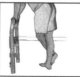

Related stretches	
6.7g stretch for short head of biceps femoris	

6.9 The Dog - active, passive and post-isometric stretches for the hamstrings, gastrocnemius and posterior fascia

6.9a Unilateral Lower Dog - an active and passive stretch

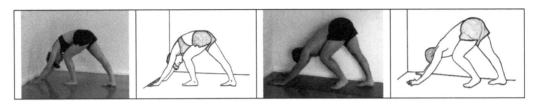

Starting position: Standing. Flex your hips and knees, and place your hands, palms down on the floor, shoulder width apart, with the ends of your fingers touching a wall. Extend your right hip, take your right foot backwards and place the sole of your foot on the floor. Extend your right knee. Your left hip, knee and ankle are flexed and relaxed, and your left foot is just in front of and to the side of your right foot. Your arms and spine are straight and in line. Adjust your stance for optimum balance.

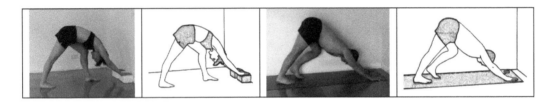

Technique: See Part A. Page 218.

6.9b Unilateral Lower Dog - a post-isometric stretch for the posterior thigh and leg

Starting position: Adopt the same starting position as in technique 6.9a
If the stretch is too difficult then it may be done with your palms on a block.

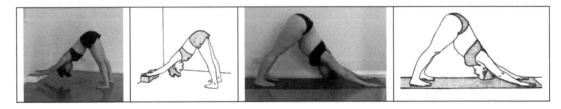

Technique: See Part A. Page 219.

6.9c Bilateral active, passive and post-isometric stretch for the hamstrings and gastrocnemius

Starting position: Only do the bilateral stretch when you can do the unilateral technique comfortably. Start using blocks and then discard them when you become more flexible. Stand on a mat or floor with your feet apart.
Flex your hips and knees and place your hands, palms down on the floor or two blocks in front of you about shoulder width apart. Walk your feet away from the blocks. Extend your knees until your legs are straight and keep your arms and spine straight.

Technique: See Part A. Page 220.

Direction and range of movement

This technique involves a combination of primary movements: hip flexion, knee extension and ankle dorsiflexion. In addition there are secondary movements which use levers to increase the stretch. These are shoulder flexion, elbow extension, and thoracic and lumbar extension.

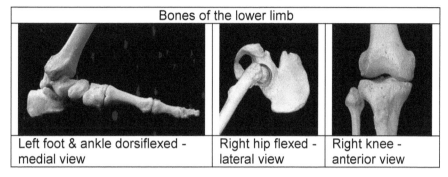

Bones of the lower limb		
Left foot & ankle dorsiflexed - medial view	Right hip flexed - lateral view	Right knee - anterior view

Target tissues

This is mainly a stretch for the hamstrings and gastrocnemius. It is also a stretch for popliteus, soleus and the posterior fascia of the thigh, leg and knee. The stretch targets popliteus and the medial head of gastrocnemius if the feet are externally rotated and targets the short head of biceps femoris and the lateral head of gastrocnemius if they are internally rotated.

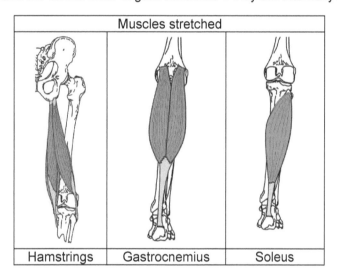

Muscles stretched		
Hamstrings	Gastrocnemius	Soleus

The angle between the trunk and the lower limb or limbs being stretched influences which muscles are stretched most. Hamstring stretch is greatest at about 45 degree and calf muscle stretch is greatest at 90 degrees hip flexion.

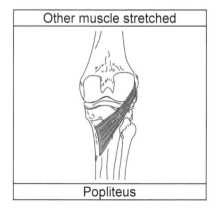

Other muscle stretched
Popliteus

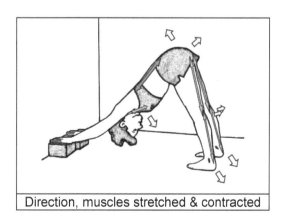

Direction, muscles stretched & contracted

The active stretch involves the contraction of tibialis anterior to dorsiflex the foot, quadriceps muscles to extend the knee, and iliopsoas and the hip flexor muscles to flex the hip.
The passive stretch involves the contraction of shoulder muscles, to produce full flexion at the glenohumeral joint, and retraction, upward rotation and backward tilting of the scapula at the scapulothoracic joint. Also, contraction of posterior spinal muscles, mainly erector spinae to extend the spine. Through a combination of shoulder and spinal levers, hip flexion is increased and the hamstrings are stretched.

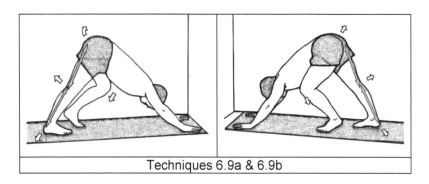

Techniques 6.9a & 6.9b

In yoga, the dog pose combines upper limb, lower limb and spinal stretching. This is an option. But a more localised stretch means your attention can be better focused, which is safer. For details on how to stretch the upper limb, and which muscles are contracted and stretched see technique 2.5, Upper dog - active extension stretches for the shoulders, thoracic and lumbar spine.

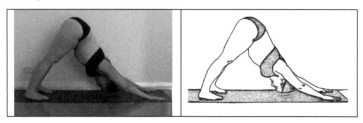

This post-isometric stretch part of this stretch, involves the contraction of gastrocnemius and soleus to plantar flex the foot, gluteus maximus to extend the hip, the hamstrings to flex the knee, and the pectoralis major and the abdominal muscles to flex the trunk.

Key:

6.9a Unilateral Lower Dog - an active and passive stretch	
6.9b Unilateral post-isometric stretch for the posterior thigh and leg	
6.9c The Dog – a bilateral active, passive and post-isometric stretch for the hamstrings and gastrocnemius	

Related stretches			
6.7f Unilateral stretch for the hamstrings standing with legs vertical		7.1a, b & c Stretches for gastrocnemius	

7.0 Forward bends - active, passive and post isometric stretches for the hamstrings, hip adductors and external rotators and gastrocnemius and strengthening trunk muscles

7.0a, 7.0b & 7.0c Active, passive and post-isometric forward bends sitting

Starting position: Sitting on a mat with your legs straight out in front and your feet together. Flex your left hip and knee and place the sole of your left foot against the inside of your right thigh, as near as possible to your groin. Place your left hand on the mat behind you and lift your body off the mat.

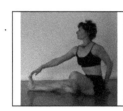 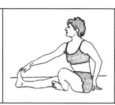 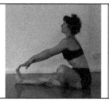 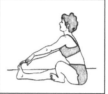

Move your anterior superior iliac spines forwards and the ischial tuberosities of your pelvis backwards. Grasp the toes of your right foot or right knee with both hands.

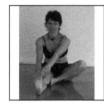 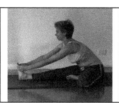 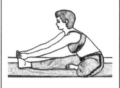

Technique: See Part A. Page 221, 222 and 223.

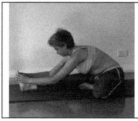 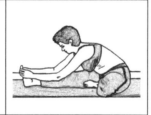

7.0d Bilateral forward bend sitting

Starting position: Sitting on a mat with your legs straight out in front and your feet together. Place one hand on the mat behind you and lift your body off the mat. Move your anterior superior iliac spines forwards and the ischial tuberosities of your pelvis backwards. Grasp the toes of your feet, leg or knee with both hands. Hamstrings flexibility plays a major role in determining where you hold in the starting position.

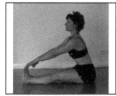 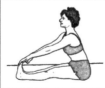 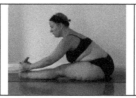 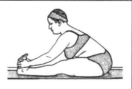

Technique: See Part A. Page 224.

Direction and range of movement

These techniques primarily involves hip flexion. The unilateral hip flexion techniques also involve hip abduction and external rotation. Hip flexion can occur from either direction, the femur can flex on the ilium, or in the case of these stretches, the ilium flexes on the femur.

The lumbar should be in extension, or held as close to extension as possible, and the sacrum held in nutation throughout the stretch. A small amount of upper limb movement is required for the execution of the technique. Ankle dorsiflexion is optional.

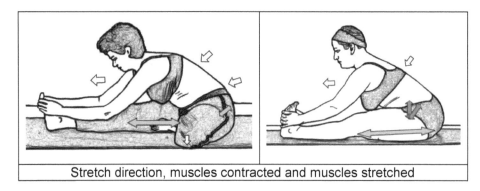

Stretch direction, muscles contracted and muscles stretched

During the passive stretches, contraction of muscles in the arms and shoulders produces elbow flexion, shoulder extension and scapula retraction, which pulls the ribs, spine and pelvis forward, and flexes the hips. The arm and shoulder work as levers, through the spine to pull the upper body forwards and flex the ilium on the femur.

During the active stretch, contraction of the iliopsoas, assisted by other hip flexor muscles, flexes the hips. Gentle isometric contraction of the hamstrings, gluteus maximus and adductor magnus facilitates the post-isometric process. Active, passive and post-isometric techniques may be done individually or combined.

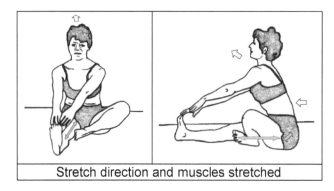

Stretch direction and muscles stretched

These stretches involve movement of the ilium, sacrum, lumbar, upper torso and head relative to the femur and the lower limbs. The head, rib cage, plus cervical, thoracic, and lumbar spine, sacrum and ilium are translated forward and slightly downward, along the mat and towards the foot, moving as a single relatively fixed unit. With the spine fixed, all forward movement of the trunk should be transferred to the hips, as hip flexion. With each movement forwards, a relocating of the hands on the foot or leg, and a repositioning of the upper limb joints is necessary to consolidate the hip flexion.

Target tissues

These are primarily stretches for the hamstrings – semimembranosus, semitendinosus and the short and long heads of biceps femoris, but only when the knee is extended. The hamstrings are stretched on the side of the straight leg or on both sides if both legs are straight. Gluteus maximus is stretched on both the straight and bent leg sides – the lower fibres are stretched the most on the bent leg side and the upper fibres are stretched the most on the straight leg side.

494

The unilateral techniques stretch the hip adductors and internal rotator muscles on the bent leg side. Gluteus minimus and the anterior fibres of gluteus medius are the primary hip internal rotators. Adductor longus, brevis, magnus and gracilis are the primary hip adductors. The fibres of adductor magnus, passing between the adductor tubercle and the ischial tuberosity, may also be stretched on the straight leg side, and especially if the hip is externally rotated. And on the straight leg side a strongly extended knee would stretch popliteus.

Primary muscle stretched - The Hamstrings		
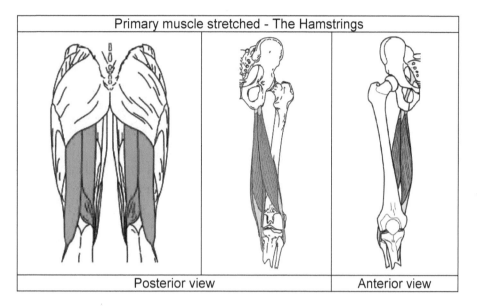		
Posterior view		Anterior view

The passive stretch involves the contraction of biceps brachii, brachialis and brachioradialis to flex the elbow; pectoralis major, latissimus dorsi, posterior deltoid and long head of triceps brachii to extend the shoulder; and rhomboids and middle trapezius to retract the scapula.

Other muscles stretched				
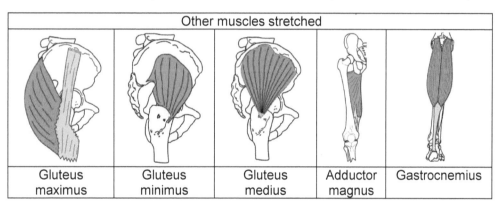				
Gluteus maximus	Gluteus minimus	Gluteus medius	Adductor magnus	Gastrocnemius

The contraction of these muscles results in movement of the head, spine and ribs forward. This movement is then carried through to the sacrum and then to the ilium, resulting in flexion of the ilium on the femur at the hip joints. In the unilateral stretches, on one side there is hip flexion, while on the other side, hip flexion is combined with abduction and external rotation.

Muscles contracted			
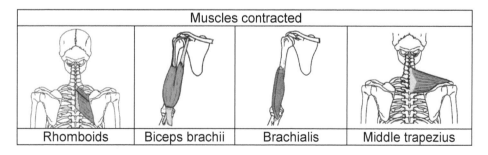			
Rhomboids	Biceps brachii	Brachialis	Middle trapezius

If you pull back on the toes with the hands or actively dorsiflex your foot and ankle, then this would stretch gastrocnemius, soleus and the overlying fascia.

The active stretch involves contraction of iliopsoas and other hip flexor muscles, the to take the top of the ilium forwards; erector spinae muscles to produce and maintain extension in the lumbar spine; hip abductor and external rotator muscles, to take the left knee downwards, towards the floor; and tibialis anterior to dorsiflex the foot at the ankle. As with the passive stretch your lumbar, lower thoracic and lower ribs move forwards with your ilium.

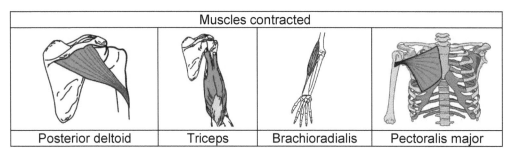

Muscles contracted			
Posterior deltoid	Triceps	Brachioradialis	Pectoralis major

Your thigh is fixed on the floor and is an anchor for iliacus. So when iliacus contracts it flexes the ilium on the femur. Psoas major also flexes the ilium on the femur but only when your lumbar and lower thoracic are held in a fixed position - in this case held in neutral or extension by the contraction of erector spinae.

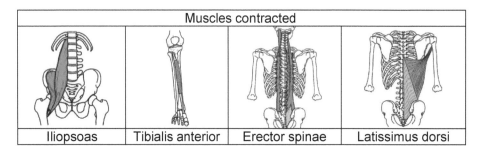

Muscles contracted			
Iliopsoas	Tibialis anterior	Erector spinae	Latissimus dorsi

Your starting position and range of forward movement depend on the flexibility of your hamstrings. If you can grasp your foot, then you have good hamstring flexibility but if you need to hold your knee when you do the stretch, then your hamstring flexibility is poor.

Safety

Although these are hamstrings stretches, they should not be done by people who have very tight hamstrings. These are potentially dangerous stretches if the hamstrings are so short the pelvis is prevent from tilting forward and the thoracic and lumbar spine is forced into flexion.

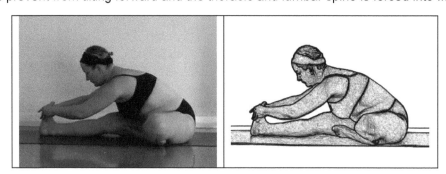

There needs to be sufficient initial flexibility in the hamstrings for the hip to flex. With one or both knees extended, short hamstrings can hold back the ischial tuberosities during forward bending, causing flexion of the thoracic, lumbar and sacrum, which can place greater strain on intervertebral discs and the posterior muscles and ligaments of the spine, including the sacroiliac ligaments.

The unilateral stretch is less of a problem than the bilateral stretch because there is less resistance offered by one sets of hamstring muscles than two, but the forward bending stretches should be avoided if you have tight hamstrings, and safer stretches adopted, such as the standing or supine hamstring stretches, which do not put the lumbar under as much strain.

Excessive lumbar flexion during forward bending in the sitting position can also put great loads on the intervertebral discs. A healthy disc will cope with an increased load from forward bends most of the time, but repetitive or abnormally high loads can cause damage. If the breath is held in inhalation during forward bending, this will increase pressure within the abdomen, resulting in greater load on the disc. When the structural integrity of a disc is compromised because of degeneration, then sitting forward bends may cause further deterioration and may lead to a disc prolapse or herniation.

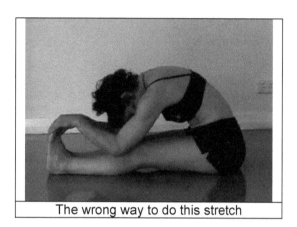
The wrong way to do this stretch

Sitting forward bending combined with short hamstrings can also cause muscle and ligament strains in the spine. Over time they can change the shape of the spine, for example increasing a thoracic kyphosis, which in turn can affect the rib cage causing rigidity, loss of rib excursion and compromised breathing. They can also cause postural problems associated with rounded shoulders.

Certain situations can exaggerated the problems associated with the sitting forward bend stretches. For example, if the stretch is done too fast or incorrectly, or without an appropriate warm-up. If there is a pre-existing weakness in the spine such as a congenital abnormality or a mild scoliosis, then these can further increases the dangers associated with forward bends.

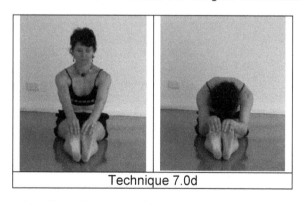
Technique 7.0d

During standing, the wedge shaped sacrum sits between both iliac bones in a relatively stable close-packed arrangement. In contrast, sitting results in the uncoupling of the sacroiliac joints, leading to a more loose-packed and less stable arrangement. During sitting, forward bending is potentially more of a problem because this increases the probability of sacroiliac joints dysfunction and posterior sacroiliac ligament strain.

It is important to keep your spine extended or as straight as possible during the forward bends and only allow flexion at the hip joints. If the lumbar spine does not extend because it has a reversed lordosis, then get as much extension into the lumbar spine as possible and maintain it during the stretch. Hip flexion is the primary goal.

To keep your spine from flexing it may be helpful to place a small pillow under your buttocks. To prevent sideways tilting of the pelvis towards the bent knee side during the unilateral stretch, a pillow may be placed under the bent knee. Sideways tilting will occur if your hip is tight and fails to drop sufficiently, resulting in a twisting of the pelvis and spine and an inefficient hamstring stretch.

If you have a pre-existing intervertebral disc problem in the lumbar spine such as a disc prolapse, herniation or a history of a reoccurring sacroiliac or lumbar ligament strain, then this technique should be avoided. Other conditions which may result in problems with this technique include: a spondylolisthesis (a pars defect) and spondylosis (osteoarthritis of the spine) or anything likely to cause a nerve impingement.

Vulnerable areas

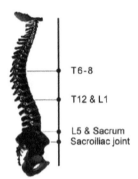

T6-8

T12 & L1

L5 & Sacrum
Sacroiliac joint

	Region	Level of Risk
1.	Thoracic	Medium
2.	Thoracolumbar	Medium
3.	Lumbar	High
4.	Sacroiliac	Medium

Key:

7.0a, 7.0b & 7.0c Unilateral forward bends sitting	
7.0d Seated bilateral forward bend for the hips	

Related stretches					
6.5c,d & h Bilateral stretches for the hip adductors		6.7a & 6.7b Unilateral stretches for the hamstrings		6.7f Unilateral stretch for the hamstrings standing	

For more detailed anatomy of the hip - sacrum, ilium and femur 6.0 - 7.0 see page 600.

7.1 Calf stretches - active, passive and post-isometric stretches for gastrocnemius, soleus and other posterior leg muscles including peroneus longus and brevis, tibialis posterior, flexor digitorum longus and flexor hallucis longus

7.1a Unilateral passive stretch for gastrocnemius

Starting position: Standing facing a wall and with your feet slightly apart. Interlace your fingers and make an angle with your forearms. Place your elbows, and the ulna side of your forearms and hands against the wall. Your elbows are shoulder width apart, and your arms are parallel to each other and perpendicular to the wall.

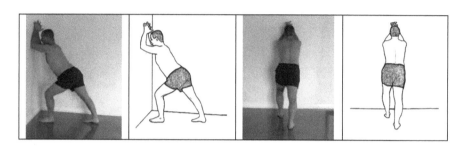

Flex your left hip and knee, and put your left foot down near the wall. Extend your right hip and place your right foot on the floor behind you. Extend your right knee and bring your right heel to the floor.

Technique: See Part A. Page 225.

7.1b Unilateral post-isometric stretch and variations for gastrocnemius

Starting position: Adopt the same starting position as in technique 7.1a.

Technique: See Part A. Page 226.

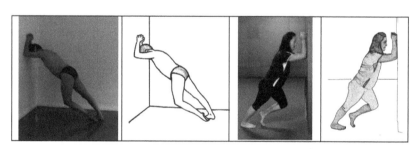

Sideshifting your pelvis right increases the stretch on tensor fasciae latae and the lateral head of gastrocnemius. Sideshifting your pelvis left increases the stretch on gracilis, sartorius and the medial head of gastrocnemius.

7.1c Bilateral passive stretch for gastrocnemius

Starting position: Standing facing a wall and with your feet slightly apart. Interlace your fingers and make an angle with your forearms. Place your elbows and ulna side of forearms and hands against the wall. Your elbows are shoulder width apart and your arms are parallel with each other. Extend your knees and bring your heels to the floor. Your feet are hip width apart and parallel and your spine and legs straight.

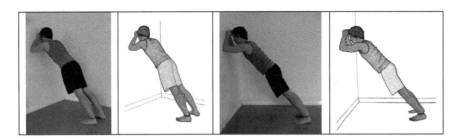

Technique: See Part A. Page 227.

7.1d Bilateral stretch for gastrocnemius using a block

Starting position: Standing facing two small blocks or bricks and a wall. Using the wall for support, place your feet on the edge of the blocks. The edge crosses your forefoot at the distal end of the metatarsals. Extend your hips and knees. Your heels hang over the side of the blocks but do not touch the floor. Keep your knees and body straight. Push against the wall and slowly move your body backwards to bring your centre of gravity further over your ankles. Stop when your body weight falls mid-point between your ankles.

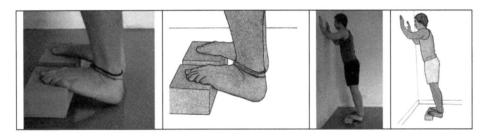

Technique: See Part A. Page 228.

7.1e Unilateral stretch for soleus and other posterior leg muscles, ankle ligaments and the Achilles tendon

Starting position: Standing facing a chair or wall, holding the chair or wall for support. Place your left foot in front of your right foot, and nearer to the wall. Flex your hips and knees. Stop when your right ankle joint is fully dorsiflexed but make sure your right heel remains in contact with the floor.

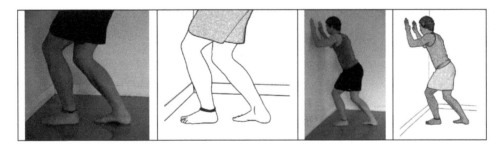

Technique: See Part A. Page 229.

7.1f Unilateral stretch for peroneus muscles, tibialis posterior, flexor digitorum longus and flexor hallucis longus on a sloping floor

Starting position: Standing facing a chair or wall, holding the chair or wall for support. Place your left foot in front of your right foot and nearer to the wall. Place your right foot along the right edge of a thin block of wood. Make sure the sharp edge of the block passes down the middle of your foot and heel, so that it makes your ankle tilt outwards. As an alternative to the edge of a thin block of wood use a board slanting downwards to the right. Flex your hips and knees. Stop when your right ankle joint is fully dorsiflexed but make sure your right heel remains in contact with the block or board on the floor.

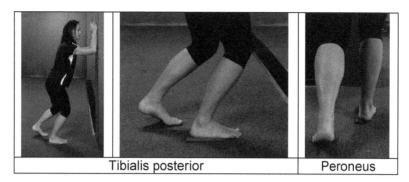

| Tibialis posterior | Peroneus |

Technique: See Part A. Page 230.

7.1g Unilateral stretch for soleus using a block or wall

Starting position: Standing next to a small block or brick between 3 cm and 8 cm thick. Flex your hips and knees. Lift your right foot and place your forefoot on the block in front of you. The distal ends of your metatarsal bones rest on the edge of the block. Your heel remains in contact with the floor. Flex your right knee until you feel the initial stages of a stretch in the back of the leg and ankle. Grasp a table, the back of a chair or a nearby wall for support if you wish. This stretch can be done with shoes on or off, or it can be done with the ball of your toes against a wall.

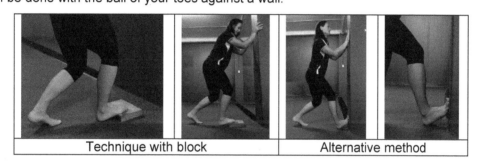

| Technique with block | Alternative method |

Technique: See Part A. Page 231.

7.1h Unilateral/ Bilateral active stretch for gastrocnemius and soleus

Starting position: Sitting or lying on the floor or a mat with your legs straight.

Technique: See Part A. Page 232.

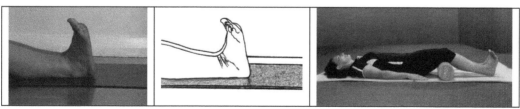

Direction and range of movement

These are a mixture of active, passive and post-isometric stretches. All the techniques involve ankle dorsiflexion. Stretches for gastrocnemius involves full knee extension and stretches for soleus involve partial knee flexion. Ankle valgus (calcaneus bent outwards) also stretches posterior compartment muscles and ankle varus (calcaneus bent inwards) also stretches the lateral compartment muscles.

There are between 20 and 30 degrees of dorsiflexion at the ankle, depending on whether the knee is flexed or extended, or whether the stretch is done actively or passively, and depending on the flexibility of the individual.

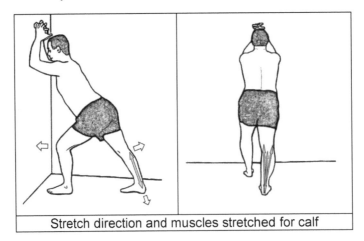

Stretch direction and muscles stretched for calf

Passive range of movement is always greater than active and ankle dorsiflexion with the knee flexed is greater than when the knee extended. Active extension of the toes is about 50 degrees.

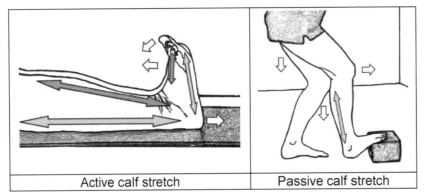

Active calf stretch	Passive calf stretch

The ankle is a hinge joint permitting motion in one plane, and is mechanically linked with the superior and inferior tibiofibular joints. During dorsiflexion the lateral malleolus moves away from the medial malleolus and the fibula moves superiorly and rotates medially.

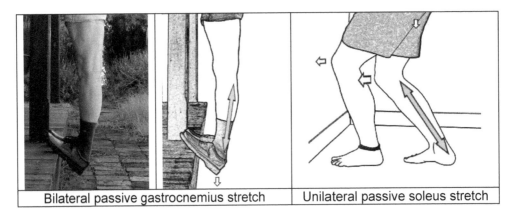

Bilateral passive gastrocnemius stretch	Unilateral passive soleus stretch

Target tissues

These are primarily stretches for gastrocnemius and soleus. Both muscles are stretched in all the techniques but the intensity of the stretch varies according to the position of the knee in each technique. Knee extension increases the stretch on gastrocnemius, while knee flexion increases the stretch on soleus and other leg muscles, and decreases it on gastrocnemius.

Combined with dorsiflexion and knee flexion, ankle valgus increases the stretch of tibialis posterior, flexor digitorum longus, flexor hallucis longus. Combined with dorsiflexion and knee flexion, ankle varus increases the stretch of peroneus longus and brevis.

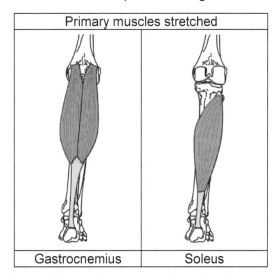

Primary muscles stretched	
Gastrocnemius	Soleus

Combined with dorsiflexion and knee extension, ankle valgus increases the stretch of the medial head of gastrocnemius. Combined with dorsiflexion and knee extension, ankle varus increases the stretch of the lateral head of gastrocnemius.

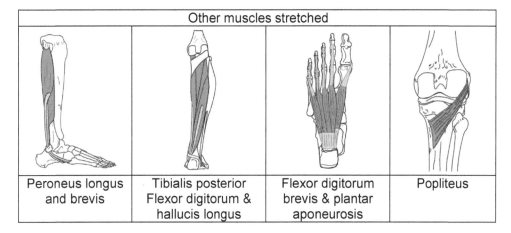

Other muscles stretched			
Peroneus longus and brevis	Tibialis posterior Flexor digitorum & hallucis longus	Flexor digitorum brevis & plantar aponeurosis	Popliteus

Technique 7.1h is an active stretch for gastrocnemius and soleus, requiring ankle dorsiflexion and toe extension. Contraction of the quadriceps muscles maintains full extension of the knee and contraction of the anterior leg muscles maintains ankle dorsiflexion.

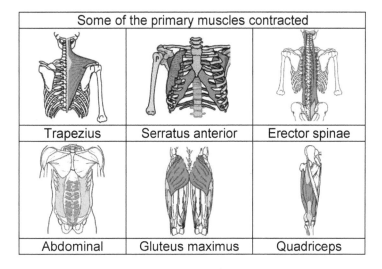

Some of the primary muscles contracted		
Trapezius	Serratus anterior	Erector spinae
Abdominal	Gluteus maximus	Quadriceps

The straight body posture, is necessary for all the gastrocnemius stretches (technique 7.1a to 7.1d) and is maintained by the contraction of muscles of the shoulder, spine, hips and knees.

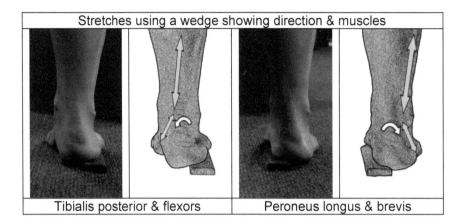

Stretches using a wedge showing direction & muscles	
Tibialis posterior & flexors	Peroneus longus & brevis

Quadriceps contraction helps maintain full knee extension, gluteus maximus and hamstrings maintain hip extension, erector spinae and the abdominal muscle maintain stability in the spine and trunk and serratus anterior, trapezius and other shoulder girdle muscles, act through the scapula to maintain shoulder stability.

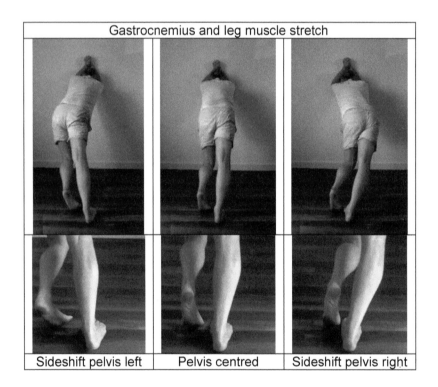

Gastrocnemius and leg muscle stretch		
Sideshift pelvis left	Pelvis centred	Sideshift pelvis right

Safety

Make sure the foot being stretched is perpendicular to the wall. Keep your spine straight and your head and neck in line with your spine. If it is passive stretch then just allow your ankle to dorsiflex. You do not need to push hard against the wall but make sure that if you are using a wall that it is solid and will support your body weight.

Make sure that any block you are using is strong enough to support your weight and has a wide base so it does not flip over and so you do not slip off the block. Make sure that there is sufficient friction between the floor and your foot so that you do not slide. There is usually good contact between bare feet and a wooden floor. Do not do the calf stretch in sock or stockings. Choose the floor surface carefully to prevent slipping.

504

Key:

7.1a Unilateral passive stretch for gastrocnemius	
7.1b Unilateral post-isometric stretch and variations for gastrocnemius	
7.1c Bilateral passive stretch for gastrocnemius	
7.1d Bilateral stretch for gastrocnemius using a block	
7.1e Unilateral stretch for soleus and other posterior leg muscles, ankle ligaments and the Achilles tendon	
7.1f Unilateral stretch for peroneus muscles, tibialis posterior, flexor digitorum longus and flexor hallucis longus on a sloping floor	
7.1g Unilateral stretch for soleus using a block	
7.1h Bilateral or unilateral active stretch for gastrocnemius and soleus	

Related stretches					
6.5d Bilateral stretch for the hip adductors sitting		6.9a, b & c Stretches for the hamstrings and calf		7.0a, b, c & d Forward bends sitting	

For more detailed anatomy of the knee - femur, tibial and fibula 6.6 - 7.1 see page 614.

7.2 Tibialis anterior stretches - active and passive stretches for tibialis anterior and the toe extensor muscles

7.2a Bilateral active stretch for the ankle dorsiflexor and toe extensor muscles

Starting position: Sitting or lying on the floor or mat with your legs straight. Bring your feet together and bring your big toes together.

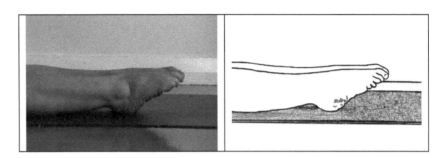

Technique: See Part A. Page 233.

7.2b Unilateral passive stretch for the ankle dorsiflexor and toe extensor muscles, standing

Starting position: Stand facing a wall and hold the wall for support. Place your left foot in front of your right foot, closer towards the wall. Flex your hips and knees. Lift your right foot off the floor, extend your hip and then place it back on the floor with your sole facing upwards and your toes pointing backwards.

Technique: See Part A. Page 234.

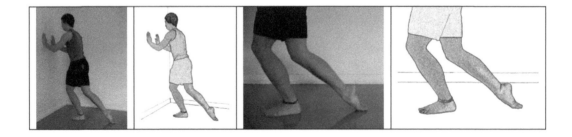

Direction and range of movement

Technique 7.2a is an active stretch and technique 7.2b is a passive stretch. Both involve ankle plantarflexion and toe flexion. Active plantarflexion at the ankle varies between individuals from 30 to 50 degrees. Approximately half occurs at the talocrural (ankle) joint and the other half occurs at the subtalar and intertarsal joints. A small amount of abduction, adduction, rotation and sideways gliding is possible at the ankle when the foot is in plantar flexion.

In the metatarsophalangeal joints flexion is between 20 and 30 degrees and in the interphalangeal joints toe flexion is about 50 degrees. Total flexion of the toes is therefore about 80 degrees.

The ankle or talocrural joint permits dorsiflexion and plantar flexion and is mechanically linked with the subtalar joint and the superior and inferior tibiofibular joints. Movement at the ankle joint is largely determined by the articulating surface of the talus, which is wider anteriorly than posteriorly.

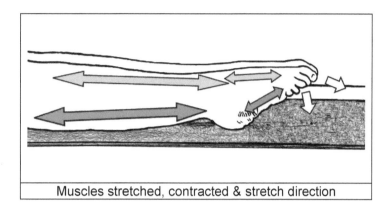

Muscles stretched, contracted & stretch direction

During plantarflexion this particular joint geometry causes the malleoli to move closer together, the fibula to move inferiorly and rotates laterally, and the joint to move into its loose-pack position with minimum joint congruence, ligamentous tension and least stability.

Target tissues

These are stretches for the ankle dorsiflexor tibialis anterior, and the toe extensor muscles, extensor hallucis longus and extensor digitorum longus.
The active stretch requires the contraction of gastrocnemius and soleus to plantar flex the ankle; tibialis posterior to plantar flex the ankle and foot; flexor hallucis longus and flexor digitorum longus to plantar flex the ankle, foot and toes.

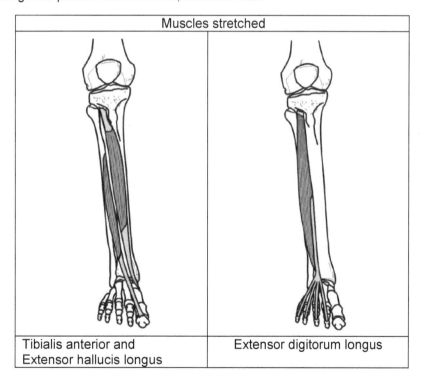

Muscles stretched	
Tibialis anterior and Extensor hallucis longus	Extensor digitorum longus

The active stretch also requires the intrinsic muscles of the foot - flexor digitorum brevis, flexor hallucis brevis, abductor hallucis, abductor digit minimi brevis, the lumbricales and the interossei to plantar flex the foot and toes. The quadriceps muscle is contracted to maintain full extension of the knee.

The passive stretch requires the contraction of the iliopsoas to fix the hip, the quadriceps to fix the knee, both muscles thus preventing hip and knee movement on the side that is being stretched. The quadriceps and calf muscles on the side not being stretched are contracted to move the pelvis and spine forwards and support the body weight.

Safety

Technique 7.2b may be contraindicated while there is an acute anterior talofibular ligament strain or if there is chronic ankle instability.

Key:

7.2a Bilateral active stretch for the ankle dorsiflexor and toe extensor muscles	
7.2b Unilateral passive stretch for the ankle dorsiflexor and toe extensor muscles, standing	

Related stretches					
1.1a Lion stretch kneeling		2.2a Thoracic and rib sidebending stretch kneeling		6.6a, b, c & d Quadriceps stretches	

7.3 Foot and toe stretches - passive and post-isometric stretches for flexor digitorum longus, flexor hallucis longus, short toe flexors, extensor hallucis longus, extensor digitorum longus, extensor digitorum brevis, peroneus longus, peroneus brevis, tibialis posterior, tibialis anterior, lumbricals, interossei and plantar fascia

7.3a Passive and post-isometric toe flexor stretch standing

Starting position: Standing facing a wall. Place your palms on the wall about shoulder height for support. Extend the toes of your right foot and place your foot against the wall so that your toes are up against to the wall, the balls of your feet are in the corner of the room, and your heel and metatarsal are on the floor. Flex your hips and knees slightly. Stop when your feel the initial stages of a stretch under your toes. Make sure your heel and metatarsals remains in contact with the floor.

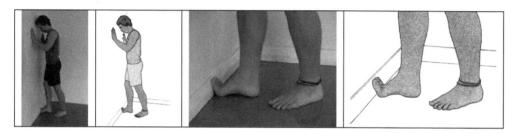

Technique: See Part A. Page 235.

7.3b Passive and post-isometric toe flexor stretch seated

Starting position: Seated in a chair. Flex your right hip and knee, and place the outside of your right ankle on your left thigh just above your knee. Allow your right knee to drop into a comfortable abducted position. Grasp the heel of your right foot with your left hand and hold it steady.

Reach under your toes and the bottom of your right foot with your right hand, and grasp your toes and the end of your foot. Hook your thumb over your big toe and fingers over your other toes. Flex your right elbow, wrist and fingers, and pull up your toes. Stop when you feel the initial stages of a stretch under your toes.

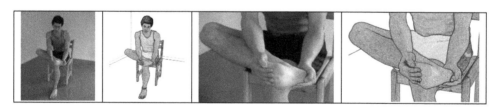

Technique: See Part A. Page 236.

7.3c Passive and post-isometric foot evertor or foot invertor stretch seated

Starting position: Seated in a chair as in technique 7.3b. Reach under your toes and the bottom of your right foot with your right hand and grasp the distal ends of your metatarsals. Contact the fourth and fifth metacarpal head (little toe side), and pull the foot into dorsiflexion and eversion to stretch the invertor muscles. Contact the first metacarpal head (big toe side), and pull the foot into dorsiflexion and inversion to stretch the foot evertor muscles.

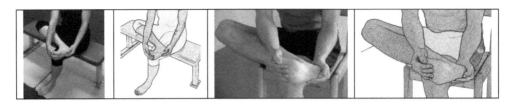

Technique: See Part A. Page 237.

7.3d Passive and post-isometric toe extensor stretch seated

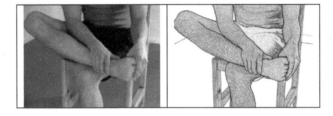

Starting position: Seated in a chair as in technique 7.3b. Grasp your right ankle with your right hand and hold your foot steady. Reach over your toes and the dorsum of your right foot with your left hand, and grasp your toes and the end of your foot. Place your thumb over your big toe and your fingers over your toes. Extend your left shoulder, flex your left wrist and fingers, and pull your toes downwards and towards you. Stop when you feel the initial stages of a stretch over the top of your foot.

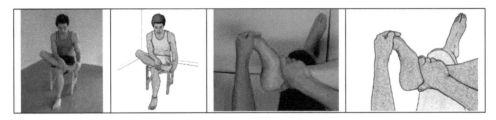

Technique: See Part A. Page 238.

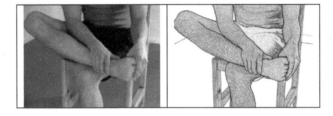

Direction and range of movement

These are passive and post-isometric stretches that involve movement in all the joints of the foot and ankle: the talocrural (ankle), subtalar, midtarsal (talonavicular and calcaneocuboid), cuneonavicular, intercuneiform, tarsometatarsal, metatarsophalangeal and interphalangeal joints.

The range of movement in the joints in the foot and ankle varies between individuals due to genetic differences affecting the shape of the bones and articulating surfaces, and the strength and elasticity of the ligaments. There is greater range of movement in the joints of the non-weight bearing foot than in the weight bearing foot because the mechanics is different.

The ankle joint (talocrural joint) is formed between the talus, tibia and fibular at the distal end of the leg. The ankle described as a 'mortise and tenon' type structure functioning as a hinge joint, with the dome shaped head of talus fitting tightly between the tibiofibular complex. The joint permits dorsiflexion or plantar flexion. In dorsiflexion, the ankle is closely packed with maximum joint contact and greatest ligament tension. In plantar flexion the opposite is true, the ligaments are more relaxed and a small amount of passive medial to lateral joint play is possible.

The ankle joint is mechanically linked with the superior and inferior tibiofibular joints. During dorsiflexion the lateral malleolus moves away from the medial malleolus, and the fibula moves superiorly and rotates medially. During plantar flexion the lateral malleolus moves towards the medial malleolus, and the fibula moves inferiorly and rotates laterally. Full ankle movement is therefore dependent on the integrity of the tibiofibular joints.

Active dorsiflexion is between 20 and 30 degrees, while plantarflexion is between 30 and 50 degrees. There are 10 degrees dorsiflexion at the ankle and 10 degrees in the intertarsal joints and 20 degrees plantarflexion at the ankle and 20 degrees in the intertarsal joints. Dorsiflexion is reduced by about 10 degrees when the knee is in extension due to the increasing tension of gastrocnemius. The tarsal joints provide a few degrees of dorsiflexion and plantar flexion. Total foot pronation is between 25 and 30 degrees and supination is about 50 degrees.

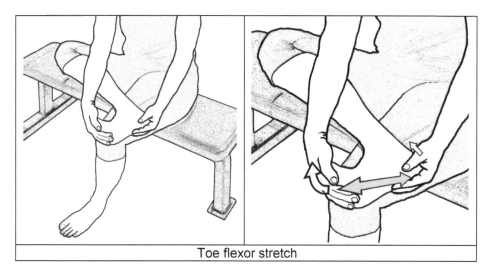

Toe flexor stretch

Dorsiflexion is first limited by tightness of the calf muscles. But if these muscles have good flexibility, then it is checked by tension of the posterior talofibular ligament, calcaneofibular ligament and the posterior and middle fibres of the deltoid ligament and by the neck of the talus coming in contact with the tibia.

Plantar flexion is first limited by tightness of the foot extensor muscles. But if these muscles have good flexibility, then it is checked by tension of the anterior talofibular ligament and anterior fibres of the deltoid ligament and by the posterior tubercule of the talus coming into contact with the tibia.

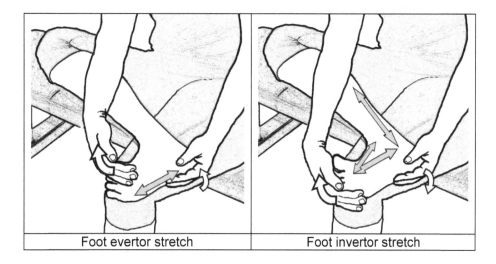

| Foot evertor stretch | Foot invertor stretch |

The subtalar joint (talocalcaneal joint) is between the inferior surface of the talus, the superior anterior surface of the calcaneus and the superior surface of the spring ligament. The joint allows a small amount of forward, backward and lateral gliding, and inversion and eversion of the foot.

The midtarsal joints form a flattened S-shape line across the foot; the talonavicular and calcaneocuboid articulations. The talonavicular joint is a shallow ball and socket joint between the head of the talus and the proximal end of the navicular bone. The joint allows movement in three planes, permitting inversion with adduction, eversion with abduction and a small amount of dorsiflexion and plantarflexion.

The calcaneocuboid joint is a flat saddle-shaped joint between the distal end of the calcaneus and the proximal end of the cuboid bone. The joint allows a small amount of gliding and rotation, which facilitates inversion and eversion in the foot.

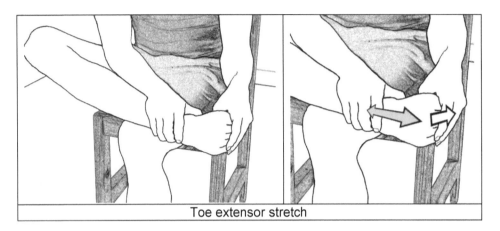

Toe extensor stretch

The subtalar and the midtarsal joints are a complex arrangement of bones and joints that are mechanically linked, acting as a single functional unit with one degree of freedom - pronation and supination. The cubonavicular joint, cubocuneiform joint, cuneonavicular joints, intercuneiform joints and the tarsometatarsal joints are plane joints that glide over one another and facilitate pronation and supination.

Pronation and supination are composite movements, components of inversion and eversion. Also adduction and abduction are components of inversion and eversion. Pronation is a combination of abduction, eversion and dorsiflexion. Supination is a combination of adduction, inversion and plantar flexion. Adduction and inversion are linked and always occur together. Similarly abduction and eversion are linked and always occur together.

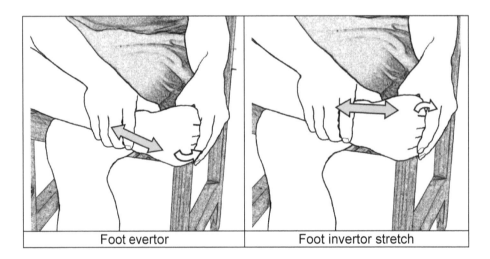

| Foot evertor | Foot invertor stretch |

Inversion is limited by tightness of the peroneal muscles and checked by the lateral part of the interosseous talocalcaneal ligament, and to a lesser extent by the calcaneofibular ligaments and lateral ligament of the foot. Eversion is limited by tightness of the tibialis anterior and tibialis posterior muscles and is checked by the deltoid ligament.

A line of tarsometatarsal joints run obliquely across the foot and facilitates dorsiflexion linked to eversion, and plantar flexion linked to inversion. In addition the line of five joints facilitates the flattening and curving of the anterior arch of the foot.

The metatarsophalangeal joints (MTP) are ovoid joints between the metatarsal bones and the proximal phalanx or toe bones. They permit 50 to 60 degrees active extension and 30 to 45 degrees active flexion. The joints can be moved about another 20 degrees passively resulting in 80 to 90 degrees passive extension and 45 degrees passive flexion. The interphalangeal joints are hinge joints formed between the short digits or toe bones. They allow significant flexion but limited extension, with most of the movement occurring between the proximal and middle phalanges of the toes.

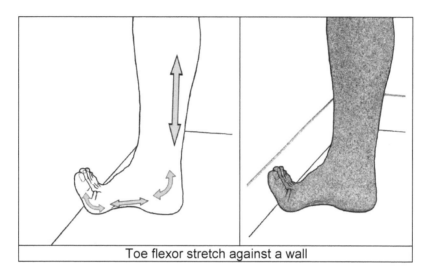

Toe flexor stretch against a wall

At the proximal interphalangeal joints (PIP) of toes 2 to 5 there is between 30 and 40 degrees active flexion and between 45 and 50 degrees passive flexion. At the distal interphalangeal joints (DIP) of toes 2 to 5 there is about 60 degrees flexion. Active extension of the toes is between 50 and 60 degrees and passive extension of the toes is about 90 degrees.

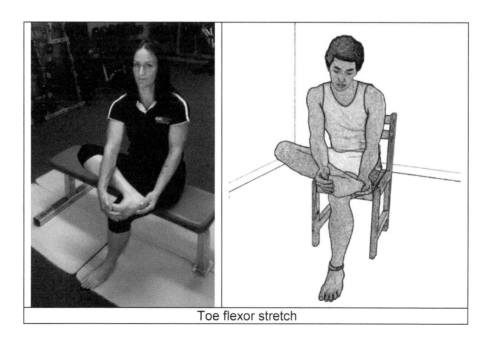

Toe flexor stretch

Target tissues

Technique 7.3a and 7.3b are stretches for the toe flexor muscles and the plantar fascia. The long toe flexors are flexor digitorum longus and flexor hallucis longus; the short toe flexors are flexor digitorum brevis, flexor hallucis brevis, flexor digiti minimi brevis, abductor hallucis, adductor hallucis, abductor digiti minimi, quadratus plantae, the lumbricales and the plantar interossei.

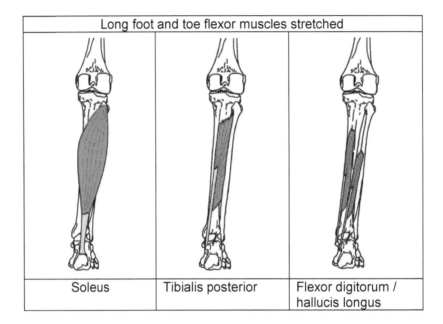

Long foot and toe flexor muscles stretched		
Soleus	Tibialis posterior	Flexor digitorum / hallucis longus

Technique 7.3c is a stretches for the foot evertor and invertor muscles, as well as soleus. The foot evertor muscles are peroneus tertius (sometimes absent), peroneus longus and peroneus brevis. The main foot invertor muscles are tibialis posterior and tibialis anterior; flexor digitorum longus and flexor hallucis longus, also assist in inversion.

Technique 7.3d is a stretch for the toe extensor muscles and ankle dorsiflexors, such as tibialis anterior; the amount of tibialis anterior stretch will depend on how much the foot is plantar flexed. The long toe extensors are extensor digitorum longus and extensor hallucis longus. The short toe extensor is extensor digitorum brevis.

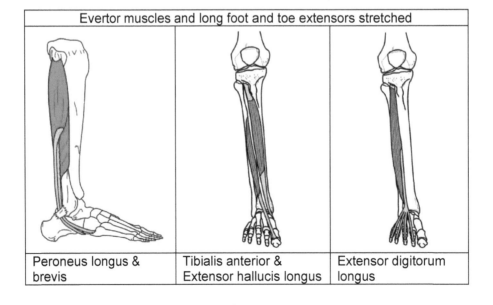

Evertor muscles and long foot and toe extensors stretched		
Peroneus longus & brevis	Tibialis anterior & Extensor hallucis longus	Extensor digitorum longus

Options

Stretch 7.3b, 7.3c and 7.3d may be done sitting on the floor if you maintain a straight spine. Alternatively they may be done sitting on the floor with your back supported against a wall.

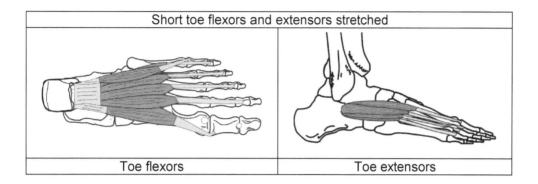

Short toe flexors and extensors stretched	
Toe flexors	Toe extensors

Key:

7.3a Unilateral toe flexor stretch standing	
7.3b Unilateral toe flexor stretch seated	
7.3c Unilateral foot evertor or foot invertor stretch seated	
7.3d Unilateral toe extensor stretch seated	

Related stretches					
1.1a Lion stretch kneeling		2.2a Thoracic & rib sidebending stretch kneeling		3.9b Supine spine stretch over a rolled towel	
6.5d Bilateral stretch for the hip adductors sitting		6.6a, b, c & d Quadriceps stretches		6.7a & 6.7b Unilateral hamstring stretch standing	
7.0a, b, c & d Forward bends sitting		7.1h Active stretch for soleus and gastrocnemius			

For more detailed anatomy of the ankle and foot - tibia, fibula, tarsals, metatarsals & phalanges 7.1 - 7.3 see page 622.

7.4 Hip and back stretches - active, passive and post-isometric stretches for the hamstrings, piriformis, gluteus medius, gluteus maximus, abdominal and lumbar muscles

7.4a Hip and back active and passive straight leg stretch

Starting position: Supine on the floor with your arms abducted about 90 degrees. Flex your right hip and then extend your knee so that your leg is straight. Keep your right leg vertical, and keep your left leg straight, horizontal and as close to the ground as possible throughout the stretch.

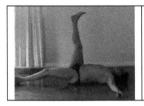 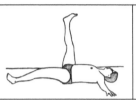 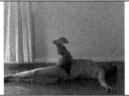 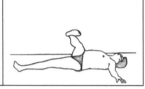

Technique: See Part A. Page 239.

7.4b Hip and back passive and isometric stretch for hip abductors and external rotators and muscles in the lumber spine

Starting position: Supine on the floor. Flex your hips and knees and place your feet on the floor slightly apart. Lift your left leg, move it over the top of your right knee and hook it around your right thigh in a cross legged position. Pull your right knee left with your left leg to adduct the hip and rotate the pelvis but stop when you feel the initial stages of muscle tension. Keep your shoulders on the floor.

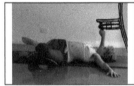 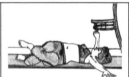 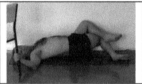 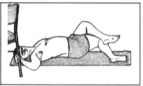

Technique: See Part A. Page 240.

Direction and range of movement

These techniques mainly involve horizontal hip adduction, lumbar and thoracolumbar rotation, and a small amount of sacroiliac movement. Technique 7.4a also involves hip flexion combined with knee extension. Technique 7.4b also involves hip internal rotation and hip flexion combined with knee flexion.

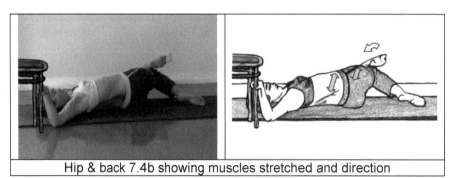

Hip & back 7.4b showing muscles stretched and direction

Horizontal adduction of the hip is about 45 degrees. Rotation of the lumbar spine is about 5 degrees in each direction or 10 degrees both ways. As there are five lumbar vertebrae this

516

means 1 degree of rotation per vertebra. The thoracolumbar spine is usually the most flexible part of the thoracic and lumbar spine but there is considerable variation in range between individuals. Between T11 and L1 there may be 10 to 20 degrees of total left-right rotation.

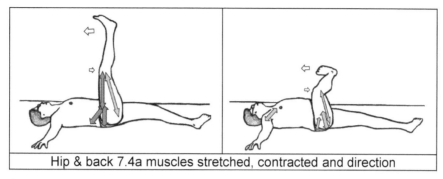

| Hip & back 7.4a muscles stretched, contracted and direction |

Target tissues

In the first part of technique 7.4a hip flexion is combined with knee extension to actively stretch the hamstrings: biceps femoris, semimembranosus and semitendinosus and the upper fibres of gluteus maximus. If dorsiflexion is added it is an active stretch for gastrocnemius.

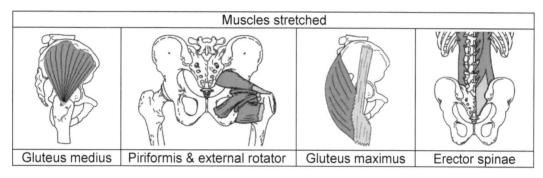

Muscles stretched			
Gluteus medius	Piriformis & external rotator	Gluteus maximus	Erector spinae

In technique 7.4b and the second part of technique 7.4a, horizontal hip adduction is added to stretch piriformis and the posterior fibres of gluteus medius and gluteus maximus. It may also be a weak stretch for the posterior fibres of gluteus minimus. In technique 7.4b some hip internal rotation is added to stretch gamellus superior, gamellus inferior, obturator internus, obturator externus and quadratus femoris.

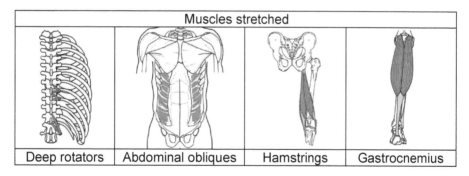

Muscles stretched			
Deep rotators	Abdominal obliques	Hamstrings	Gastrocnemius

In technique 7.4b and the third part of the technique 7.4a pelvic and spinal rotation is added to stretch erector spinae and the deep rotator muscles of the lumbar and thoracolumbar spine. They also both stretch the abdominal oblique muscles, thoracolumbar fascia, quadratus lumborum and serratus posterior inferior.

The technique helps strengthen iliopsoas and the quadriceps muscles on the side that is primarily being stretched and it may stretch iliopsoas on the opposite side. Pelvic and spinal rotation may occur from the middle of the thoracic spine to the ilium. The area that is stretched most will depend on the structure of the spine, the history of pathology and how the stretch is done. It is useful to try and identify which vertebral levels are flexible and which are restricted and then localise the stretch on the restricted part of the spine.

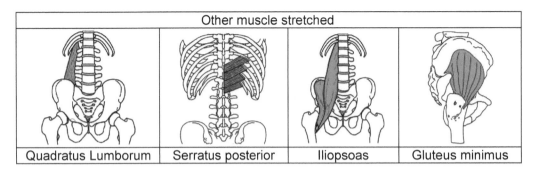

Other muscle stretched			
Quadratus Lumborum	Serratus posterior	Iliopsoas	Gluteus minimus

As a general rule greatest flexibility occurs in the thoracolumbar spine, while the least flexibility occurs in the mid lumbar spine. One side of the spine will usually be more flexible in rotation than the other. Spinal degeneration is common between L5 and S1 after the age of about 40 years, and then all movement ceases at this level.

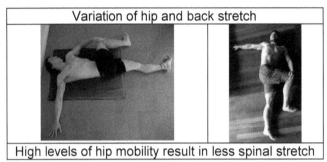

Variation of hip and back stretch
High levels of hip mobility result in less spinal stretch

Safety

Avoid any overstretching with these techniques because it may result in ligament strain in the lumbar or sacroiliac spine. If there is pre-existing degeneration in the joints of the lower lumbar spine, overstretching may result in unwanted hypermobility in other areas. Find out if your lumbar spine is in good health before attempting these stretches.

If there is a pre-existing intervertebral disc problem in the lumbar spine then avoid these techniques because rotation may cause further damage. Also avoid using these techniques to cavitate the facet joints in the lumbar spine. Cavitation is the popping of the joints and if this is done repeatedly as a form of self manipulation for the relief of muscle tension it will result in overstretching of capsular ligaments and hypermobility.

Vulnerable areas

Key:

	Region	Level of Risk
1.	Lumbar spine	Medium
2.	Sacroiliac joints	Low

7.4a	
Unilateral active and passive straight leg stretch	

7.4b	
Unilateral passive and isometric stretch for hip abductors and external rotators and muscles in the lumber spine	

Related stretches					
3.0d Active knees to chest stretch with rotation supine		3.1a, b & c Spinal twists seated		6.2a Unilateral stretch for the hip external rotators	

7.5 Squats – active stretches and strengthening exercises for the whole body but especially the spine, thighs and legs

7.5a Squat with palms together above head

Starting position: Standing with your feet together or apart and your arms at your sides. Abduct your arms until your hands are above your head. Bring your palms together but keep your elbows straight.

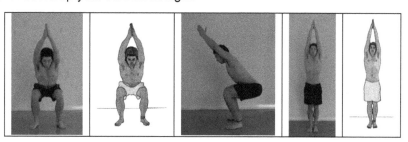

Technique: See Part A. Page 241.

7.5b Squat with arms in front of body

Starting position: Standing with your feet parallel and approximately hip width apart. Flex your arms until they are level with your shoulders and horizontal. Keep your elbows straight. Bend both hips and knees, and lower your body towards the floor. Stop before your heels come off the floor and before there is any strain on your body. Hold this easy squatting position.

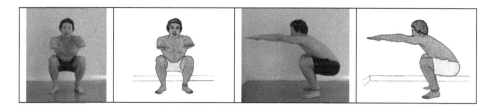

Technique: See Part A. Page 242.

Direction and range of movement

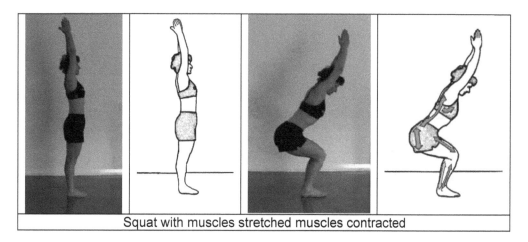

Squat with muscles stretched muscles contracted

In technique 7.5a shoulder abduction is 180 degrees, a combination of glenohumeral and scapulothoracic joint movement. In technique 7.5b shoulder flexion is 90 degrees and there may be up to 10 cm of scapula protraction. These techniques also involve elbow extension, finger extension, hip flexion, knee flexion and ankle dorsiflexion.

Target tissues

This is an active stretch which also strengthens muscles important for the maintenance of good posture.

This technique stretches the sternal and abdominal fibres of pectoralis major, latissimus dorsi and the lumbodorsal fascia, the most superior fibres of gluteus maximus and the overlying superficial fascia, soleus and the overlying deep fascia merging with the Achilles tendon.

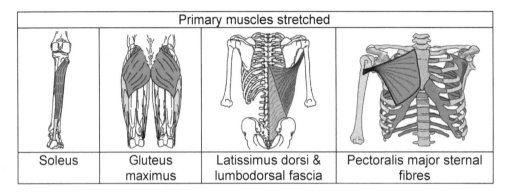

Primary muscles stretched			
Soleus	Gluteus maximus	Latissimus dorsi & lumbodorsal fascia	Pectoralis major sternal fibres

To a lesser extent it also stretches the anterior intercostal muscles, the abdominal muscles, lateral pectoral fascia, brachialis, pronator teres, vastus medius, lateralis and intermedius, the long and short finger flexor muscles and the palmar aponeurosis.

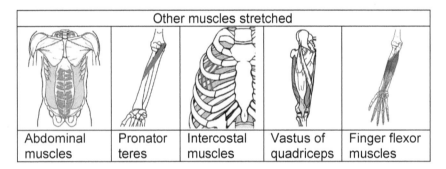

Other muscles stretched				
Abdominal muscles	Pronator teres	Intercostal muscles	Vastus of quadriceps	Finger flexor muscles

The muscles most contracted in the execution of this technique include the erector spinae, trapezius, rhomboids, serratus anterior, triceps brachii, finger extensor muscles, gluteus maximus, tensor fasciae latae, quadriceps femoris and tibialis anterior.

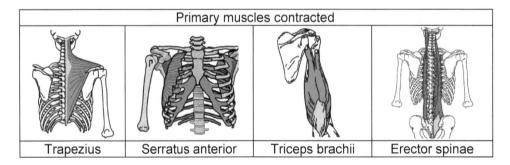

Primary muscles contracted			
Trapezius	Serratus anterior	Triceps brachii	Erector spinae

These are assisted by coracobrachialis, supraspinatus, infraspinatus, deltoid, clavicular fibres of pectoralis major, anconeus, biceps brachii, supinator, iliopsoas, gastrocnemius and the toe extensor muscles.

520

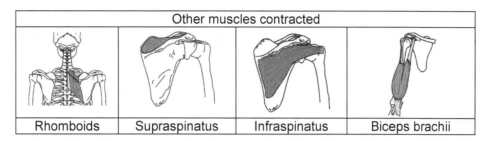

Other muscles contracted			
Rhomboids	Supraspinatus	Infraspinatus	Biceps brachii

Other muscles act as stabilisers holding body parts in position, and synergists neutralising and countering unwanted actions of the prime movers. These include teres major, wrist flexor muscles, gluteus medius, rectus abdominis, abdominal obliques, hip adductors, hamstrings and peroneus longus and brevis.

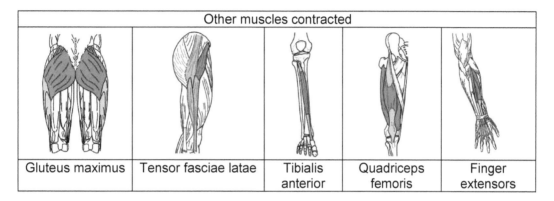

Other muscles contracted				
Gluteus maximus	Tensor fasciae latae	Tibialis anterior	Quadriceps femoris	Finger extensors

The full squat

The full squat is a natural posture for nearly half of the world's population, who are able to relax their body in a locked-in squat posture close to the ground. But the other half of the population who grow up sitting in chairs will find the full squat difficult. The flexibility of your lower limbs and in particular your ankles will determine whether you can do this technique.

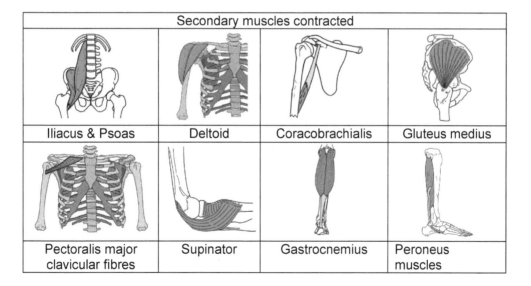

Secondary muscles contracted			
Iliacus & Psoas	Deltoid	Coracobrachialis	Gluteus medius
Pectoralis major clavicular fibres	Supinator	Gastrocnemius	Peroneus muscles

If you find technique 7.5a difficult then start with technique 7.5b, reaching out in front of you and use the weight of your upper limbs to help maintain your centre of gravity forwards and to help keep you balance. Alternatively try the squatting techniques 4.9b and 4.9c, holding onto a post to gain some lower limb flexibility.

Safety

Although this is a strenuous technique it is relatively safe because the body is not put in any extreme positions. Do not do the squat if you have a rotator cuff strain, subacromial bursitis, torn meniscus or knee degeneration. The knees and shoulders are put under load and need to be structurally sound.

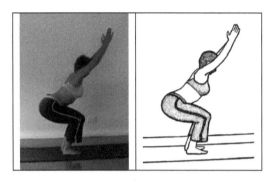

The main danger in doing the squat is falling over and injuring yourself. Until you are confident you can keep your balance do techniques 4.9b and 4.9c or a similar squatting technique supported.

Key:

7.5a Squat with palms together above head	
7.5b Squat with arms in front of body standing	

Related stretches					
2.5a & 2.5b Upper Half Dog		2.7a The Locust		4.9b & 4.9c Shoulder retractor stretch squatting	
3.0a, b & c Knees to chest stretches supine		3.7 Longitudinal stretch over a towel		4.6a Palms above head forearms supinated	
4.9e Scapula active retractor stretch standing		5.2a & 5.2b Bilateral biceps stretch on a ledge			

7.6 Pelvic tilt - active stretch for posterior muscles of the lumbar and cervical spine and strengthening exercise for the abdomen

7.6 Pelvic tilt supine

Starting position: Supine on the floor, preferably on a carpet or mat, with your hips and knees flexed, and your arms on the floor abducted to about shoulder height. If after you lie down your head drops backwards into extension, tuck your chin in, flatten your cervical lordosis, lengthening the back of your neck. If you have an exaggerated thoracic kyphosis, with an inflexible thoracic spine and your head drops into extension, you may need to support your head on a pillow or book.

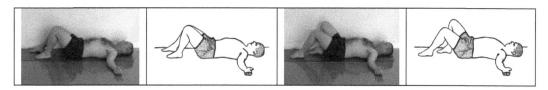

Technique: See Part A. Page 243.

Direction and range of movement

Total head and neck flexion is about 45 degrees. This technique involves full flexion of the head (about 20 degrees) and partial flexion of the neck. If the head is maintained in a position horizontal with the floor, then any flexion that does occur is converted to posterior translation.

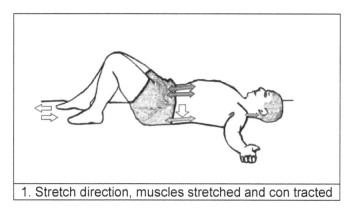

1. Stretch direction, muscles stretched and con tracted

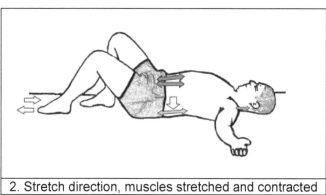

2. Stretch direction, muscles stretched and contracted

And posterior translation of the head and neck is compensated by extension in the upper thoracic spine. Total lumbar flexion is about 45 degrees and most occurs in the middle lumbar between L4 and L5. This technique involves flattening the lumbar which requires partial flexion of the lumbar spine - about 25 degrees.

Target tissue

This primarily stretches the muscles, ligaments and fascia of the posterior lumbar and cervical spine. In the cervical spine these include the suboccipital muscles, posterior cervical muscles, anterior and middle scalene, and upper fibres of erector spinae. In the lumbar spine these include the posterior lumbar ligaments, quadratus lumborum and lower fibres of erector spinae.

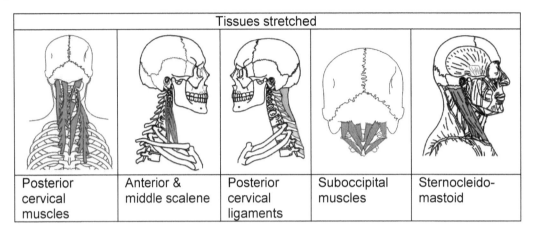

Tissues stretched				
Posterior cervical muscles	Anterior & middle scalene	Posterior cervical ligaments	Suboccipital muscles	Sternocleido-mastoid

In addition to stretching tissues involved in maintaining poor posture, this techniques is useful in strengthening the rectus abdominis muscles involved in maintaining good posture.

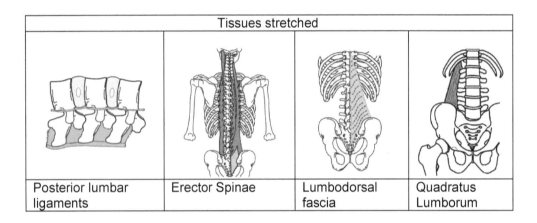

Tissues stretched			
Posterior lumbar ligaments	Erector Spinae	Lumbodorsal fascia	Quadratus Lumborum

When the head is held in the chin tuck position, sternocleidomastoid and anterior scalene are stretched, while the cervical prevertebral muscles, longus colli, longus capitis and rectus capitis anterior are strengthened, which helps maintain good cervical and head posture.

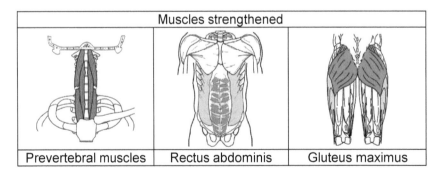

Muscles strengthened		
Prevertebral muscles	Rectus abdominis	Gluteus maximus

Safety

Vulnerable areas

Occiput, C1 and C2 - the occipito-atlanto-axial joints of the sub-occipital region.

Care should be taken not to over extend the neck and put pressure on the muscles or ligaments of the suboccipital region. These can be strained if the head is allowed to drop back too far into extension. As you progress with this technique, reposition your head in progressively greater amounts of flexion by tucking your chin in.

If you have an increased thoracic kyphosis or inflexible spine, support your head on a pillow or book. Adjust the height of the pillow or book so that your head remains horizontal, while at the same time, challenges the muscles and ligament in the back of the neck with a mild stretch.

Do not permit your head to drop back into extension and place the suboccipital spine under stress. Caution should also be applied if there is degeneration in the lower cervical spine by using a support for the head.

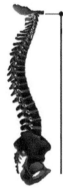

Occiput, C1 & C2

	Region	Level of Risk
1.	Occiput, C1 & C2	Low

Key:

7.6 Supine Pelvic tilt	

Related stretches			
3.0d Active knees to chest stretch with rotation supine		4.9c Scapula retractor stretch squatting	

The mechanics of stretching

Musculoskeletal system

Terminology

The musculoskeletal system is made up of both contractile and non-contractile components. The contractile component is the muscle cell or fibre, in particular the actin-myosin cross-bridges. The non-contractile component is made up of connective tissue which includes bone, cartilage, fasciae, tendons and ligaments, as well as endomysium and perimysium, which runs through the muscle, binding the fibres together, while the epimysium, the outermost layer surounds the muscle, and together they join the muscle to the tendons at either end and then the tendons attach to the bone.

Connective tissue

Structure

Connective tissue is made up of a cellular and an extracellular component. The cellular component includes: osteoblasts in bone; chondroblasts in cartilage; and fibroblasts in fasciae, ligaments and tendons; and the cells actually make the extracellular component. The extracellular component is made up of two components: a fibrous and a non-fibrous component; both of which contribute to physical properties of the different connective tissues. Many different types of proteins contribute to the fibrous component, including elastin and many different types of collagen. A non-fibrous component, also known as a ground substance or extrafibrillar matrix, includes: glycoproteins and glycosaminoglycans (GAGs); with the GAGs combining to form larger molecules called proteoglycans. Examples include: chondroitin sulphate, dermatan sulphate, keratan sulphate, heparin, heparan sulphate, and hyaluronan (hyaluronic acid). About 20 per cent of tendons and ligaments is cellular, while about 80 per cent is extracellular; the extracellular component which is about 70 per cent water and 30 per cent solid, is mainly collagen proteins or fibres, with some elastin.

Function

Collagens provide tensile strength, resisting forces that tend to lengthen connective tissues. Elastin provides elasticity, allowing some connective tissues to return to their resting or ideal length. Ground substance acts as a lubricant, allowing collagen fibres to slide over one another and giving some pliability to the tissue; glue or filler holding the collagen fibres in place and adding to their strength; sponge pulling in water, and as the water is contained by the collagen fibres it helps resist compressive forces, especially useful in joint cartilage which needs to withstand weight bearing loads. Connective tissues that are subjected to large compressive forces have more proteoglycans, whereas connective tissues that resist tensile forces have less.

Collagens

Collagens are the most extensive proteins in the human body and are extremely strong. There are over 20 types of collagens in the body, but the most common are type I and type II, found in ligaments, tendons, menisci, joint capsules and intervertebral discs. Collagen fibres vary in size, shape and arrangement. They are not elastic but the arrangement of the collagen can give them elastic properties. Some collagens when relaxed form a wave like configuration called a crimp, which straighten when they are stretched out. The orientation of the collagen in the ligaments and tendons determines the ease at which the crimping will unravel and influences movement by limiting fibre elongation to only one direction before tensile stresses are experienced.

Deformation of collagen

During the first phase of stretching, the crimp phase, there is a considerably large amount of elongation or deformation for the amount of force applied but this progressively decreases as stretching continues. Similarly, when a muscle contracts with sufficient force, it straightens out the crimps in the tendon; when force is applied to a tendon it undergoes a linear elongation or

526

deformation. At the end of the crimp phase the amount of elongation decreases and thereafter a much greater force is required to produce the further elongation. Eventually the tendon fails. Initially, the straight parallel fibres fail and later the diagonally arranged fibres fail. First there is slippage between the molecules, then between the fibrils and eventually disruption of the collagen fibres.

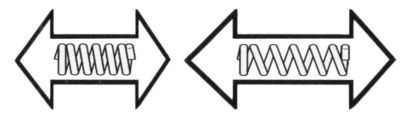

Collagen crimping orientation determines primary movement direction

Any slack in a tendon that is the result of the crimp, must be taken up by the muscle before the muscle can produce any movement at a bone through the tendon. During the second phase of stretching, the elastic phase, there is there is some give in the tendon but it is less than in the crimp phase. The elongation has an almost linear relationship with the force until the end of the elastic phase when any further force results in progressively less elongation. At this point, if the force is removed, the tendon or ligament will return to its initial length. In the third phase of deformation, the plastic phase, there is very little give in the tendon or ligament, and their ability to recovery will depend on their unique structure and the load applied. Ligaments in particular, but also cartilage, tendons and other types of fasciae, have viscoelastic properties, in that they regain their original shape following deformation. Depending on the viscoelastic properties of the individual tissue, the speed at which it returns to its pre-stretched length will vary.

Creep is a type of deformation that occurs in connective tissues and other viscoelastic materials when prolonged forces are applied slowly. The amount of deformation that is possible before failure occurs will depend on the amount, duration and speed of loading, the duration of rest, the type of tissue and where it is found in the body. It is greatest in ligaments, followed by tendons, deep fasciae, cartilage and bone. Creep is a time-dependent elongation of a tissue when subjected to a constant stress. It occurs as a result of a loss of fluid from within these tissues and the movement of long GAG chains in the solid matrix.

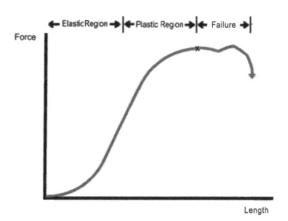

Viscoelastic deformation of tendons and ligaments

If any further force is applied, the tendon or ligament will move into the 'plastic' phase, where there is progressive failure of the collagen arrangement and they will no longer be able to return to their original length. Microfailure will eventually be followed by a macrofailure, where there is a tear in the tissue, a rupture in the middle of a tendon or ligament or an avulsion at the junction with a bone.

Elastin

Elastin is a yellow coloured protein, which as its name suggests is elastic and deforms when a force is applied and returns to its original state when the force is removed. Compared with collagen it makes up a much smaller part of the total amount of fibrous component of connective tissues, depending on the type of tissue and the location of that tissue. Elastin is most commonly found in the ligamentum nuchae and ligamentum flavum of the spine, the skin and the walls of arteries.

ELASTIN FIBRE

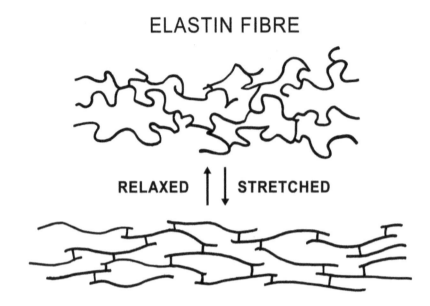

RELAXED ↑↓ STRETCHED

Elastin fibres and how they behave when relaxed or stretched

Ligaments

Ligaments connect bones to bones, enhance joint stability and guide joint motion in the correct direction. Like all connective tissue they have a cellular component and an extracellular component (about 80 per cent and is mainly type I collagen). They are usually distinct but sometimes they blend with joint capsules. They are named according to their location, shape, structures they connect, or sometimes after the person who discovered them.

The arrangement of the collagen in particular, but also other fibres and other materials within ligaments permits the ligament to resist forces from many different directions, including shearing and torsional forces, and for different parts of the ligament to tighten when the joint is in different positions. As a ligament merges with a bone, the materials, including the relative amount of materials, progressively change to allow for strength transition at these junctions.

Tendons

Tendons connect muscle to bone, transmit the force of muscle contraction to the bone and absorb and release energy. There is a progressive mineralisation of the tendon as it attaches onto the bone, and a progressive change into muscle at the myotendinous junction. Tendons have a small cellular component mostly of fibroblasts and a larger extracellular component, mainly type I collagen and small amounts of elastin and other collagens. The collagen is grouped together into bundles, and these are grouped together with small nerves and capillaries, to form larger bundles, which in turn are grouped together to form the tendon. Finally, the tendon may be surrounded by a synovial-filled sheath for reducing friction as the tendon moves over bone.

Tendons are made from long cylindrical structures with a tightly packed parallel arrangement of longitudinally running collagen fibres, which enables them to deal with strong unidirectional forces. They are usually very strong and rarely torn but they are weakest and most vulnerable to strain at the extremities such as myotendinous and osteotendinous junctions.

Tendons compared with ligaments

Both ligaments and tendons have a similar hierarchical structure of splitting into fascicles, fibrils, sub-fibrils and microfibrils but ligaments have smaller diameter collagen fibres than tendons. The collagen content in tendons is relatively high and is organised in a long axis direction, in contrast to ligaments where the collagen content is relatively low and is organised more randomly or in a cross weaving pattern. Elastin is found in varying amounts in ligaments but there is very little in tendons. Ligaments are more variable than tendons. Ligaments exhibit viscous and elastic behaviour which allows them to better deal with a range of different loads before failure. In addition to dealing with tensile forces like tendons they are also able to deal with compressive and shear forces.

The properties of tendons and ligaments and especially their ability to resist stretching depends on their location, use or lack of use, level of crimp, level of hydration, the relative amounts of different collagens and their organisation, including their level of cross-linking, the relative amounts of other materials in the matrix, the levels of hormones in the body, the age of the person and the presence of disease such as diabetes. The length, thickness and size of a ligament or tendon will determine the amount of force that it can resist and the amount of elongation that it can undergo. A ligament or tendon will grow thicker and stronger when subjected to regular stress.

Fascia

There are three types of fasciae: superficial fascia (subcutaneous tissue), deep fascia and visceral fascia. Sometimes the terms muscular fascia and visceral fascia are used in place of deep fascia and as subdivisions of deep fascia. When I am discussing fasciae in this book, then unless it is clearly stated as either superficial fascia or visceral fascia, then I am referring to the deep or muscular fascia, which surrounds muscles and other structures.

Superficial fasciae forms the deepest part of the subcutaneous layer of the skin. It is made up of a thin layer of loose fatty tissue, which helps to define the shape of a body including the outward features of the face and bind the skin to the reticular dermis layer below. It supports and helps protect glands, capillaries, lymph vessels and small nerves and acts as a padding to cushion and insulate. It stores fat and water and acts as a filler of otherwise unoccupied space. Visceral fascia is a thin, fibrous membrane that supports and suspends organs and glands, forms partitions between them and binds them together, as well as surrounding and connecting them to each other.

Deep fasciae is dense fibrous connective tissue that stabilises, encloses, and separates muscles, joins muscles to each other and assist tendons to attach muscles to bones. Deep fasciae contributes to a body wide tensional network of fibres forming many different types of connecting structures - tendons, ligaments, aponeurosis, retinaculae, muscle envelopes, septi and intramuscular fascia.

Fasciae in a general sense is continuous throughout the body, covering and penetrating every muscle, bone, nerve, artery, vein, lymph vessel, gland or organ in the body including the brain and spinal cord. It is made up of a combination of loose and/or dense fibres, mostly made from collagen, plus elastin and a small amount of other structural proteins.

The fibres within the dense fascia can be either unidirectional, like tendons or ligaments or multidirectional like aponeuroses and retinaculae; whereas the fibres in the loose fascia are usually multidirectional only. Fasciae requiring great strength in one direction are made from unidirectional dense fascia, fasciae requiring strength in multiple directions, are made from multidirectional dense fascia, whereas all other fascial structures are usually made from multidirectional loose fascia. Both types of dense fasciae are stronger and usually resistant to short term stretching, than multidirectional loose fascia, which has much greater variability in the different directions it can be stretched.

Healthy fasciae are elastic, storing kinetic energy, which is released as a dynamic recoil action with movement. The density and the directional alignment of the collagen fibres affect the strength and the flexibility of the fascia. Like with the crimping of ligaments and tendons, the collagen fibres are organised in a wavy pattern, oriented towards the direction of pull and it is this orientation which determines the elasticity of the facia. When the wavy pattern has been straightened out by the pulling force, the collagen fibres become aligned in a tight parallel orientation and any further lengthening of the fascia is resisted with great strength.

Fasciae has mainly a passive role of support and the transmission of forces. It serves as an expansive attachment for muscles to produce efficient joint movement, reduces friction between muscles, tendons and other structures, supports nerves and blood vessels as they pass through and between muscles, acts as a scaffolding supporting muscles and internal organs and helps maintain posture. Fascia may also have a weak dynamic role. Contractile cells have been found within fascia which may enable it to actively contract in an involuntary smooth muscle-like manner and influence musculoskeletal function.

Fasciae is adaptable and will change if there is demand placed upon it. Fibroblast cells remodel fasciae according to the mechanical loading and in general, greater loading will produce stronger and thicker fasciae. The rate of fibre replacement in fasciae is relatively high, with perhaps half of the fibres replaced in one year. So there is good potential for remodelling of fasciae.

A large volume of fasciae is made of water and the integrity of this tissue and other connective tissues is dependent on their levels of hydration. The amount of water in the tissues for example, determines their resistance to compressive forces. During exercise there is an exchange of water, some is pushed out and some returns, bringing with it essential nutrients and oxygen for the benefit of the fasciae. Rehydration and cellular nourishment is one of the great benefits of exercise, not only for fasciae, but for all tissues that are dependent on passive mechanisms of fluid and nutrient exchange, including intervertebral discs and cartilage.

The response of fasciae and other tissues to loading is dependent on the magnitude, speed and duration of loading and the history of prior loading. Loading includes both tissue compression and elongation; and beyond a specific threshold of increased loading there will be tissue failure. Tissue compression and elongation are time-dependent, and after a specific length of time, even moderate loading will cause tissue failure. This time-dependent loading is of course influenced by whether the compression and elongation stress is cyclic or constant.

Practical considerations

Exercise including stretching, helps maintain the viscous plasticity and elasticity of the fasciae and other tissues, but to get the greatest benefit from exercise, loading needs to be varied so that the fasciae can adapt appropriately. For example, a walk periodically during a running session will change the loading; by periodically resting the fasciae, it will permit rehydration, so that it can remain healthy and elastic for continued running. By avoiding continuous loading and varying the stresses on the fasciae, it regenerates better and maintains its structural integrity for longer, ultimately functioning better.

Proprioception is an essential component in movement. Fasciae is well endowed with proprioceptive cells, providing the brain with important feedback about the position of the body in space and the direction of movement; and these cells are essential for normal function. Proprioceptive cells tend to become less responsive during movements which are repetitive, as is common in many exercise systems such as running for example, hence it is important to vary the load, the speed and the direction of movement. When the brain is able to predict the loading situation being applied, the result is less benefit for fascial development. For optimal fascial stimulation, vary the type of loading, use a combination of slow and fast movements, and vary the direction of stress.

Exercises involving high velocity and moderately high loads are required for strengthening fasciae. This is in contrast to muscles which are strengthened with low velocity muscle contractions, such as in active stretching and light weight training. Fasciae needs to be sufficiently stressed in order to become stronger and more durable, and dynamic stretching which involves a bouncing action at the end of a quick movement is more appropriate for this. Dynamic stretching is better for developing fascial strength and elasticity, whereas static stretching is better for stretching muscles. Dynamic exercises, where the muscle is in a lengthened position are preferable for unidirectional fasciae, whereas multidirectional movements; varying the direction, and utilising sideways, rotational, spiral or diagonal forces, are better for stimulating the other types of fasciae found in the body.

Tennis is a good exercise for fascial development, and especially for the lateral fascia of the body. Sudden changes in direction, a focus on a difficult to predict external object (the ball), and a variety of movement directions (forward, backward, rotation and sideways) make tennis ideal for developing strength and elasticity in lateral fascia such as the abdominal aponeurosis, iliotibial band and the collateral ligaments of the lower limb.

Fast movements for fascial development have safety issues. Static stretches or slow dynamic movements should be used to warm up before attempting faster movements. Extreme jerky ballistic movements should be avoided in favour of more moderate techniques. Collagen remodelling does not need long periods of exercise – a few minutes of appropriate training a couple of times a day is sufficient, but it should be consistent. Remodelling is slow, and may take anywhere from a few months to one or two years, for more resilient fasciae to develop. The ultimate goal is to get the fascia to become stronger, more durable and adaptable to loading, and better able to maximise the storage of elastic energy and hence its recoil action, so muscles don't have to work as hard.

Muscle

A single muscle is made from many thousands of muscle fibres or cells forming the contractile part of the muscle and many different cells and materials forming the non-contractile part of the muscle. The number, size, type and arrangement of muscle fibres varies between muscles. The amount and type of collagen, as well as other materials that make up the non-contractile part of a muscle also varies between muscles, as does the ratio of contractile and non-contractile tissues. These as well as other structural differences, influence the mechanical properties of each muscle including its strength, how quickly it contracts and fatigues, its degree of elasticity and how it responds to stretching.

SKELETAL MUSCLE (cross section)

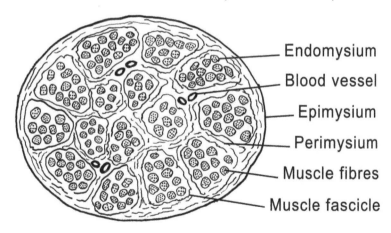

Transverse section of a muscle

Structure

Like most cells, muscles fibres have a cell membrane (sarcolemma) and a cytoplasm (sarcoplasm) with several nuclei. Muscle fibres contain mitochondria, ribosomes, glycogen, and various proteins such as enzymes for cell metabolism, and myofibrils, which are the contractile part of the cell.

The myofibrils are made up of two main proteins: actin and myosin. Two other proteins, tropomyosin and troponin work with actin to facilitate muscle contraction by regulating the binding of myosin cross-bridges to the actin filaments. Tropomyosin, with energy from ATP and the cyclic movement of calcium, enables the binding and breaking of the actin-myosin bonds, allowing the myosin head to 'walk' along the actin filament, thus producing muscle contraction. Titin (connectin) functions as a molecular spring and is a particularly important for the passive elasticity of muscle. The non-contractile components of muscle include: proteins such as elastin, dystrophin, fibronectin, talin, vinculin, desmin and structural glycoproteins such as collagen and laminin.

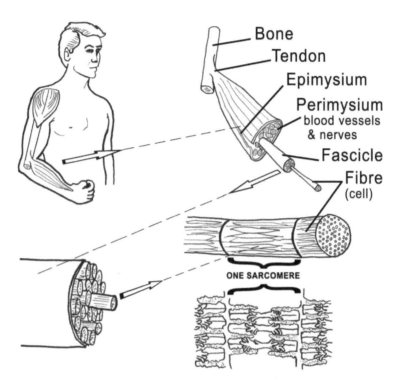

Muscle from macroscopic to microscopic level

Muscle fibres are surrounded by connective tissue called endomysium, which gives them support. In a pattern similar to tendons, muscle fibres and their surrounding endomysium are grouped together into bundles and covered by connective tissue called perimysium and in turn these are grouped together with nerves, capillaries and lymph vessel, to form larger bundles covered by connective tissue called epimysium. These envelop the entire muscle and merge with the deep fasciae, the aponeuroses and the tendon, all of which attach then attach to bones. Aponeuroses are sheets of dense white compact collagen fibres, which through their invagination within, and attachment around muscles and to bones, serve to more evenly distribute the forces generated by muscle contraction.

Function

Muscle is different from other tissues because it can generate force by itself. The functioning part of the muscle fibres are the interlocking actin and myosin cross-bridges already mentioned. During muscle contraction, these slide over one another making the fibre shorter and generating tension in the muscle. The tension may cause the muscle to lengthen, shorten, or remain the same depending on whether the contraction is concentric or eccentric, isotonic or isometric. Contractile muscle tissue also has the property of irritability, which is its ability to respond to chemical, electrical and mechanical stimuli.

The myosin molecule is shaped like a hockey stick, with the shaft of the hockey stick forming the sliding filament and the end of the hockey stick that hits the ball forming the head. It is this myosin head which interacts with the actin protein. The head is able to swivel and bind to different points along the actin molecule. At cellular level, the binding, breaking and rebinding of the myosin head enables the myosin to slide along the actin molecule; it is the combined effect of many of these actin-myosin molecules sliding on each other that produces the muscle contraction.

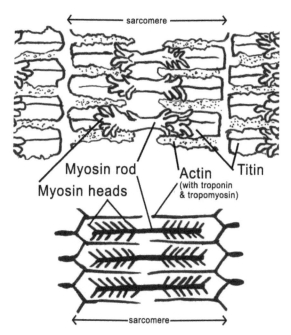

The functional unit of muscle contraction

Fast and slow fibres

Muscles fibres have been divided into slow-twitch and fast twitch, depending on how quickly they are able to convert energy into contraction. All muscles contain a mixture of slow-twitch and fast-twitch fibres, but some contain more of one type than another. For example soleus contains more slow-twitch fibres, while biceps brachii contains more fast-twitch fibres. As a consequence, muscles with greater numbers of one type of fibre will tend to exhibit more extremes of function and thus dysfunction.

Actin sliding on myosin filament

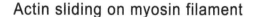

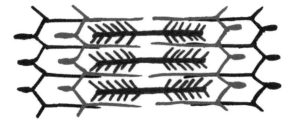

Muscles with a greater numbers of slow-twitch fibres are called tonic muscles. They are slow to contract but do not fatigue rapidly and as a result are better for stability and postural support. They are best suited to be continually active during erect standing and to make fine adjustments in body balance against the effects of gravity. Muscles with a greater numbers of fast twitch fibres are called phasic muscles. These are fast acting initially but fatigue rapidly and recover slowly, they are better for mobility; i.e. they generate large ranges of movement of body parts and non-postural activities.

As well as fibre type, many other factors also influence muscle function including fibre length, muscle length and cross sectional area, as well as the architecture of the muscle itself, for example, strap, pennate, fusiform and circular.

A muscle fibre is able to shorten to approximately half of its length. A long muscle fibre is able to shorten over a relatively greater distance than a short muscle fibre. But while this may be true for a strap or fusiform muscles whose fibres are organised parallel or nearly parallel, it does not hold true for pennate or spiral muscles, whose fibres are organised diagonally. The obliquity of these fibres will diminish the range of contraction because only a proportion of the force of a pennate muscle will go towards producing motion. Similarly, muscles with oblique fibres will be less able to elongate and therefore stretch.

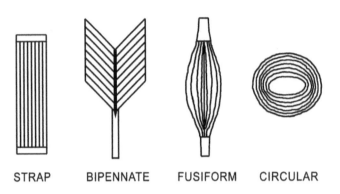

STRAP   BIPENNATE   FUSIFORM   CIRCULAR

Types of muscles by shape

Although the diagonal arrangement of the fibres reduces the total strength of a muscle, this is compensated for by the fact that more fibres can be packed into a pennate arrangement. Also when a muscle fibre contracts it acts via a bony lever and the length of the moment arm will also diminish the distance it is able to contract or elongate.

Muscle stretched/relaxed

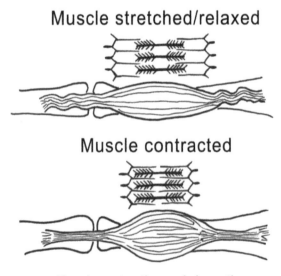

Muscle contracted

Muscle contraction and elongation

Other factors influencing the strength of a muscle contraction and the capacity of the muscle to lengthen through stretching, is the size of the muscle fibres and how many muscle fibres are packed side by side. The larger the muscle fibres and the more they are arranged in parallel, the stronger the contraction and the greater the resistance to elongation.

The connective tissue around muscle fibres is interconnected and forms the passive elastic component, a parallel system that shortens as the muscle fibres shorten with concentric contraction, or lengthen as the muscle fibres lengthen with eccentric contraction or active or passive stretching. In addition, there is the connective tissue at either end of the muscle fibres that forms the tendon and which functions in series with the contractile element.

When a muscle is at rest, the collagen fibres in the parallel connective tissue are slack. When a muscle is shortened, either through active concentric contraction or passive movement, the collagen fibres crimp and the parallel connective tissue becomes even slacker than in the resting position. When the muscle is lengthened through eccentric contraction or stretching, they become taut. When the elastic limit of the collagen has been reached, it becomes resistant to any further elongation. This passive resistance is one of several mechanism which helps to prevent injury from overstretching.

Types of muscle

1. Tonic or postural muscles – static muscles that maintain posture. Fibres are called upon constantly for ongoing activity. They contract slowly, are slow to fatigue but quickly recover. Slow-twitch speed and slow to fatigue (Type 1 fibres)
Metabolism is oxidative. Capillary density is high
React to disturbance by shortening or tightening – facilitation and hypertonicity
Colour is red (dark) because of large amounts of myoglobin
There is a greater number of mitochondria
Examples: Pelvis/Hip = Hamstrings, Iliopsoas, Rectus femoris, TFL and Piriformis
Trunk = Erector spinae, especially lumbar and cervical, Quadratus lumborum and Scalenes
Legs Gastrocnemius, Soleus. Shoulder = Pectoralis major, Levator Scapulae, Sternocleidomastoid, Latissimus dorsi, Subscapularis, Upper trapezius and Biceps brachii
Dysfunctional tonic or postural muscles tend to become hypertonic, short and tight.

2. Phasic muscles – dynamic muscles that provide movement. Fibres are at rest a lot of the time but are frequently called on for brief bouts of intense activity. They can contract quickly but are fast to fatigue and slow to recover.
Fast-twitch speed and quick to fatigue (Type2A and 2B fibres)
Metabolism is glycolytic. Capillary density is low
React to disturbance by weakening – inhibition and hypotonicity.
Colour is lighter red because there is less myoglobin. Also there are fewer mitochondria.
Examples: Pelvis/Hip = Vastus medialis and lateralis, Gluteus maximus, medius and minimus. Trunk = Erector spinae, especially thoracic, Rectus abdominis and obliques
Legs = Tibialis anterior and Peroneus muscles. Shoulder = Rhomboid, Lower trapezius, Triceps brachii. Dysfunctional phasic muscles tend to become weak and inhibited.

The tendon is that part of the connective tissue in series with the muscle. So when muscle fibres contract eccentrically, concentrically, or isometrically or are stretched, this exerts a pull on the tendon. Only about 3 per cent of the muscle contraction takes up slack in the tendon, the rest pulls on or actually moves the bone. In other words, there is very little muscle contraction lost stretching the tendon and most of the muscle force is used moving the bony lever. Only when a muscle is relaxed in a shortened position is there no tension on the tendon.

Stretching muscle

Stretching involves a combination of biomechanical and neurological mechanisms.

Biomechanical mechanisms

When a muscle is loaded, it can have passive or active tension or a combination of both. Passive tension is the result of the viscoelastic properties of the non-contractile part of the muscle, whereas active tension is the result of the resistance offered by actin and myosin filaments in the contractile part of the muscle.

Passive tension

If a tissue is subjected to brief periods of relatively light loading such as with safe stretching, the tissue will return to its original length when the force is no longer applied. One of the benefits of stretching is as a result of this passive uncoiling of muscle and its surrounding connective tissue. Short periods of stretching or isometric contraction, also affects the water content of connective tissue, acting like squeezing a sponge, which stimulates the movement of water and nutrients into the tissue, and wastes out of the tissue.

When a tissue is subjected to strong forces or long periods of loading, such as during prolonged holding of a poor posture, then this may result creep. There is slow elongation or permanent deformation of the tissues depending on the viscoelastic properties of the individual material. Creep results in loss of energy or hysteresis and repeated loading before the tissue has recovered will result in deformation. Continued loading will result in plastic changes and eventual remodelling of the tissue at a longer length. Depending on the magnitude of the applied stress and its duration, the deformation may become so large that a tissue can no longer perform its function.

Active tension

When a muscle is actively stretched, the overlapping actin-myosin filaments move apart. They slide apart following the normal physiological mechanism of eccentric isotonic muscle contraction, facilitated by reciprocal inhibition. When a muscle is passively stretched the actin-myosin filaments are physically pulled apart. Neurological and mechanical resistance to stretching is countered using slow movement or the use of isometric contraction prior to stretching to inhibit or help neutralise the stretch reflex so that the actin-myosin filaments are not damaged. This is the typical short-term reversible mechanism for stretching tense muscles.

In order to bring a very short muscle to a longer resting length it may be necessary to stretch the muscle more strongly. Micro-tearing of the muscle fibres will occur as the actin-myosin bonds are broken, forcing these filaments are forced apart. This may sound drastic but micro-tearing and cellular repair is the classical longer-term mechanism for stretching chronically short muscles. Micro-tearing is a natural process and part of many exercise systems, for example the pain after a workout at the gym. After strong stretching, the actin-myosin filament regrow with the muscle remaining in a longer resting state.

The sarcomere is the basic functional unit of a muscle. In most muscles repeated or prolonged stretching causes proteins to be synthesised within the muscle, leading to the formation of additional sarcomeres. This means the muscle grows or hypertrophies and becomes stronger. Muscle remodelling not only allows the muscle to grow longer but there can be changes in muscle cell metabolism in some muscles. In contrast, prolonged shortening of a muscle causes the loss of sarcomeres, muscle atrophy and weakness.

When a muscle is in an elongated or stretched state, there is minimal overlapping between the actin-myosin filaments and little cross-bridging can occur. When a muscle is in a fully shortened or contracted state, there is full overlapping between the actin-myosin filaments and there is saturated cross-bridging. Maximum muscle tension and active muscle contraction are only possible between the two extremes of muscle elongation and shortening, in other words, when there is sufficient overlap between the actin-myosin filaments for more cross-bridging to occur but not complete overlap so no more cross-bridging is possible.
In contrast to the contractile component where maximum tension is midway between full contraction and full stretch, in the noncontractile part of the muscle maximum passive tension increases progressively as the muscle is elongated. So when the contractile and noncontractile parts of the muscle are combined, the point of maximum tension and contraction would lie between these two points. This is also the point with the greatest resistance to stretching.

Active insufficiency occurs when a muscle has a diminishing capacity to develop isometric tension and power, either because it is too short or because it is too long. Other factors affecting the tension that can be developed within a muscle include the total length of the fibre within the muscle, the shape of the muscle, the changing angle between muscle and bone, whether the contraction is concentric or eccentric, and whether it is acting over a single or multiple joints.

Neurological mechanism

Sensory receptors like Golgi tendon organs and muscle spindles are feedback mechanisms protecting muscles against injury. Golgi tendon organs are located in the tendon, close to the myotendinous junction and are sensitive to tension either from active muscle contraction or stretching. Muscle spindles are located within muscles and are sensitive to changes in muscle length, and the rate of change of length or its velocity. A muscle spindle is a special type of muscle fibre known as an intrafusal fibre, in contrast to extrafusal fibres, which are muscle cells responsible for primary muscle contaction.

When a muscle is lengthened as it is stretched, these sensory receptors monitor the changes that take place within the muscle and tendon, sending messages to the brain so that the muscle can respond appropriately. If stretching is too strong, too quick or unexpected, then the muscle spindle can activate a stretch reflex in the muscle. The stretch reflex, also known as the myotatic reflex, is an involuntary muscle contraction in response to stretching of the muscle and is for preventing injury.

As stretching increases, the resistance offered by a muscle increases. Some of this resistance is due to the elastic recoil of the noncontractile passive structures within the muscle and some is due to neurological mechanisms such as the stretch reflex within the contractile structures of the muscle.

The stretch reflex can be a problem for fitness programs like stretching, where it is necessary to lengthen a muscle to restore range of movement. Stretch receptors can impede effective stretching, especially when there is a high level of irritability in a muscle such as in a spastic torticollis.

Post isometric theory

Post-isometric relaxation is the reduction in tone of a muscle after an isometric contraction. It is a natural, protective mechanism that may help prevent injury. Isometric contraction is sometimes used before stretching because it relaxes muscles thus enabling greater lengthening of muscles and increased range of movement at joints. It may also help decrease local swelling and pain and increase strength in weak muscles. Precise positioning at the point of initial resistance and at the pain free barrier is important, as is the intensity of isometric muscle contraction, which should be between 10 per cent and 20 per cent of maximum contraction force, depending on the joints.

Various mechanisms by which post-isometric contraction facilitate relaxation and stretching have been proposed. Although these theories have been used by multiple sources, there is no evidence or published proof to support them. The most promising explanation is the post-synaptic theory, also known as the autogenic inhibition or refractory theory, which says that immediately after an isometric contraction the neuromuscular mechanism is in a refractory or relaxed state and passive stretching may be done without triggering the stretch reflex.

According to this theory, the isometric muscle contraction activates the Golgi tendon organs causing them to override the impulses from the muscle spindle. This causes a type of reflex relaxation and this neuromuscular inhibition can reduce the tone of the muscle for up to five seconds. The resisted muscle contraction results in an increased electromyographic (EMG) response followed by an electrical silent period.

During a mild isometric contraction, only a small proportion of the muscle fibres contract. There is no partial contraction of muscle fibres, muscle fibres either contract fully or they don't contract. The few muscle fibres that fully contract increase tension in the tendon, thereby activating the Golgi tendon organ which is situated at the muscle-tendon junction in series with the muscle. This causes a reduction in tension in the non-contractile connective tissue and the majority of muscle fibres that do not contract, causing an inhibition of the muscle spindles, which are all situated in the muscle in parallel with the contracting muscle fibres.

According to theory, post-isometric relaxation works because of the difference in tension between the tissues arranged in parallel with the contacting muscle fibres and the tissues arranged in series with the contacting muscle fibres. The difference is compensated for by the Golgi tendon organ inhibiting the muscle spindle, thereby relaxing the muscle. The logic also extends to additional receptors being involved: as resistance to movement would have stimulated other receptors in muscles, joints, connective tissues and cutaneous tissues, these may also be involved in the post-isometric relaxation mechanism.

Anatomy of the face, head and jaw 1.1 – 1.2

Muscles of facial expression

Occipitofrontalis covers the dome of the skull and is formed by two thin broad muscles, frontalis and occipitalis connected to an aponeurotic sheet, the galea aponeurotica.

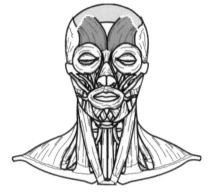

Frontalis is formed by two quadrilateral muscles. Their posterior border attaches to the anterior aponeurosis just in front of the coronal suture. Anteriorly they merge with the muscles of the superior orbit: the procerus, corrugator supercilii and orbicularis oculi. There are no bony attachments.

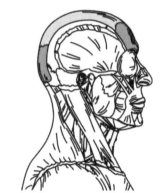

Occipitalis is formed by two quadrilateral muscles attached to the posterior aponeurosis and to the lateral two thirds of the highest nuchal line of the occiput and to the mastoid of the temporal bone.

Actions: Pulls scalp forwards and backwards, raises brow and wrinkles forehead.
Clinical indications: Headaches, scalp injuries, eye strain.

Nerve supply: The facial nerve.

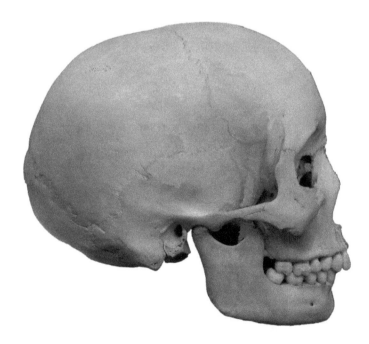

The skull – lateral view of mandible maxilla, frontal, parietal, temporal, sphenoid, occiput, ethmoid, lacrimal, nasal and zygomatic bones

538

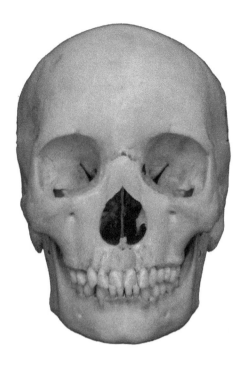

The skull – anterior view of mandible, maxilla, frontal, ethmoid, lacrimal, nasal and zygomatic bones

Orbicularis oculi has orbital, palpebral and lacrimal parts. Fibres encircle the orbit and occupy the upper cheek, temple, eyelids and lacrimal bone. The orbital part arises on the frontal process of the maxilla and the nasal part of the frontal bone. The palpebral part arises on the medial palpebral ligament and inserts into the corner of eye. The lacrimal part arises on the orbital surface of the lacrimal bone and inserts on the superior and inferior tarsi.

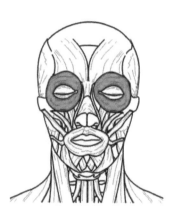

Actions: The muscle closes the eyes and eyelids. The parts can work independently of each other. The palpebral portion can act voluntarily or involuntarily, as in blinking.

Levator palpebræ superioris raises the upper eyelid and exposes the eyeball and is the antagonist to orbicularis oculi.

Orbicularis oris is a complex of muscles in the lips that encircle the mouth. The muscle arises from other muscles some of which attach on the maxilla and mandible bones.

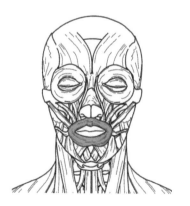

Actions: The muscle is responsible for bringing the lips together, puckering the lips and pressing the lips against the teeth. It is sometimes referred to as the kissing muscle and it is involved in playing music instruments such as the trumpet.

539

Zygomaticus minor and **major** arise from the zygomatic bone and pass inferiorly and medially and to merges into the fibres of orbicularis oculi and the other muscles in the outer part of the upper lip and the angle of the mouth.

Actions: These muscles draw the upper lip backward, upward, and outward.

Nerve supply: All the muscles of facial expression are innervated by branches of the facial nerve (CN VII).

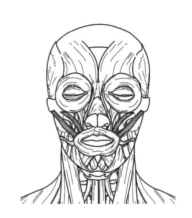

Muscles of mastication

Temporalis arises from most of the temporal fossa and from the deep surface of temporal fascia. The fibres from this fan-shaped muscle converge on a tendon which passes under the zygomatic arch and attaches on the coronoid process and the anterior border of the ramus of the mandible. Strong temporal fascia covers the muscle.

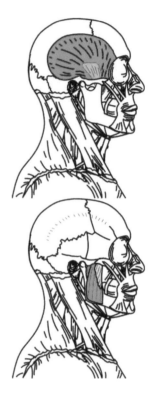

Masseter arises on the zygomatic arch and attaches to the lateral ramus and angle of the mandible. The quadrilateral muscle has three layers and is covered by and connected to a layer of fascia, the parotid fascia. Some of the deep fibres also attach on the coronoid process. The strong overlying fascia makes temporalis and masseter difficult to palpate unless they are contracted.

Actions: Closes jaw in biting, chewing and speech.
Clinical indications: Dental treatment, malocclusion, neurosis, bruxism and other overuse syndromes.

Nerve supply: Trigeminal nerve mandibular division

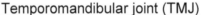
Temporomandibular joint (TMJ)

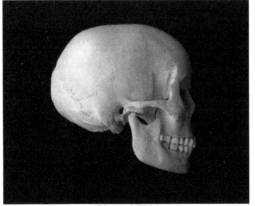
Closed TMJ

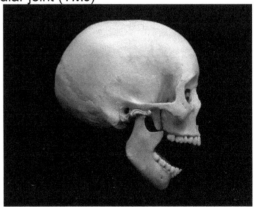
Open TMJ

Lateral pterygoid lies superiorly to the medial pterygoid and is just palpable deep in the buccal cavity. The muscle has two heads. The upper head arises on the infratemporal crest of the greater wing of the sphenoid bone and the lower head arises on the lateral surface of the lateral pterygoid plate. The muscle attaches on the neck of the condyle of the mandible and the articular disc of the temporomandibular joint.

Actions: The muscle acts to open the jaw, protrude the jaw and move the jaw from side to side and controls the disc during opening and closing.

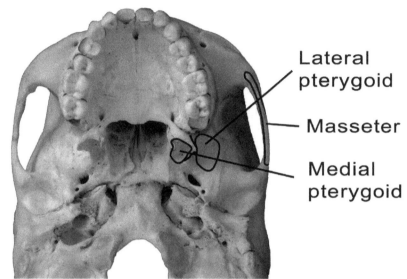

The skull - inferior view with mandible removed showing maxilla, palatine, sphenoid, zygomatic, occipital and temporal bones and muscle attachments

Medial pterygoid arises on the medial surface of the lateral pterygoid plate of the sphenoid bone, the pyramidal process of the palatine bone and the tuberosity of maxilla. It attaches on the posterior and inferior part of the medial surface of the ramus of the mandible and the angle of the mandible. It assists in closing the jaw.

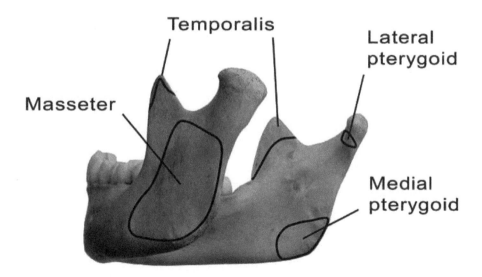

The mandible – posterior inferior and lateral view showing muscle attachments

The tongue

Muscles fibres attach on the hyoid, mandible, styloid process of the temporal bone and the soft palate and the pharynx.

Actions: The intrinsic muscles alter the shape of the tongue for deglutition, taste and speech. The superior longitudinal muscle fibres shorten the tongue and turn the tip and sides upwards, the inferior longitudinal muscle fibres shorten the tongue and pull the tip downwards, the transverse muscle fibres narrow and elongate the tongue and the vertical muscle fibres flatten and widen the tongue.

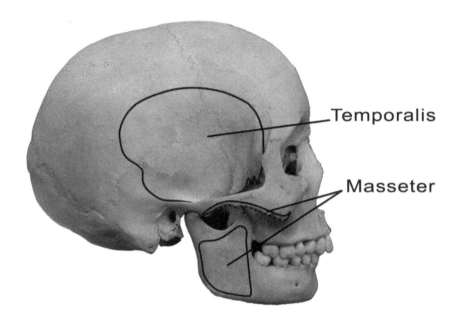

The skull – lateral view showing muscle attachments

The temporomandibular joint

An articular disc sits within the temporomandibular joint and during movement the mandibular condyles roll and glide over the disc and across the mandibular fossa of the temporal bone. The disc facilitates movement between each condyle and the articulating surfaces of the temporal bones. The discs sits behind articular tubercles and movement ceases as the condyles approach the articular tubercles.

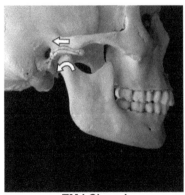 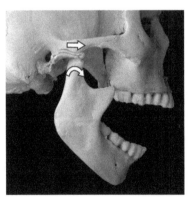 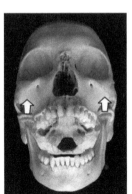

TMJ Closed   **TMJ Open**

Anatomy of the suboccipital and cervical spine 1.3 – 1.9

The suboccipital spine

The suboccipital muscles are a group of small muscles covered by semispinalis capitis and trapezius medially and sternocleidomastoid and splenius and longissimus capitis laterally and by fascia and dense adipose tissue

From medial to lateral these consist of:
1. **Rectus capitis posterior minor** running from the inferior nuchal line of the occiput to the tubercle of the posterior arch of the atlas.

2. **Rectus capitis posterior major** running from the inferior nuchal line of the occiput to the spinous process of the axis (C2).

3. **Obliquus capitis inferior** running from the posterior margin of the transverse process of the atlas to the spinous process of the axis.

4. **Obliquus capitis superior** running from the inferior nuchal line of the occiput to posterior margin of the transverse process of the atlas.

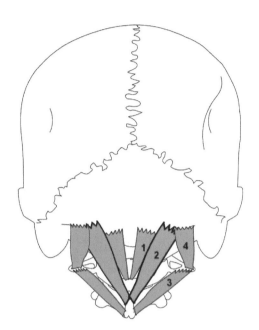

Actions: Extension of the head is produced by rectus capitis posterior major and minor and rotation is produced by obliquus capitis superior and inferior. The atlas has a large transverse process which provides a good mechanical advantage for obliquus capitis inferior to rotate the atlas on the axis.
Nerve supply: Dorsal ramus of the first spinal nerve (C1).

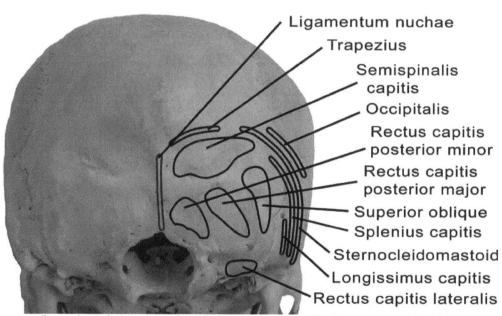

Posterior inferior view of skull showing muscle attachments on occiput for sternocleidomastoid, trapezius and posterior cervical muscles

Atlas and axis

Atlas (C1) and Axis (C2) as individual vertebrae and shown articulating
Top row – Atlantoaxial combination   Middle row – Atlas   Bottom row – Axis

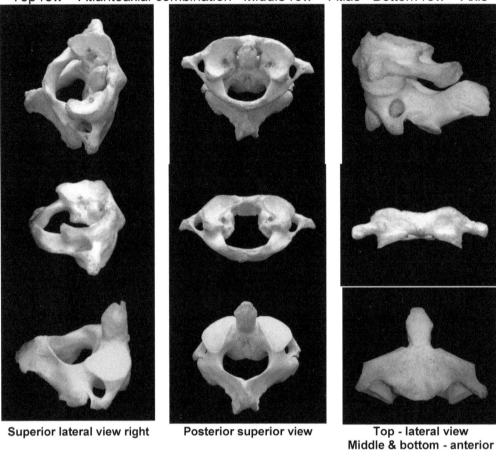

Superior lateral view right   **Posterior superior view**   **Top - lateral view**
Middle & bottom - anterior

Cervical prevertebral structures

The carotid tubercle is the anterior tubercle of the transverse process of C6. It is a useful landmark on the anterior aspect of the cervical spine and relatively easy to palpate. Palpate unilaterally so as not to occlude the carotid arteries. Trachea rings descend until disappearing under the suprasternal notch.

Suboccipital spine – occiput, atlas and axis

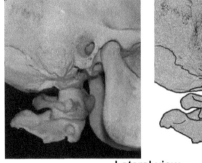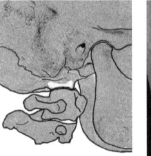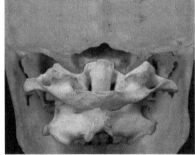

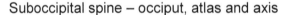

Lateral view   **posterior view**

The transverse process of C1 is palpable between the mastoid process and the angle of the mandible. The transverse process of C2 is level with the angle of the jaw. Except for C1 the cervical transverse processes are not easily palpable. Anterior and posterior tubercles follow a line down the lateral cervical spine from C1 down to the middle of the clavicle.

Prevertebral muscles

The **longus capitis** arise on the anterior tubercles of the transverse processes of C3 to C6. The fibres run superiorly and medially over the anterior bodies of the cervical spine and attach onto the basilar part of the occipital bone. The muscle flexes the head.
Nerve supply: Branches from the ventral rami of C1, C2 and C3 spinal nerves.

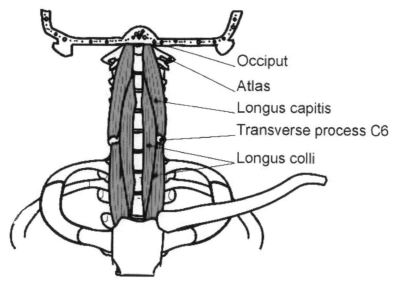

Occiput
Atlas
Longus capitis
Transverse process C6
Longus colli

Prevertebral muscles

The **longus colli** is in three parts. The *inferior oblique fibres* arise on the bodies of T1 to T3 and run superiorly and laterally over the anterior bodies of the cervical spine to attach on the anterior tubercles of the transverse processes of C5 and C6. The *superior oblique fibres* arise on the anterior tubercles of the transverse processes of C3 to C5 and run superiorly and medially over the anterior bodies of the cervical spine and attach on the tubercle of the anterior arch of C1. The *vertical fibres* arise from in front of the bodies of C5 to T3 and run superiorly to attach in front of the bodies of C2 to C4.

Actions: The muscle flexes the cervical spine. The oblique fibres may have a weak sidebending action and the inferior oblique fibres produce contralateral rotation of the spine.
Nerve supply: Branches from the ventral rami of C3, C4, C5 and C6 spinal nerves.

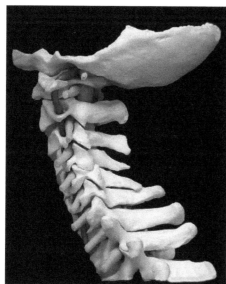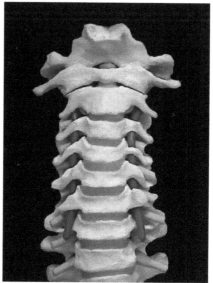

Cervical spine - lateral view (left) anterior view (right)

545

The **rectus capitis anterior** arises on the lateral mass and the root of the transverse process of the atlas and attaches on the basilar part of the occipital bone. The **rectus capitis lateralis** arises on the upper surface of the transverse process of the atlas and attaches on the jugular process of the temporal bone.

Actions: Rectus capitis anterior produces head flexion and rectus capitis lateralis produces ipsilateral sidebending of the head
Nerve supply: Branches from the ventral rami of C1 and C2 spinal nerves.

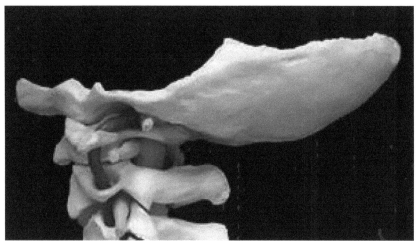

Suboccipital spine - occiput, upper cervical spine, cord, nerves and artery

The cervical prevertebral muscles are thin and deep to the larynx and not easily palpable. These small anterior suboccipital and prevertebral muscles may be strained when subject to whiplash injuries such as from car accidents.

Superior and inferior hyoid muscles

The hyoid muscles arise on the mandible, mastoid process and styloid process, and attach on the clavicle and manubrium via the hyoid. The superior hyoid muscles are palpable in the soft area within the U shape of the mandible, and between the mandible and hyoid. The inferior hyoid muscles are palpable as a thin superficial layer on the anterior of the neck.

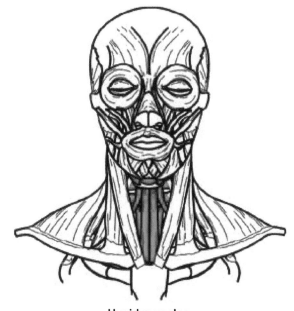

Hyoid muscles

The hyoid bone is U shaped and level with C3. The lateral cornua is palpable under the mandible. Thyroid cartilage is level with C4 and C5. It is more prominent in males and easily palpable. The cricoid cartilage is level with C6 and is palpable. The hyoid muscles are covered by a layer of deep fascia, the sheet-like platysma muscle and by superficial fascia. The deep fascia invests the vessels, glands and muscles in the region.

Actions: The hyoid muscles are involved in speech, mastication and swallowing. Digastric and mylohyoid depress the mandible or elevate the hyoid; stylohyoid elevates the hyoid or in combination with other muscles, fixes the hyoid; omohyoid depresses the hyoid; and thyrohyoid depresses the hyoid or raises the larynx.
Clinical indications: Whiplash, singing or speaking overuse and the local effects of infection.

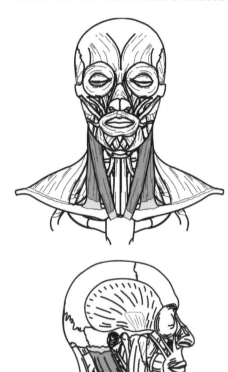

Sternocleidomastoid arises by two heads, one from the manubrium part of the sternum and the other from an upper area of the medial third of the clavicle. Fibres from the two heads spiral and merge but much of the clavicular part attaches on the mastoid process as a strong tendon and much of the sternal part attaches on the lateral half of the superior nuchal line of the occiput as a thin aponeurosis. Platysma and deep cervical fascia cover the muscle.

Actions: Acting with longus colli bilateral contraction of sternocleidomastoid produces head and neck flexion. When longus colli is relaxed bilateral contraction produces head extension and neck flexion. When one sternocleidomastoid contracts it sidebends the head and neck to one side and rotates them to the other. When acting with other muscles, sternocleidomastoid produces level rotation.

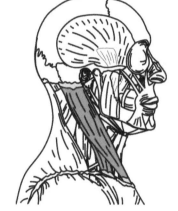

Nerve supply: Accessory nerve and ventral rami of the second, third and sometimes fourth cervical spinal nerves.
Clinical indications: Torticollis.

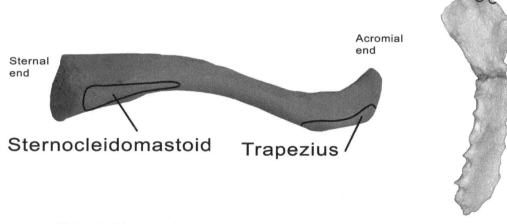

Right clavicle - superior view and muscle attachments　　**Sternum**

Scalene

Anterior Scalene arises from the anterior tubercles of transverse processes of C3 to 6 and attaches on the scalene tubercle and on a ridge on the upper surface of rib 1. It lies behind sternocleidomastoid and in front of the brachial plexus and subclavian artery.

Middle Scalene arises from the posterior tubercles of transverse processes of C2 to 7 and attaches on the upper surface of rib 1. Sometimes fibres arise from the atlas. The brachial plexus and subclavian artery lie between it and the anterior scalene. The posterior scalene and levator scapulae are posterolateral to it.

Posterior Scalene arises from the posterior tubercles of transverse processes of C5 to 7 and attaches on rib 2.

The scalene muscles exhibit some variation in the number and levels of cervical vertebrae to which they attach.

Actions: The scalene raise the upper ribs and sidebend the cervical spine to the same side.

Clinical indications: Chronic respiratory diseases such as asthma or bronchitis. Changes in the muscles may compromise the function of nerves derived from the brachial plexus and circulation to the upper limb.

Nerve supply: Cervical nerves from the cervical plexus C1-4 supplies neck muscles and skin.

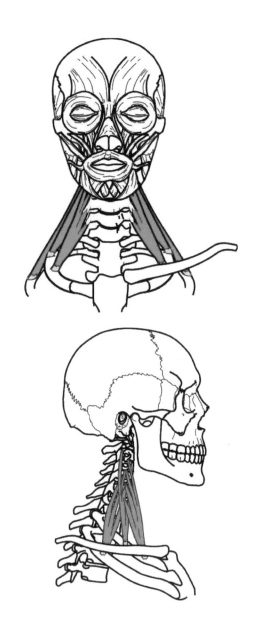

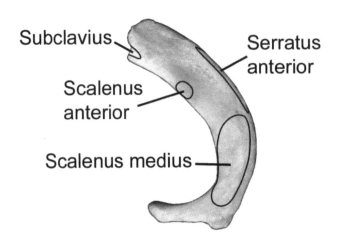

Right Rib 1 – superior view and muscle attachments

548

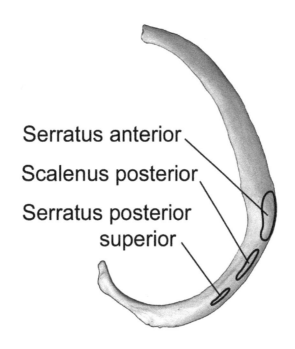

Right Rib 2 – superior view and muscle attachments

Posterior cervical muscles

Splenius capitis arises on the ligamentum nuchae and spinous processes of C7 to T3 and attaches under the lateral part of the superior nuchal line of the occiput and on the mastoid process of the temporal bone.
Nerve supply: Lateral branches of the dorsal rami of the middle cervical spinal nerves.

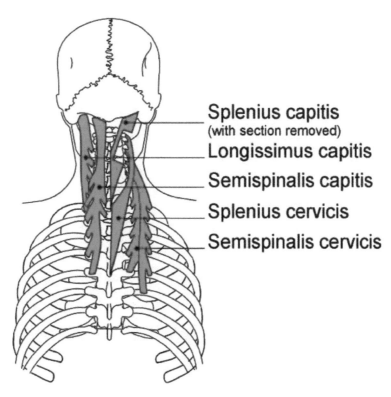

Posterior head, ribs, cervical and thoracic spine

Splenius cervicis arises on the spinous processes of T3 to T6 and attach on the posterior tubercles of the transverse process C1 to T3.

Splenius capitis and splenius cervicis lie deep to sternocleidomastoid, trapezius and the rhomboids and superficial to the segmental muscles, interspinales, intertransversarii and transversospinalis.

Nerve supply: Lateral branches of the dorsal rami of the lower cervical spinal nerves.
Actions: Splenius capitis and splenius cervicis contracting bilaterally extend the head and neck, contracting unilaterally they sidebend and slightly ipsilaterally rotate the head and neck.

Transversospinalis
Semispinalis thoracis arises on the transverse processes of T6 to T10 and attaches on the spinous processes of C6 to T4. More tendinous in form.
Semispinalis cervicis arises on the transverse processes of T1 to T6 and attaches on the spinous processes of C2 to C5. More muscular especially the fibres that attach on the axis.
Semispinalis capitis arises on the transverse processes of C7 to T6 and the articular processes of C4 to C6 (sometimes C7 and T1) and attaches either side of the mid-sagittal line between the superior and inferior nuchal lines on the occiput.

Action: Extension of the head and cervical spine.
Nerve supply: Dorsal rami of cervical and thoracic nerves.

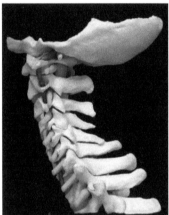 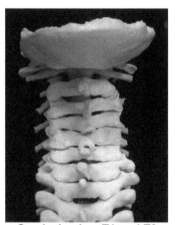

Cervical spine, T1 and T2
side view

Cervical spine, T1 and T2
posterior view

Multifidus arise on the sacrum down as far as S4, the aponeurosis of the erector spinae, posterior superior iliac spine, posterior sacroiliac ligament, mamillary processes of L1 to L5, transverse processes of T1 to T12 and articular processes of C4 to C7. The muscle runs obliquely superiorly and medially and attaches along the length of a spinous process one to four vertebral segments above, as high up as C2.
Nerve supply: Dorsal rami of the spinal nerves.

Interspinales (interspinalis) run from one spinous process to the spinous process above. They are present between C2 and T3, and between T11 and L5. They are more distinct in the cervical spine. Sometimes they occur between L5 and the sacrum.
Nerve supply: Dorsal rami of the spinal nerves.

Intertransversarii run from a transverse process to the transverse process above. They are present between C1 and T1, and between T10 and the sacrum. In the cervical and lumbar, pairs of muscles lie either side of the spine.
Nerve supply: Dorsal and ventral rami of the spinal nerves.

Erector spinae
Upper erector spinae muscles with cervical attachment include **iliocostalis cervicis, longissimus cervicis and spinalis cervicis.** Muscle fibres run between ribs, transverse

process and spinous processes of cervical and upper thoracic vertebra. Deep cervical fascia covers the erector spinae and separates the individual muscle. The fascia attaches to the superior nuchal line of the occipital bone and the ligamentum nuchae and is a continuation of the thoracolumbar fascia inferiorly.

The ligamentum nuchae is the continuation of the supraspinous ligaments connecting the spinous processes of the thoracic and lumbar vertebrae below. It arises on the external occipital protruberance and external occipital crest runs inferiorly and attaches onto the spinous process of the C7 vertebra. It also attaches on the posterior tubercle of the atlas and the all cervical spinous processes. It is a fibro-elastic membrane and septum for the attachment of muscles on both side of the neck. It is not distinctly palpable but in flexion is on tension.

Some or all of the spinous processes of the vertebrae between C2 and C7 may be bifid. C7 is known as vertebra prominens and has a large spine and is easily palpable. C6 is usually just palpable but disappears in extension.

The articular pillars are palpable running down the posterior cervical spine lateral to the spinous processes. Facet joints run down the length of the articular pillars at about finger-width spacings and are useful as diagnostic landmarks.

Clinical indications: Whiplash, postural changes, torticollis, degenerative arthritic changes and congenital defects.

Upper shoulder muscles

Trapezius arises on aponeurosis firmly anchored at the midline to the occipital bone and the external occipital protuberance, the medial one third of the superior nuchal line of the occiput, the ligamentum nuchae, and the spinous processes and supraspinous ligaments of vertebra C7 to T12.

Posterior view of skull, ribs, scapula, upper humerus, cervical and upper thoracic spine

Lateral view of skull, ribs 1 & 2 cervical & upper thoracic spine

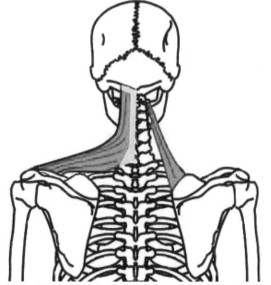

Upper Trapezius (left) & Levator Scapulae (right)

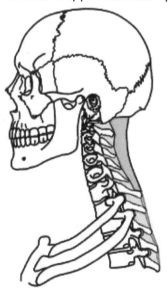

Supraspinous and interspinous ligaments & ligamentum nuchae

The triangular sheet of trapezius wraps around the shoulder and converges on a U shaped area of the clavicle acromion and spine of the scapula. The superior fibres attach on the posterior border of the lateral third (sometimes half) of the clavicle; the middle fibres attach on the medial side of the acromion and a superior line along the spine of scapula. The inferior fibres merge into an aponeurosis which converges to attach on a tubercle near the medial end of the spine of the scapula. During scapulothoracic movement this aponeurosis slides over the flat triangular surface at the medial end of the spine as the scapula rotates around the tubercle.

Actions: When the scapula is fixed and the upper fibres contract bilaterally they extend the head, when they contract unilaterally they produce ipsilateral sidebending and contralateral rotation of the head and neck. When the head is fixed they elevate the scapula. The middle and lower fibres stabilise, retract or rotate (upward tilt) the scapular and this is covered in 4.0 Anatomy of the shoulder.
Nerve supply: Accessory nerve (Cranial nerve 11).

Levator scapulae lies deep to trapezius. Its tendons arise from the transverse processes of the atlas and axis, and the posterior tubercles of the transverse processes of C3 and C4. The muscle attaches to the medial border of the scapula, between the superior angle and the spine of scapula. Vertebral attachments vary and fibres may attach onto the occiput, mastoid process, rib 1 and 2 and merge with adjacent muscles.

Actions: The muscle moves the scapular and stabilises it when the upper limb is active. It strongly elevates the scapula and is active when carrying a load. With other muscles it draws the scapula medially and rotates the scapula so that the glenoid points down. Levator scapulae extends, ipsilaterally rotates, sidebends and helps stabilise the cervical spine.
Nerve supply: C3 and C4 and via the dorsal scapular nerve to C5.
Clinical indications: Overuse, headaches, whiplash injuries, torticollis.

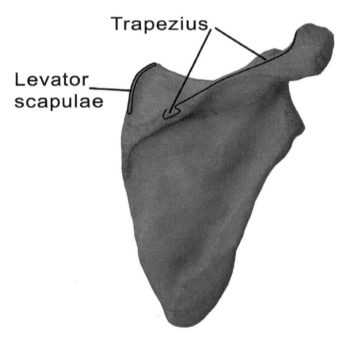

Scapula – posterior view and muscle attachments

Joint movement

Upper cervical spine

The shape of a joint determines its range of movement and the type of movement that it can produce. The atlantoaxial and the atlanto-occipital joints are uniquely structured to facilitate fine movements of the head, and can compensate for unwanted movements and postural imbalances from below.

The atlantoaxial joint is mainly concerned with the rotation of the head, and a small amount of flexion and extension. The atlanto-occipital joint is mainly concerned with flexion and extension of the head such as in nodding yes, and some sidebending and rotation.

The atlanto-occipital joint is between the condyle of the occipital bone and the superior articular facet of the lateral mass of the atlas. They are like two curved bowls sitting snugly within one other. The inferior facing convex occipital joints or condyles sit on the superior facing concave joints of the atlas.

As the head nods forward into flexion the condyles of the occiput slide backward on the atlas. As the head nods backward into extension the condyles of the occiput slide forward on the atlas. This sliding action also occurs during sidebending of the head.

Lateral view of the occiput, atlas and axis

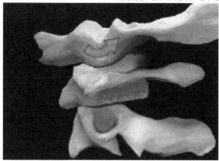 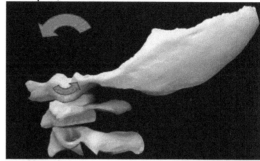

Flexion or Nutation

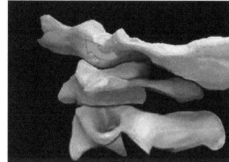 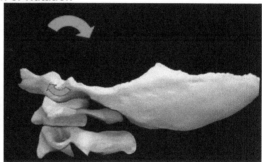

Extension or Counter Nutation

The atlantoaxial joint is between the atlas and the axis. At the front of the atlas and axis are two interlocking cylindrical structures. The odontoid process is the inside cylinder. It projects upwards like a peg from the front of the axis. The outer cylinder is formed by the anterior arch of the atlas and the transverse ligament. The odontoid process sits in the cartilage lined ring formed by the atlas and ligament and when the obliquus capitis inferior muscle contracts it turns the atlas on the axis and this produced rotation of the atlas and the head - the two cylinders turn around each other.

Atlantoaxial joint and rotation

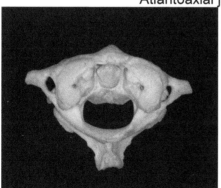 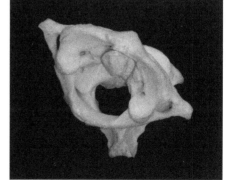

Superior view neutral   **Superior view atlas rotated right**

The inferior facet joint of the atlas and the superior facet joint of the axis are both convex in shape. This convex to convex articulation results in the atlas rising and falling on the axis during rotation. During flexion and extension the convex inferior facets of the atlas roll and slide on the convex superior facets of the axis.

Lower cervical spine

The lower cervical spine is between C2 and C7. The orientation of the facet joints of these vertebrae, as well as their angle of incline and relatively large size facilitates good range of movement in all direction in this part of the spine – flexion, extension, sidebending and rotation.

Flexion of the spine is a forward downward bending movement in the sagittal plane about a frontal horizontal axis. During flexion the lower facets of the vertebrae above slide upwards on the upper facets of the vertebra below and then tilt forwards until ligament tension and disc compression prevents any further movement. This may be described as an opening of the facet joints. The vertebra slides and then tilts and the joints open posteriorly and by the end of flexion the articular pillars of the vertebra above are more superior and anterior to those below

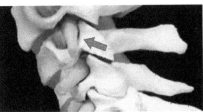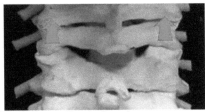

Lateral view – Cervical flexion – Posterior view

Flexion is limited by the tension of the capsular ligaments, posterior longitudinal ligaments, ligamentum flavum, ligamentum nuchae and by compression of the anterior part of the intervertebral disc.

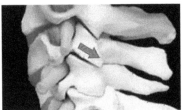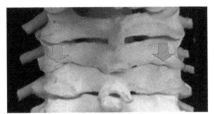

Lateral view – Cervical extension – Posterior view

Extension or hyperextension of the spine is a backward downward movement in the sagittal plane about a frontal horizontal axis. During extension the lower facets of the vertebrae above slide downwards on the upper facets of the vertebra below and then tilt backward until ligament tension, disc compression or bony approximation prevents any further movement. This may be described as a closing of the facet joints. The vertebra slides and tilts and the joints closes posteriorly and by the end of extension the articular pillars of the vertebra above are more posterior and inferior to the ones below.

Extension is limited by the tension of the anterior longitudinal ligaments, the compression of the intervertebral disc posteriorly and the approximation of the facet joints and the spinous processes.

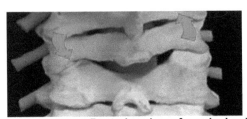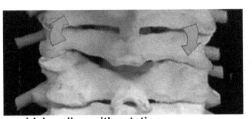

Posterior view of cervical spine - sidebending with rotation

Sidebending or lateral flexion of the spine is a sideways movement in the frontal plane about a sagittal horizontal axis. During sidebending a facet on one side of the spine slides upwards and forward and a facet on the other side slides downwards and backwards. There is no tilting but there is an opening of a facet on one side of the spine and a closing of a facet on the other side. Ligament and muscle tension and disc compression limit movement.

Although the mechanics differ in different parts of the spine, pure sidebending and pure rotation do not occur in the thoracic, lumbar or lower cervical spine. Sidebending is always combined with rotation, and rotation is always combined with sidebending. At the atlanto-occipital joint, in the lumbar spine and down most of the thoracic spine sidebending results in automatic rotation to the opposite side. In the lower cervical spine and down the thoracic spine as far as about T3, sidebending produces automatic rotation to the same side.

This means that for the head to remain straight, and not rotate during sidebending, the upper cervical spine must compensate for the rotation by rotating in the opposite direction. Similarly when the head is rotated the lower cervical spine produces unwanted sidebending and the upper cervical spine must compensate for this by sidebending in the opposite direction.

Because the facet joints at the top of the lower cervical spine have a more horizontal angle of incline and the facet joints at the bottom have a steeper angle of incline there is a greater amount of combined sidebending and rotation at the top and a tendency towards more pure rotation at the bottom.

In addition to unwanted rotation during sidebending of the cervical spine there is also some unwanted extension produced. If this unwanted extension was not neutralised the head would drop backward during sidebending. But the lower and upper cervical spine compensate for it by flexing. So in addition to producing the major head movements of flexion, extension and rotation the suboccipital muscles are responsible for producing small movements which fine tune the position of the head so that it always remains vertical, and they compensate for the unwanted movements for the lower cervical spine as described and imbalances below from unequal leg length and curvatures in the spine such as scoliosis.

Flexion, extension and sidebending are greatest in the cervical and lumbar spine and rotation is greatest in the cervical spine. The upper thoracic spine permits a small amount of flexion and middle to lower thoracic spine permits a small amount of rotation. The thoracic spine has smaller intervertebral discs and is surrounded by the rib cage which limits movement. The sacroiliac joint permits a small amount of flexion and extension of the sacrum during backward and forward movement of the torso and some torsion during walking.

Muscles according to function

Prime movers, also known as **agonists** are muscles that produce most of the movement at a joint when they contract. They continue the movement until **antagonists** act to decelerate the joint in the final stages of the movement. For example brachialis flexes the forearm and triceps slow down the flexion toward the end of movement. Gravity can assists movement or oppose it. For example when falling asleep in a seat, the rapid head flexion of the head falling forwards is the result of gravity.

Lifting the head from the flexed position back to a vertical position requires the concentric contraction of trapezius and posterior cervical muscles to counter gravity. When the head is slowly lowered from a vertical position to a flexed position this involves the eccentric contraction of trapezius and some posterior cervical muscles, assisted by gravity.

Sometimes prime movers and antagonist contract together as **fixators** to stabilise a bone while other muscles act to move another bone attached to the fixed bone. When the head is lowered or lifted into or away from a flexed position, muscles fix the scapula to the rib cage so that it can act as a stable base for the trapezius to contract effectively. **Neutralisers** and **synergists** may contract to counter unwanted movements produced by a prime mover. For example during finger flexion wrist extensors contract to prevent wrist flexion. In addition **shunt muscles** have an important stabilising function by increasing compression on the articulating surfaces of joints while prime movers, also know as **spurt muscles**, produce movement.

Anatomy of ribs, thoracic, lumbar and sacroiliac 2.0 – 3.9

Erector spinae

The erector spinae, also known as sacrospinalis or the paravertebral muscles is made up of many different muscles of varying lengths, size and attachments, and the composition of these muscles and their tendon varies throughout the spine.

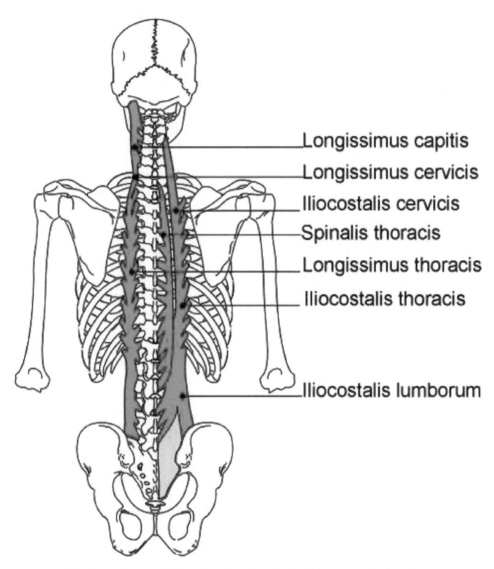

Longissimus capitis

Longissimus cervicis

Iliocostalis cervicis

Spinalis thoracis

Longissimus thoracis

Iliocostalis thoracis

Iliocostalis lumborum

Erector spinae, pelvis, spine, head and shoulders – posterior view

Erector spinae arises on the sacrum as a broad thick tendon, and in the lumbar it becomes a thick muscle. In the thoracic it separates into three distinct columns, from lateral to medial they are the iliocostalis (iliocostocervicalis), longissimus and spinalis. A depression, the paravertebral gutter, runs the length of the thoracic and lumbar spine between the bulk of the muscle mass and the spinous processes. Interspinales, rotatores and multifidus may be palpable here.

Erector spinae attaches on the spinous processes of T11 and T12, all lumbar vertebrae and their supraspinous ligaments, the median and lateral sacral crests and a medial area on the iliac crest. Its fibres merge with the sacrotuberous and posterior sacroiliac ligaments and with gluteus maximus.

Iliocostalis
Iliocostalis lumborum arises on the iliac crest and attaches onto the inferior borders of the angles of ribs 6 to 12.

Iliocostalis thoracis arises on the superior border of the angles of ribs 6 to 12, and it attaches onto the superior border of the angles of ribs 1 to 6 and the transverse process of C7.

Iliocostalis cervicis arises on the superior border of the angles of ribs 3 to 6 medial to iliocostalis thoracis attachments, and it attaches onto the posterior tubercles of the transverse process of C4 to C6.

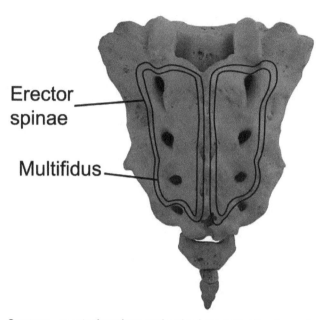

Erector spinae

Multifidus

Sacrum - posterior view and spinal muscle attachments

Longissimus
Longissimus thoracis arises on the iliocostalis lumborum, posterior transverse processes of lumbar vertebrae and the thoracolumbar fascia. It attaches onto the tips of the transverse processes of all thoracic vertebrae and between the tubercles and angles of ribs 3 to 12.

Longissimus cervicis arises on the transverse processes of T1 to T5 medial to longissimus thoracis and to the posterior tubercles of the transverse processes of C2 to C6.

Longissimus capitis arises on the transverse processes of T1 to T5 and the articular processes of C4 to C7. It attaches onto the posterior mastoid process, deep to splenius capitis and sternocleidomastoid.

Thoracic and Lumbar vertebrae – lateral view

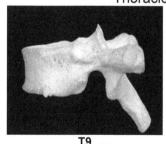

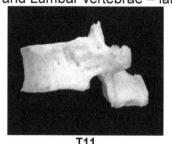

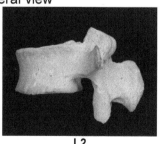

| T9 | T11 | L2 |

Spinalis
Spinalis thoracis arises on the spinous processes of T11 to L2 and the tendons unite into a small muscle and this later separates into distinct tendons which attach on the spinous processes of between four and eight upper thoracic vertebrae. It merges anteriorly with semispinalis thoracis and laterally with longissimus thoracis.

Spinalis cervicis arises on the spinous processes of C7 to T2 and the ligamentum nuchae and attaches onto the spinous processes of C2 to C4. It exhibits variation in its attachments and may be absent.

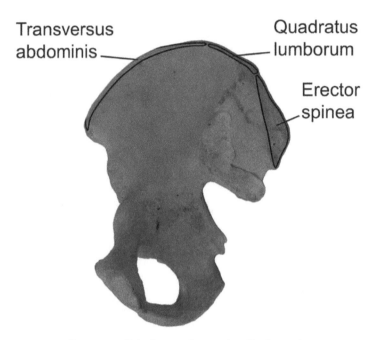

Transversus abdominis

Quadratus lumborum

Erector spinea

Ilium - medial view and muscle attachments

Spinalis capitis arises with semispinalis capitis, blends with it and attaches on the occiput.
Actions: Bilateral contraction of spinalis cervicis produces extension of the cervical spine and bilateral contraction of spinalis capitis produces extension of the head and cervical spine. Unilateral contraction produces sidebending and rotation.
Nerve supply: Dorsal rami of cervical, thoracic and lumbar spinal nerves.

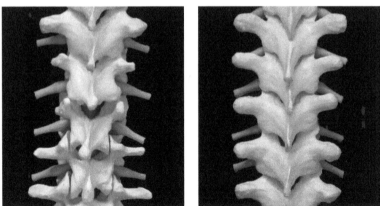

Thoracolumbar and Thoracic spine – posterior view

Transversospinalis
Semispinalis thoracis arises on the transverse processes of T6 to T10 and attaches onto the spinous processes of C6 to T4. More tendinous in form.
Semispinalis cervicis arises on the transverse processes of T1 to T6 and attaches onto the spinous processes of C2 to C5. More muscular, especially the fibres that attach on the axis.
Semispinalis capitis arises on the transverse processes of C7 to T6 and the articular processes of C4 to C6 (sometimes C7 and T1) and attaches either side of the mid-sagittal line, between the superior and inferior nuchal lines on the occiput.

Nerve supply: Dorsal rami of cervical and thoracic nerves.
Actions: Extension of the head and cervical spine.

558

Multifidus arises on the sacrum as low as S4 level, on the aponeurosis of the erector spinae, posterior superior iliac spine, posterior sacroiliac ligament, mamillary processes of L1 to L5, transverse processes of T1 to T12 and articular processes of C4 to C7. The muscle runs obliquely superiorly and medially and attaches along the length of a spinous process one to four vertebral segments above, as high up as C2.
Nerve supply: Dorsal rami of the spinal nerves.

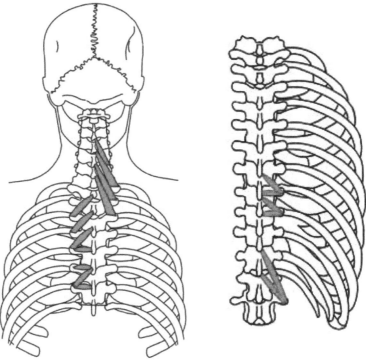

Rotatores and multifidus

Rotatores are the deepest muscles and are most developed in the thoracic spine. They arise on the upper posterior part of a transverse process and attach on a lower lateral area on a lamina and the root of a spinous process of a vertebra above.
Nerve supply: Dorsal rami of the spinal nerves.

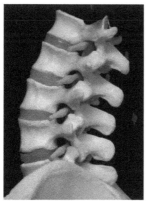 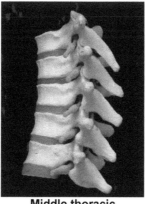 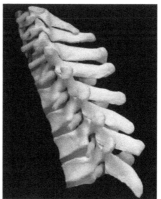

| Lumbar spine | Middle thoracic | Upper thoracic |

Interspinales (interspinalis) run from one spinous process to the spinous process above. They are present between C2 and T3, and between T11 and L5. They are more distinct in the cervical spine. Sometimes they occur between L5 and the sacrum.
Nerve supply: Dorsal rami of the spinal nerves.

559

Intertransversarii run from one transverse process to the transverse process above. They are present between C1 and T1, and between T10 and the sacrum. In the cervical and lumbar, pairs of muscles lie either side of the spine.
Nerve supply: Dorsal and ventral rami of the spinal nerves.

Actions: The short muscles of the back show intermittent contractions in the upright position and have a mainly postural function. They protect the spine from injury by finetuning the movements of individual vertebrae. They prevent the longer muscles exerting buckling forces on the spine. They produce extension, sidebending and rotation.

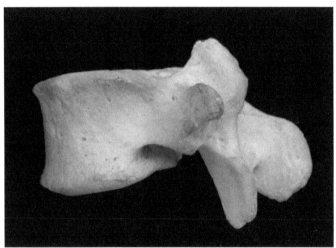

Lumbar L5 vertebra – lateral view

The **thoracolumbar fascia** extends from the ligamentum nuchae in the cervical spine to the medial crest of the sacrum. It is continuous with the deep cervical fascia and it extends laterally to the rib angles, abdominal aponeurosis and iliac crest. In the cervical spine it also attaches onto the cervical transverse processes. In the thoracic it attaches onto the tips of all thoracic spinous processes and supraspinous ligaments, and to the rib angles laterally. It is thin and lies between the erector spinae and the muscles connecting the spine to the upper limb.

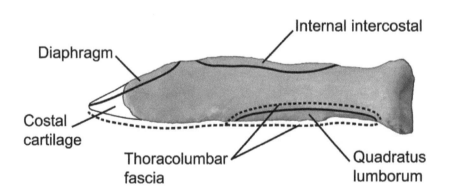

Right Rib 12 - anterior view and muscle attachments

In the lumbar it is thick and strong and has three layers. The posterior layer is the most superficial layer and attaches on the spines of lumbar and sacral vertebrae and supraspinous ligaments. The middle layer attaches onto the tips of all lumbar transverse processes, intertransverse ligaments, iliac crest and anterior part of the inferior border of rib 12 and its costal cartilage. The anterior layer attaches medially onto the anterior surface of all lumbar transverse processes, and the iliolumbar ligament, and inferiorly on the iliac crest. The upper part forms the lateral arcuate ligament superiorly.

560

The thoracolumbar fascia encloses and intermeshes with muscles in the lumbar region. The posterior and middle layers pass behind and in front of erector spinae. The middle and anterior layer passes behind and in front of, quadratus lumborum. The posterior and middle layers unite at the lateral side of erector spinae and then unite with the anterior layer at the lateral side of quadratus lumborum and all three layers become continuous with the aponeurosis of the transversus abdominis.

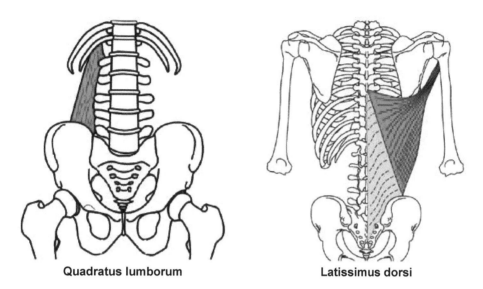

Quadratus lumborum   **Latissimus dorsi**

Quadratus lumborum arises on the posterior iliac crest and the iliolumbar ligament. Some fibres run vertically and attach on the medial half of the inferior border of rib 12 and other fibres run more obliquely and attach on the tip of transverse processes of lumbar vertebrae L1 to L4. A third layer may be present running obliquely from L1 to L4 transverse processes to the lower border of rib 12. The muscle has an irregular quadrilateral shape and apart from a small lateral area arising from the iliac crest the muscle lies deep to erector spinae.

Actions: Unilaterally quadratus lumborum produces sidebending of the lumbar spine. Bilaterally it helps with inspiration by fixing the lower ribs for the action of the diaphragm. Nerve supply: The ventral rami of spinal nerve T12 to L3.

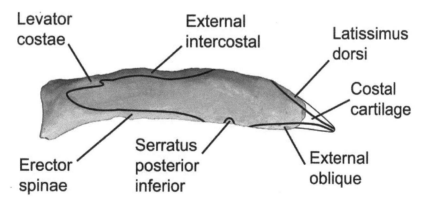

Right Rib 12 - posterior view and muscle attachments

Costal muscles

Serratus posterior inferior arises from the spinous processes of T11 to L2 and the adjacent supraspinous ligaments and passes obliquely superiorly and laterally to attach on the inferior border and anterior surfaces of the lower four ribs.
Actions: Depresses lower four ribs.
Nerve supply: The ventral rami of spinal nerve T9 to T12.

Serratus posterior superior arises from a lower part of the ligamentum nuchae and the spinous processes and supraspinous ligaments from C7 to T3 and attaches on the upper surface of ribs 2 to 5, just lateral to their angles. It covers a layer of fascia and lies deep to the rhomboids. The number of vertebral attachments may vary or the muscle may be absent. Nerve supply: Intercostal nerves from T2 to T5.

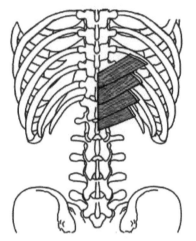

Serratus posterior inferior

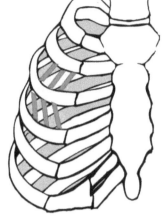

Anterior intercostal muscles

The **intercostal muscles** arise from the inferior border of ribs 1 to 11. The **external intercostal muscles** are the most superficial and run obliquely, inferiorly and anteriorly, to attach on the superior border of the adjacent rib below. Their action is to produce inspiration. The **internal intercostal muscles** are deeper and run obliquely, inferiorly and posteriorly, to attach on the superior border of the adjacent rib below. Their action is to produce expiration. Nerve supply: Segmental nerves (anterior division T2 to L1).

The abdominal muscles

The abdominal wall consists of a corset of three sheets of muscle and fascia attached to the lateral margin of two long muscles running parasagittally, which attach at the midline. It is important for posture, digestion, defecation, venous return, urination, vomiting, breathing, parturition and fine control of vocal actions such as singing. It works in balance with the erector spinae to support the spine.

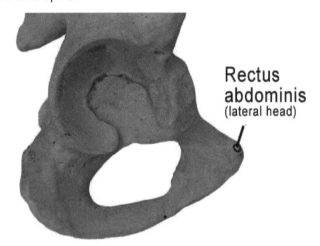

Rectus abdominis (lateral head)

Ilium - lateral view and rectus abdominis attachment

Superficial fascia covers most of the abdominal wall. It is made up of two layers, with blood vessels, nerves, lymph nodes and variable levels of fat in between. It passes over the inguinal ligament and below, is continuous with the fascia latae. The deeper of the two layers merges with the linea alba.

562

Rectus abdominis arises inferiorly by a lateral tendon from the pubic crest and pubic tubercle, and by a medial tendon which merges with the lateral tendon, the interpubic ligament of the symphysis pubis and occasionally with the linea alba. It attaches superiorly on the cartilages of ribs 5, 6 and 7, and occasionally ribs 3 and 4 and the xiphoid process.
Action: It compresses and supports the abdomen and flexes the spine.
Nerve supply: Intercostal nerves T7 to T12.

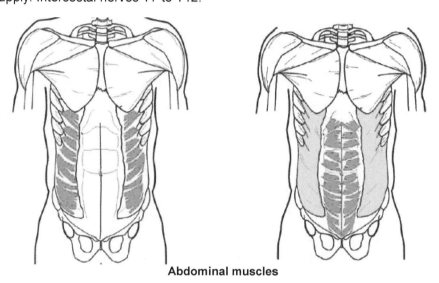

Abdominal muscles

Deep and superficial layers of fascia envelop the rectus abdominis muscle forming the rectus sheath. The fascia attaches at the midline as the linea alba. Laterally the sheath attaches to the oblique muscles. Three tendinous intersections run transversely or zigzag obliquely across the muscle. One occurs at the level of the umbilicus and two occur above it. One or two more may also occur below the umbilicus. They may be incomplete. The tendinous intersections divide the rectus abdominis along its length into bands with distinct segmental innervation, giving the muscle greater control.

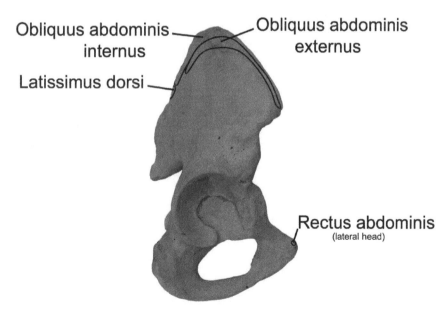

Obliquus abdominis internus

Obliquus abdominis externus

Latissimus dorsi

Rectus abdominis
(lateral head)

Ilium - lateral view and muscle attachments

The **external abdominal oblique** muscle arises on the lower 8 ribs directly as muscle and interdigitate with the fibres of serratus anterior and latissimus dorsi. It runs inferiorly and medially to attach onto the anterior half of the iliac crest and a strong tendinous sheet of aponeurosis covering the anterior abdomen. The external oblique fibres extend to the linea alba at the midline, and to the pubic symphysis, pubic crest, pubic tubercle and inguinal ligament, inferiorly. The inguinal ligament is a thickening of the aponeurosis, folded internally and with fibres from the rectus sheath forms the floor of the inguinal canal.

The external oblique is the most superficial and largest of the group of muscles, which form the lateral abdominal wall and is palpable, lateral to rectus abdominis. The muscle and aponeurosis are covered in fascia. Digitations of the muscle may be absent or duplicated.

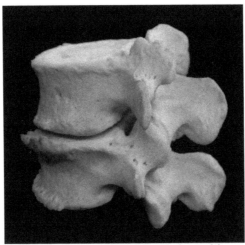

Lumbar L3 and L4 - lateral view with osteophytes on side of vertebral body

The **internal abdominal oblique** is thinner and deep to the external oblique and so is not directly palpable. It arises on the anterior two-thirds of the iliac crest, the lateral two-thirds of the inguinal ligament and on the thoracolumbar fascia.

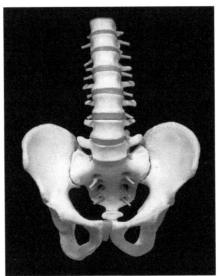

Lumbar and pelvis – anterior view

The fibres arising from the posterior part of the iliac crest run superiorly and laterally to attach onto the lower 4 ribs and are continuous with the internal intercostals. The fibres arising from the anterior part of the iliac crest diverge, the more posterior fibres running superiorly and medially and the more anterior fibres running horizontally and medially to attach on an aponeurosis.

At the lateral border of the rectus abdominis the aponeurosis separates into two layers which wrap around the muscle, reuniting at the linea alba. The aponeurosis of the internal oblique joins with the aponeurosis of the external oblique to form the anterior part of the rectus sheath, and joins with the aponeurosis of the transversus abdominis to form the posterior part of the rectus sheath. The fibres arising from the inguinal ligament run inferiorly and medially

564

and form a tendon, which attaches onto the pubic crest. The internal oblique and transversus abdominis may be fused, and the lower parts of these muscles may be replaced by fascia.

Actions: The oblique muscles compress the abdomen, flex and sidebend the spine and depress the ribs.
Nerve supply: The ventral rami of spinal nerves T7 to T12 with the internal oblique also being supplied by L1.

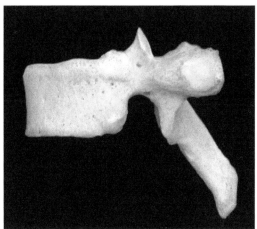
Thoracic T3 - lateral view

Transversus abdominis is the deepest layer and not directly palpable; It arises on the lateral third of the inguinal ligament, the anterior two thirds of the iliac crest, thoracolumbar fascia and cartilages of the lower 6 ribs. It attaches onto aponeurosis and linea alba, pubis and pectineal line. The transversus abdominis may be absent.

Actions: Depresses ribs and acts to constrict the abdomen.
Nerve supply: Intercostal nerves T7 to T12 and spinal nerve from L1.

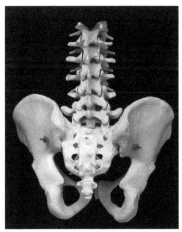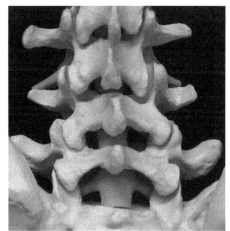
Lumbar, sacrum and ilium - posterior views

The **supraspinous and interspinous ligaments** are small ligaments running from one vertebra to the next, from the seventh cervical vertebrae to the sacrum. The supraspinous ligaments are stronger, thicker and more superficial than the interspinous ligaments and are more easily palpable.

In the lumbar the sacrospinous and interspinous ligaments are thicker and connected to thick, broad spinous processes that are directed posteriorly and are proportionally larger. In the thoracic they are connected to long spinous processes directed inferiorly and posteriorly, and they are exposed in flexion. In the cervical spine they continue as the ligamentum nuchae.

Clinical indications: In the cervical region these ligaments may be damaged by motor vehicle accidents and other whiplash injuries. In the lumbar the ligaments may be strained from the lifting of heavy objects by unprepared or weak muscles.

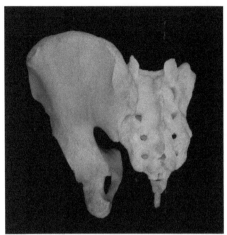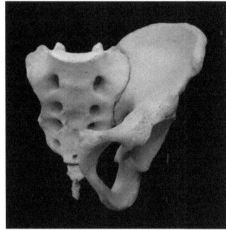

Sacrum, ilium and sacroiliac joint - posterior view (left) and anterior view (right)

The sacroiliac ligaments
The primary ligaments of the sacroiliac joint are the posterior sacroiliac ligament, interosseous sacroiliac ligament, sacrotuberous ligament and the sacrospinous ligament

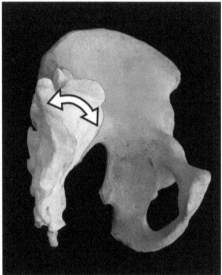

Sacroiliac joint movement

The **sacrotuberous ligament** is a thick ligament that arises on the posterior iliac spine, lateral margin of the sacrum and upper coccyx. It runs inferiorly, laterally and anteriorly to attach on the ischial tuberosity. At the posterior iliac spine it merges with the sacroiliac ligament and at the sacrum it merges with the sacrospinous ligament. Its posterior border serves as an attachment for gluteus maximus and some of its superficial fibres merge with the tendon of the long head of biceps femoris.

The **sacrospinous ligament** arises on the lateral margin of the sacrum and coccyx just anterior to the sacrotuberous ligament. It runs inferiorly, laterally and anteriorly to attach on the ischial spine.

Actions: The sacrotuberous and sacrospinous ligaments passively oppose the forward tilting (nutation) of the sacrum on the ilium.

The **posterior sacroiliac ligaments** are long and short ligaments running between the sacrum and ilium. They are superficial to the stronger interosseous sacroiliac ligaments and the sacroiliac joints. The short posterior sacroiliac ligament arises on an inner lip of the dorsal iliac crest and attaches on an area on the superior posterior sacrum. The long posterior sacroiliac ligament arises on posterior superior iliac spine and attaches on the third and fourth segments of the lateral sacrum. They are easily palpable unless they are covered by a fibrolipoma. The ligaments may be strained from the lifting of heavy objects by unprepared or weak muscles.

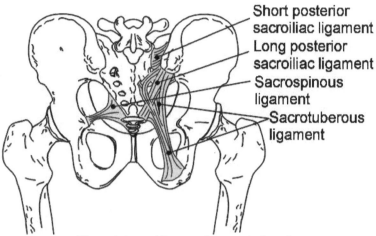

Short posterior sacroiliac ligament
Long posterior sacroiliac ligament
Sacrospinous ligament
Sacrotuberous ligament

The pelvis and ligaments - posterior view

The sacroiliac joints

The sacroiliac joints are strong, L-shaped, weight bearing synovial joints between the sacrum and the two ilium bone of the pelvis. The joints are covered by two different kinds of cartilage; the sacral surface has hyaline cartilage and the iliac surface has fibrocartilage. The joint is supported by strong ligaments which maintain the stability of the joint. There is a small amount of movement at the SI joints, ranging between individuals from 2 to10 degrees.

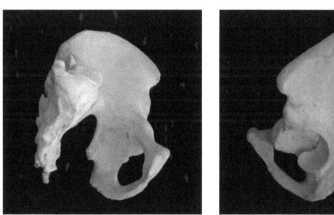

Sacrum, Ilium and sacroiliac joint - medial view (left) and lateral view (right)

The sacroiliac joints function as a shock absorber dampening forces from the lower extremity to the spine and from the weight of the body through the spine to the both lower limbs. Like some other joints it has an important locking mechanism where the joint adopts a more stable close pack position during standing and during the push-off phase of walking. In flexion and when seated the sacroiliac joint can unlock into a lose pack position and this is where it is most vulnerable to injury and locking in an unwanted position,

There are several types of motion available at the sacroiliac joint. The sacroiliac joint moves during walking. The ilium tilts backwards at the heel strike phase of walking and forwards at the push off phase. Also during the walking cycle the sacrum rotates obliquely on a diagonal axis between both ilium. The sacrum also moves with the torso – during spinal backward bending the sacrum flexes (nutation) between the ilium and during spinal forward bending the sacrum extends (counter-nutation).

The sacroiliac joint can become hypermobile or hypomobile. Ligament laxity may be caused genetically, by overstretching or from a single injury or repeated injury or hormonal changes such as in pregnancy. It may lead to hypermobility and instability and the joint can get stuck in a range of different positions, but usually in a forwards tilting position, and become a source of pain. Overly stretched, sprained or torn ligament are a major problem and stretching can be part of a solution for fixing it or it can be part of the problem. Do not go beyond a joints normal range and do not over stretch lax ligaments. The posterior sacroiliac ligaments are a common site for lower back pain usually from a strain.

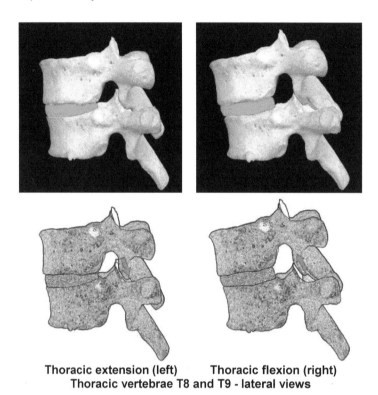

Thoracic extension (left)   Thoracic flexion (right)
Thoracic vertebrae T8 and T9 - lateral views

There are genetic differences between the sacroiliac joints of different people. Lifestyle and environmental factors also act on the joint and change it structurally throughout life. The surfaces of the sacroiliac joint are flat in early life but develop irregular elevations and depressions that interlock the sacrum between the two iliac bones as we get older. The sacroiliac joint usually gets stiffer as we get older.

Sacroiliac hypomobility may be the consequence of biomechanical factors acting on the joints, such as extremes of kyphosis, scoliosis or reversed lordosis, an anatomical or physiological short leg, altered gait patterns, muscle length imbalances hip or knee osteoarthritis and surgical spinal fusion. These may cause changes within the joint, which may lead to dysfunction and pain. Hypomobility in the sacroiliac joint can also be caused by ankylosing spondylitis, rheumatoid arthritis or infection.

Joint movement

Range of joint movement in the spine is determined by the angle and size of the facet joints, the width and thickness of the intervertebral discs, the presence or absence of ribs, the size and elasticity of ligaments and the tightness of supporting muscles.

In the thoracic spine the strongly backward sloping coronal alignment of the facet joints facilitates movement in all direction but the discs are thinner and the attachment of ribs acts to significantly limit movement. In the cervical spine a more moderately backward sloping coronal alignment of the facet joints and thicker intervertebral discs facilitates good levels of

568

flexion, extension sidebending and rotation. In the lumbar the sagittal alignment of the facet joints limits rotation but wide and thick intervertebral disc facilitates good levels of other movements.

Thoracic T8 and T9 - posterior views

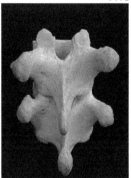 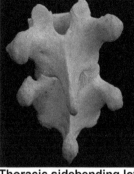 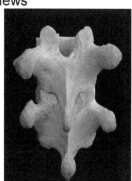

| **Thoracic extended** | **Thoracic sidebending left** | **Thoracic flexed** |

Compared with other joints, such as the shoulder or hip joints there is relatively little movement in the spine, especially with respect to individual vertebrae. Only when the spine as a whole is taken into consideration is there a moderate amount of overall movement.

The primary function of the spine is not intrinsic movement, it is to protect the spinal cord and nerves, support the head for eating and other sensory activities, support the rib cage for respiration, anchor muscles for movement of the upper and lower limbs, and stabilize the upright body for locomotion and other activities. Also the large vertebral bodies of the lumbar support the weight of the upper body and transfer the weight through the pelvis to the lower limbs.

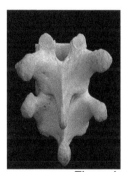 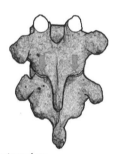 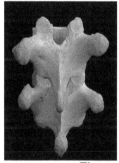 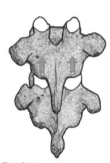

Thoracic extension　　　　　　　**Thoracic flexion**

Variation in the structure of the spine between different individuals influences their range of movement. An increased thoracic kyphosis may reduce thoracic extension whereas an extended thoracic may reduce flexion. In the lumbar an increased lordosis will reduce flexion and a reverse lordosis will reduce extension. Loss of movement in one part of the spine may be compensated for in another part of the spine. The thoracolumbar spine can make up the difference for some of the losses, such as in the lumbar spine, or there may be little or no compensation until the upper cervical spine when the suboccipital muscles must contract to compensate for everything by attempting to keep the head level.

Genetic and lifestyle factors combine to cause degeneration in the lower lumbar and lower cervical spine after about the age of 40 years, reducing the range of movement in these areas. Loss of disc height causes greater load on the facet joints resulting in cartilage loss, and over time, osteophyte formation around the disc and joints. When this level of degeneration has occurred, this is osteoarthritis, and there is defacto vertebrae fusion and all movement is lost. The C5/6 and C6/7 and the L4/5 and L5/S1 joints are most affected. Safe stretching is especially important whenever there is degeneration because of the danger of overstretching the area unaffected by the osteoarthritis.

In the spine flexion is limited by the tension of the capsular ligaments, posterior longitudinal ligaments, ligamentum flavum, supraspinous ligament and interspinous ligaments and by compression of the anterior part of the intervertebral disc. Extension is limited by the tension of the anterior longitudinal ligaments, compression of the intervertebral disc posteriorly and the approximation of the facet joints and the spinous processes.

Lumbar L3 and L4 - posterior views

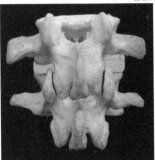 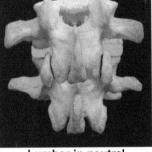 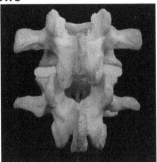

| **Lumbar in neutral** | **Lumbar sidebending left** | **Lumbar flexed** |

There are several natural factors acting on joints to limit movement, the most important of which is the tension of ligaments. Other factors include the passive viscous and elastic tension of muscles; the active reflex tension of muscles, joint apposition, especially of congruent joint surfaces by synovial fluid and internal pressure and assisted by shunt muscles, gravity adding compression or distraction to a joint, the approximation of body parts and the inertia of the body part being moved.

Apposition is the tightly packed position of joints, which occurs when two joint surfaces are in maximum contact or congruent. When this occurs the capsule and surrounding ligaments are maximally tense. Usually they are twisted in such a way that they form a tightly compressed lock screw mechanism around the joint, resulting in the two articulating surfaces being so locked together that even strong distractive forces cannot separate them and no movement is possible. This is the close packed position.

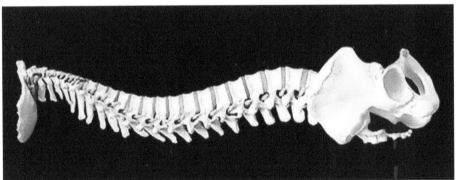

Spine and pelvis – lateral view

In contrast the least packed position occurs when a joint is in its least congruent position, the capsule and ligaments are at their lowest tension, and the joint is freer to move and can be more easily distracted.

Joints have little or no mobility when they are in a close packed position but they are more stable and the joint is better protected against injury. The close packed arrangement is a more energy conserving state for the body and is usually the best option for joints that have a supporting or stabilising role such as the knees, hips and sacroiliac joints. In an activity such as a stretching exercise, choosing to positioning a joint in a close packed position or a least packed position is an important consideration influencing the safety.

Anatomy of the shoulder: scapula, clavicle and humerus 4.0 – 5.2

Trapezius arises on aponeurosis, firmly anchored at the midline to the occipital bone and skin, the external occipital protuberance, the medial one third of the superior nuchal line of the occiput, the ligamentum nuchae, the spinous processes and supraspinous ligaments of vertebra C7 to T12.

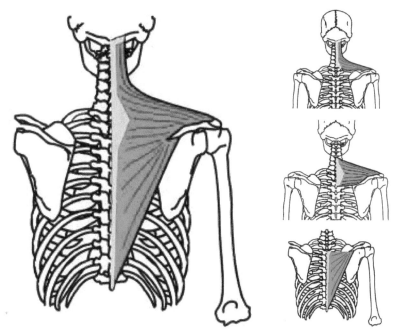

Upper, middle and lower trapezius - posterior view

The superior fibres attach on the posterior border of the lateral third of the clavicle; the middle fibres attach on the medial side of the acromion and a superior line along the spine of scapula. The inferior fibres merge into an aponeurosis that attaches onto the medial end of the spine of the scapula. The middle fibres arise from a broad aponeurosis between C6 and T3. The muscle may merge with the sternocleidomastoid. It may be absent at the occiput and after T8.

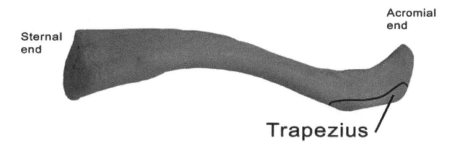

Clavicle - superior view and trapezius attachment

Actions: The muscle supports and stabilises the scapular when the upper limb is active. Working with levator scapulae its upper fibres elevate the scapula, with the rhomboids its middle fibres retract the scapula and working with serratus anterior it rotates the scapular to assist with arm elevation. Its upper fibres also extend and sidebend the head when the scapula is fixed. The upper trapezius is covered in 1.3 the anatomy of the cervical spine. Nerve supply: Accessory nerve (Cranial nerve 11).

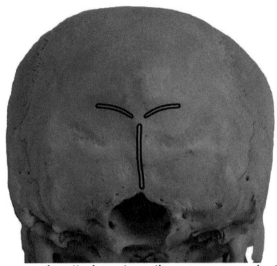

Trapezius superior attachments on the squamous occiput - posterior inferior view 1. Horizontal lines - Superior nuchal lines 2. Vertical line - external occipital crest via ligamentum nuchae

Levator scapulae arises from the transverse processes of the atlas and axis and the posterior tubercles of the transverse processes of C3 and C4 and attaches to the medial border of the scapula, between the superior angle and the spine of scapula. The fibres twist so that the lowest fibres on the scapula become the highest on the spine. The muscle lies deep to trapezius

The muscle is variable in its attachments and may have additional slips to the occiput, mastoid process, first or second rib or merge with other muscles such as trapezius, scalene and serratus muscles.

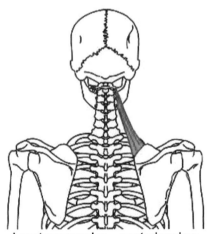

Levator scapulae – posterior view

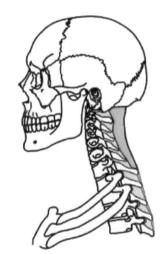

Supraspinous ligaments & ligamentum nuchae (trapezius origin – lateral view)

Actions: When the neck is fixed, levator scapulae strongly elevates the scapula and is active when carrying a load. It stabilises and moves the scapular when the upper limb is active. With other muscles it draws the scapula medially and rotates the scapula so that the glenoid points down. When the scapula is fixed levator scapulae extends, ipsilaterally rotates and sidebends the cervical spine and it helps stabilise the cervical spine.
Nerve supply: C3 and C4 and via the dorsal scapular nerve to C5.

572

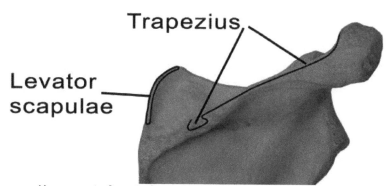

Upper part of posterior scapula and muscle attachments

Rhomboid minor arises from the ligamentum nuchae and spinous processes of C7 and T1 and **rhomboid major** arises from the spinous processes of T2 to T5. Both muscles run inferiorly and laterally to attach onto the medial border of the scapula. Rhomboid minor attaches at the medial end of the spine of the scapula. Rhomboid major attaches on the medial border of the scapula between the spine and the inferior angle.

The muscles are variable in there attachments. Rhomboid major may split into on two tendons, one inserting near the inferior angle and the other near the spine of the scapula. Fibres of rhomboid minor may extend superiorly to the occiput.

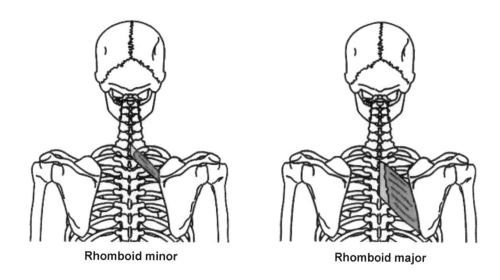

Rhomboid minor   Rhomboid major

Actions: Retraction and downward rotation of the scapula.
Nerve supply: Dorsal scapular nerve C4 and **C5**.
Clinical indications: Overuse, postural fatigue, headaches, whiplash injuries, torticollis.

Supraspinatus arises from the medial two thirds of the supraspinatus fossa, passes under the acromion and its tendon attaches on the top of the greater tubercle of the humerus. The muscle is deep to trapezius. The tendon merges with the capsule of the shoulder joint and is the most frequently strained of the shoulder muscles.

Actions: Starter of abduction and stabiliser.
Clinical indications: Partial or complete rupture of the tendon, and subacromial bursitis.
Nerve supply: Suprascapular nerve C4, **C5** and C6.

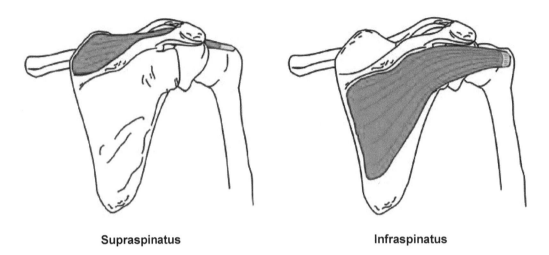

Supraspinatus   **Infraspinatus**

Infraspinatus arises from the medial two thirds of the infraspinatus fossa and infraspinous fascia that covers it and the tendon attaches to the middle facet of the greater tubercle of the humerus. The tendon merges with the capsule of the shoulder joint.

The muscle is palpable but the medial fibres are deep to trapezius and the lateral fibres are covered by posterior deltoid. Sometimes it is merged with teres minor and the tendon may be is separated from the capsule by a bursa.

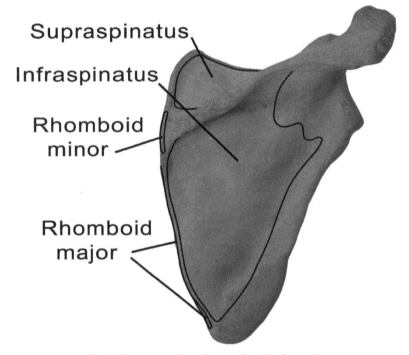

Posterior scapula and muscle attachments

Actions: External rotation and horizontal extension of the shoulder. A stabiliser of the shoulder joint.
Clinical indications: Overuse, bursitis and tendon strain.
Nerve supply: Suprascapular nerve **C5** and C6

574

Teres minor arises as a muscle from the upper two thirds of a flat strip which runs along the posterior surface on the lateral side of the scapula and from aponeurosis separating it from infraspinatus and teres major. The tendon attaches to a facet on the lower part of the greater tubercle of the humerus and to a small area of the humerus below this.

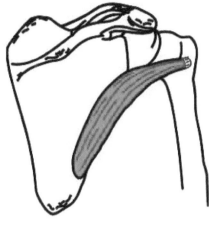

Teres minor

The muscle is palpable but laterally its upper part is covered by posterior deltoid. The tendon merges with the capsule of the shoulder joint.

Actions: External rotation and horizontal extension of the humerus.
Nerve supply: Axillary nerve **C5** and C6.

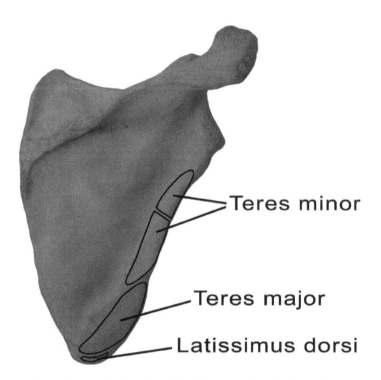

Scapula - posterior view showing muscle attachments

Teres major arises as muscle from the lateral side of the posterior surface of the scapula near the inferior angle and from aponeurosis separating it from infraspinatus and teres minor. The flat tendon attaches on the crest of the lesser tubercle and medial lip of the intertubercular sulcus, which is the groove for the biceps tendon. It is palpable as it passes laterally from under latissimus dorsi

575

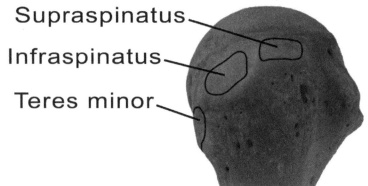

Head of humerus - lateral view and muscle attachments

Actions: Teres major acts with latissimus dorsi to adduct, extend and medially rotate the humerus.
Nerve supply: Subscapular nerve **C6** and C7.

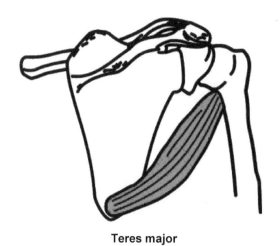

Teres major

Latissimus dorsi is a triangular muscle which arises on thoracolumbar fascia, from the sacrum, iliac crest and spinous processes of thoracic vertebrae T6 to T12 and all lumbar vertebrae. Between T6 and T12 it is deep to trapezius.

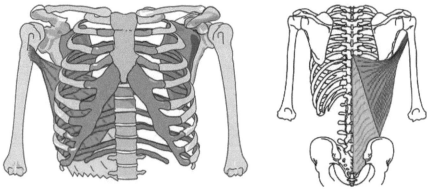

Latissimus dorsi - anterior view (left) and posterior view (right)

Latissimus dorsi arises directly as muscle from ribs 9 to 12, from a small area on the iliac crest and usually from the inferior angle of the scapula. The muscle fibres run superiorly and laterally, pass over the lower part of teres major posteriorly then twist around it so that the

576

anterior surface faces backwards, and is in contact with the anterior surface of teres major. Together they form the posterior axillary fold.

The tendon attaches onto a lower part intertubercular sulcus of humerus. The highest midline fibres form the lowest tendon attachment and the lowest midline fibres form the highest tendon attachment on the humerus.

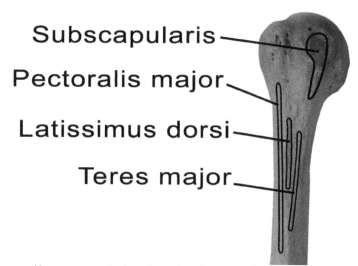

Humerus - anterior view showing muscle attachments

Actions: Latissimus dorsi extends, adducts and medially rotates the humerus. It depresses the shoulder as in climbing and is active in forced exhalation as in coughing. Fibres that arise from the inferior angle of the scapula contribute towards stabilisation of the scapula.
Nerve supply: Thoracodorsal nerve **C6, C7** and C8 from brachial plexus.

Subscapularis arises from the medial two-thirds of the subscapular fossa and from aponeurosis covering the muscle. Its tendon attaches on the lesser tubercle of humerus and the anterior of the shoulder joint capsule. Its fibres are deep and run laterally as part of the posterior axilla. It is not palpable but in flexible individuals some of its medial fibres may be accessible.

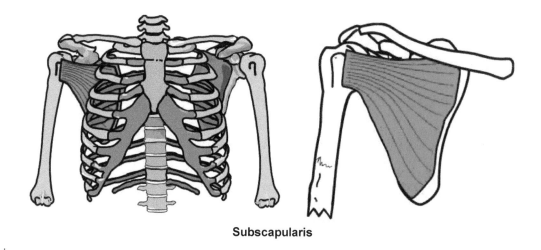

Subscapularis

Actions: Internal rotation and horizontal flexion of the humerus.
Nerve supply: Subscapular nerve C5 and **C6**.

577

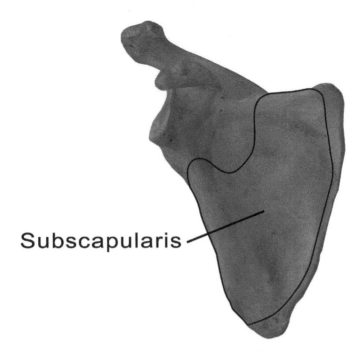

Scapula - anterior view and subscapularis attachment

Pectoralis major is a thick triangular muscle which defines the anterior axillary fold. It can be emphasised by pressing the hands on the hips. Its upper part, the clavicular fibres, arises from the medial half of the clavicle. Its lower part, the sternocostal fibres, arises from the anterior surface of the sternum, costal cartilages of ribs 2 to 6 and the aponeurosis of the external oblique muscle.

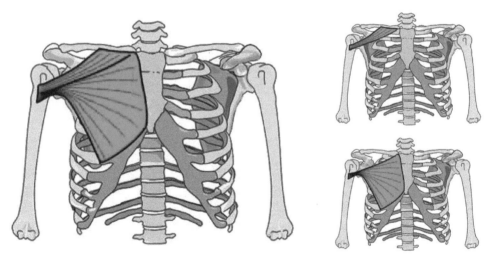

Pectoralis major - clavicular and sternal costal fibres

The two heads unite on a narrow flat tendon about 5 cm wide, which passes deep to the deltoid to insert on the lateral lip of the intertubercular sulcus of the humerus. The tendon combines with fibres from the transverse ligament to form a cover over the sulcus and create a fibro-osseous tunnel for the tendon of the long head of the biceps. Some of the tendon merges with the fascia of the upper arm and the capsular ligaments.

The tendon has two layers anterior and posterior which usually blend inferiorly. The anterior layer receives its fibres from the upper parts of the muscle and the posterior layer receives its fibres from the lower parts of the muscle and the front of the sternum. The sternal and abdominal fibres twist so that the lowest fibres attach highest on the intertubercular sulcus and the highest fibres attach lowest.

The number of costal attachments varies. Overlying pectoralis major are deep and superficial layers of fascia, platysma, supraclavicular nerves and mammary glands. Deep to pectoralis major is the sternum, ribs, costal cartilages, clavipectoral fascia, subclavius, serratus anterior, intercostal and pectoralis minor muscle.

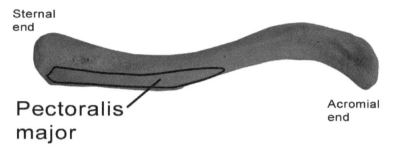

Sternal end

Pectoralis major

Acromial end

Clavicle - inferior view and pectoralis major attachment

Actions: Clavicular fibres: From a position of extension these fibres produce flexion of the humerus. In addition they produce medial rotation and horizontal flexion of the humerus. Sternocostal fibres: From a position of flexion these fibres produce extension of the humerus. In addition they produce adduction, medial rotation and horizontal flexion of the humerus, especially against resistance. When the upper limb is fixed above the head the muscle pulls the torso upwards and forwards as in climbing. The muscle may be involved in forced inhalation.

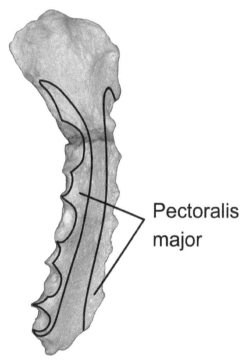

Pectoralis major

Sternum - anterior and lateral view

Nerve supply: Medial and lateral pectoral nerves. Nerves from C5 and **C6** supply the clavicular fibres and nerves from **C7**, **C8** and T1 supply the sternocostal fibres.

Pectoralis minor arises from the upper margins and outer surface of ribs 3 to 5, near the costochondral junction and from fascia covering the external intercostals. The fibres run superiorly and laterally to attach onto the medial border and upper surface of the coracoid process. Part of the tendon or the whole tendon of pectoralis minor may bypass the coracoid process and attach onto the acromion or humerus. Sometimes the muscle arises from rib 2, and on rare occasions from rib 1 or it may be limited to ribs 3 and 4.

Pectoralis minor is a thin muscle deep to pectoralis major and is best palpated with the arm relaxed and using resisted protraction. The muscle lies over the upper ribs, external intercostals, and serratus anterior and forms the posterior part of the anterior axillary fold.

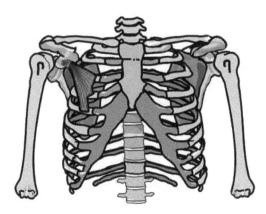

Pectoralis minor

Actions: Stabilization, depression, protraction, forward tilt and downward rotation of the scapula. When the ribs are fixed the muscle brings the scapula forward and down around the chest; and when the scapula is fixed, it lifts up the rib cage.
Nerve supply: Medial and lateral pectoral nerves C6, **C7** and C8. The brachial plexus passes between pectoralis minor and rib 1

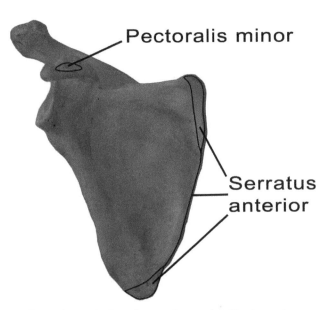

Scapula - anterior view and muscle attachments

Clinical considerations: A short hypertonic pectoralis minor, for example from a prolonged slumping posture pulling the shoulders forward, can cause postural distortions in the upper body and compress the neurovascular structures that lie deep to it, resulting in symptoms of numbness and tingling in the hand, especially when the arm is abducted and extended.

Serratus anterior arises as interdigitations from the outer surface and superior border of ribs 1 to 8 and from fascia covering the intercostal muscles. It runs back and around the thoracic as a muscular sheet, passing under the scapula to attach on two triangular areas on the medial anterior surface of the scapula and along the medial border of the scapula. The first digitation arises from ribs 1 and 2 and attach on the upper anterior surface of the scapula near the superior angle. Digitations from ribs 3 and 4 attach along the medial border of the scapula and digitations from ribs 5 to 8 attach on the lower anterior surface of the scapula near the inferior angle. Serratus anterior may attach as far down as rib 10, or may be absent from rib 1, rib 8 or the middle part of the muscle.

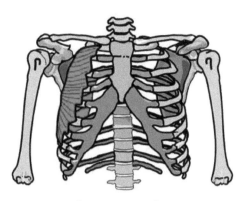

Serratus anterior

Actions: Protraction and upward rotation of the scapula. All the fibres working together protract the scapula and steady it while the deltoid abducts the arm. The upper fibres assist with suspension of the scapula. The more powerful lower four or five digitations converge onto the inferior angle of the scapula like a fan and act in producing upward rotation so the glenoid fossa faces more vertically. The muscle is involved in reaching or pushing actions and for taking the arm above the head.

Nerve supply: Long thoracic nerve C5, **C6** and **C7**, which descends along the external surface of the muscle. Damage leads to weakness of serratus anterior and winging of the scapula.

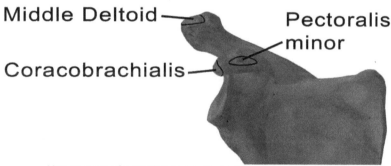

Upper part of anterior scapula and muscle attachments

Coracobrachialis arises from the apex of the coracoid process where it shares a common tendon with the short head of biceps. The rope-like muscle passes down the upper medial shaft of humerus and attaches onto a broad area half way down the medial shaft of the humerus.

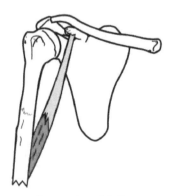

Coracobrachialis

581

The muscle may also attach above on the lesser tubercle of the humerus, or below on the medial epicondyle or merge with the medial intermuscular septum. It can be palpated as a round ridge just medial to the short head of biceps and close to the brachial artery.

Actions: It is a flexor, horizontal flexor and adductor of the humerus, especially from a position of extension and acts as a stabiliser of the shoulder.
Nerve supply: Musculocutaneous nerve C5, **C6** and C7.

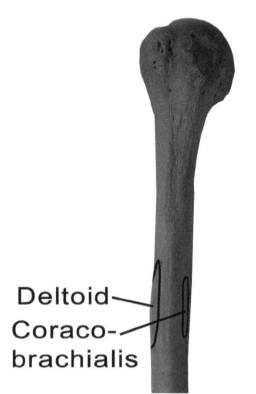

Deltoid—
Coraco-
brachialis

Proximal anterior humerus and muscle attachments

Deltoid gives the shoulder its rounded shape. It has three parts, anterior, posterior and middle or intermediate which are separated by deep fascia.

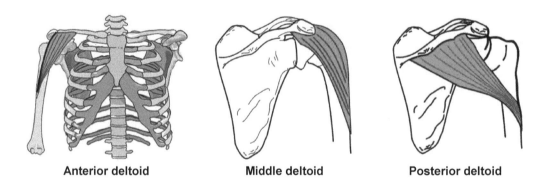

Anterior deltoid   **Middle deltoid**   **Posterior deltoid**

Anterior deltoid arises on the anterior superior border of the distal clavicle; **middle deltoid** arises on the lateral margin of the superior acromion; and **posterior deltoid** arises on the lower border of the spine of the scapula.

All insert on the deltoid tuberosity on the lateral shaft of the humerus via a short thick tendon. The anterior and posterior deltoid attach on the tendon directly. The middle deltoid is multipennate and attaches on the tendon via four intramuscular tendinous septa which makes

582

it by far the strongest part of the muscle. Some fibres from the tendon merge with deep brachial fascia.

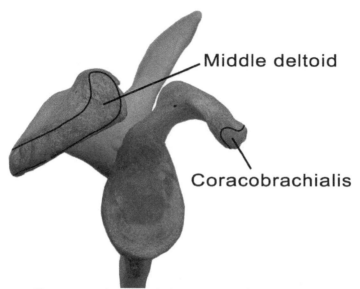

Upper scapula - lateral view and muscle attachments

Superficial and deep fascia and platysma cover the deltoid. The deep fascia is continuous with the pectoral, infraspinous and brachial fascia and attaches to the clavicle, acromion and spine of the scapular.

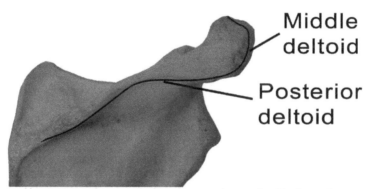

Upper scapula – posterior view and muscle attachments

Clinical indications: Shoulder injuries such as to the rotator cuff tendon may result in compensatory structural changes in the middle deltoid and symptoms of pain.

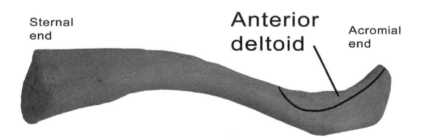

Clavicle - superior view and deltoid attachment

Actions: Anterior deltoid is an arm flexor, horizontal flexor and medial rotator. Middle deltoid is an arm abductor. Posterior deltoid is an arm extensor, horizontal extensor and lateral rotator. Nerve supply: Axillary nerve **C5** and C6.

583

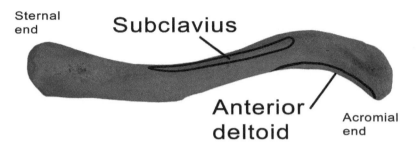

Clavicle - inferior view and muscle attachments

Subclavius arises on the superior aspect of rib 1 on the costal cartilage and the medial part of the rib. It passes obliquely upwards and laterally and attaches on the middle third of the underside of the clavicle. Sometimes it attaches on the coracoid process.

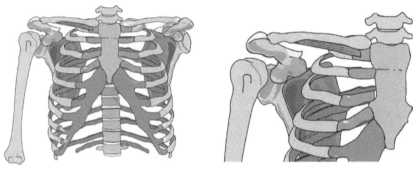

Subclavius

Actions: It pulls down on the clavicle, depresses the shoulder and stabilise the clavicle during movement of the upper limb.
Nerve supply: A branch of the brachial plexus **C5** and C6.

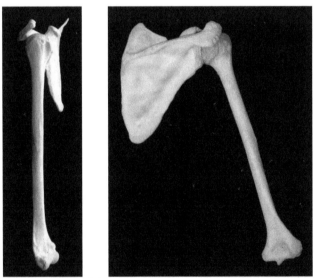

Shoulder joint - lateral view (left) and posterior view (right)

The glenohumeral joint is a multi-axial spheroidal joint between the larger head of the humerus and the smaller glenoid fossa of the scapula. A shallow cavity permits good range of movement but at the expense of stability. A fibrocartilagenous glenoid labrum provides congruence as the head rolls in one direction and slides in the other.

Anatomy of the elbow and forearm: humerus, radius and ulna 5.3 – 5.6

The tendon of the **long head** of **triceps brachii** arises from the infraglenoid tubercle of the scapula and from the capsule of the glenohumeral joint. The **lateral head** arises from a flattened tendon which attaches on a ridge and on the lateral border of the posterior shaft of the humerus, above the radial groove, and from the lateral intermuscular septum.

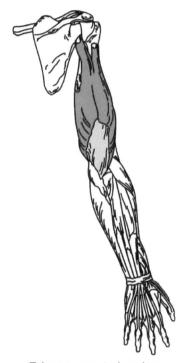

Triceps - posterior view

The **medial or deep head** arises from the posterior surface of the shaft of the humerus, below the radial groove, and from the posterior surface of the medial intermuscular septum and a lower part of the lateral intermuscular septum. A common tendon inserts onto the posterior and upper olecranon, blending with the antebrachial fascia of the forearm.

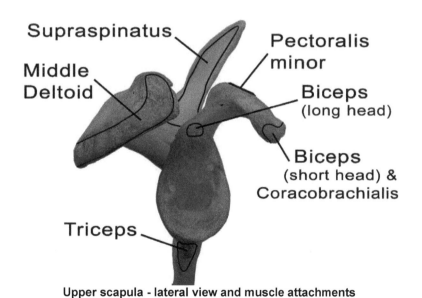

Upper scapula - lateral view and muscle attachments

The brachial fascia is thickest where it covers the triceps and epicondyles of the humerus and is continuous with the deep fascia overlying pectoralis major, deltoid, latissimus dorsi and the antebrachial fascia. It attaches to the epicondyles and the olecranon process of the ulna. An olecranon bursa may be palpable when inflamed or thickened.

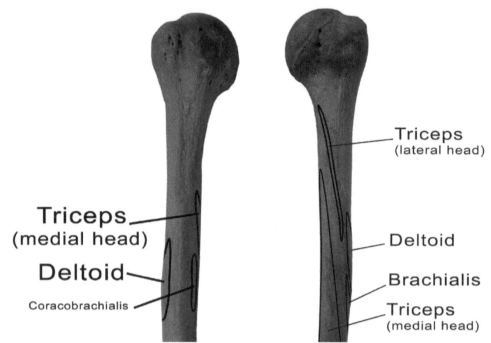

Humerus - anterior view (left) and posterior view (right) showing muscle attachments

Actions: Forearm extension is consistently produced by the medial head and by the long and lateral heads when acting against resistance. The long head of triceps assists with arm extension when the arm moves from a position of flexion.
Nerve supply: Radial nerve C6, **C7** and **C8**.

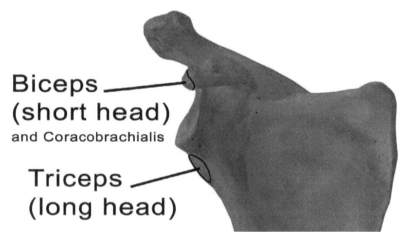

Upper scapula - anterior view and muscle attachments

The **short head** of **biceps brachii** arises on the apex of the coracoid process. It shares a common tendon origin with coracobrachialis. **The long head** arises from glenoid labrum and the supraglenoid tubercle of the scapular, above the glenoid cavity. The tendon is within the shoulder joint capsule and passes over the shoulder through a synovial lined sheath. The long slender tendon passes over a groove on the head of the humerus, the intertubercular sulcus of the humerus under cover of the transverse ligament and fibres of the pectoralis major tendon. The groove is palpable between the greater and lesser tuberosity.

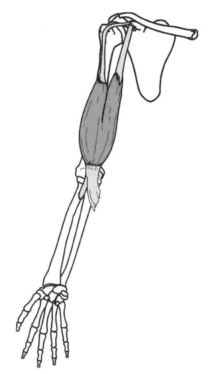

Biceps - anterior view

The two muscles from each head join as a tendon that attaches onto the posterior of the radial tuberosity and the bicipital aponeurosis. This aponeurosis, also known as lacertus fibrosus, is a broad fibrous expanse, which merges with the deep fascia of the flexor muscles of the forearm. It provides greater flexor pull and protects the brachial artery and the median nerve in the cubital fossa. The biceps tendon twists before attaching on the radial tuberosity so that its anterior surface faces laterally.

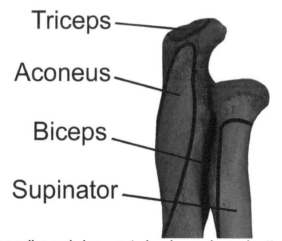

Triceps
Aconeus
Biceps
Supinator

Upper radius and ulna - posterior view and muscle attachments

Other heads may arise from the upper part and medial side of the brachialis muscle and elsewhere in the arm.

Actions: Forearm flexion and supination, and arm flexion.
Clinical indications: Partial rupture of the muscle and tendonitis at the intertubercular sulcus.
Nerve supply: Musculocutaneous nerve to both heads C5 and **C6**.

587

Brachialis arises on the anterior surface of the lower half of the shaft of the humerus and the intermuscular septum, especially the medial intermuscular septum. It narrows to a thick broad tendon which attaches on the tuberosity of the ulna and an anterior area on the coronoid process of the ulna. The muscle lies deep to biceps.

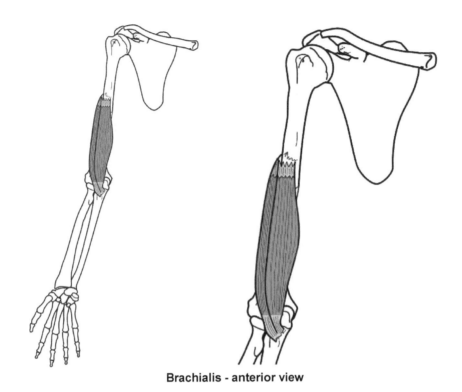

Brachialis - anterior view

The muscle may be split into two or more parts, fuse with biceps, brachioradialis or pronator teres or attach on the radius or bicipital aponeurosis.
Actions: Forearm flexion.
Nerve supply: Musculocutaneous nerve C5 and **C6**.

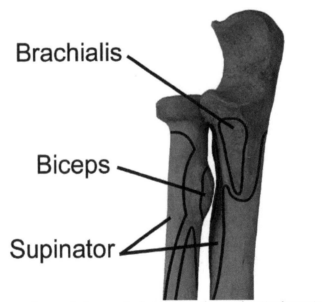

Upper radius and ulna - anterior view and muscle attachments

Brachioradialis arises on the lateral supracondylar ridge and lateral intermuscular septum. The muscle ends in the middle of the forearm as a long flat tendon which attaches onto the lateral side of the distal radius near the styloid process. The muscle is the most lateral and superficial muscle in the forearm, and is easily observed with resisted elbow flexion half way between pronation and supination.

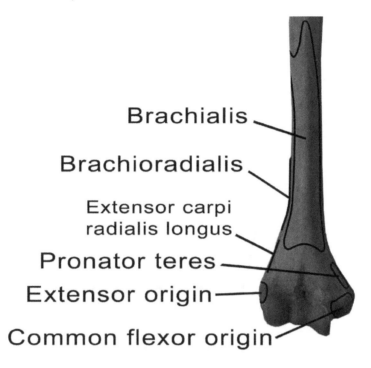

Brachialis

Brachioradialis

Extensor carpi
radialis longus

Pronator teres

Extensor origin

Common flexor origin

Distal humerus - anterior view and muscle attachments

Actions: Brachioradialis is a forearm flexor especially in mid-pronator. It is a shunt muscle helping to stabilise the elbow during rapid forearm flexion.
Nerve supply: Radial nerve C5, **C6** and C7.

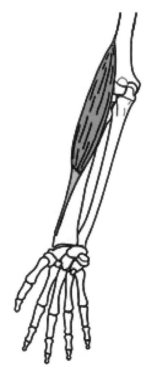

Brachioradialis

Supinator is made up of a deep part and a superficial part. The superficial part arises on the lateral epicondyle of the humerus, the lateral collateral ligament of the elbow joint and annular ligament and the deep part arises on the ulna, below the radial notch. The muscle winds around the radius to insert on the lateral surface of the proximal third of the radius. This is a deep muscle, which surrounds the proximal radius and forms the lateral floor of the cubital fossa.

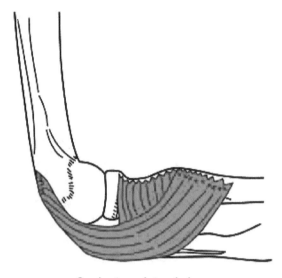

Supinator – lateral view

Actions: Supination of the forearm in all positions of the elbow. When the forearm is in flexion the muscle works with biceps to produce forceful supination
Nerve supply: Posterior interosseous branch of the radial nerve C5 and **C6**.

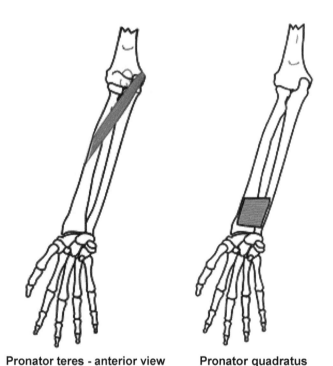

Pronator teres - anterior view   **Pronator quadratus**

Pronator teres has two heads, the larger humeral head arises from an area just above the medial epicondyle of the humerus, on the common flexor tendon, the antebrachial fascia and from the intermuscular septum between it and flexor carpi radialis. The humeral head is palpable between the medial epicondyle and biceps tendon.

590

The smaller ulnar head arises on the medial side of the coronoid process of the ulna. The muscle runs diagonally across the anterior forearm and attaches on a flat tendon attaching about half way down the lateral side of the radius. Fibres may attach onto the biceps, brachialis or the medial intermuscular septum of the arm, and the ulnar head may be absent. This muscle forms the medial border of the cubital fossa.

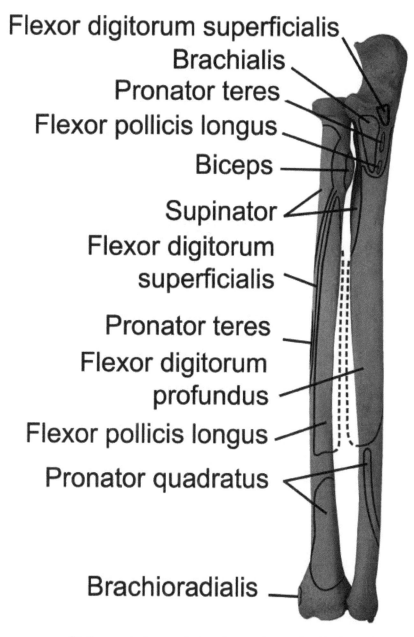

Flexor digitorum superficialis
Brachialis
Pronator teres
Flexor pollicis longus
Biceps
Supinator
Flexor digitorum superficialis
Pronator teres
Flexor digitorum profundus
Flexor pollicis longus
Pronator quadratus
Brachioradialis

Radius and ulna - anterior view and muscle attachments

Actions: Resisted and rapid pronation of the forearm. It is also a weak flexor of the forearm. Nerve supply: The median nerve C6 and **C7**

Deep fascia, the **antebrachial fascia** covers the muscles of the forearm and its internal surface serves as attachment for some of these muscles. It is attached to the olecranon and posterior ulna. It gives off transverse septa, which separate the deep and superficial layers of muscle. It is continuous with the brachial fascia and strengthened by fibres extending from the biceps and triceps. At the wrist it has two thickenings the flexor and extensor retinacula.

Pronator quadratus arises on a line running diagonally across the distal quarter of the anterior shaft of the ulna and attaches on a broad area on the distal quarter of the anterior shaft of the radius. This flat rectangular muscle lies deep to all the long forearm flexor tendons and is not palpable.

Actions: This is the main pronator of the forearm.
Nerve supply: The median nerve **C8** and T1.

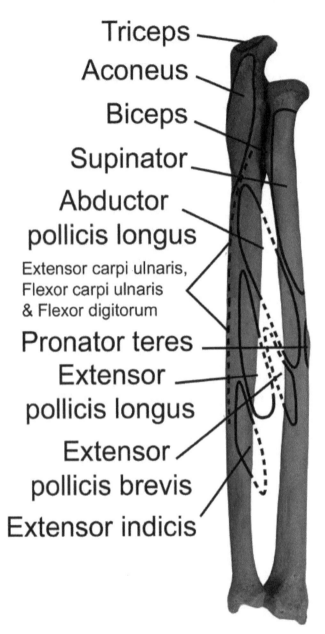

Triceps
Aconeus
Biceps
Supinator
Abductor pollicis longus
Extensor carpi ulnaris, Flexor carpi ulnaris & Flexor digitorum
Pronator teres
Extensor pollicis longus
Extensor pollicis brevis
Extensor indicis

Radius and ulna - posterior view and muscle attachments

The elbow consists of three joints, the humeroulnar and humeroradial joints, which are concerned with forearm flexion and extension, and proximal radioulnar joint which is concerned with pronation and supination. At the proximal radioulnar joint the head of the radius pivots within an osseoligamentous ring formed by the radial notch of the ulna and the annular ligament. At the humeroulnar joint the trochlear notch of the ulna hinges on the trochlea of the humerus. At the humeroradial joint the head of the radius moves relative to the capitulum of the humerus.

When the elbow is in full flexion the coronoid process of the ulna sits within the coronoid fossa of the humerus and when the elbow is in full extension the olecranon process of the ulna sits within the olecranon fossa of the humerus.

Elbow joint

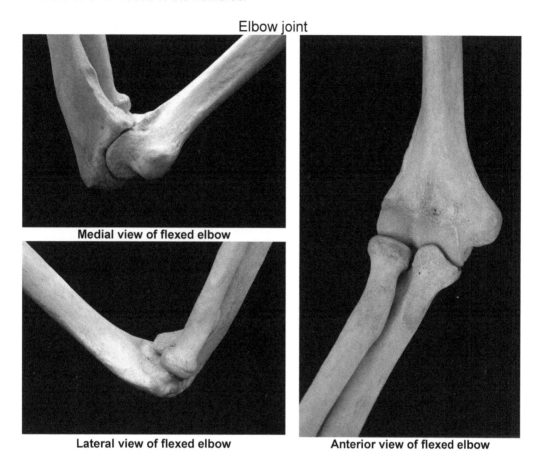

Medial view of flexed elbow

Lateral view of flexed elbow

Anterior view of flexed elbow

Strong collateral ligaments prevent medial and lateral movement at the elbow. On the ulnar side the medial collateral ligament joins the medial epicondyle of the humerus with the coronoid process and the olecranon process of the ulna. On the radial side the lateral collateral ligament joins the lateral epicondyle of the humerus with the head of the radius and the annular ligament.

When the elbow is fully extended and supinated the long axis of the forearm forms a slight lateral angle with the long axis of the humerus, called the carrying angle and this varies from 15 to 20 degrees. In congenitally hypermobile people the elbow may also extend by 5 or 10 degrees but normally the elbow is straight.

Anatomy of the hand: radius, ulna, carpals, metacarpals and phalanges 5.7 – 5.9

Flexor carpi ulnaris arises on the medial epicondyle of the humerus as the common flexor tendon and through a larger head arising on the medial olecranon and the proximal two-thirds of the posterior border of the ulna. It also arises proximally on an intermuscular septum between it and flexor digitorum superficialis and from an aponeurosis in the forearm common to it and extensor carpi ulnaris and flexor digitorum profundus. It primarily attaches on the pisiform bone. It also has distal attachments on the flexor retinaculum, hamate and fifth metacarpal bone, via carpal ligaments, and thenar muscles.

Actions: Wrist flexion and adduction and stabilisation of the wrist during thumb abduction and movement of the little finger.
Nerve supply: The ulnar nerve C7 and **C8.**

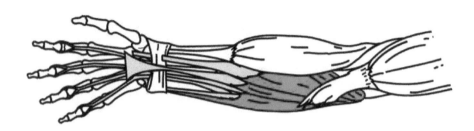

Wrist flexor muscles: Palmaris longus, flexor carpi ulnaris and flexor carpi radialis

Flexor carpi radialis arises on the medial epicondyle as the common flexor tendon, antebrachial fascia and intermuscular septum between it and other muscles. Its long tendon starts about half way along the forearm and attaches onto the base of the second metacarpal, with slips to the third metacarpal. It may be absent or have additional slips to the biceps tendon or biceps aponeurosis, coronoid process, radius, flexor retinaculum, trapezium, or fourth metacarpal. It is palpable.

Actions: Wrist flexion and abduction.
Nerve supply: The median nerve C6 and **C7**.

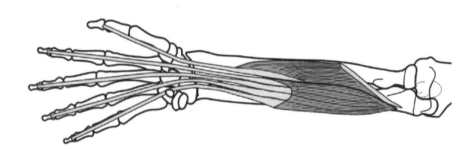

Finger flexor muscles: Flexor pollicis longus, flexor digitorum profundus and superficialis

Palmaris longus arises on the medial epicondyle of the humerus as the common flexor tendon, antebrachial fascia and intermuscular septa. It lies between flexor carpi radialis and flexor carpi ulnaris. Its long tendon bisects the wrist, runs superficial to the flexor retinaculum and attaches onto the palmar aponeurosis. It exhibits variation in its attachments and form. It may attach on adjacent muscles, carpal ligaments or carpal bones. It may be absent unilaterally or bilaterally or double or its tendon devoid of muscle fibres.

Actions: Wrist flexion and it tenses the palmar fascia.
Nerve supply: The median nerve C7 and C8.

Flexor digitorum superficialis lies deep to brachioradialis and pronator teres. It has two heads. The humero-ulnar head arises from the medial epicondyle of the humerus as the common flexor tendon, the medial collateral ligament and the medial side of the coronoid process of ulna. The radial head arises as a thin sheet of muscle, from an oblique line running from the radial tuberosity to a point about half way down the anterior radius.

The muscle separates into deep and superficial layers and gives rise to four tendons, which diverge after passing under the flexor retinaculum. Over the digits the tendons pass through fibrous sheaths lined by synovial membrane. At the level of the proximal phalanx each tendon splits to form a channel for the passage of the flexor digitorum profundus tendon to the distal phalanx. The two tendon slips then insert onto either side of the middle phalanx of all four fingers. The tendons may exhibit variation in number and form. The radial head may be absent.

Actions: Flexion of the middle and then proximal phalange. Fast and resisted finger flexion.
Nerve supply: The median nerve C7, **C8** and T1.

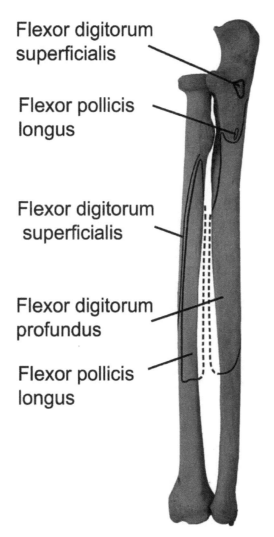

Radius and ulna - anterior view and muscle attachments

Flexor digitorum profundus arises on the proximal three quarters of the anterior and medial ulna, on an aponeurosis running down the posterior border of the ulna in common with flexor carpi ulnaris and extensor carpi ulnaris, and on the anterior side of the medial part of the interosseous membrane. The muscle and its four tendons lie deep to flexor digitorum superficialis and its tendons. The tendons pass under the flexor retinaculum and then diverge. Over the digits the tendons pass through fibrous sheaths lined by synovial membrane. At the level of the proximal phalanges the individual tendons pass through a groove formed by a split in the flexor digitorum superficialis tendon. They attach onto the anterior surface of the base of the distal phalanges. The muscle exhibits variations in its attachments and may have fibres arising on the medial epicondyle, coronoid process, radius, flexor digitorum superficialis or flexor pollicis longus.

Actions: Flexion of the distal phalanges and wrist.
Nerve supply: The ulnar nerve supplies the medial half of the muscle and the median nerve supplies the lateral half of the muscle **C8** and T1.

Flexor pollicis longus arises just distal to the radial tuberosity on the anterior two-thirds of the shaft of the radius and a lateral part on the anterior side of the interosseous membrane. The tendon passes under the flexor retinaculum and attaches on the base of distal phalanx of the thumb. Fibres may arise from the coronoid process, the medial epicondyle of the humerus, pronator teres and the flexor digitorum superficialis or profundus. The muscle may be completely absent or may not have an interosseous attachment.

Actions: Flexion of the distal phalanx of the thumb. It assists with flexion and adduction of the first metacarpal and flexion of the wrist.
Nerve supply: The median nerve **C8** and T1.

Extensor carpi ulnaris arises on the lateral epicondyle by the common extensor tendon, from antebrachial fascia and aponeurosis attached to the posterior ulna shared with extensor carpi ulnaris and flexor digitorum profundus. It attaches onto the medial side of the base of the fifth metacarpal bone. This is the most medial of the extensor muscles and its tendon is situated along the ulnar border of the wrist between the ulnar head and the styloid process.

Actions: Wrist extension and adduction and wrist stabilisation when grasping objects.
Nerve supply: Posterior interosseous nerve arising from the radial nerve C7 and **C8**.

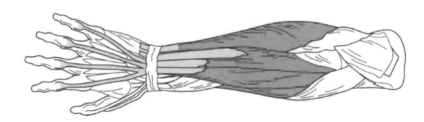

Wrist and finger extensor muscles

Extensor carpi radialis longus arises on the lateral supracondylar ridge of humerus and lateral intermuscular septum and a few fibres arise from the common extensor tendon. It passes under the extensor retinaculum and attaches onto the posterior base of the second metacarpal. It may send slips to the first and third metacarpal bone.

Actions: Wrist extension and abduction and wrist stabilisation when grasping objects.
Nerve supply: Radial nerve C6 and C7.

596

Extensor carpi radialis brevis arises on the lateral epicondyle of humerus by the common extensor tendon and from an intermuscular septum, the lateral collateral ligament of the elbow and from the strong aponeurosis that covers it. It attaches onto the dorsal surface of the base of the third metacarpal bone. The tendons of extensor carpi radialis longus and brevis pass over the wrist on the radial side of the radial tubercle and is prominent at the back of the wrist when the fist is clenched.

Actions: Wrist extension and abduction and wrist stabilisation when grasping objects.
Nerve supply: Posterior interosseous nerve arising from the radial nerve **C7** and C8.

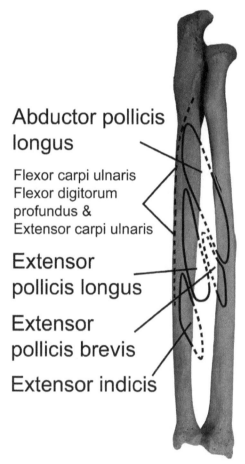

Abductor pollicis longus

Flexor carpi ulnaris
Flexor digitorum profundus &
Extensor carpi ulnaris

Extensor pollicis longus

Extensor pollicis brevis

Extensor indicis

Radius and ulna - posterior view and muscle attachments

Extensor digitorum (communis) arises on the lateral epicondyle of the humerus by the common extensor tendon, from an intermuscular septum and from antebrachial fascia. It attaches onto the base of the second and third phalanges of all fingers. The tendon has a dorsal digital expansion to which attaches lumbricals and interosseous muscles.

Actions: Extension of hand and fingers.
Nerve supply: Posterior interosseous nerve arising from the radial nerve **C7** and C8.

Extensor indicis (proprius) arises on a distal part of the posterior ulna and interosseous membrane. The tendon of extensor indicis passes under the extensor retinaculum with the tendon of extensor digitorum communis, the two tendons join and then attach onto the index finger. The tendon is medial to extensor pollicis longus and lateral to the radioulnar joint. It is prominent when extending the index finger.

Extensor digiti minimi arises from the common extensor tendon by a tendinous slip and from an intermuscular septum and its tendon attaches onto the posterior aspect of first phalanx of the little finger via the dorsal digital expansion. The tendon is situated on the lateral side of the ulnar styloid process and overlying the radioulnar joint.

Abductor pollicis longus arises on the lateral posterior ulna, interosseous membrane and posterior radius and attaches to the lateral side of the base of the first metacarpal bone. The tendon passes over a groove just behind the radial styloid process, and at the lateral side of the distal radius, with the tendon of extensor pollicis brevis and together they form the radial border of the anatomical snuffbox.

Extensor pollicis longus arises in the lateral posterior ulna and the interosseous membrane and attaches to the base of the distal phalanx of the thumb. The tendon makes a 45 degree turn at the radial tubercle and forms the ulnar border of the anatomical snuffbox.

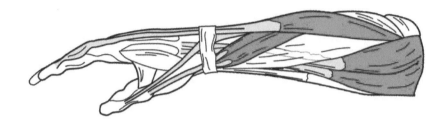

Thumb and finger extensors

Extensor pollicis brevis arises on the posterior radius and interosseous membrane and attaches to the base of the first phalanx of the thumb. The muscle may be absent or fused with abductor pollicis longus.

Three synovial sheaths prevent friction as finger tendons act around angles. Six osseofascial dorsal tunnels are formed by extensor retinaculum over bone. Retinacula and transverse ligaments hold the extensor tendons in place.

Short muscles of the hand

Thenar eminence
Abductor pollicis brevis mostly arises on the flexor retinaculum, but a few fibres arise from the scaphoid and trapezium and attaches onto the lateral base of the first phalanx. It is the most superficial muscle of the group.

Opponens pollicis arises on the flexor retinaculum and trapezium and attaches onto the lateral side of the first metacarpal bone.

Flexor pollicis brevis arises on the flexor retinaculum and trapezium and attaches onto the lateral sides of the base of the first phalanx. A deeper head sometimes arises from the trapezoid and capitate bones and carpal ligaments.

Adductor pollicis arises on the capitate, second and third metacarpal and attaches onto the medial side of the base of the first phalanx. It is deep to the other muscles.

Actions: Abduction, opposition, flexion and adduction of the thumb.
Nerve supply: Median nerve **C8** and T1 except adductor pollicis and the deep head of flexor pollicis brevis which are supplied by the ulnar nerve.

Hypothenar eminence
Abductor digiti minimi, opponens digiti minimi and **flexor digiti minimi** arise on the flexor retinaculum, pisiform and hamate and attach onto the first phalanx and metacarpal of the little finger.

Actions: Abduction, opposition and flexion of the little finger.
Nerve supply: Deep branch of the ulnar nerve C8 and **T1**.

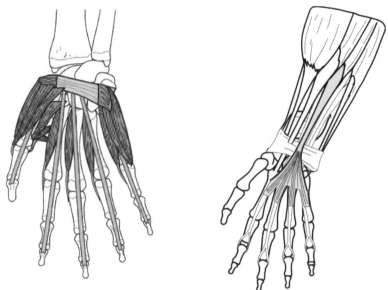

Short finger flexor muscles: thenar, hypothenar, interossei muscles and flexor digitorum profundus tendons (left) Palmar aponeurosis (right) - anterior view

Other structures in the hand

The **skin** on the palmar creases of the hand is fixed to fascia, which binds it to the structures beneath and allows for objects to be held securely in the hand. The skin of the fingers is fixed to the lateral and medial sides of the carpal bones, via septa and small ligaments. The skin on the dorsum of the hand is loose to permit the making of a fist.

On the palmar surface of the metacarpophalangeal joints are fleshy mounds containing **neurovascular bundles** which supply the fingers. The valleys are where the flexor tendons cross the joint.

A **palmar aponeurosis** covers the metacarpal bones, finger flexor tendons, lumbricals and interosseous muscles and superficial and deep palmar arches.

The joints of the wrist and hand

The hand has 27 bones, including 14 proximal, intermediate and distal phalanges forming the fingers, 5 metacarpals bones and 8 carpal bones. Movement in the hand occurs at the carpometacarpal joints, the intermetacarpal joints, metacarpophalangeal joints and interphalangeal joints.

The wrist is made up of 10 bones, the radius and ulna, the proximal row of carpal bones, including the scaphoid, lunate, triquetrum and pisiform, and the distal row of carpal bones including the trapezium, trapezoid, capitate, and hamate.

The wrist joints are formed between the distal radius articulating with the proximal row of carpal bones at the radiocarpal joint, and the proximal row of carpal bones articulating with the distal row of carpal bones at the midcarpal joint. The radiocarpal joint is formed between the radius, an articular disc and the scaphoid, lunate, and triquetral bones. The carpal bones on the ulnar side of the wrist only make contact with the ulnar during extreme wrist abduction.

The midcarpal joint is formed between the scaphoid, lunate, and triquetral bones articulating with the trapezium, trapezoid, capitate, and hamate bones. Intercarpal joints also exist between the various carpal bone and all these are supported by strong ligaments.

Anatomy of the hip: sacrum, ilium and femur 6.0 – 7.0

Iliacus arises on the iliac fossa, iliac crest, anterior sacroiliac ligament and a small area at the base of the sacrum. A few fibres of iliacus attach directly onto the femur just below the lesser trochanter but most of iliacus merges with the lateral side of the psoas tendon which attaches on the lesser trochanter. It is not directly palpable.

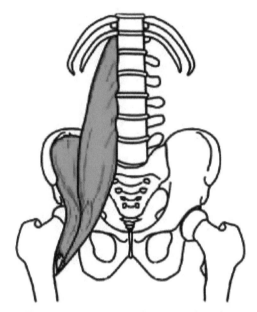

Iliacus and psoas major - anterior view

Psoas major arises on the transverse processes and bodies of vertebrae L1 to L5 and intervertebral discs T12 to L5 and attaches onto the lesser trochanter of the femur. It is not directly palpable. Iliac fascia covers the iliacus and psoas, which becomes thicker inferiorly. The tendon sits over a bursa, which may become inflamed.

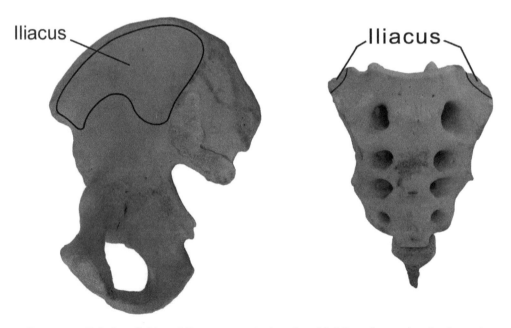

Ilium – medial view (left) and Sacrum – anterior view (right) and muscle attachments

Actions: Acting from above iliacus and psoas major flex the thigh and acting from below they flex the trunk and when acting unilaterally psoas sidebends the spine. They may exert a weak lateral rotation of the thigh. When seated the iliopsoas assists in balancing the trunk but when standing the hip joint is in a close-packed position and the muscle has a lower level of activity.

Nerve supply: Psoas major is supplied by the ventral rami of **L1**, **L2** and L3. Iliacus is supplied by branches of the femoral nerve **L2** and L3.

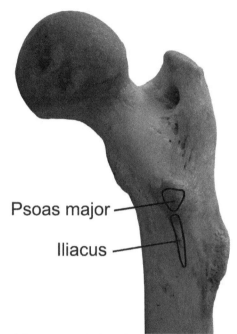

Proximal femur - posterior view and muscle attachments

The Gluteal muscles

Gluteus maximus arises on the posterior gluteal line of the ilium and on a small area of the ilium just behind it, the posterior surface of the inferior sacrum, the side of the coccyx, the aponeurosis of the erector spinae and the gluteal aponeurosis covering gluteus medius, and the sacrospinous and sacrotuberous ligaments.

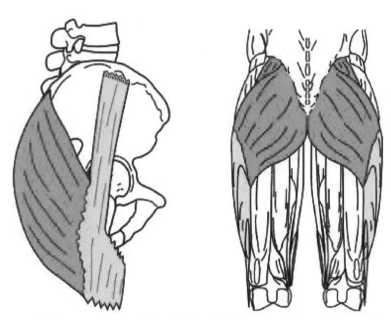

Gluteus maximus - lateral view (left) and posterior view (right)

601

Most of the muscle, including the upper fibres and the superficial fibres attach on a thick tendinous laminar which attaches onto the iliotibial tract and the deeper fibres of the lower part of the muscle attach onto the gluteal tuberosity. The muscle and adipose tissue define the characteristic roundness of the buttock.

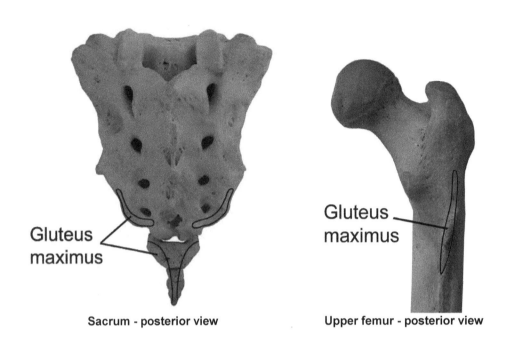

Sacrum - posterior view

Upper femur - posterior view

Actions: Gluteus maximus is a hip extensor and lateral rotator, and its' upper fibres are involved in hip abduction. It adds tension to the iliotibial tract and helps balance the femur on the tibia when the quadriceps are relaxed. It is important in climbing and coming up from a flexed position but it is not active during standing.
Nerve supply: Inferior gluteal nerve L5, **S1** and **S2**.

Short posterior sacroiliac ligament
Long posterior sacroiliac ligament
Sacrospinous ligament
Sacrotuberous ligament

Femur, ilium, sacrum and lumbar L5 vertebra – posterior view

Gluteus minimus is deep to gluteus medius. It arises on the outer ilium between the anterior and inferior gluteal lines and around the greater sciatic notch. It attaches onto the deep surface of an aponeurosis that ends on a tendon on the lateral side of the anterior surface of the greater trochanter. Some fibres attach onto the joint capsule and some may merge with the piriformis, gemellus superior and vastus lateralis.

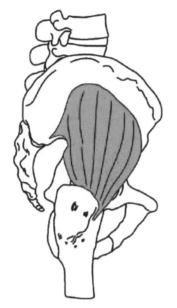 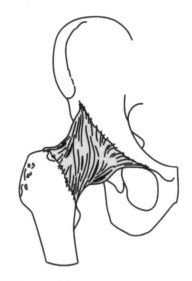

Gluteus minimus - lateral view   **Iliofemoral ligament - anterior view**

Actions: Medial rotation and abduction of the hip. With gluteus medius it counters the tendency of the pelvis to drop when the foot is lifted off the ground, such as in walking.
Nerve supply: Superior gluteal nerve **L5** and S1

Gluteus medius arises on the outer ilium between the crest and the posterior gluteal line and from the deep fascia that covers it. It attaches onto the lateral greater trochanter by a flat tendon. Its anterior two third is directly palpable below the iliac crest but its posterior third is covered by gluteus maximus.

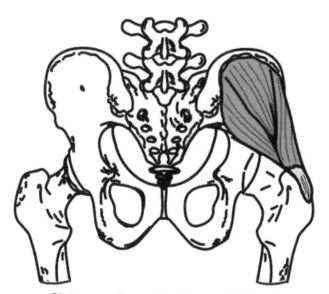 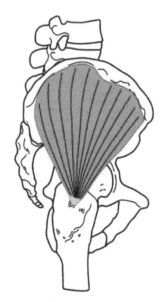

Gluteus medius and pelvis – posterior view   **Lateral view**

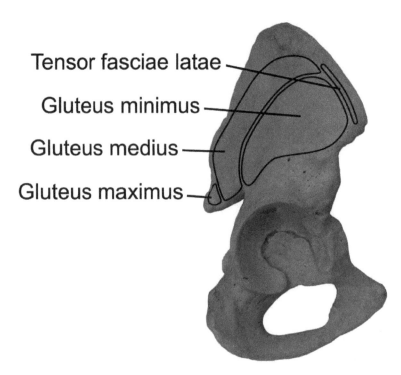

Tensor fasciae latae

Gluteus minimus

Gluteus medius

Gluteus maximus

Ilium - lateral view and muscle attachments

Actions: Gluteus medius is primarily a hip abductor. Its anterior fibres rotate the hip medially, and its posterior fibres weakly rotator it laterally. It is important in gait and supporting the weight bearing leg.

Nerve supply: Superior gluteal nerve **L5** and S1.

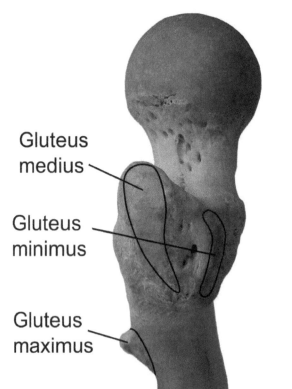

Gluteus medius

Gluteus minimus

Gluteus maximus

Upper femur - superior lateral view and muscle attachments

Tensor fasciae latae arises on the anterior iliac crest, anterior superior iliac spine and the deep surface of the fascia lata and attaches about one third of the way down the iliotibial tract. The iliotibial tract inserts onto the lateral condyle of the tibia. The muscle and iliotibial tract are palpable.

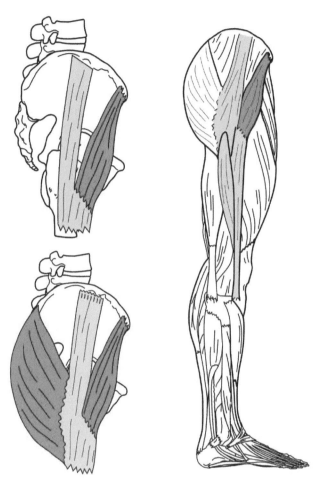

Tensor fascia latae - lateral view

Actions: The tensor fascia lata extends the knee and abducts and medially rotates the hip. It is most efficient when the knee is in extension. In the erect position it acts to stabilise the pelvis on the head of the femur and the condyles of the femur on the tibia and works with gluteus maximus to help control posture.
Nerve supply: Superior gluteal nerve L4 and L5.

The **fascia lata** is the deep fascia of the thigh and surrounds the thigh like a stocking. It attaches on all the bones of the pelvis including the coccyx, the condyles of the femur and tibia and head of the fibula and to the linea aspera via two intermuscular septa. It attaches on the inguinal ligament and sacrotuberous ligament and serves as partial attachment for some muscles in the thigh. It varies in thickness and splits into layers which envelop some of the muscles in the thigh.

On the lateral aspect of the thigh the fascia lata is thickened as the **Iliotibial tract**. It is thicker in the proximal thigh where gluteus maximus and tensor fascia lata attach and around the knee where biceps femoris, sartorius and quadriceps attach.

The iliotibial tract runs the length of the thigh and may function as a ligament and as a tendon. When the dense fascial sheet is taut it assists with the maintenance of an erect posture. It also acts as a shock absorber between the pelvis and the leg. When one side becomes hypertonic, its stabilising postural function becomes distorted and it may cause the pelvis to tilt anteriorly and inferiorly, increase the lumbar lordosis and create a functional short leg.

The hip external rotator muscles

Piriformis arises on the anterior sacrum but a few fibres arise from a small area on the gluteal surface of the ilium near the posterior inferior iliac spine and from the capsule of the sacroiliac joint. The muscle passes through the greater sciatic foramen and attaches by a rounded tendon onto the superior greater trochanter. The tendon may merge with the common tendon of the obturator internus and gamelli. The muscle may be partly or completely absent, divide or merge with gluteus medius.

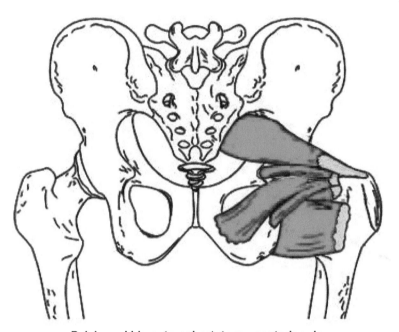

Pelvis and hip external rotators - posterior view
Muscles from top to bottom: piriformis, gamellus superior, obturator
internus, gamellus inferior, obturator externus and quadratus femoris

The **gamellus superior** arises on the posterior surface of the ischial spine and attaches onto the medial surface of the greater trochanter, via the tendon of obturator internus. It may be absent.

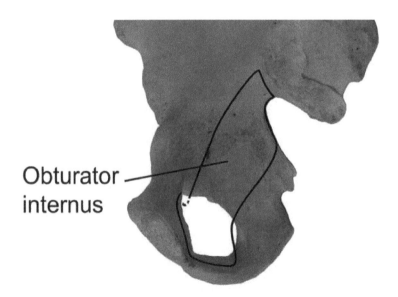

Lower ilium - medial view and obturator internus attachment

Obturator internus arises from within the true pelvis on the inner surface of the anterolateral wall of the pelvis, inferior pubic ramus, ischial ramus, and the medial surface of the obturator membrane.

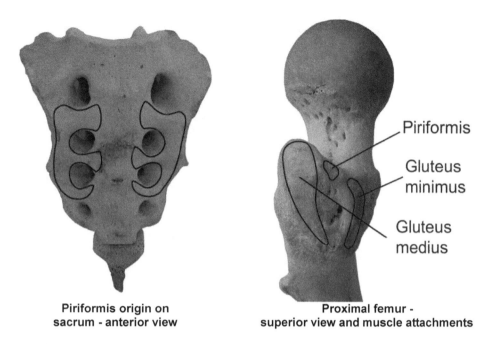

Piriformis origin on sacrum - anterior view

Proximal femur - superior view and muscle attachments

The muscle fibres converge onto four tendinous bands which makes a 90 degree bend over the ischium, between its spine and tuberosity and exits the pelvis through the lesser sciatic foramen. The bands merge into a single, flat tendon which receives fibres from the gamelli and then attaches onto the medial surface of the greater trochanter.

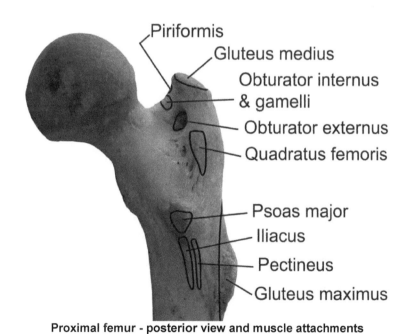

Proximal femur - posterior view and muscle attachments

The **gamellus inferior** arises on the upper ischial tuberosity and attaches onto the medial surface of the greater trochanter, via the tendon of obturator internus.

Actions: The piriformis, obturator internus and gamelli laterally rotate the extended thigh and abduct the flexed thigh.
Nerve supply: Piriformis - L5, **S1** and S2. Obturator internus and the gamelli - L5 and S1.

Obturator externus arises from the pubic ramus, ischial ramus and the outer surface of the obturator membrane. The muscle fibres converge onto a tendon which passes over the back of the neck of the femur and then attaches on the trochanteric fossa of the femur.

Actions: Lateral rotation of the thigh.
Nerve supply: L3 and **L4**.

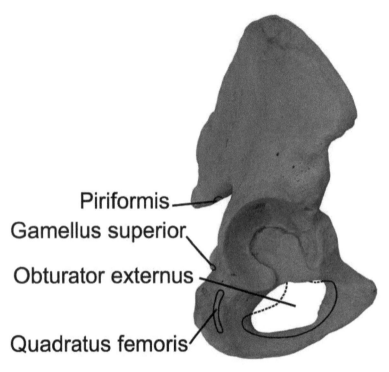

Piriformis
Gamellus superior
Obturator externus
Quadratus femoris

Ilium - lateral view and muscle attachments

The **quadratus femoris** arises from the upper lateral ischial tuberosity. The muscle passes posterior to the hip joint and the neck of the femur between gamellus inferior and adductor magnus and attaches onto the upper trochanteric crest of the femur. It may be absent.

Actions: Lateral rotation of the thigh.
Nerve supply: L5 and S1.

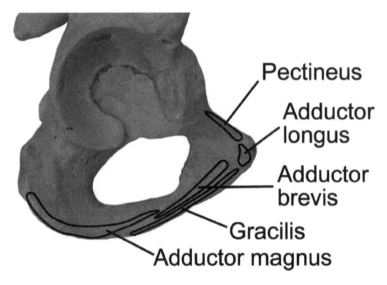

Pectineus
Adductor longus
Adductor brevis
Gracilis
Adductor magnus

Lower ilium - lateral view and muscle attachments

Piriformis, obturator internus and externus, quadratus femoris and the gamelli are deep and not easily palpable. They are important postural muscles and help to stabilise the hip joint.

The **Sciatic nerve** is derived from the lumbosacral plexus L4, L5, S1, S2 and S3. The sciatic nerve passes out of the pelvis through the greater sciatic foramen. It normally passes under the piriformis but it may pass over the piriformis or it may pierce the piriformis or it may divide early and the division, usually the common peroneal nerve, passes over or through the muscle. If hypertonic, the piriformis may then result in sciatica.

A hypertonic piriformis also has the ability to displace the sacrum anteriorly and laterally, distorting the sacroiliac joint and stretching the ligaments which pass over the joint, and creates the possibility of nerve impingement of the sacral plexus. A hypertonic obturator externus can irritate the **obturator nerve** as it passes through the obturator foramen, and there may be symptoms of pain, burning and tingling in the anterior and medial thigh and groin.

The hip adductor muscles

Adductor longus arises as a flat narrow tendon on the anterior pubis. The muscle runs inferiorly, posteriorly and laterally to attach along the middle third of the medial linea aspera of femur by an aponeurosis. Fibres of the muscle usually merge with those of adductor magnus, and the muscle may be doubled. It forms the medial border of the femoral triangle and is easily palpable in abduction, especially at its tendon origin.

Actions: Adduction, flexion and rotation of the thigh, depending on the position of the limb. Nerve supply: Obturator nerve L2, **L3** and L4.

Hip adductor muscles - anterior view

Pectineus and
adductor longus

Adductor brevis and
gracilis - layer 2

Adductor magnus -
posterior layer

Adductor brevis arises on the external aspect of the inferior pubic ramus and body of the pubis. The muscle runs inferiorly, posteriorly and laterally to attach by an aponeurosis to the upper medial linea aspera of the femur from as high up as the lesser trochanter. The muscle may be split into separate parts or merge with adductor magnus. It is deep to adductor longus and pectineus and is not directly palpable.

Actions: Hip adduction and it is a weak hip flexor.
Nerve supply: Obturator nerve L2, **L3** and L4.

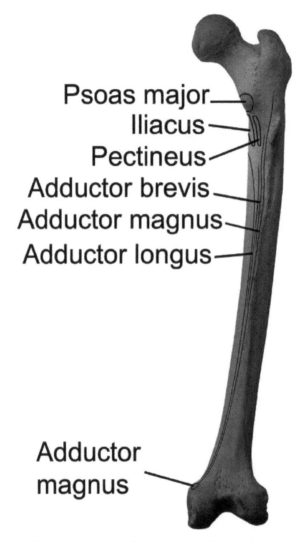

Psoas major
Iliacus
Pectineus
Adductor brevis
Adductor magnus
Adductor longus

Adductor magnus

Femur - posterior view and muscle attachments

Adductor magnus arises on the anterior surface of inferior ramus of pubis and ischium and inferolateral part of the ischial tuberosity. Its fibres fan out from their origin to attach on an aponeurosis with short fibres running horizontally to the medial edge of the gluteal tuberosity, intermediate fibres running diagonally to attach along most of the whole length of the linea aspera and to a proximal part of the medial supracondylar line.

The longest ischiocondylar fibres run almost vertically from the ischial tuberosity to a round tendon attaching onto the adductor tubercle on the medial condyle of the femur. The aponeurotic attachment is broken at several places by tendinous arches, the most significant of which is the large adductor hiatus which allows the femoral vessels to pass between the anterior thigh and the popliteal fossa.

610

Adductor magnus is a large triangular sheet of muscle covered anteriorly by adductor longus and adductor brevis and posteriorly by the hamstrings. Although its tendons are palpable, the muscle is only directly palpable along its thicker medial border between the hamstrings and gracilis.

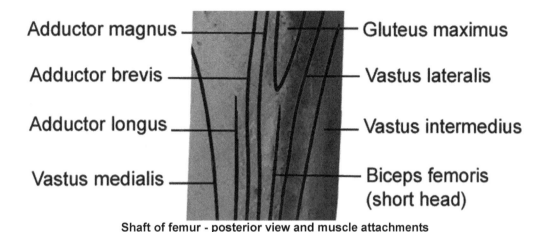

Shaft of femur - posterior view and muscle attachments

Actions: Adductor magnus adducts, flexes, extends and may rotate the thigh, depending on the position of the limb. Because of its posterior placement and attachment on the ischial tuberosity the muscle functionally acts like a hamstring.
Nerve supply: Obturator nerve L2, **L3** and **L4**. The tibial division of the sciatic nerve supplies the ischiocondylar part of the muscle.

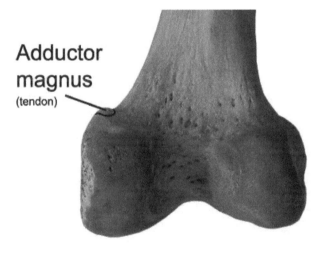

Distal femur - posterior view and muscle attachment

Gracilis arises on a thin aponeurosis running along a line of the inferior pubic arch. It arises on the lower half of the body of the pubis, the ramus of the pubis and a small part of the ramus of the ischium. Its tendon merges with the tendon of sartorius and attaches onto the medial surface of the tibia, distal to the condyle and just proximal to the semitendinosus tendon. Some of its fibres merge with the deep fascia of the leg. It is palpable as a thin flat muscle running down the medial thigh.

Actions: Gracilis flexes and medially rotates the leg. It is a weak adductor of the thigh.
Nerve supply: Obturator nerve **L2**, L3 and L4 supplies the gracilis and the adductors and the skin of the upper medial thigh. The nerve descends through obturator foramen and is not palpable.

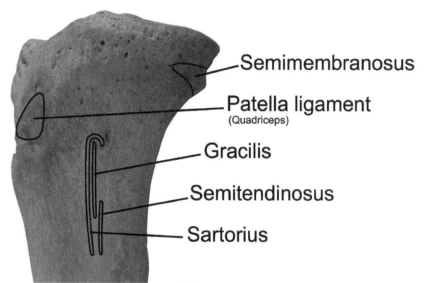

Semimembranosus

Patella ligament
(Quadriceps)

Gracilis

Semitendinosus

Sartorius

Proximal tibia - anteromedial view and muscle attachments

Pectineus arises on the crest of the pubis, along a line running between the iliopubic eminence and the pubic tubercle and from the fascia covering its anterior surface. Its fibres run inferiorly, posteriorly and laterally to attach along a line between the lesser trochanter and the linea aspera. The muscle has a flat quadrangular shape and forms part of the floor of the femoral triangle. It may be two-layered and may attach onto the capsule of the hip joint.

Nerve supply: Femoral nerve **L2** and L3 and sometimes the accessory obturator nerve L3. Actions: Pectineus flexes the thigh and assists with adduction, especially when the hip is flexed. During normal standing it has minimal activity. Its major role is as synergists in controlling posture, particularly during gait.

Hip joint - anterior view

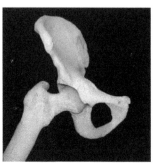
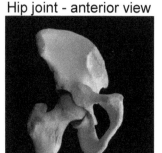
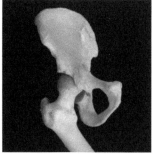

| **Hip abduction** | **Hip in neutral** | **Hip adduction** |

The hip joint

The hip joint is a spheroidal or ball and socket type joint between the head of the femur and acetabulum of the pelvis, augmented by a ring-shaped fibrocartilagenous rim, the acetabular labrum. The synovial joint is covered by cartilage except near the centre where the ligamentum teres joins the head to acetabulum.

612

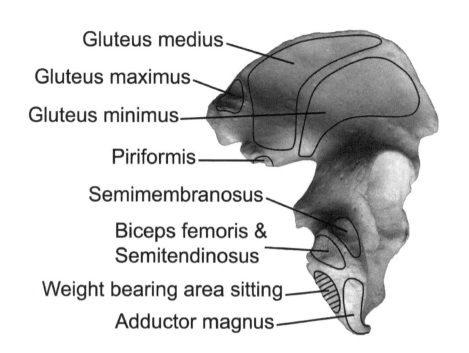

Ilium - inferior lateral view and muscle attachments

A joint capsule is supported by the iliofemoral, ischiofemoral, and pubofemoral ligaments. Of these, the iliofemoral ligament is the strongest, and with the ischiofemoral prevents the trunk from falling backward when in the upright standing position. In the sitting position, it relaxes, and permits the pelvis to tilt forward or backward. The iliofemoral ligament also prevents excessive adduction and internal rotation, and the ischiofemoral ligament also prevents internal rotation. The pubofemoral ligament restricts abduction and internal rotation.

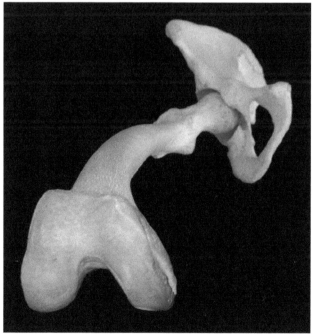

Hip flexion - anterior view

The hip joint supports the weight of the body and enables locomotion, balance and normal posture. It is a multiaxial joint permitting movement in three planes.

Anatomy of the knee: femur, tibial and fibula 6.6 – 7.1

Quadriceps femoris

The four muscles that make up quadriceps femoris are rectus femoris, vastus lateralis, vastus medialis and vastus intermedius.

Rectus femoris arises by two tendinous heads. The straight head arises from the anterior inferior iliac spine of the ilium and the reflected head arises from an area just above the acetabulum and from the hip joint capsule. The two heads form an aponeurosis and the muscle arises from this. Inferiorly another thick aponeurosis emerges from the posterior part of the muscle which becomes a flat tendon attaching onto the base of the patella. Rectus femoris is the most superficial quadriceps muscle running down the anterior thigh and is easily palpable.

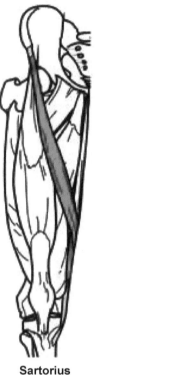 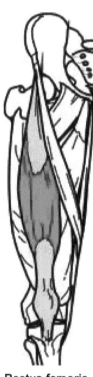 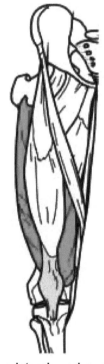

| **Sartorius** | **Rectus femoris** | **Vastus laterals and medialis** |

Vastus lateralis arises on a broad aponeurosis attached to the intertrochanteric line, the greater trochanter, and the lateral lip of the gluteal tuberosity and the upper linea aspera. The aponeurosis covers a large part of the muscle. The muscle also arises on the tendon of gluteus maximus and on the lateral intermuscular septum. Inferiorly a thick aponeurosis emerges from the deep part of the muscle which becomes a flat tendon attaching onto the lateral patella. Some fibres of the tendon also blend with the capsule of the knee joint and the iliotibial band.

Vastus medialis arises on a lower area of the intertrochanteric line, the medial lip of the linea aspera and the medial supracondylar line. The muscle also arises on the tendons of adductor longus and magnus and the medial intermuscular septum. The muscle attaches onto an aponeurosis emerging from a deep part of the muscle which attaches on the medial border of the patella and the quadriceps tendon. Some fibres of this aponeurosis blend with the capsule of the knee joint and the medial tibial condyle. The muscle is prominent just above the medial aspect of knee and is important for knee stability.

Vastus intermedius arises on the upper anterior and lateral shaft of the femur and a lower part of the lateral intermuscular septum. The muscle attaches on an aponeurosis which forms the deep layer of the quadriceps tendon, and on the lateral border of the patella and the lateral condyle of the tibia. The muscle is deep to rectus femoris.

Actions: Quadriceps femoris extends the leg on the thigh. Rectus femoris is also a weak hip flexor, flexing the thigh on the pelvis or, if the thigh is fixed, flexing the pelvis on the thigh. The lowest fibres of vastus medialis are important in maintaining the patella in its groove during the final phase of knee extension. Both vastus medialis and lateralis may help with knee stability.
Nerve supply: Femoral nerve L2, **L3** and **L4**.

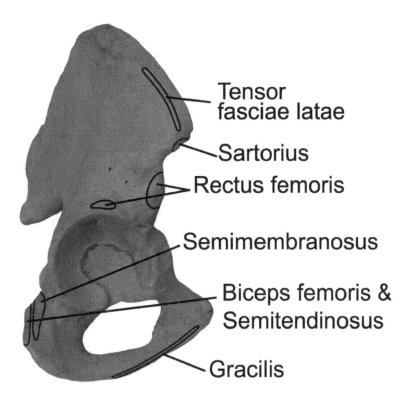

Ilium - lateral view and muscle attachments

The tendons from the four parts of the quadriceps muscle unite to form a single quadriceps tendon. Some of the fibres of the tendon attach onto the base of the patella and other fibres pass over the patella and attach on the tibial tuberosity. The patella is a sesamoid bone within the quadriceps tendon. The quadriceps tendon from the patella to the tibial tuberosity is known as the patella ligament. Fibrous expansions of the quadriceps tendon extend into and provide support to the capsule of the knee, and other fibres attach on the tibial condyles and merge with fascia of the leg. Fibrous slips of rectus femoris may attach on the anterior superior iliac spine and the reflective head may be absent.

Sartorius arises on the anterior superior iliac spine of the ilium and a small area of the notch below it. The muscle passes obliquely down the whole length of the medial thigh and then medial to the knee. It is palpable as a long narrow strap muscle forming the lateral border of the femoral triangle. Below the knee it passes inferiorly and then anteriorly to attach on the medial surface of the upper tibia as a broad aponeurosis. Its muscle fibres cover the tendons of gracilis and semitendinosus and the upper part of its aponeurosis wraps around gracilis.

At the medial side of the knee the sartorius muscle is medial to the gracilis tendon, and the semitendinosus tendon is lateral and slightly posterior to gracilis. The semimembranosus is muscular to its insertion and lies deep between the semitendinosus and gracilis tendons.

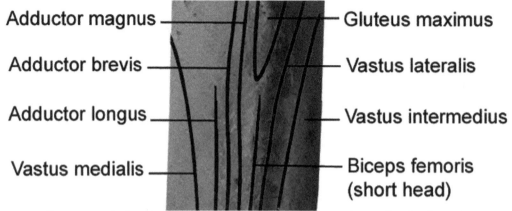

Femur - posterior view of upper part of linea aspera and muscle attachments

Actions: Sartorius flexes, abducts and laterally rotates the thigh and flexes and medially rotates the leg. It is usually called on to combine simultaneous flexion, abduction and lateral rotation of the thigh with flexion of the leg, as in bringing the foot up towards the upper body. Nerve supply: Femoral nerve L2, L3 and L4.

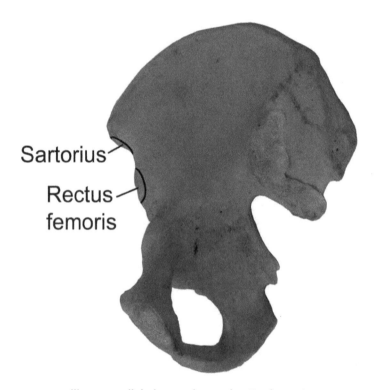

Ilium - medial view and muscle attachments

Hamstrings

The four muscles that make up hamstrings are semimembranosus, semitendinosus and biceps femoris.

Semimembranosus tendon arises on a superolateral area of the upper ischial tuberosity. It also receives fibres inferiorly and medially from the semitendinosus, biceps femoris and adductor magnus. Muscle fibres arise from an aponeurotic expansion of its upper tendon and a second aponeurosis emerges distally to narrow into its tendon of insertion. The muscle and aponeurosis are deep to semitendinosus in the posteromedial thigh.

616

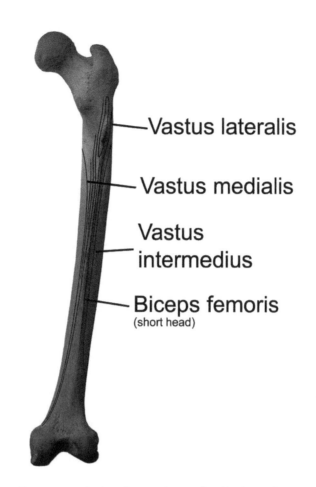

Femur - posterior view and muscle attachments

Semimembranosus remains a muscle to its insertion on the tubercle on the posterior aspect of the medial tibial condyle. Fibres also attach onto the medial tibia, just posterior to the lateral collateral ligament, onto the fascia overlying popliteus, and merge with the oblique popliteal ligament which attaches onto the lateral femoral condyle.

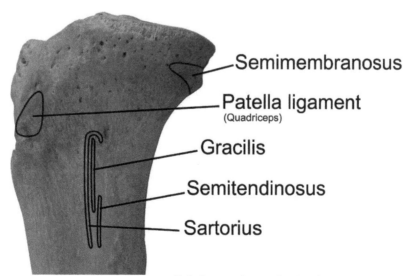

Proximal tibia - anteromedial view and muscle attachments

Variations: Fibres may attach on the sacrotuberous ligament or femur. The muscle varies in size and may be absent.

Semitendinosus arises on a medial area of the upper ischial tuberosity by a short tendon, which it shares with the long head of biceps femoris and by an aponeurosis joining the two muscles. The fusiform muscle ends about half way down the posteromedial thigh as a long round tendon. The tendon curves around the medial tibial condyle and attaches onto the anteromedial tibia, posterior and inferior to the tendons of gracilis and sartorius. Its tendon merges with the tendon of gracilis and extends into the deep fascia of the leg.

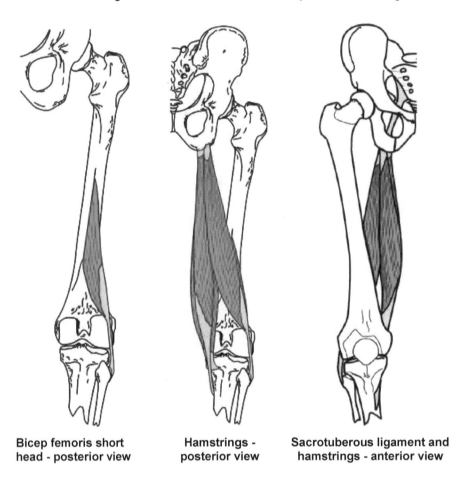

| Bicep femoris short head - posterior view | Hamstrings - posterior view | Sacrotuberous ligament and hamstrings - anterior view |

Biceps femoris has two heads. The long head of arises on a medial area of the upper ischial tuberosity by a tendon, which it shares with semitendinosus and from an inferior area of the sacrotuberous ligament.

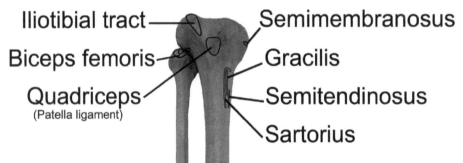

Iliotibial tract — Semimembranosus

Biceps femoris — Gracilis

Quadriceps — Semitendinosus
(Patella ligament)

— Sartorius

Proximal tibia and fibula - anterior view and muscle attachments

The short head arises on the lateral lip of the linea aspera and the lateral supracondylar line of the femur and the lateral intermuscular septum. The short heads is connected to the long head by an aponeurosis which covers the posterior surface of the long head of biceps femoris.

Most of the tendon attaches onto the head of the fibula. Part of the tendon attaches on the lateral condyle of the tibia and part of it merges with fibres of the lateral collateral ligament. The short head may be absent.

Actions: Acting from above the hamstrings flex the leg. Semimembranosus, semitendinosus and the long head of biceps femoris extend the thigh and assist in stabilisation of the hip joint. In the semiflexed position semimembranosus and semitendinosus internally rotate the leg, and biceps femoris externally rotates the leg. When the hip is extended semimembranosus and semitendinosus medially rotate the thigh, and the long head of biceps femoris laterally rotates the thigh. The hamstrings may also give collateral support to the knee joint.

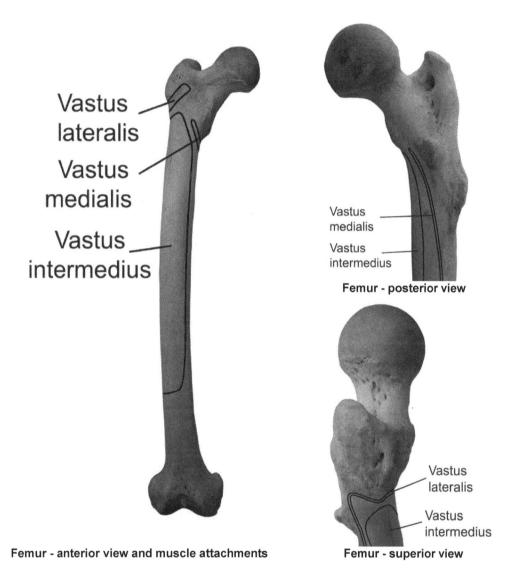

Femur - anterior view and muscle attachments **Femur - superior view**

Nerve supply to the hamstrings: Sciatic nerve **L5, S1** and S2. The common peroneal nerve supplies the short head of biceps femoris. The tibial nerve supplies the long head of biceps femoris, semimembranosus and semitendinosus.

Popliteus arises on the anterior end of a depression on the lateral side of the lateral condyle of the femur by a broad tendon. This depression also forms a groove for the tendon to slide in when the knee is in flexion. The muscle also arises on the arcuate popliteal ligament which merges with the capsule and the outer part of the lateral meniscus. The lower part of the muscle is attached on a triangular area on the posterior tibia just above the soleal line.

619

Popliteus is a flat triangular muscle covering part of the floor of the popliteal fossa deep behind the knee. It is covered by a layer of strong fascia derived mainly from semimembranosus

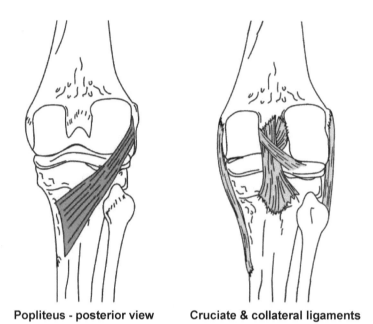

Popliteus - posterior view   **Cruciate & collateral ligaments**

Nerve supply: Tibial nerve L4, L5 and S1.
Actions: Popliteus medially rotates the tibia on the femur or if the tibia is fixed laterally rotated the femur. The muscle unlocks the extended knee at the beginning of knee flexion. It acts on the posterior part of the lateral meniscus and may protect it from being crushed by the condyle of the femur during knee flexion and rotation.

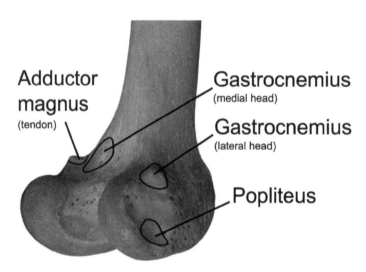

Distal femur - posterolateral view and muscle attachments

The knee joint

The knee joint is a hinge type joint, made up of three articulating parts. The femoropatellar joint is a saddle joint between the patellar, a sesamoid bone within the quadriceps tendon, and the patellar groove, the articulating surface in font of the femur. During knee flexion or extension the patella slides on the patella groove. Two femorotibial joints are between the corresponding medial and lateral condyles of the femur and tibia. These pivotal condylar joints each have a meniscus, synovial membrane, joint capsule and supporting ligaments.

The medial and lateral menisci contain extensive collagen fibres which act as shock absorbers, stop the ends of the bones from rubbing against each other, deepen the tibial joint surface for the femoral condyles to sit and maintain congruency between the articulating surfaces.

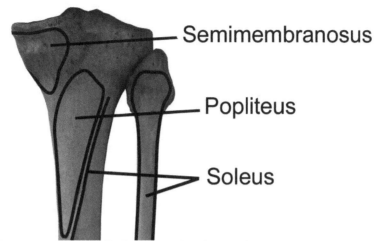

Proximal tibia and fibula - posterior view and muscle attachments

Ligaments stabilize the knee. Medial and lateral collateral ligaments prevent lateral and medial knee movements and anterior and posterior cruciate ligaments prevent the tibia from sliding to far forward or backward. The knee permits flexion and extension and a small amount of internal and external rotation when the knee is in the semi-flexed position.

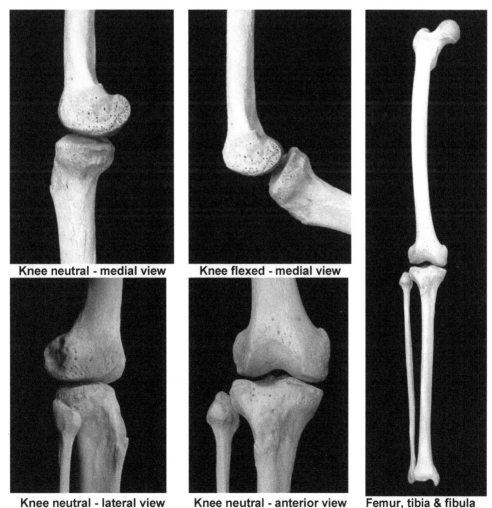

Knee neutral - medial view   **Knee flexed - medial view**

Knee neutral - lateral view   **Knee neutral - anterior view**   **Femur, tibia & fibula**

Anatomy of the ankle and foot: tibia, fibula, tarsals, metatarsals and phalanges 7.1 – 7.3

The calf muscles

The most superficial muscles of the posterior leg, the gastrocnemius and soleus, known as the calf muscles, are separated from the deeper muscles of the posterior compartment by deep transverse fascia.

Gastrocnemius forms the bulk of the calf and arises by two heads attached to the medial and lateral femoral condyles by strong flat tendons and from adjacent parts of the knee joint capsule. The larger medial head arises from an area behind the adductor tubercle, just above and behind the medial femoral condyle. The lateral head arises from the lateral surface of the lateral femoral condyle. Fibrous expansions from the tendons of both heads extend inferiorly over the posterior surface of the muscles. The heads are separated by an aponeurosis which attaches to its posterior surface, and this tendinous expansion forms the tendo calcaneus also known as the Achilles tendon.

Actions: Plantar flexion, knee flexion, stability and balance.
Nerve supply: Tibial nerve **S1** and S2.

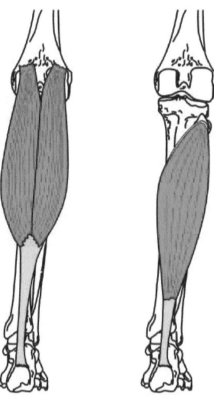

Gastrocnemius   **Soleus**

Soleus arises from a posterior area of the upper fibula, the head of the fibula, the soleal line and the upper medial tibia, and from the posterior surface of an aponeurosis which spans between the tibia and fibula. The muscle fibres insert on the anterior surface of the tendo calcaneus. The tendo calcaneus inserts onto the middle of the posterior calcaneus. Soleus is deep to gastrocnemius and only directly palpable at the distal aspect of the medial and lateral sides of the leg.

Actions: Plantar flexion and balance. During standing, soleus is continuously active whereas gastrocnemius exhibits only intermittent contraction.
Nerve supply: Tibial nerve S1 and **S2**.

Tendo calcaneus (the Achilles tendon) extends about half the length of the leg. It is broad and flat superiorly and becomes thicker and rounded as it descends. Its fibres spiral and give the tendon elastic properties which facilitate gait. The tendon is strong but may be ruptured.

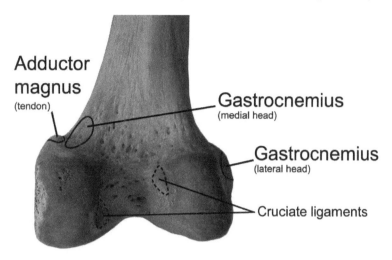

Distal femur - posterior view

The posterior compartment

Tibialis posterior arises on the lateral side of the proximal half of the posterior shaft of the tibia, along the medial side of the proximal two thirds of the posterior shaft of the fibula and the posterior interosseous membrane, and from the deep transverse fascia and intermuscular septa. It is the deepest of the flexor muscles.

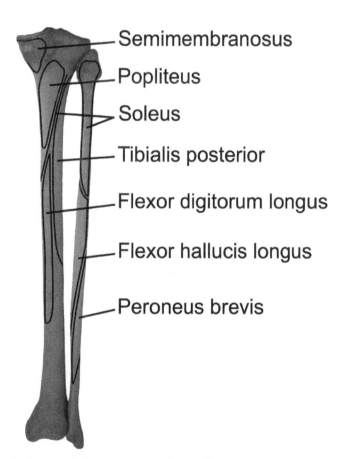

Tibia and fibula - posterior view and muscle attachments

The tendon passes over a groove behind the medial malleolus, with the flexor digitorum longus tendon just posterior to it and separated from it by a fibrous septum and its own synovial sheath. After passing over the plantar calcaneonavicular ligament the tendon splits into a larger, direct branch which runs more superficially to attach onto the navicular tuberosity. From this fibres continue to the first cuneiform and the sustentaculum tali of the calcaneus. The deeper branch sends fibrous expansions laterally to the second cuneiform and the bases of metatarsals 2, 3, and 4. The cuboid and third cuneiform may also receive slips. In the foot the tendon encloses a sesamoid fibrocartilage. The tendon is prominent below the malleolus with resisted inversion and plantar flexion of the foot.

Actions: The muscle produces inversion of the foot and assists with plantar flexion and adduction. It supports the arch during gait.
Nerve supply: Tibial nerve L4 and L5.

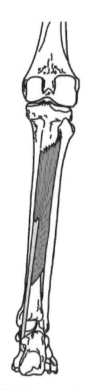
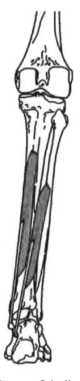

Tibialis posterior   **Flexor digitorum & hallucis longus**

Flexor Digitorum longus arises along the medial side of the posterior shaft of the tibia, medial to tibialis posterior and just below the soleal line, on the fascia covering tibialis posterior. The tendon passes over a groove behind the medial malleolus and over the medial side of the sustentaculum tali. More distally it crosses the tendon of flexor hallucis longus and receives a slip from it. It also receives slips from flexor accessorius. It attaches onto the bases of the distal phalanges of the lateral four toes. The tendon is palpable posterior and inferior to the medial malleolus and is prominent with resisted toe flexion.

Actions: It flexes toes and assists in inversion, adduction and plantar flexion of the foot.
Nerve supply: Tibial nerve **S2** and S3.

Flexor Hallucis longus arises along two thirds of the medial side of the posterior shaft of the fibula, the interosseous membrane and the fascia covering tibialis posterior. It lies deep to soleus and the Achilles tendon and is separated from it by the deep transverse fascia. The tendon runs the whole length of the muscle. As it descends it passes over grooves on the posterior tibia, posterior talus and the inferior side of the sustentaculum tali of the calcaneus. More distally it crosses over the tendon of flexor digitorum longus. It attaches onto the plantar surface of the base of the distal phalanx of the big toe.

624

Actions: It flexes the big toe and assists in inversion, adduction and plantar flexion of the foot. It is most active in the push off phase of gait
Nerve supply: Tibial nerve **S2** and S3.

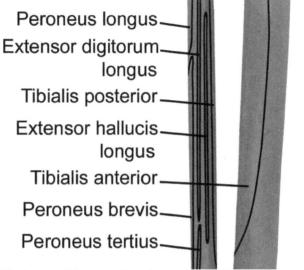

Fibula and tibia - anterior view and muscle attachments

The tendons of the deep posterior muscles pass behind the medial malleolus, deep to the flexor retinaculum but superficial to the deltoid ligament. From medial to lateral the structures passing behind the medial malleolus and into the foot are: tibialis posterior tendon, flexor digitorum longus tendon, the posterior tibial artery and tibial nerve and the flexor hallucis longus tendon.

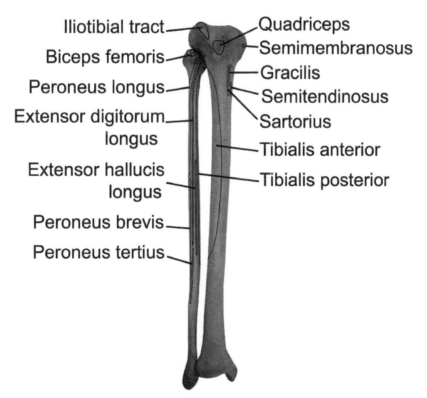

Fibula and tibia - anterior view and muscle attachments

The deltoid ligament or medial collateral ligament is broad and strong. It runs from the medial malleolus to the talus and calcaneus. The deep transverse fascia divides the superficial and deep muscles of the posterior compartment of the leg. At the ankle it forms a thickening, the flexor retinaculum, which supports the flexor tendons, blood vessels and nerves as they pass into the foot. The flexor retinaculum runs from the tip of the medial malleolus to the medial process of the calcaneal tuberosity. It also attaches on the sustentaculum tali above and below the flexor hallucis longus tendon and merges with the deep fascia of the dorsum of the foot and the plantar aponeurosis.

The anterior compartment

Tibialis anterior arises on the lateral tibial condyle and proximal two thirds of the anterolateral surface of the tibia, the interosseous membrane, the intermuscular septum between it and extensor digitorum longus, and on the deep surface of the deep fascia (fascia cruris) of the leg. The tendon attaches on the medial and inferior side of the first cuneiform and the base of the first metatarsal. Tibialis anterior is the most superficial muscle in the anterior compartment and lies lateral to the sharp subcutaneous border of the tibia. Its tendon is prominent with resisted dorsi flexion of the foot.
Variations: Attachments may occur on the talus, first metatarsal head or proximal phalanx.

Actions: It dorsiflexes and inverts the foot. It is active during gait.
Clinical indications: When the tibialis anterior becomes extremely hypertonic, its muscle attachment may pull away the periosteum from the tibia, resulting in shin splints and periostitis. Hypertonicity of the muscles of the anterior compartment can result in ischaemia of the deep peroneal nerve, causing toe drop.
Nerve supply: Deep peroneal nerve **L4** and L5.

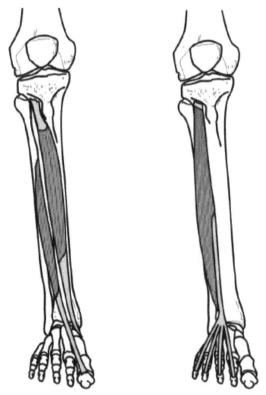

Extensor hallucis longus   **Extensor digitorum longus**
and tibialis anterior

Extensor hallucis longus arises on the middle of the fibula shaft and interosseous membrane and attaches onto the base of the distal phalanx of the big toe. A slip usually attaches on the base of the proximal phalanx. The muscle lies deep in the anterior compartment. The tendon is prominent with resisted extension of the big toe.

Actions: It extends the big toe, dorsiflexes the foot.
Nerve supply: Deep Peroneal nerve L5 and S1

626

Extensor digitorum longus arises on the lateral tibial condyle, upper 2/3 of the anterior fibula, interosseous membrane, the intermuscular septum, between it and tibialis anterior and on the deep surface of the deep fascia (fascia cruis) of the leg. It may be palpated lateral to tibialis anterior but part of it lies deep to tibialis anterior. The tendon passes under the extensor retinaculum, lateral to extensor hallucis longus and on the dorsum of the foot splits into four tendons which attach onto the bases of the middle and distal phalanges of the lateral four toes. The tendon is prominent with resisted extension of the toes. Variations include attachment on the metatarsals or big toe.

Actions: It extends the toes and dorsiflexes the foot.
Nerve supply: Deep peroneal nerve L5 and S1

Peroneus tertius is part of extensor digitorum longus. It arises on a lower part of the fibula, interosseous membrane and anterior crural intermuscular septum. The tendon passes under the extensor retinaculum with extensor digitorum longus and attaches on the base of the fifth metatarsal. It may be absent.

Actions: It dorsiflexes the foot and may aid eversion of the foot.
Nerve supply: Deep peroneal nerve L5 and S1.

Peroneus muscles

Peroneus longus arises on the head of the fibula and upper two-thirds of the lateral shaft of the fibula, the deep fascia of the leg (the fascia cruris) and from the anterior and posterior crural intermuscular septum. A few fibres may arise on the lateral tibial condyle.

The tendon is long and passes over a groove on the posterior aspect of the lateral malleolus, which it shares with the peroneus brevis tendon. It runs over the lateral calcaneus going anteriorly and inferiorly and passing below the peroneal tubercle, also known as the peroneal trochlea. A sesamoid fibrocartilage or bone is present in a thickening of the tendon as it changes direction at the cuboid. It goes deep, passing over a groove running under the cuboid and is covered by the long plantar ligament. It stays hard up against the tarsals, running diagonally under the plantar surface of the foot, over the third cuneiform and second metatarsal bone. It attaches onto the lateral side of the base of the first metatarsal and onto the anterolateral corner of the first cuneiform. Slips may also attach onto the bases of the other metatarsals or adductor hallucis and sometimes peroneus longus and brevis may be fused.

Action: Plantar flexion and eversion of the foot. It helps supports the arch, especially during toe off. It may act on the leg from its distal attachment during side swaying.
Nerve supply: Superficial peroneal nerve **L5**, **S1** and S2.

Peroneus brevis arises on the middle third of the lateral shaft of the fibula and on the anterior and posterior crural intermuscular septum. It lies deep to peroneus longus. Behind the lateral malleolus the peroneus brevis tendon lies anterior to the peroneus longus tendon. Both tendons run close together under the superior peroneal retinaculum where they share a common synovial sheath.

On the lateral side of the calcaneus the tendons diverge, the peroneus longus tendon passing below the peroneal tubercle and then under the foot, and the peroneus brevis tendon passing above the peroneal tubercle and attaching on the dorsal lateral side of the tuberosity of the fifth metatarsal, also known as the styloid process.

Actions: Eversion and plantar flexion of the foot. It may give support to the lateral ligaments and steady the leg on the foot.
Nerve supply: Superficial peroneal nerve **L5**, **S1** and S2.

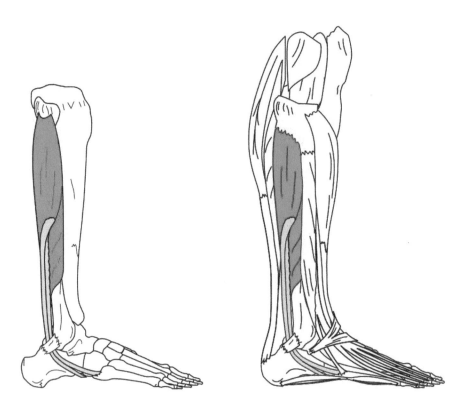

Peroneus longus and peroneus brevis

The peroneus longus and brevis tendons are held in place against the lateral side of the ankle by fibrous bands, the superior and inferior peroneal retinaculum. The superior peroneal retinaculum attaches onto the lateral surface of the calcaneus and the posterior lateral malleolus and merges with the deep transverse fascia of the leg. It forms a canal for peroneus longus and brevis tendons as it covers the groove behind the lateral malleolus. The inferior peroneal retinaculum attaches onto the lateral calcaneus and merges with the inferior extensor retinaculum anteriorly. Some fibres attach on the periosteum of the peroneal tubercle of the calcaneus, thereby forming a septum, which separates the peroneus longus and brevis tendons. A common synovial sheath encloses the tendons for a distance of about 4 cm proximal to the tip of the lateral malleolus. When the tendons split they pass through separate osseo-aponeurotic canals formed by inferior peroneal retinaculum and the calcaneus and have independent synovial sheaths. The peroneus longus tendon passes through a second synovial sheath as it runs obliquely under the sole of the foot.

Clinical considerations
Pain in front of the lateral malleolus is commonly due to a sprained anterior talofibular ligament. If untreated this may leave the peroneus longus and peroneus brevis muscles in a hypertonic state causing tendonitis or tenosynovitis.

Short muscles of foot

Dorsal aspect
Extensor digitorum brevis arises on the distal, lateral and superior surface of the calcaneus and the inferior extensor retinaculum. The medial tendon attaches onto the dorsal aspect of the base of the proximal phalanx of the big toe. The other three tendons attach onto the lateral side of the long extensor tendons of the second, third and fourth toes. The muscle is subject to significant variation including additional slips arising from the talus, navicular and dorsal interosseous muscles, missing tendons and additional tendons.

Actions: Extension of the medial four toes.
Nerve supply: Deep peroneal nerve S1 and S2.

628

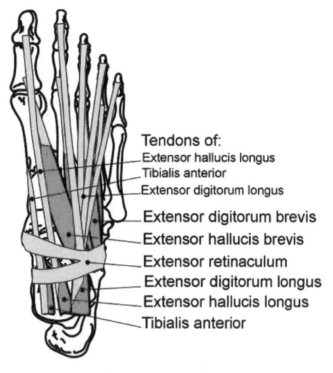

Tendons of:
Extensor hallucis longus
Tibialis anterior
Extensor digitorum longus

Extensor digitorum brevis
Extensor hallucis brevis
Extensor retinaculum
Extensor digitorum longus
Extensor hallucis longus
Tibialis anterior

Foot - superior view

The **dorsal interossei** lie between the metatarsal bones. They arise by two heads on adjacent sides of two metatarsal bones and attach onto the base of the proximal phalanx of the toes.

Actions: These muscles abduct and flex the toes. They act at the metatarsophalangeal joints on the proximal phalanx of the toes.
Nerve supply: Deep branch of the lateral plantar nerve S2 and **S3**.

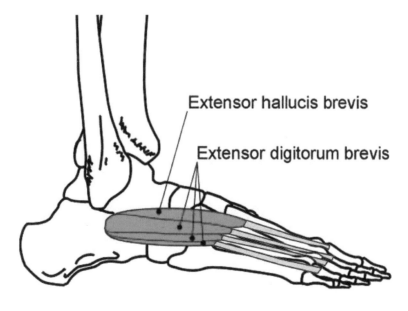

Extensor hallucis brevis

Extensor digitorum brevis

Foot - lateral view

The deep fascia is thin. Proximally it arises on the inferior extensor retinaculum. On each side of the foot it merges with the plantar aponeurosis. Distally it form a sheath around the extensor tendons.

Plantar aspect
Flexor digitorum brevis arises as a tendon on the medial process of the calcanean tuberosity, plantar aponeurosis and fascia attached to adjacent muscles. It splits into four tendons which attach onto the middle phalanx of the lateral four toes. The tendon to the fifth toe is frequently absent.
Actions: Flexes toes.
Nerve supply: The medial plantar nerve S2 and **S3**.

Flexor hallucis brevis arises on the plantar surface of the cuboid and third cuneiform bone and on the tibialis posterior tendon and plantar fascia. It attaches onto the base of the proximal phalanx and onto the abductor tendon. A sesamoid bone is found within the tendon.
Actions: Flexes proximal phalanx of big toe.
Nerve supply: The medial plantar nerve S2 and **S3**.

Abductor hallucis arises on the flexor retinaculum, medial process of the calcanean tuberosity, plantar aponeurosis and fascia between it and flexor digitorum brevis. It attaches, via a tendon, onto the medial side of the base of the proximal phalanx of the big toe. A slip may attach onto the medial sesamoid bone. The muscle lies on the medial side of the foot.
Actions: Flexes and abducts the big toe.
Nerve supply: The medial plantar nerve S2 and **S3**.

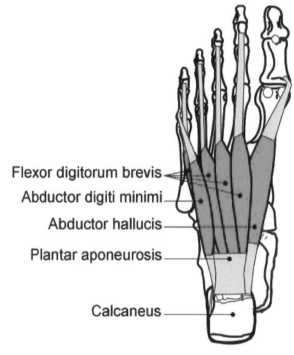

Flexor digitorum brevis
Abductor digiti minimi
Abductor hallucis
Plantar aponeurosis
Calcaneus

Foot - inferior view

Adductor hallucis arises by two heads. The oblique head arises from the base of the second, third and fourth metatarsal bones and the sheath of the peroneus longus tendon. The transverse head arises from capsules and overlying ligaments of the third, fourth and fifth metatarsophalangeal joints. It attaches onto the lateral side of the base of the proximal phalanx of the big toe and merges with flexor hallucis brevis and lateral sesamoid bone. It is important for the internal strength of the foot. Variations include additional attachments on the first metatarsal and the proximal phalanx of the second toe.
Actions: Adducts and flexes the proximal phalanx of the big toe.
Nerve supply: The lateral plantar nerve S2 and **3**.

Flexor digiti minimi brevis arises on the medial side of the plantar surface of the base of the fifth metatarsal bone and the sheath of the peroneus longus tendon. It attaches onto the lateral side of the base of the proximal phalanx of the fifth toe. Some of its fibres may attach onto the lateral and distal area on the fifth metatarsal bone.

Actions: Flexes the proximal phalanx of the little toe.
Nerve supply: The lateral plantar nerve S2 and **3.**

Abductor digiti minimi arises on the lateral and medial processes of the calcanean tuberosity and the area of bone between, plantar aponeurosis and fascia between it and flexor digitorum brevis. It attaches by a single tendon onto the lateral side of the base of the proximal phalanx of the fifth toe. The muscle runs down the lateral side of the foot, frequently with intermediate attachments on the base of the fifth metatarsal bone.
Actions: It is more a flexor than an abductor of the little toe.
Nerve supply: The lateral plantar nerve S2 and **S3**.

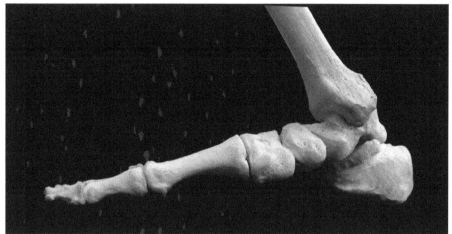

Foot, ankle and distal tibia - medial view

The **plantar interossei** lie below the metatarsal bones. They arise on the base and proximal shaft on the medial sides of the third, fourth and fifth metatarsal bones and attach to the base on the medial sides of the proximal phalanx of the toes.
Actions: Abducts toes and flexes proximal phalanx of the toes. They work together with the dorsal interossei to strengthen the metatarsal arch
Nerve supply: Deep branch of the lateral plantar nerve S2 and **S3**.

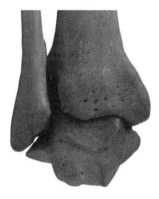

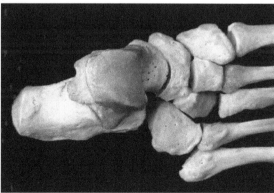

Ankle - posterior view   **Ankle and midtarsal area of foot**

The calcaneus
The medial tubercle of the calcaneus is the weight bearing medial part of the heel. As well as serving as the attachment for muscle, the medial tubercle also serves as the attachment for the plantar aponeurosis, which lies superficially and acts as a tie-beam to support the longitudinal arch of the foot. From the medial calcaneal tuberosity the plantar aponeurosis fans out to attach onto the metatarsal heads. The skin of the heel is thickened and supported with subcutaneous fibro-fatty tissue.

Clinical indications: Pes planus and other structural variations, shortness, strains and spasms. Heel spurs and plantar fasciitis can develop at or near the medial tubercle.

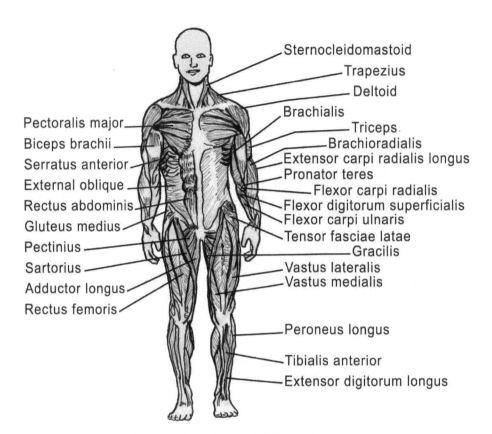

Anterior view of superficial muscles

Sternocleidomastoid
Trapezius
Deltoid
Brachialis
Triceps
Brachioradialis
Extensor carpi radialis longus
Pronator teres
Flexor carpi radialis
Flexor digitorum superficialis
Flexor carpi ulnaris
Tensor fasciae latae
Gracilis
Vastus lateralis
Vastus medialis
Peroneus longus
Tibialis anterior
Extensor digitorum longus

Pectoralis major
Biceps brachii
Serratus anterior
External oblique
Rectus abdominis
Gluteus medius
Pectinius
Sartorius
Adductor longus
Rectus femoris

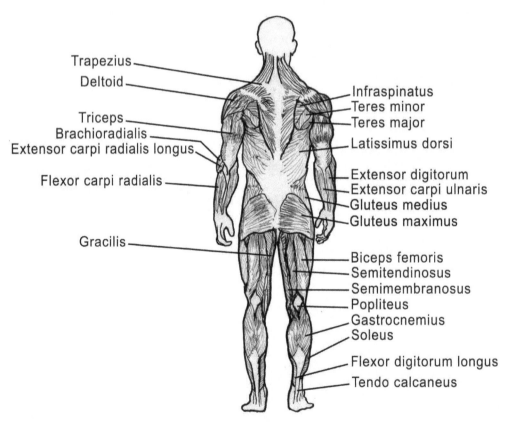

Posterior view of superficial muscles

Trapezius
Deltoid
Triceps
Brachioradialis
Extensor carpi radialis longus
Flexor carpi radialis
Gracilis

Infraspinatus
Teres minor
Teres major
Latissimus dorsi
Extensor digitorum
Extensor carpi ulnaris
Gluteus medius
Gluteus maximus
Biceps femoris
Semitendinosus
Semimembranosus
Popliteus
Gastrocnemius
Soleus
Flexor digitorum longus
Tendo calcaneus

Part C. Tables Routines, Combinations and Appendix

Regional tables - stretches based on anatomical region

No	Description	Title	Icon
1.1a (1)	The Lion - active stretches for the face, tongue, jaw, shoulders, cervical and thoracic spine	Lion stretch kneeling	
1.1b (2)		Lion stretch seated	
1.1c (3)		Lion stretch standing	
1.2 (4)	The Shrug - an active, post-isometric and passive stretch for the face, jaw, shoulders, arms and hands	The Shrug standing	
1.3a (5)	Chin tuck - active stretches for the suboccipital, cervical and upper thoracic spine	Chin tuck prone	
1.3b (6)		Chin tuck standing or seated	
1.3c (7)		Chin tuck supine	
1.4a (8)	Neck flexion stretches - active, passive and post-isometric flexion stretches for the suboccipital, cervical and upper thoracic spine	Head & neck active flexion stretch seated	
1.4b (9)		Head & neck post-isometric flexion stretch supine	
1.4c (10)		Head & neck post-isometric flexion, sidebending and rotation stretch supine	

No	Description	Title	Icon
1.5 (11)	Neck extension stretch - an active and passive extension stretch for the cervical, upper thoracic and suboccipital spine	Head & neck extension stretch seated	
1.6 (12)	Neck rotation stretch - an active rotation stretch for the suboccipital, cervical and upper thoracic spine	Head & neck active rotation stretch seated	
1.7a (13)	Neck sidebending stretches - active, passive and isometric sidebending stretches for the suboccipital, cervical and upper thoracic spine and shoulders	Head & neck active sidebending stretch seated with both arms free for anterior and lateral neck muscles	
1.7b (14)		Head, neck & shoulder active sidebending stretch seated with one shoulder fixed for the upper trapezius & lateral neck	
1.7c (15)		Head, neck & shoulder active sidebending stretch seated with one shoulder fixed for posterolateral fibres of trapezius & the neck	
1.7d (16)		Head, neck & shoulder active sidebending stretch standing with one shoulder fixed for upper trapezius & muscle of the neck	
1.7e (17)		Head & neck active sidebending rotation stretch seated with both arms free for anterior and lateral neck muscles	
1.7f (18)		Head, neck & shoulder active sidebending and rotation stretch seated with one shoulder fixed for levator scapulae and neck muscles	
1.7g (19)		Head, neck & shoulder post-isometric sidebending and rotation technique seated with one shoulder fixed	
1.7h (20)		Trapezius and levator scapulae post-isometric stretch seated with one shoulder fixed	

No	Description	Title	Square Icon
1. 7i (21)		Levator scapulae active, passive or post-isometric stretch sidelying	
1.8 (22)	Active stretch for sternocleidomastoid and the cervical spine	Head & neck extension, sidebending and reverse rotation stretch seated or standing for sternocleidomastoid	
1.9 (23)	Post-isometric stretches for the atlanto-occipital joints	Atlanto-occipital post-isometric technique seated / Head flexion stretch seated	
2.0a (24)	Active sidebending stretch for the thoracic, lumbar and hip	Standing lumbar and hip sidebending stretch / Standing sidebending stretch	
2.0b (25)		Standing middle and lower thoracic and thoracolumbar sidebending stretch	
2.1a (26)	Passive sidebending stretch for the thoracic, lumbar and hip	Wall supported passive lumbar & hip sidebend stretch / Wall supported sidebend stretch	
2.1b (27)		Wall supported passive thoracic sidebend stretch	
2.1c (28)		Wall supported post-isometric hip or spine sidebend stretch	

No	Description	Title	Icon
2.2a (29)	Active sidebending stretches for the thoracic and ribs	Thoracic and rib sidebending stretch seated	
2.2b (30)		Thoracic and rib sidebending stretch kneeling	
2.3 (31)	Active stretch for the shoulder, lateral trunk and hip	Kneeling lateral stretch / Kneeling side stretch	
2.4a (32)	Passive and post-isometric stretches for latissimus dorsi, the thoracolumbar fascia, quadratus lumborum and the lateral fibres of erector spinae	Hanging stretch erect	
2.4b (33)		Hanging stretch flexed unilateral	
2.4c (34)		Hanging stretch flexed bilateral	
2.4d (35)		Hanging passive stretch unilateral sidebending	
2.5a (36)	Active stretch for the shoulders, thoracic and lumbar spine	Upper Dog extension stretch kneeling	
2.5b (37)		Upper Dog extension stretch standing	
2.5c (38)		Latissimus stretch kneeling 2.5c	

636

No	Description	Title	Icon
2.6a (39)	Active and passive extension stretches for the neck, shoulders, thoracic, lumbar and hips	Half Cobra	
2.6b (40)		Full Cobra	
2.6c (41)		Sidebending Cobra	
2.6d (42)		Rotation Cobra	
2.7a (43)	Active stretch for the shoulders, thoracic, lumbar and hips	Diagonal Locust	
2.7b (44)		Full Locust arms at side	
2.7c (45)		Full Locust arms abducted	
2.8 (46)	Active extension stretch for the shoulders, hips, and cervical, thoracic and lumbar spine	Extended Cat	
2.9a (47)	Active flexion stretch for the shoulders, hips, and cervical, thoracic and lumbar spine	Flexed Cat	
2.9b (48)		Flexed Cat standing	

No	Description	Title	Icon
3.0a (49)	Passive, active and post-isometric flexion stretches for the lower thoracic, lumbar and hips	Passive knees to chest stretch supine	
3.0b (50)		Post-isometric knees to chest stretch supine	
3.0c (51)		Active knees to chest stretch supine	
3.0d (52)		Active knees to chest stretch with rotation supine	
3.0e (53)		Unilateral stretch for the lumbar and gluteus maximus	
3.1a (54)	Active and passive rotation stretch seated for the head, shoulders and cervical, thoracic and lumbar spine	Passive spinal twist seated	
3.1b (55)		Active spinal twist seated	
3.1c (56)		Spinal twist sitting on the floor	
3.2a (57)	Active and passive rotation stretch standing for the head, shoulders and cervical, thoracic and lumbar spine	Passive spinal twist standing wall supported	
3.2b (58)		Active spinal twist standing	

638

No	Description	Title	Icon
3.3 (59)	Active rotation stretch standing flexed at the hips, for the shoulders and thoracic and lumbar spine	Active spinal twist standing flexed at the hips	
3.4 (60)	Active rotation stretch kneeling for shoulders and thoracic and lumbar spine	Active spinal twist kneeling	
3.5 (61)	Passive and active rotation stretch prone for the head, shoulders and cervical, thoracic and lumbar spine	Passive and active spinal twist prone	
3.6 (62)	Active, post-isometric and passive stretch over a rolled up towel for pectoralis major, the ribs, thoracic and cervical spine	Supine pectoralis stretch over a rolled up towel	
3.7 (63)	Active, post-isometric and passive stretch over a rolled-up towel for the shoulders, ribs, thoracic and cervical spine	Supine longitudinal stretch over a rolled up towel	
3.8a (64)	Active, post-isometric and passive stretch over a rolled-up towel for shoulders, arms, forearms, wrist, hands and fingers	Supine bilateral anterior forearm and hand stretch	
3.8b (65)		Supine unilateral anterior forearm and hand stretch	
3.8c (66)		Supine unilateral anterior finger and hand stretch	
3.8d (67)		Supine unilateral posterior forearm and hand stretch over a rolled towel	
3.8e (68)		Supine unilateral posterior finger and hand stretch over a rolled towel	

No	Description	Title	Icon
3.9a (69)	Active and passive stretch for one side of the body - shoulder, spine, ribs and hip	Supine hip and spine stretch over a rolled towel	
3.9b (70)		Supine lumbar and thoracic spine stretch over a rolled towel	
4.0a (71)	Active, passive and post-isometric stretches for pectoralis major and other anterior shoulder muscles	Easy pectoralis stretch sitting on the floor	
4.0b (72)		Easy pectoralis stretch standing	
4.0c (73)		Pectoralis stretch seated in a chair	
4.0d (74)		Pectoralis stretch prone	
4.0e (75)		Unilateral passive and post-isometric pectoralis stretch standing and wall supported	
4.0f (76)		Bilateral passive and post-isometric pectoralis stretch standing and doorway supported	
4.0g (77)		Bilateral pectoralis stretch standing walls supported	
4.0h (78)		Bilateral active pectoralis and latissimus dorsi stretch standing with pole or towel	

640

No	Description	Title	Icon
4.1 (79)	Passive and post-isometric stretch for subscapularis and other anterior shoulder muscles	Unilateral passive and post-isometric subscapularis stretch	
4.2 (80)	Passive and post-isometric stretch for the scapula depressor muscles	The shoulder drop	
4.3 (81)	Active stretch for muscles responsible for scapular elevation	Active scapular elevator stretch	
4.4 (82)	Passive and post-isometric stretch for the muscles responsible for shoulder abduction and scapula retraction	Shoulder abductor front stretch	
4.5 (83)	Passive and post-isometric stretch for the shoulder abductors	Shoulder abductor stretch behind	
4.6a (84)	Active stretch for shoulder muscles and strengthening technique for muscles of the spine, thighs and legs	Palms together above head with forearms supinated	
4.6b (85)		Palms together above head with forearms pronated	
4.7 (86)	Active stretch for pectoralis minor and a passive stretch for the anterior forearm, wrist and finger flexor muscles and fascia	Palms together behind back	
4.8 (87)	Active and passive stretch for shoulder muscles	Multi shoulder stretch	

No	Description	Title	Icon
4.9a (88)	Active, passive and post-isometric stretches for the shoulder, spine and scapula retractor muscles	Scapula retractor stretch standing	
4.9b (89)		Scapula retractor stretch squatting unilateral	
4.9c (90)		Scapula retractor stretch squatting bilateral	
4.9d (91)		Scapula wrap stretch standing	
4.9e (92)		Scapula active retractor stretch standing	
5.0a (93)	Passive, post-isometric and active stretches for muscles responsible for shoulder external rotation and scapular retraction	Shoulder external rotator stretch	
5.0b (94)		Active scapular retractor & shoulder external rotator stretch	
5.1a (95)	Passive and post-isometric stretch for the shoulder flexor muscles	Shoulder flexor drop	
5.1b (96)		Standing winged anterior deltoid stretch	

No	Description	Title	Icon
5.2a (97)	Passive and post-isometric stretch for anterior shoulder muscles and fascia	Bilateral passive biceps stretch against a ledge	
5.2b (98)		Bilateral post-isometric biceps stretch against a ledge	
5.2c (99)		Unilateral passive and post-isometric biceps stretch against a ledge	
5.3a (100)	Passive and post-isometric stretches for muscles responsible for forearm flexion	Passive elbow flexor stretch	
5.3b (101)		Post-isometric elbow flexor stretch	
5.4 (102)	Passive stretch for the triceps and muscles responsible for shoulder adduction	Passive triceps stretch	
5.5 (103)	Active and post-isometric stretch for the muscles responsible for forearm supination	Supinator stretch	
5.6a (104)	Active, passive and post-isometric stretch for pronator teres	Pronator stretch using a doorframe	
5.6b (105)		Pronator stretch assisted by the hand of the other limb	

No	Description	Title	Icon
5.7a (106)	Passive and post-isometric stretches for the extensor muscles of the wrist and hand	Kneeling unilateral wrist extensor stretch	
5.7b (107)		Kneeling bilateral wrist extensor stretch	
5.7c (108)		Kneeling wrist extensor and ulna deviator stretch	
5.7d (109)		Kneeling wrist extensor and radial deviator stretch	
5.8a (110)	Passive and post-isometric stretches for the flexor muscles of the wrist and hand	Kneeling unilateral wrist flexor stretch	
5.8b (111)		Kneeling bilateral wrist flexor stretch	
5.8c (112)		Kneeling wrist flexor and radial deviator stretch	
5.8d (113)		Kneeling wrist flexor and ulnar deviator stretch	
5.8e (114)		Standing unilateral wrist flexor stretch	
5.9 (115)	Post-isometric and passive stretch for the forearm, wrist, hand and fingers	Standing finger flexor muscle stretch on a table	

No	Description	Title	Icon
6.0a (116)	Passive stretches for iliacus, psoas and other hip flexor muscles	The lunge	
6.0b (117)		The forwards splits	
6.0c (118)		The hanging hip stretch	
6.1a (119)	Passive and post-isometric stretches for piriformis and gluteus minimus, medius and maximus in hip flexion and external rotation	Unilateral passive stretch for hip extensors and rotators	
6.1b (120)		Unilateral post-isometric stretch for hip extensors and rotators	
6.1c (121)		Unilateral passive cross leg stretch for hip extensors and rotators	
6.1d (122)		Unilateral post-isometric cross leg stretch for hip extensors and rotators	
6.1e (123)		Unilateral passive and post-isometric stretch for hip extensors and rotators over a table	
6.1f (124)		Unilateral passive and post-isometric stretch for hip extensors, rotators and abductors over a table	
6.1g (125)		Unilateral post-isometric stretch for gluteus minimus with your hips in flexion and sitting on a chair	

No	Description	Title	Icon
6.2a (126)	Passive and post-isometric stretch for hip external rotators	Unilateral stretch for the hip external rotators	
6.2b (127)		Unilateral stretch for piriformis	
6.2c (128)		Unilateral stretch for the hip external rotators	
6.3a (129)	Active, passive and post-isometric stretches for gluteus minimus and the anterior fibres of gluteus medius	Unilateral gluteus minimus stretch supine	
6.3b (130)		Unilateral active and post-isometric stretches for gluteus minimus sidelying	
6.3c (131)		Unilateral post isometric stretch for gluteus minimus prone	
6.3d (132)		Unilateral gluteus minimus stretch standing using a chair	
6.4a (133)	Passive and post-isometric stretches for tensor fasciae latae, gluteus medius, minimus and the upper fibres of gluteus maximus	Unilateral passive stretch tensor fasciae latae standing	
6.4b (134)		Unilateral passive stretch gluteus maximus and medius kneeling	
6.4c (135)		Unilateral passive stretch tensor fasciae latae standing	

646

No	Description	Title	Icon
6.4d (136)	Passive and post-isometric stretches for tensor fasciae latae, gluteus medius, minimus and the upper fibres of gluteus maximus	Unilateral passive or post-isometric hip abductor stretch supine	
6.4e (137)		Unilateral passive stretch for quadratus lumborum, tensor fasciae latae and gluteus maximus sidelying on a table	
6.4f (138)		Unilateral post-isometric stretch for quadratus lumborum, tensor fasciae latae and gluteus maximus sidelying on a table	
6.4g (139)		Unilateral passive and post-isometric stretch for tensor fasciae latae and gluteus maximus sidelying with the knee straight	
6.4h (140)		Unilateral passive and post-isometric stretch for gluteus medius and gluteus minimus sidelying with the knee bent	
6.5a (141)		Bilateral stretch for the hip adductors and internal rotators sitting	
6.5b (142)		Bilateral active stretch for the hip adductors, extensors and internal rotators sitting	
6.5c (143)		Bilateral passive stretch for the hip adductors and extensors sitting	
6.5d (144)		Bilateral post-isometric stretch for the hip adductors and extensors sitting	
6.5e (145)		Bilateral active and passive stretch for the hip adductors supine and with legs against a wall	

647

No	Description	Title	Icon
6.5f (146)	Passive, active and post-isometric stretches for the hip adductors	Bilateral stretch for the hip adductors and internal rotators supine and with knees flexed and heels against a wall	
6.5g (147)		Bilateral stretch for the hip adductors and internal rotators supine with knees flexed and feet against a wall	
6.5h (148)		Bilateral stretch for the hip adductors standing	
6.5i (149)		Unilateral passive stretch for the hip adductors standing	
6.5j (150)		Bilateral stretch for the hip adductors and internal rotators supine	
6.5k (151)		Bilateral stretch for the hip adductors kneeling with knees flexed and hips externally rotated	
6.5l (152)		Bilateral stretch for the hip adductors kneeling with hips extended and knees flexed	
6.5m (153)		Bilateral stretch for the hip adductors standing with hips and knees extended	
6.5n (154)		Unilateral stretch for the hip adductors sidelying with your back against a wall and your hips and knees extended	
6.6a (155)	Active and passive stretches for quadriceps, tibialis anterior and the toe extensor muscles	Standing quadriceps stretch	

648

No	Description	Title	Icon
6.6b (156)	Active and passive stretches for quadriceps, tibialis anterior and the toe extensor muscles	Standing passive knee, ankle & toe stretch	
6.6c (157)		Standing post-isometric knee, ankle and toe stretch	
6.6d (158)		Supine quadriceps stretch	
6.6e (159)		Prone passive and post-isometric quadriceps stretch	
6.6f (160)		Sidelying quadriceps stretch	
6.7a (161)	Passive, active and isometric stretches for the hamstrings	Unilateral easy passive and active stretch for the hamstrings standing with one leg horizontal	
6.7b (162)		Unilateral combined active and passive stretch for the hamstrings standing with one leg horizontal	
6.7c (163)		Unilateral passive stretch for the hamstrings supine	
6.7d (164)		Unilateral post-isometric stretch for the hamstrings supine	
6.7e (165)		Unilateral active and post-isometric stretch for the hamstrings supine with your leg vertical and against a post or wall	

No	Description	Title	Icon
6.7f (166)	Passive, active and isometric stretches for the hamstrings	Unilateral passive or post-isometric stretch for the hamstrings standing with legs vertical	
6.7g (167)		Unilateral active and passive stretch for the short head of biceps femoris standing with legs vertical	
6.8a (168)	Popliteus stretch - active, passive, and post-isometric stretches for popliteus	Unilateral active and passive stretch for the popliteus standing with legs vertical	
6.8b (169)		Unilateral post-isometric stretch for the popliteus standing with legs vertical	
6.9a (170)	Active, passive and post-isometric stretch for the hamstrings and gastrocnemius muscles and posterior fascia	Unilateral active and passive stretch for the hamstrings and gastrocnemius	
6.9b (171)		Unilateral post-isometric stretch for the posterior thigh and leg	
6.9c (172)		Bilateral active, passive and post-isometric stretch for the hamstrings and gastrocnemius	
7.0a (173)	Active, passive and post isometric stretches for the hamstrings, hip adductors and external rotators and gastrocnemius and strengthening major trunk muscles	Active forward bend sitting	
7.0b (174)		Passive forward bend sitting	
7.0c (175)		Post-isometric forward bend sitting	

650

No	Description	Title	Icon
7.0d (176)	hamstrings, hip adductors, rotators gastrocnemius and strengthening trunk muscles continued	Bilateral forward bend sitting	
7.1a (177)	Passive, active and post-isometric stretch for the calf muscles	Unilateral passive stretch for gastrocnemius	
7.1b (178)		Unilateral post-isometric stretch and variations for gastrocnemius	
7.1c (179)		Bilateral passive stretch for gastrocnemius	
7.1d (180)		Bilateral stretch for gastrocnemius using a block	
7.1e (181)		Unilateral stretch for soleus and other posterior leg muscles, ankle ligaments and the Achilles tendon	
7.1f (182)		Unilateral stretch for peroneus muscles, tibialis posterior, flexor digitorum longus and flexor hallucis longus on a sloping floor	
7.1g (183)		Unilateral stretch for soleus using a block or wall	
7.1h (184)		Bilateral or unilateral active stretch for gastrocnemius and soleus	
7.2a (185)	Active and passive stretch for tibialis anterior and the toe extensor muscles	Bilateral active stretch for the ankle dorsiflexor and toe extensor muscles	

No	Description	Title	Icon
7.2b (186)	Active and passive stretch for tibialis anterior and the toe extensor muscles	Unilateral passive stretch for the ankle dorsiflexor and toe extensor muscles standing	
7.3a (187)	Passive and post-isometric stretches for the foot and toes	Unilateral toe flexor stretch standing	
7.3b (188)		Unilateral passive and post-isometric toe flexor stretch seated	
7.3c (189)		Unilateral passive and post-isometric foot evertor or foot invertor stretch seated	
7.3d (190)		Unilateral toe extensor stretch seated	
7.4a (191)	Active, passive and isometric stretches for the hamstrings, piriformis, gluteus medius, gluteus maximus, abdominal and lumbar muscles	Unilateral active and passive straight leg stretch	
7.4b (192)		Unilateral passive and isometric stretch for hip abductors and external rotators and muscles in the lumber spine	
7.25a (193)	Active stretch and strengthening technique for the whole body	Squat with palms together above head	
7.5b (194)		Squat with arms in front of body	
7.6 (195)	Strengthening exercise for the abdomen lumbar and cervical spine	Supine pelvic tilt	

Movement tables - stretches based on direction of movement and secondarily according to anatomical region

Head and upper cervical movements

Anterior occiput

1.1a	1.1b	1.1c	1.5	1.8	2.5c	2.6b	2.8

6.5d	6.5h	6.5i	6.6e	7.0a-c	7.0d	7.5b

Posterior occiput

1.3a	1.3b	1.3c	1.4a	1.4b	1.4c	1.9	2.7a
2.7b	2.7c	2.9a	2.9b	3.0a	3.0b	3.0c	3.0d
3.0e	3.6	3.7	3.8a	3.9a	3.9b	4.0c	4.0d
4.2	4.3	6.5b	7.6				

Face and jaw

1.1a	1.1b	1.1c	1.2

Head and cervical movements

Cervical rotation with sidebending (rotation is primary movement)

1.6	2.6d	3.1a	3.1b	3.1c	3.2a	3.2b	3.3

3.5	4.9b

Cervical sidebending with rotation (sidebending is primary movement)

1.4c	1.7a	1.7b	1.7c	1.7d	1.7e	1.7f	1.7g
1.7h	1.7i	1.8	2.0a	2.0b	2.1a	2.1b	2.1c
2.2a	2.2b	2.4d	2.6c	2.6d	3.9a	3.9b	

Cervical flexion

1.3a	1.3b	1.3c	1.4a	1.4b	1.4c	2.9a	2.9b

Cervical extension

1.5	2.5c	2.6b	2.8	6.5d	6.5h	6.5i	6.6

Thoracic and lumbar movements

Upper thoracic sidebending with rotation

1.7b	1.7c	1.7d	1.7e	1.7f	1.7g	1.7h	1.7i

1.8	2.1a	2.1b	2.1c	2.2a	2.2b	2.6c	2.6d

3.9a	3.9b

All thoracic sidebending with rotation

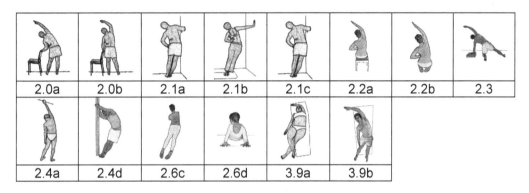

2.0a	2.0b	2.1a	2.1b	2.1c	2.2a	2.2b	2.3

2.4a	2.4d	2.6c	2.6d	3.9a	3.9b

Thoracolumbar and lumbar sidebending

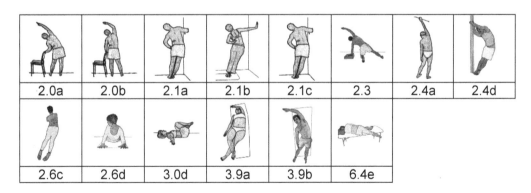

2.0a	2.0b	2.1a	2.1b	2.1c	2.3	2.4a	2.4d

2.6c	2.6d	3.0d	3.9a	3.9b	6.4e

Longitudinal sidebending

2.3	2.4a	2.4b	2.4c	2.4d	3.7	3.8a	3.9a

3.9b	6.4d	6.4e	6.4f

Upper thoracic flexion

1.4a	1.4b	1.4c	2.9a	2.9b

Mid or all thoracic flexion

2.9a	2.9b	7.5b

Lumbar or thoracolumbar flexion

2.9a	2.9b	3.0ab	3.0c	3.0d	3.0e	6.1ab	6.1cd

6.1e	6.5b	7.5b	7.6

Thoracolumbar and lumbar rotation

3.0d	3.1a	3.1b	3.1c	3.2a	3.2b	3.3	3.4

3.5	7.4a	7.4b

Upper thoracic extension

1.1a	1.1b	1.1c	1.3a	1.3b	1.3c	1.5	1.8

2.5a	2.5b	2.5c	2.6b	2.6c	2.6d	2.7a	2.7b

2.7c	2.8	6.9ab	6.9c

Mid thoracic extension

1.1a	1.1b	1.1c	1.3a	1.3b	1.3c	2.4c	2.5a

2.5b	2.5c	2.6b	2.6c	2.6d	2.7a	2.7b	2.7c

2.8	4.0a	4.0b	4.0c	4.0d	4.0e	4.0f	4.0g

4.0h	6.9ab	6.9c	7.0abc	7.0d	7.5a

Lumbar or thoracolumbar extension

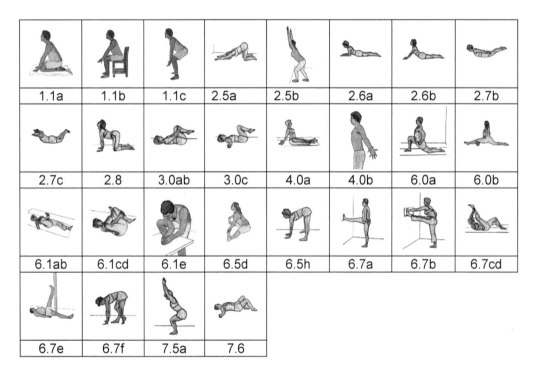

1.1a	1.1b	1.1c	2.5a	2.5b	2.5c	2.6a	2.6b
2.6c	2.6d	2.7a	2.7b	2.7c	2.8	6.5d	6.5h
6.9ab	6.9c						

Sacral nutation/ flexion/ anterior rotation/ posterior iliac rotation, unilateral or bilateral

1.1a	1.1b	1.1c	2.5a	2.5b	2.6a	2.6b	2.7b
2.7c	2.8	3.0ab	3.0c	4.0a	4.0b	6.0a	6.0b
6.1ab	6.1cd	6.1e	6.5d	6.5h	6.7a	6.7b	6.7cd
6.7e	6.7f	7.5a	7.6				

Sacral counter nutation/ extension/ posterior rotation/ anterior iliac rotation, unilateral or bilateral

2.9a	2.9b	4.9b	4.9c	6.5b	6.6abc	6.6d	6.6e
6.6f	7.5b						

Upper and lower limb movements

Scapula retraction

2.0b	2.1a	2.1b	2.1c	2.5a	2.5b	2.5c	2.6a
2.6b	2.6c	2.6d	2.7a	2.7b	2.7c	2.8	3.1a
3.1b	3.1c	3.2a	3.2b	3.3	3.4	3.5	4.0a
4.0b	4.0c	4.0d	4.0e	4.0f	4.0g	4.0h	4.1
4.5	4.7	4.8	5.1a	5.1b	5.2ab	5.2c	5.3ab
6.5d	6.5h						

Scapula elevation

1.2	2.0a	2.0b	2.2a	2.2b	2.3	2.4a	2.4b
2.4c	2.4d	2.5a	2.5b	2.5c	3.7	3.8a	3.8b
3.8c	3.8d	3.8e	3.9a	3.9b	4.2	4.6a	4.6b
5.1a	5.4	7.5a					

Scapula protraction

1.1a	1.1b	1.1c	2.0a	2.2a	2.2b	2.3	2.4a
2.4b	2.4c	2.4d	2.5a	2.5b	2.5c	2.9a	3.1a
3.1b	3.1c	3.2a	3.2b	3.3	3.4	3.5	3.7
3.8a	3.8b	3.8c	3.8d	3.8e	3.9a	3.9b	4.4
4.6a	4.6b	4.8	4.9a	4.9b	4.9c	4.9d	4.9e
5.0a	5.0b	5.4	7.5a	7.5b			

Scapula depression

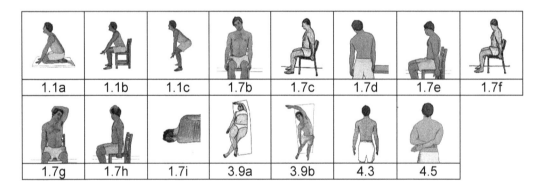

1.1a	1.1b	1.1c	1.7b	1.7c	1.7d	1.7e	1.7f
1.7g	1.7h	1.7i	3.9a	3.9b	4.3	4.5	

Shoulder extension

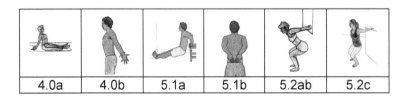

4.0a	4.0b	5.1a	5.1b	5.2ab	5.2c

Shoulder flexion

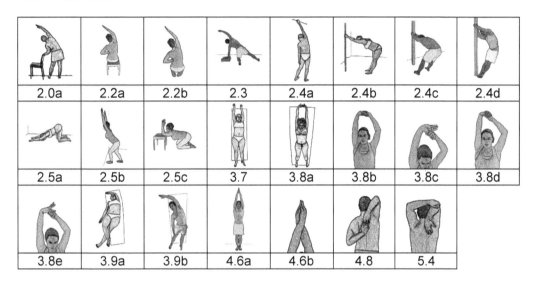

2.4b	2.4c	2.5a	2.5b	2.5c	2.7a	6.9ab	6.9c

7.5a

Shoulder abduction

2.0a	2.2a	2.2b	2.3	2.4a	2.4b	2.4c	2.4d

2.5a	2.5b	2.5c	3.7	3.8a	3.8b	3.8c	3.8d

3.8e	3.9a	3.9b	4.6a	4.6b	4.8	5.4

Shoulder external rotation

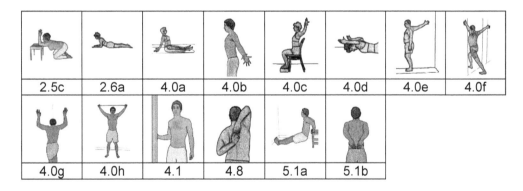

2.5c	2.6a	4.0a	4.0b	4.0c	4.0d	4.0e	4.0f

4.0g	4.0h	4.1	4.8	5.1a	5.1b

Shoulder internal rotation

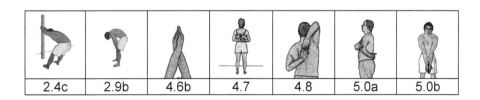

2.4c	2.9b	4.6b	4.7	4.8	5.0a	5.0b

Shoulder adduction and horizontal adduction

1.4b	4.4	4.5	4.8	4.9a	4.9b	4.9d	5.0b

Shoulder horizontal abduction

4.0c	4.0d	4.0e	4.0f	4.0g	4.0h

Elbow extension

1.1a	1.1b	1.1c	2.0a	2.1b	2.3	2.4a	2.4b
2.4c	2.5a	2.5b	2.6b	2.6c	2.6d	2.7b	2.8
2.9a	3.1c	3.4	3.7	3.8a	3.8b	3.8c	3.8d
3.8e	4.0a	4.0b	4.0e	4.0f	4.0h	4.2	4.3
4.6a	4.6b	4.9a	4.9b	4.9c	5.0b	5.2ab	5.2c
5.3ab	5.5	5.6a	5.7a	5.7b	5.7c	5.7d	5.8a
5.8b	5.8c	5.8d	5.8e	7.5a			

662

Elbow flexion

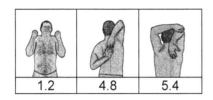

| 1.2 | 4.8 | 5.4 |

Forearm pronation

| 5.5 |

Forearm supination

| 5.3ab | 5.6a | 5.6b |

Wrist flexion

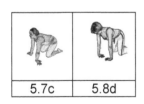

| 3.8d | 3.8e | 5.2ab | 5.7a | 5.7b | 5.7c | 5.7d |

Wrist extension

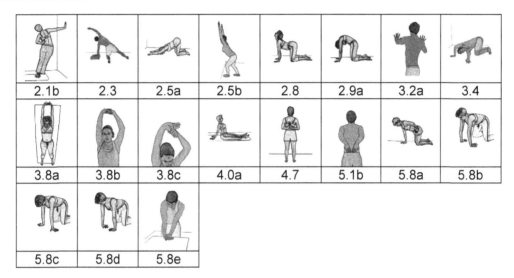

2.1b	2.3	2.5a	2.5b	2.8	2.9a	3.2a	3.4
3.8a	3.8b	3.8c	4.0a	4.7	5.1b	5.8a	5.8b
5.8c	5.8d	5.8e

Wrist abduction

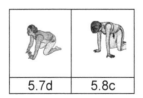

| 5.7c | 5.8d |

Wrist adduction

| 5.7d | 5.8c |

Finger flexion

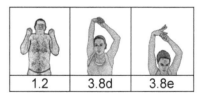

| 1.2 | 3.8d | 3.8e |

Finger extension and abduction

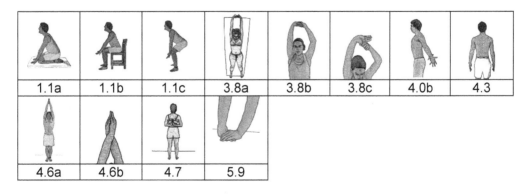

| 1.1a | 1.1b | 1.1c | 3.8a | 3.8b | 3.8c | 4.0b | 4.3 |
| 4.6a | 4.6b | 4.7 | 5.9 |

Hip flexion

2.4b	2.4c	2.9a	2.9b	3.0ab	3.0c	3.0d	3.0e
4.9b	4.9c	6.0c	6.1ab	6.1cd	6.1e	6.1f	6.5h
6.7a	6.7b	6.7cd	6.7e	6.7f	7.0abc	7.0d	7.4
7.5b							

Hip extension

2.6b	2.6c	2.6d	2.7a	2.7b	2.7c	6.0a	6.0b
6.0c	6.6abc	6.6f					

Hip adduction

2.0a	2.0b	2.1a	2.1b	2.1c	2.4d	3.1	3.9a
6.4a	6.4b	6.4c	6.4d	6.4e	6.4f	6.4g	6.4h

Hip horizontal adduction

3.0d	7.4a	7.4b

664

Hip abduction

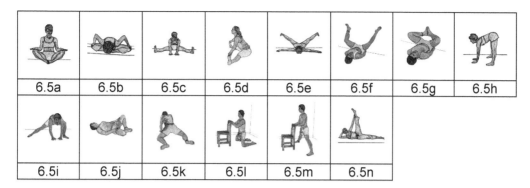

6.5a	6.5b	6.5c	6.5d	6.5e	6.5f	6.5g	6.5h

6.5i	6.5j	6.5k	6.5l	6.5m	6.5n

Hip internal rotation

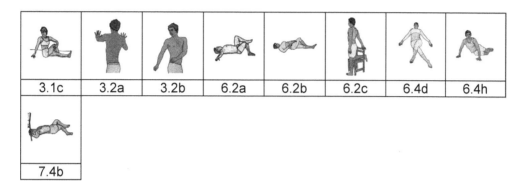

3.1c	3.2a	3.2b	6.2a	6.2b	6.2c	6.4d	6.4h

7.4b

Hip external rotation

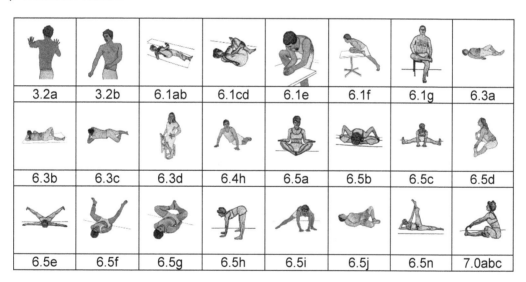

3.2a	3.2b	6.1ab	6.1cd	6.1e	6.1f	6.1g	6.3a
6.3b	6.3c	6.3d	6.4h	6.5a	6.5b	6.5c	6.5d
6.5e	6.5f	6.5g	6.5h	6.5i	6.5j	6.5n	7.0abc

Hip and thoracolumbar sidebending

2.0a	2.0b	2.1a	2.1b	2.1c	2.3	2.4a	2.4d
2.6c	3.9a	3.9b	6.3a	6.4a	6.4b	6.4c	6.4d
6.4e	6.4f	6.4g	6.4h				

Knee extension

2.0a	2.0b	2.1a	2.1b	2.1c	2.3	2.4b	2.4c
2.4c	3.7	3.8	4.2	4.3	4.6a	4.6b	4.9a
5.1a	6.2b	6.2c	6.3a	6.3b	6.3c	6.3d	6.4a
6.4b	6.4c	6.4e	6.4f	6.4g	6.5c	6.5d	6.5e
6.5h	6.5i	6.5n	6.6abc	6.6d	6.7a	6.7b	6.7e
6.7f	6.7g	6.8ab	6.9ab	6.9c	7.0abc	7.0d	7.1a
7.1b	7.1c	7.1d	7.1h	7.2a	7.4a		

Knee flexion

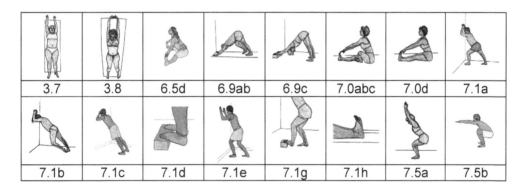

1.1a	2.2b	3.0ab	3.0c	3.0d	3.0e	4.9b	4.9c
6.0c	6.1ab	6.1cd	6.1f	6.5a	6.5b	6.5g	6.6abc
6.6d	6.6e	6.6f	7.5b				

Ankle dorsiflexion

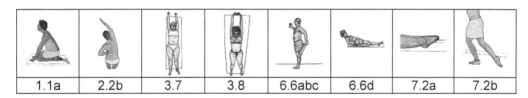

3.7	3.8	6.5d	6.9ab	6.9c	7.0abc	7.0d	7.1a
7.1b	7.1c	7.1d	7.1e	7.1g	7.1h	7.5a	7.5b

Ankle plantarflexion

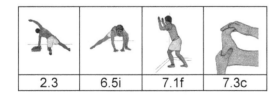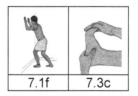

1.1a	2.2b	3.7	3.8	6.6abc	6.6d	7.2a	7.2b

Foot inversion

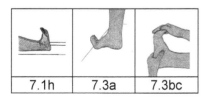

2.3	6.5i	7.1f	7.3c

Foot eversion

7.1f	7.3c

Toe extension

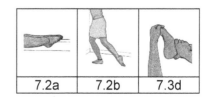

7.1h	7.3a	7.3bc

Toe flexion

7.2a	7.2b	7.3d

Day stretches for pain

Pain can have many causes and an accurate diagnosis is necessary to establish if there is a biomechanical basis for the pain. Stretching may be inappropriate if there is pathology such as a malignancy, infection, active inflammation, joint hypermobility, instability or strain such as immediately after trauma and if the pain is acute. Stretching is appropriate for joint and muscle stiffness caused by inactivity, postural fatigue or emotional tension and if the pain is chronic or intermittent.

Low back pain								
2.0a	2.0b	2.5b	3.1a	3.0e	6.2b	6.6a	6.7f	7.1a

Low back pain may be mechanical, non-mechanical or referred. It is acute if less than 6 weeks, sub-acute between 6 and 12 weeks and chronic if greater than 12 weeks duration. If the pain is mechanical it may be from a muscle, tendon, joint, ligament or intervertebral discs. An acute back should be treated with ice, analgesic and rested for a day - or a few days if required. Stretching may be helpful when pain levels subside if the lower back pain is mechanical and caused by a muscle or ligament strain. Lower back pain is usually gone within one week and does not need treatment but ongoing or intermittent pain should be properly assessed and treated.

Neck and shoulder pain								
1.2	1.3b	1.4a	1.7c	1.6	1.7f	2.0a	4.0g	6.9a

Neck and shoulder pain may be the result of muscle strain, spasm or trauma such as a whiplash injury, prolonged sitting, faulty habits, bad posture, stress, psychoemotional and occupational factors and genetic susceptibility. Osteoarthritis is a degenerative disease that results in high levels of stiffness and pain in the lower lumbar and lower cervical spine after the age of about 40 years of age.

Tension headaches								
1.2	1.1a	1.4b	1.7d	1.7e	1.7f	1.9	3.1b	4.0b

Tension headaches may be associated with neck and shoulder pain. They are usually caused by stress and anxiety but may be caused by eye strain, hunger, lack of sleep, poor posture or overuse and tension in muscles of the face, jaw, occiput, neck or shoulders.

Wrist pain								
2.4b	3.8b	3.8c	3.8d	3.8e	5.5	5.6b	5.7c	5.7d

668

Wrist pain may be from a tendon or ligament strain caused by overuse (repetition) or overload (trauma). Osteoarthritis may develop years after injury or from frequent impact (boxing). Tendonitis or tenosynovitis are common. Acute injuries need rest, ice and a compression bandage. Pain after a fall may indicate a fracture and require X-ray. After 24 hours or when swelling has gone stretch using light pressure and increase the stretching and begin strengthening exercises after a few days

Rotator cuff pain								
1.7c	1.7f	4.0a	4.1	4.3	4.4	4.5	5.0a	5.1b

Rotator cuff pain may be from a mild tendonitis or bursitis, calcific tendonitis, partial tear or a more severe full thickness tear. Rotator cuff impingement syndrome occurs when the supraspinatus tendon is squeezed as it passes through an osseous tunnel. The degree of damage will determine the prognosis and influence whether stretching will help or exacerbate the problem and which stretches are appropriate. A single injury or repeated minor trauma may trigger the cuff strain but a postural problem is usually the underlying cause.

Calcaneal spurs or heel spurs are the result of a calcium build-up on the underside of the calcaneal bone of the foot. It is frequently associated with plantar fasciitis, a painful inflammation of the plantar fascia that runs along the bottom of the foot and connects the heel bone to the ball of the foot.

Calcaneal spurs and plantar fasciitis								
6.2b	6.5h	6.6a	6.7c	6.9a	6.7b	7.1b	7.1f	7.3b

Heel spurs may be caused by repeated strain of the foot muscles, ligaments and plantar fascia. They may be associated with flat feet or high arches, stiff hip joints placing stress on the heel bone during gait, running or jogging on hard surfaces, poorly fitting or old worn shoes, badly designed shoes that lack an arch support, excess weight, loss of plantar fascia flexibility and thinning of the fat pad under the heel with increasing age, long hours standing and inactivity followed by short bursts of intense physical activity.

Day stretches for pregnancy

During pregnancy hormonal changes cause the ligaments to become more elastic in preparation for the birth of the baby. Although this is to enable the baby's head to pass through pelvis the hormonal action is on ligaments throughout the whole body. As pregnancy progresses the weight of the foetus acting in front of the body's centre of gravity can put strain on muscles of the spine and behind the shoulders and cause postural fatigue and pain. Although it is important not to overstretch already lax ligaments during pregnancy but there is benefit from stretching muscles in the shoulders, back, pelvis and calf.

Pregnancy								
1.7c	2.0a	3.1a	6.5a	6.2b	6.9c	6.7e	7.1b	7.6

Day stretches for gym exercises

Squats are used in powerlifting, gymnastics, aerobics workouts, martial arts and other exercise systems. They strengthen the whole body, but especially work the lower limb muscles gluteus maximus, quadriceps and hamstrings.

Squats								
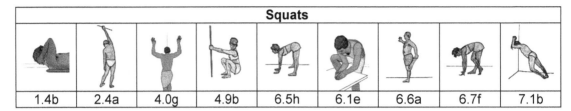								
1.4b	2.4a	4.0g	4.9b	6.5h	6.1e	6.6a	6.7f	7.1b

Squats also strengthen supporting muscles (synergists, neutralisers and stabilizers) including erector spinae in the lumbar and thoracic spine, gluteus medius and minimus, the hip adductors, gastrocnemius, soleus and the abdominal muscles. Squatting mainly involves head, cervical, thoracic and lumbar extension, sacroiliac flexion, scapula retraction, shoulder flexion and abduction, elbow flexion, hip flexion extension and abduction, knee flexion and extension and ankle dorsiflexion and plantar flexion.

Jumping jacks or star jumps are a jumping exercise performed by jumping to a position with the legs spread wide and the hands touching overhead, and then returning to a position with the feet together and the arms at the sides. Jumping jack may be used in aerobic classes or as a warm up exercise.

Jumping jacks work the calf muscles, quadriceps, hamstrings, hip abductors, adductors, flexors and extensors, shoulder abductors and adductors and core muscles. These include gastrocnemius and soleus, gluteus maximus, medius and minimus, gracilis, adductor brevis, longus and magnus, middle deltoid, supraspinatus, latissimus dorsi, teres major, pectoralis major, rectus abdominis, transversus abdominis, the obliques, iliacus, psoas major and lower part of erector spinae. The return of the arms to the side of the body is assisted by gravity.

Jumping jacks								
2.4b	4.0f	4.5	6.4d	6.5m	6.6a	6.7f	7.1b	7.1f

The key features of jumping jacks are: starting with feet together and arms at your side bend your knees, jump into the air and move your legs apart while simultaneously raising your arms over your head. As your feet land on the ground your hands meet above your head with your arms slightly bent. Return to the start position by jumping and bring your feet together and arms back to your side and repeat the movement in cycles.

 Calf raises are a group of exercises for strengthening gastrocnemius, soleus, tibialis posterior and other muscles of the lower leg. They can be done sitting or standing, in knee flexion or knee extension and with one or both feet and they involved repeated cycles of plantar flexion and dorsiflexion.

Calf raises								
6.7f	6.9a	6.9c	7.1b	7.1c	7.1f	7.1g	7.3a	7.3b

Push-ups are done prone by raising and lowering the body with the arms while holding the body in a straight line from head to heels. It mainly works triceps and pectoralis major. The exercise starts with the elbows flexed and the hands beside the body and in line with the shoulders and the palms flat on the ground. It involves repeating cycles of shoulder flexion and elbow extension followed by shoulder extension and elbow flexion. If the hands are close to the body the push-up mainly works triceps and if the hands are away from the side of the body the push-up mainly work pectoralis major. On the way up the muscles contract concentrically and shorten and on the way down they contract eccentrically and lengthen.

Push-ups								
1.7c	2.4a	4.0g	5.2a	4.8	6.1c	6.6c	6.7b	7.1b

Muscles contracting isotonically and assisting the prime mover muscles to raise the body off the ground are anterior deltoid, serratus anterior, coracobrachialis, pectoralis minor and subscapularis. In some parts of the body there is isometric muscle contraction stabilising the body, fixing the scapula, holding the body straight and countering gravity but there is no joint movement. Muscles contracting isometrically include the cervical extensors, erector spinae, iliopsoas, gluteus maximus, medius and minimus, the abdominals, trapezius, the rhomboids and quadriceps and tibialis anterior.

The isotonic part of the push-up involves shoulder flexion and extension, elbow flexion and extension, and a small amount of wrist flexion and extension. The isometric part of the push-up involves head, cervical, thoracic and lumbar extension, scapula retraction, hip extension, knee extension and ankle dorsiflexion.

Dips strengthen triceps and other upper limb muscles. Dips are done by raising and lowering the body with the arms while holding the head, spine and the lower limbs in a fixed position. In a repeating cycle the elbows are flexed about 90 degrees and the shoulders are extended and then the elbows are extended to a straight position and the shoulders are flexed and brought closer to the side of the body. Dips may be modified so that they are easier or more difficult for example wearing a weighted belt or changing the body position relative to gravity. But as a general rule during the dip the spine remains straight and vertical, the hip remain flexed and the heels of rest on the ground or a bench. The knees may be flexed or extended but remain in a fixed position throughout the exercise. The palms of both hands are placed downwards flat on a chair, table, bench or ledge or grasp parallel bars or rings

Dips								
1.7c	2.4a	4.0g	5.2a	4.2	5.1a	4.8	5.3a	5.4

In addition to working triceps the dip also work pectoralis major. Doing the dip with the upper limbs close to the side of the body increases the demand on triceps and decreases it on pectoralis major, and vice versa, doing the dip with the upper limbs away from the body increases the demand on pectoralis major and decreases it on triceps. This fact is also true for bench presses and push ups. Dips also work anterior deltoid. Other muscles have a scapula stabilising function including levator scapulae, rhomboid major and minor, trapezius and serratus anterior. Infraspinatus, teres minor and major and latissimus dorsi contract to neutralise the actions of other muscles. Which muscles are contracted depends on how the dips are done.

Sit-ups, crunches and curl-ups are abdominal strengthening exercises which involve flexing the head and spine against gravity from a supine position. Sit-ups, crunches and curl-ups all involve lifting the head off the floor and then flexing the spine one vertebra at a time from above down. They differ by the amount of spinal flexion involved. In the curl-up there is head, cervical and thoracic flexion. The crunch increases flexion to include the lumbar but the lower back remains on the floor. The sit-up may increase flexion to include the sacrum and pelvis.

The starting position is lying on the back on the floor. In sit-ups and crunches the forearms may be crossed in front of the chest or flexed with the hands beside the head and both knees are flexed. In the curl-up the hands may be placed palms down under the lumbar spine to prevent lumbar flexion.

Sit-ups, crunches and curl-ups								
1.4b	2.0a	3.0a	4.0g	6.0a	6.4a	6.4d	6.6a	6.7c

These exercises strengthen rectus abdominis and to a lesser extent the abdominal oblique muscles. Combining rotation with flexion by lifting one shoulder increases strengthening of the abdominal oblique muscles. Sit-ups also strengthen iliopsoas, tensor fasciae latae, rectus femoris and sartorius and muscles that stabilise the trunk such as quadratus lumborum.

Variations include lying on a declined bench or exercise ball, holding a weight, placing arms by the side of the body or over the head, flexing one or both legs or crossing legs. Reverse crunches are done with the upper thoracic and shoulders on the floor and lifting the hips up.

Pull-ups strengthen the torso and upper limb muscles. The pull-up begins with the hands gripping a bar with the full weight of the body suspended by the arms. In a repeating cycle the body is first raised by concentric muscle contraction and then using the same muscles is lowered by eccentric muscle contraction. An upward movement involving scapular retraction, elbow flexion and shoulder extension and/or adduction is followed by a downward movement involving scapular protraction, elbow extension and shoulder flexion and/or abduction.

Good muscle strength is required to raise the body and take the head over the bar until the chin is about level with the bar and bring the elbows to the side of the body. Pull-ups counter gravity. They are usually done using an underhand grip with the forearms supinated but people who climb may prefer an overhand grip with the forearms pronated. The head, spine and hips remain straight, vertical and in a fixed position but the knees may be bent to reduce pendulum-type swinging.

Pull-ups								
1.7d	2.4a	2.5c	3.8c	3.8d	4.9a	5.2a	4.8	5.0a

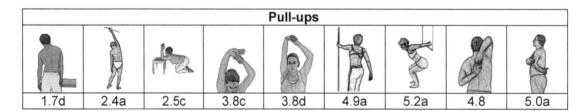

Pull-ups mainly strengthen latissimus dorsi which extends and adducts the shoulder. Shoulder and elbow movement is assisted by the contraction of biceps, brachialis, brachioradialis, posterior deltoid, coracobrachialis, teres major and pectoralis major. Finger flexor and wrist extensor muscles enable the hands to grasp the bar and support the weight of the body during the pull-up and the long head of triceps assists in shoulder adduction.

Levator scapula, rhomboid major and minor, trapezius and serratus anterior stabilise the scapula. The abdominal muscles - rectus abdominis, transversus abdominis and external and internal obliques stabilise the torso and hip muscles stabilise the hips and pelvis and prevent the legs from swinging during the exercise. Infraspinatus and teres minor are neutralisers. Doing the pull-ups with the hands wide apart increases resistance on latissimus dorsi and decreases it on biceps and doing the pull-ups with the hand close together increases the resistance on biceps and decreases it on latissimus dorsi.

Day stretches for musicians

The use of the wrist, hand and fingers to play musical notes is common to playing all the string instruments listed below, guitar cello and violin, as well as the piano and other keyboard instruments. Wrist and hand flexibility are important for finger independence, dexterity, speed and coordination of fine movements.

Playing with the hands involves finger flexion, extension, abduction and adduction as a result of the contraction of flexor digitorum profundus and superficialis, the lumbricals, palmar and dorsal interossei, extensor digitorum and extensor and abductor muscles of the thumb. Flexor carpi ulnaris and radialis and palmaris longus flex the wrist and extensor carpi ulnaris and extensor carpi radialis longus and brevis extend and stabilise the wrist during finger flexion. String instruments also use the muscles responsible for thumb flexion, opposition and adduction to press against the back of the neck to counter finger pressure.

Guitar								
1.7d	2.0a	4.8	4.0c	5.2a	3.8b	3.8c	3.8d	3.8e

The Guitar is a string instrument played by strumming, plucking or finger picking with the right hand while holding the strings against the fret board with the fingers of the left hand. The strings of the classical guitar are nylon and the strings of the acoustic guitar are steel. Both are played acoustically with the sound produced by the vibration of the strings and amplified by the body of the guitar.

Electric and electric bass guitars use an amplifier to convert the sound into an electrical signal which can be manipulated by effects. Although there are many different types of guitar and styles of playing and other string instruments such as the banjo and ukulele these stretches apply equally to all.

The Violin is a string instrument played with a bow. Playing a violin involves holding the instrument under the chin and over the left shoulder and drawing the bow across the strings or sometimes by plucking the strings with the right hand. The left hand produces different notes and alters the length of the notes by holding the string against the fingerboard with the fingers.

Violin								
1.4c	1.7b	1.7f	2.0a	4.0c	4.8	5.2a	5.7b	5.8b

The left wrist should be relaxed and mostly straight for free finger motion. The bow is held in the right hand between the thumb and fingers and the bowing action is produced with combined movement of the right hand, forearm, arm or shoulder. A chinrest or shoulder rest is sometimes used by the violin player.

When playing the violin the right side involves shoulder abduction with horizontal flexion and extension, elbow flexion and extension, finger flexion and a small amount of wrist flexion. On the left side the shoulder is adducted and slightly flexed, the elbow flexed and the fingers are flexed. Movement of the wrist and fingers of the left hand are described above. The head may be flexed, sidebent and rotated – usually to the left.

The Cello is a bowed string instrument with four strings played while seated. It is steadied between the knees and chest and by a spike fixed to the floor. The neck of the cello is above and in front of the player's left shoulder and held by the left hand. The fingers and the thumb of the right hand hold the bow perpendicular to the strings and draw it horizontally across the strings.

The right arm, forearm and wrist work together to draw the bow across the strings. The arm may be raised or lowered to control the bow and maintain the correct angle with the strings. Movement of the bow across the strings is mainly a mixture of shoulder adduction and internal rotation and elbow flexion and pronation. The return movement is shoulder abduction and external rotation and elbow extension and supination.

Cello								
4.8	4.0c	5.2a	5.3a	5.5	5.6b	5.7b	5.8b	5.9

Good wrist flexibility is necessary to play the cello well. The wrist is used in very fast bow movements and to change the direction of the bow, and the arm, forearm and wrist are used for longer strokes. Muscles also contract to maintain an erect spine and stabilise the scapula.

The fingers of the left hand flex push and hold down the strings at various points along their length. Usually the thumb rests on the back of the neck but it can be used to press on the strings alongside the fingers to generate higher notes. Movement of the fingers is described above.

The Piano is a musical instrument made up of a soundboard and metal strings surrounded by a protective wooden case. The piano is played by pressing down on a keyboard made up of rows of black and white keys. When the keys are pressed the strings inside the piano are hit by a padded hammer and sounded and when the keys are released the sound stops. The soundboard and wooden case amplify the vibration of the strings and the sound and the note can be sustained by holding down pedals at the bottom of the piano.

The electric keyboard and piano have the same keyboard layout and are played the same way but the electric keyboard produces sound using an electric circuit and uses electronics to produce a much wider range of sounds than the piano.

Piano								
1.2	1.4a	1.7d	2.5b	3.1a	4.0g	5.8c	5.8d	3.8e

In addition to the wrist and hand actions listed above playing a piano also involves shoulder flexion, extension, internal and external rotation, elbow flexion, extension, pronation and supination, and wrist abduction and adduction. There is also some scapula protraction and retraction, head flexion and rotation and cervical and thoracic flexion and rotation and thoracolumbar rotation.

Drums can be played seated using drum sticks and foot pedals to hit a collection of different types of drums (the drum kit) or they can be played standing using the palms of both hands to strike a stretched membrane such as on a bongo drum. Playing a bongo may also be done sitting on the floor such as in playing an Indian tabla.

674

Drums								
2.5c	4.0g	5.2a	5.4	5.3a	5.7c	5.7d	3.8b	3.8c

The standard drum kit contains a snare, hi-hat, cymbals and tom-toms played with sticks and a bass drum played with a foot pedal and a second foot pedal is often present. Many drummers extend the standard acoustic drum kit to include more drums, cymbals and other percussion instruments as well as electronic drums.

Playing a drum kit involves head extension and cervical and thoracic flexion, shoulder abduction, adduction, flexion and extension, elbow flexion and extension, wrist extension, abduction and adduction and finger flexion.

Singing is the act of producing musical sounds with the voice. A singer or vocalist combines tonality and rhythm to produce song, either alone or with other singers and usually accompanied by musical instruments. Singing is a form of sustained speech. It may be done for pleasure or professionally.

Singing								
1.1a	1.2	1.7a	1.7c	2.4a	3.1b	4.0g	4.9b	7.6

Singing depends on the lungs to supply air; diaphragm for its bellows action; bronchi and trachea as a tubular instrument; larynx as a vibrator or reed instrument; vocal cords to change pitch; chest and sinuses for resonance and amplification; oral cavity, nasal cavity, soft palate, tongue, teeth and lips to articulate and amplify the sound. Singing requires a high degree of muscle coordination involving the abdominal muscles, intercostal muscles, pelvic diaphragm, scalene, sternocleidomastoid, hyoid muscles and muscles of the face, jaw and throat.

Good posture, muscle tone and flexibility are necessary for singing. All the muscles involved must be relaxed to allow free movement of air into and out of the lungs and must remain relaxed throughout the act of singing. Singing requires pectoralis major and minor, intercostals and the abdominals to work in coordinated way with the diaphragm.

Wind instruments are musical instruments that include the flute, trumpet, saxophone, clarinet, trombone and oboe. A wind instrument consists of a mouthpiece, tube and some sort of mechanism for adjusting the pitch.

Wind instrument								
1.1c	1.2	1.7e	1.7c	2.0a	3.1a	3.8a	4.0g	7.6

Playing involves blowing into the mouthpiece with the cheeks and lips while simultaneously either moving a tuning slide, pushing down on piston valves or pressing keys with the fingers or changing the aperture and tension of your lips. All these actions change the length of the tube which changes the length of the vibrating column of air and this changes the pitch of the sound the instrument produces. Playing a wind instrument involves head and upper cervical extension, lower cervical and upper thoracic flexion, shoulder adduction and flexion, elbow flexion, wrist extension and coordinated flexion of the fingers.

Day stretches for workers and professionals

These stretches only involve standing or sitting and can be done at work. None of them require lying on the floor supine which might be impractical if the floor is hard or dirty. At work the cook usually stands so requires a calf stretching exercise. But a jeweller is usually seated and so the stretches focus on the upper limb and spine. Painters and decorators only have stretches for the spine and the upper limb whereas shop assistants and waiters have more lower limb stretches because there is more standing involved.

The stretches focus on one type of work, but with only nine stretches to choose from compromises were necessary and stretches for some muscles may have been omitted from the selection. In order to stretch all tense muscles the reader is advised to combine these stretches with day, weekly or individual stretches from other parts of the book for example the weekly stretching programs for heavy manual labour and for sedentary work sitting in a chair.

Boilermaker Welder								
1.9	1.7c	1.8	2.0a	4.8	3.1a	4.9a	4.0c	5.9

Carpenter								
1.7d	2.0a	2.4b	3.3	3.8b	3.8d	4.0c	5.4	5.2a

Carpet layer and Tilers								
1.4a	1.7c	2.0a	3.1a	4.0c	6.0a	6.9a	3.8c	3.8d

Cleaners								
1.7d	4.0f	5.2c	5.4	5.8b	6.0a	6.6a	6.7a	7.1a

Computer Gamer								
1.7d	2.0a	3.2b	2.5b	3.8b	3.8c	3.8d	3.8e	4.5

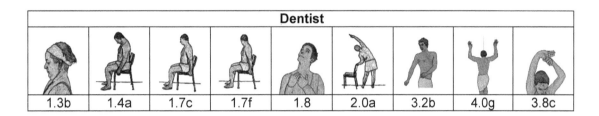

Cook								
1.7c	2.0a	2.5b	4.8	3.1b	5.8e	5.9	4.0g	7.1a

Counsellor Psychotherapist								
1.3b	1.4a	1.5	1.7d	2.0a	3.2a	4.0g	6.7f	7.1a

Dentist								
1.3b	1.4a	1.7c	1.7f	1.8	2.0a	3.2b	4.0g	3.8c

Electrician								
1.2	1.7d	2.1a	2.5b	3.2a	3.8b	4.0b	6.7f	7.1a

Fine Artist								
1.3b	1.7b	2.0a	3.3	4.0c	4.5	5.2a	5.4	5.8b

Gaming, Cards and Board Games								
1.4a	1.7c	2.0a	3.3	4.0g	4.1	4.5	4.9a	5.2a

Gardener Landscaper								
1.7d	2.4a	3.3	4.0h	4.5	5.2c	6.4b	6.5h	7.1a

Hairdresser

1.2	1.7b	1.7f	2.0a	3.2a	3.8c	3.8e	4.5	4.0g

Jeweller

1.3b	1.4a	1.7b	2.4b	4.1	4.0c	3.8d	3.8b	3.8d

Knitting

1.4a	1.7b	1.7f	2.5b	3.2b	4.0b	4.5	3.8b	3.8d

Masseur and Manual Therapist

1.7d	2.0a	3.2a	2.5b	4.9a	4.0c	5.4	5.2a	5.8b

Mechanic

1.9	1.4a	1.7d	2.0a	4.0f	5.2c	5.4	5.8b	6.9a

Painter and Decorator

1.3b	1.7c	2.0a	3.2a	3.8b	4.0g	4.5	5.2a	5.4

Plasterer

1.7d	2.4d	2.5b	3.2a	3.8b	4.0g	4.8	6.7a	7.1b

Plumber								
1.7c	2.0a	4.0g	5.4	5.2a	5.8e	6.0a	6.7f	7.1c

Receptionist using telephone								
1.7c	1.7f	2.0a	2.1b	3.2a	4.0g	4.3	5.2a	4.9a

Salesperson and Shop Assistant								
1.7d	4.0f	4.8	6.0a	6.5h	6.6a	6.7f	7.1b	7.3c

Seamstress, Tailor and Sewing								
1.7b	1.7f	2.4b	2.1b	3.1a	3.8b	3.8c	3.8d	4.0g

Waiter and Waitresses								
3.2a	4.0g	6.0a	6.5m	6.6a	6.7a	6.9a	7.1a	7.3d

679

Criteria to determine which muscles need to be stretched

In the stretch assessment tables provided for the weekly stretching programs for sports or other activities, three symbols are used: (**X**) refers to maximum or full, (**.**) refers to partial and (**O**) refers to zero or none.

There are four headings in the rows of the table: Direction, Range, Contraction and Stretch. Depending on the row heading the symbols in the table (**X**), (**.**) and (**O**) refer to different quantifiable things.

For Direction they pertain to whether there is movement or no movement.
For Range they pertain to whether there is full, partial or no range of movement.
For Contraction they pertain to whether there is full, partial or no muscle contraction.
For Stretch the symbols pertain to whether there should be full, partial or no stretch.

The columns are divided into the different regions of the body: Head, Cervical, Thoracic, Lumbar, Scapula, Shoulder, Elbow, Wrist, Hand (Fingers), Sacroiliac, Hip, Knee, Foot (Ankle) and Toes. The abbreviations for the movements in the different regions are listed below.

The criterion to determine which muscles are selected for stretching for a particular sport or activity depends on:

1. **Direction** of movement:

Flexion (F), Extension (E), Sidebending (S), Rotation (R), Abduction (Ab), Adduction (Ad), Internal rotation (Ir), External rotation (Er), Retraction (Re), Protraction (Pr), Elevation (El), Depression (De), Plantar flexion (Pf), Dorsi flexion (Df), Inversion (In), Eversion (Ev), Pronation (P) and Supination (Su)

In this category there are only two options: X or O.

(a) There is movement (**X**)
(b) There is no movement. (**O**)

If there is no direction of movement (O) then there is no range of movement.

2. **Range** of movement:

(a) Full range of movement (**X**)
(b) Partial range of movement (**.**)
(c) Very little or no range of movement (**O**)

3. The type of movement:

(a) Controlled and under isotonic muscle contraction
(b) Ballistic and ending at the elastic limit of the ligaments and fascia
(c) No movement and under isometric muscle contraction

4. When there is partial or no range of movement the joint may be in:

(a) The inner part of its range which will result in a shortened muscle.
(b) The outer part of its range which will result in a longer muscle
(c) The middle part of its range which will result in a muscle of medium length.

5. **Contraction** level:

(a) Full strong muscle contraction (**X**)
(b) Partial muscle contraction (**.**)
(c) Little or no muscle contraction (**O**)

6. **Contraction** type:

(a) Concentric isotonic contraction – muscle shortens during contraction.
(b) Eccentric isotonic contraction – muscle lengthens during contraction.
(c) Isometric muscle contraction – muscle stays the same length.

Some muscles the prime mover (agonists) contract to produce movement, while other muscles (stabiliser) contract to stabilise body parts so that they can act as a platform for other muscles to produce movement. Other muscles (neutralisers) contract to neutralise unwanted movements and some muscle contract to fine tune movements or prevent injury. When selecting the right stretching technique for a particular sport or activity all these muscle actions are considered, including their influence on the body, especially in terms of their ability to shorten muscles, and the dangers they present to the individual.

Most contraction is as a result of the action of agonist muscles and these are given an (X) rating in the table under the heading contraction, and usually an (X) rating under the heading stretch because they need to be stretched. Neutralisers and stabilisers are given an (X) rating under the heading contraction if they exert a sufficient high level of muscle contraction and shorten. Neutralisers and stabilisers usually need to be stretched less than agonists but because they contribute to overall function and protect against injury they still need to be considered important. Depending on other factors neutralisers and stabilisers may be given an (X) rating or a (.) rating under the stretch heading. If muscles exert a low to moderate level of contraction then they are given a (.) rating under the contraction heading, and if they exert a no contraction or very little contraction then they are given an (O) rating. Antagonists need to be stretched because they need to elongate without straining, so they may be given an (X) rating or a (.) rating under the stretch heading, depending on other factors.

It is important to prioritise which muscle should be stretched. Muscles are prone to shortening if they contract strongly or repeatedly or are held in a prolonged shortened state or if they contract isometrically or if they move a joint over of a limited range or if they only move a joint over the inner part of its range. It is especially important to stretch these types of muscles. Muscles involved in eccentric isotonic contraction, slowing down and eventually stopping movement, will also need stretching. Fascia and ligaments will need stretching when they are involved in stopping ballistic type movements such as throwing or kicking a ball.

7. The number of muscles and joints involved in the sport or activity.

When a sport is a team event involving players with different roles then that sport is broken down into the different roles. For example cricket is broken down into bating, catching, running and over arm bowling. If a sporting role or activity involves multiple movements, the contraction of many muscles or the involvement of the whole body, then that role or activity is broken down into smaller units. For example basketball is broken down into catching, running and throwing and soccer is broken down into kicking, running and sprinting.

8. **Stretch** level required.

The need to stretch a muscle or muscles is determined by the combination of (O), (.) and (X) ratings under the respective headings: Direction, Range and Contraction. The level of stretch required for a specific region of the body can be:

(a) Full strong stretch (**X**)
(b) Moderate stretch (**.**)
(c) Little or low level of stretch (**O**)

The highest level of importance for stretching a muscle (X) is given to those contracting strongly isotonically over the inner part of a given joint range or held in a shortened state and the lowest level of importance (O) is given to those not contracting. Muscles with a low level of contraction (.) or contracting over the outer part of its joint range or over a full range are of middle level importance for stretching.

Abseiling

Abseiling is the controlled descent down a rock face using a rope. Abseiling mainly involves the lower limb muscles When waking down the rock face or pushing off and returning to the rock face there is strong contraction of hip and knee extensor muscles such as gluteus maximus and the quadriceps, ankle plantar flexor muscles such as gastrocnemius and soleus and toe flexor muscles. Shoulder, elbow, wrist and finger muscles are involved in controlling the rope.

During abseiling the body remains straight and is leaning backwards in an almost horizontal position. The anterior muscles of the body have to work against gravity with a sustained isometric contraction. For example the muscles of the anterior cervical spine contract against gravity to maintain the head in the same plane as the rest of body. In addition to head and neck flexion abseiling also requires active thoracic, lumbar and hip flexion.

Abseiling	Head		Cervical				Thoracic				Lumbar			
	F	E	F	E	S	R	F	E	S	R	F	E	S	R
Direction	X	O	X	O	O	O	X	.	O	O	X	O	O	O
Range	.	O	.	O	O	O	.	.	O	O	.	.	.	.
Contraction	X	O	X	.	.	.	X	.	.	.	X	.	.	.
Stretch	X	.	X	.	.	.	X	.	.	.	X	.	.	.

	Scapula				Shoulder					
	Re	Pr	El	De	F	E	Ab	Ad	Ir	Er
Direction	O	X	.	.	X	O	.	.	.	.
Range	O	.	.	.	.	O	.	.	.	.
Contraction	.	X	.	.	X	X	.	.	.	.
Stretch	.	X	.	.	X	X	.	.	.	.

	Elbow				Wrist				Hand		SI	
	F	E	P	Su	F	E	Ab	Ad	F	E	F	E
Direction	X	O	O	O	X	X	O	O	X	.	.	.
Range	.	O	O	O	.	O	O	O	X	.	.	.
Contraction	X	O	O	O	X	X	O	O	X	.	.	.
Stretch	X	.	O	O	X	X	O	O	X	.	.	.

	Hip						Knee		Foot				Toes	
	F	E	Ab	Ad	Ir	Er	F	E	Pf	Df	In	Ev	F	E
Direction	X	X	.	.	.	.	.	X	X	.	O	O	X	O
Range	.	X	.	.	.	.	.	X	X	.	.	.	.	O
Contraction	.	X	.	.	.	.	.	X	X	.	.	.	X	O
Stretch	.	X	.	.	.	.	.	X	X	.	.	.	X	O

Key: None (O) partial (.) full (X) Range = Range of joint movement, Contraction = Level of muscle contraction, Direction = Direction of movement Direction may be Flexion (F), Extension (E), Sidebending (S), Rotation (R), Retraction (Re), Protraction (Pr), Elevation (El), Depression (De), Abduction (Ab), Adduction (Ad), Internal rotation (Ir), External rotation (Er), Pronation (P), Supination (Su), Plantar flexion (Pf), Dorsi flexion (Df), Inversion, (In), Eversion (Ev)

Weekly stretching program for abseiling

Day 1	Day 2	Day 3	Day 4	Day 5	Day 6	Day 7
1.4a	1.3a	1.3b	1.4b	1.4c	1.9	1.2
1.5	1.8	1.7c	3.0e	4.0c	2.9b	2.9a
1.7a	2.5b	1.7f	6.9c	2.5a	4.0d	2.8
2.5c	6.5d	2.3	6.5i	7.0a	2.6b	6.5h
3.0a	4.0a	6.9a	4.2	2.7a	4.5	2.4b
2.0a	5.3a	5.2a	4.0b	4.0e	2.4a	4.0f
3.8b	3.8c	5.7b	5.8a	5.8b	5.8e	5.9
6.0a	6.0c	6.6a	6.7a	6.7b	6.7c	6.7f
6.1c	7.1h	7.3a	7.3c	7.1b	7.1c	7.1d

Aerobics classes

Aerobics is a type of exercise that combines rhythmic movement and dance-like exercises with music with the goal of improving flexibility, strength, and cardio-vascular fitness. It is usually performed in a group setting led by an instructor, although it can be done solo and without musical accompaniment.

Aerobics mainly involves the upper and lower limbs and lumbar spine. All the joints listed in the table below are used during an aerobics class. The face and jaw are not commonly associated with aerobics but in all other respects aerobics is a whole body exercise system and involves many different movements.

Aerobics mostly requires lumbar flexion, extension, sidebending and rotation, scapula retraction, protraction, elevation and depression, shoulder flexion, extension, abduction, adduction, internal rotation and external rotation, elbow flexion and extension, hip flexion, extension, abduction, adduction, internal rotation and external rotation, knee flexion and extension and ankle dorsiflexion and plantar flexion.

In addition to stretching the prime movers also stretch their antagonists and the joint stabiliser and neutraliser muscles.

Aerobics classes	Head		Cervical				Thoracic				Lumbar			
	F	E	F	E	S	R	F	E	S	R	F	E	S	R
Direction	X	X	X	X	X	X	X	X	X	X	X	X	X	X
Range	.	.	.	.	.	.	.	.	.	.	X	X	X	X
Contraction	X	X	X	X	X	X	X	X	X	X	X	X	X	X
Stretch	X	X	X	X	.	.	X	X	X	X	X	X	X	X

	Scapula				Shoulder					
	Re	Pr	El	De	F	E	Ab	Ad	Ir	Er
Direction	X	X	X	X	X	X	X	X	X	X
Range	X	X	X	X	X	X	X	X	X	X
Contraction	X	X	X	X	X	X	X	X	X	X
Stretch	X	X	X	X	X	X	X	X	X	X

	Elbow				Wrist				Hand		SI	
	F	E	P	Su	F	E	Ab	Ad	F	E	F	E
Direction	X	X	X	X	X	X	X	X	X	X	X	X
Range	X	X	.	.	X	X	.	.	X	X	.	.
Contraction	X	X	.	.	X	X	.	.	.	.	.	.
Stretch	X	X	.	.	.	.	.	.	X	X	.	.

	Hip						Knee		Foot				Toes	
	F	E	Ab	Ad	Ir	Er	F	E	Pf	Df	In	Ev	F	E
Direction	X	X	X	X	X	X	X	X	X	X	X	X	X	X
Range	X	X	X	X	X	X	X	X	X	X	.	.	X	X
Contraction	X	X	X	X	X	X	X	X	X	X	X	X	X	X
Stretch	X	X	X	X	X	X	X	X	X	X	.	.	.	.

Key: None (O) partial (.) full (X) Range = Range of joint movement, Contraction = Level of muscle contraction, Direction = Direction of movement Direction may be Flexion (F), Extension (E), Sidebending (S), Rotation (R), Retraction (Re), Protraction (Pr), Elevation (El), Depression (De), Abduction (Ab), Adduction (Ad), Internal rotation (Ir), External rotation (Er), Pronation (P), Supination (Su), Plantar flexion (Pf), Dorsi flexion (Df), Inversion, (In), Eversion (Ev)

Weekly stretching program for aerobics

Day 1	Day 2	Day 3	Day 4	Day 5	Day 6	Day 7
1.3b	2.0a	2.1b	2.2a	1.9	1.7c	1.4a
2.6a	2.5b	2.4a	2.5c	2.4b	1.7f	1.5
1. 7i	3.0e	2.7a	2.9a	2.8	2.5a	2.9b
3.0a	3.5	3.3	3.2b	3.2a	3.1a	3.1b
3.4	4.0d	3.8a	3.9a	4.0h	4.0c	3.7
4.0e	4.4	4.5	4.0g	4.7	4.2	4.1
4.3	5.1a	5.3a	4.6a	5.2a	4.8	4.9a
5.0a	6.0a	6.1a	6.2a	6.3a	6.4a	6.5a
6.6a	6.7f	6.7a	6.9ab	7.1b	7.2b	7.1e

685

Archery

Archery is the practice of propelling arrows with the use of a bow to a target. Traditionally, archery has been used for hunting and warfare but it is now a major competitive sport and recreational activity.

Head flexion and cervical flexion, sidebending and rotation are necessary for positioning the head and lining up the eye with the arrow and the target. Thoracic and lumbar sidebending and rotation place the spine and body in the correct position for controlling the bow. Pulling on the bow involves scapula retraction, shoulder abduction and horizontal extension, and elbow flexion in one limb and elbow extension in the other and finger flexion. Hip extension and external rotation as well as knee extension and foot plantar flexion stabilise the lower limb for upper limb execution.

Stretching the muscles that contract, stretch their antagonists to allow movement and stretch the joint stabiliser and neutraliser muscles. For example stretch the wrist extensor muscles because they contract to stabilise the wrist during finger flexion.

Archery	Head		Cervical				Thoracic				Lumbar			
	F	E	F	E	S	R	F	E	S	R	F	E	S	R
Direction	X	O	X	O	X	X	O	O	X	X	O	O	X	X
Range	.	O	.	O	X	X	O	O	.	.	O	O	.	X
Contraction	X	.	.	.	X	X	O	.	.	.	.	.	X	X
Stretch	X	X	.	.	X	X	.	.	X	X	.	.	X	X

	Scapula				Shoulder					
	Re	Pr	El	De	F	E	Ab	Ad	Ir	Er
Direction	X	O	O	O	O	X	X	O	O	X
Range	X	O	O	O	O	.	X	O	O	.
Contraction	X	.	.	.	O	.	X	O	O	.
Stretch	X	.	.	.	.	.	X	.	.	.

	Elbow				Wrist				Hand		SI	
	F	E	P	Su	F	E	Ab	Ad	F	E	F	E
Direction	X	X	O	X	O	X	O	O	X	O	O	O
Range	X	X	O	.	O	X	O	O	X	O	O	O
Contraction	X	X	O	.	.	X	.	.	X	.	O	O
Stretch	X	X	O	.	.	X	.	.	X	.	O	O

	Hip						Knee		Foot		Toes	
	F	E	Ab	Ad	Ir	Er	F	E	Pf	Df	In	Ev	F	E
Direction	O	X	X	O	O	X	O	X	X	O	O	O	O	O
Range	O	O	O	O	O	.	O	X	O	O	O	O	O	O
Contraction	O	X	.	.	O	.	O	X	.	O	O	O	O	O
Stretch	.	X	X	.	.	.	.	X	X	.	O	O	O	O

Key: None (**O**) partial (.) full (**X**) Range = Range of joint movement, Contraction = Level of muscle contraction, Direction = Direction of movement Direction may be Flexion (F), Extension (E), Sidebending (S), Rotation (R), Retraction (Re), Protraction (Pr), Elevation (El), Depression (De), Abduction (Ab), Adduction (Ad), Internal rotation (Ir), External rotation (Er), Pronation (P), Supination (Su), Plantar flexion (Pf), Dorsi flexion (Df), Inversion, (In), Eversion (Ev)

Weekly stretching program for archery

Day 1	Day 2	Day 3	Day 4	Day 5	Day 6	Day 7
1.3a	1.1c	1.3b	2.9a	1.4c	1.9	1.4a
2.6a	1.7e	2.6b	2.8	1.7c	3.1a	1.5
1.7i	2.0a	3.6	1.7d	1.7f	1.7b	1.7a
2.1b	2.0b	3.9a	4.2	2.3	2.4d	1.6
4.5	3.2b	3.8b	3.4	3.2a	4.9a	4.1
2.4a	5.7b	3.8c	3.3	5.7c	5.5	3.1b
4.0e	4.0d	4.0g	4.9e	5.7d	5.2a	4.0c
5.0b	6.1a	6.6a	5.9	5.3a	6.5m	4.9b
4.8	6.4b	6.7f	5.4	7.1b	6.2a	7.1g

Arm wrestling

Arm wrestling is a combat sport with two participants. Each participant places the elbow of one bent arm (usually the right) on a table surface and grasps the other participant's hand. The goal is to pin the opponents forearm and hand onto the table surface with the arm.

Arm wrestling involves thoracic and lumbar sidebending and rotation, shoulder extension, adduction and internal rotation, elbow flexion and pronation, wrist and hand flexion,

In addition to stretching the prime movers you will need to stretch their antagonists and joint stabiliser such as the muscles of scapula retraction and protraction, hip extension and abduction and knee extension.

Arm wrestling	Head		Cervical				Thoracic				Lumbar			
	F	E	F	E	S	R	F	E	S	R	F	E	S	R
Direction	O	O	O	O	O	O	O	O	X	X	O	O	X	X
Range	O	O	O	O	O	O	O	O	O	O	O	O	.	O
Contraction	.	.	.	.	.	O	.	.	X	.	.	.	X	.
Stretch	.	.	.	.	.	O	.	.	X	X	.	.	X	X

	Scapula				Shoulder					
	Re	Pr	El	De	F	E	Ab	Ad	Ir	Er
Direction	X	X	O	O	O	X	O	O	X	O
Range	O	O	O	O	O	O	O	O	X	O
Contraction	X	X	.	.	.	.	.	.	X	O
Stretch	X	X	.	.	.	X	X	X	X	.

	Elbow				Wrist				Hand		SI	
	F	E	P	Su	F	E	Ab	Ad	F	E	F	E
Direction	X	O	X	O	X	O	O	O	X	O	O	O
Range	.	O	.	O	.	O	O	O	.	O	O	O
Contraction	X	.	.	.	X	.	O	O	X	.	O	O
Stretch	X	X	X	X	X	X	.	.	X	.	O	O

	Hip						Knee		Foot				Toes	
	F	E	Ab	Ad	Ir	Er	F	E	Pf	Df	In	Ev	F	E
Direction	O	O	O	O	O	O	O	O	O	O	O	O	O	O
Range	O	O	O	O	O	O	O	O	O	O	O	O	O	O
Contraction	.	X	X	.	.	.	.	X	X	.	.	.	O	O
Stretch	.	X	X	.	.	.	.	X	X	.	.	.	O	O

Key: None (**O**) partial (.) full (**X**) Range = Range of joint movement, Contraction = Level of muscle contraction, Direction = Direction of movement Direction may be Flexion (F), Extension (E), Sidebending (S), Rotation (R), Retraction (Re), Protraction (Pr), Elevation (El), Depression (De), Abduction (Ab), Adduction (Ad), Internal rotation (Ir), External rotation (Er), Pronation (P), Supination (Su), Plantar flexion (Pf), Dorsi flexion (Df), Inversion, (In), Eversion (Ev)

Weekly stretching program for arm wrestling

Day 1	Day 2	Day 3	Day 4	Day 5	Day 6	Day 7
1.2	1.3a	1.4a	2.1b	1.7d	2.0a	2.3
1.8	1. 7i	1.5	2.4c	2.4a	2.0b	2.5b
2.4d	3.4	1.7a	3.2b	2.6b	2.5c	3.0a
2.9a	3.9b	1.7c	4.0c	4.0e	3.1a	4.0d
2.8	4.0f	4.0g	4.2	4.3	4.1	4.5
4.7	4.8	5.0a	5.1a	5.2a	4.9a	5.3a
5.5	5.8c	5.8e	5.7b	6.0a	5.6a	6.1a
6.2b	5.8d	5.9	6.4d	6.1c	6.5h	6.6a
6.7f	6.9c	7.1b	7.1g	7.5a	7.5b	7.6

Batting

Batting requires good spine and shoulder flexibility as well as strength, and skill, and especially good eye, muscle, bat, ball coordination.

Batting primarily involves a combination of head extension, cervical flexion, extension, sidebending and rotation, thoracic and lumbar flexion, extension, sidebending and rotation, scapula retraction and protraction, shoulder flexion, extension, abduction, adduction, internal rotation and external rotation, elbow flexion, supination and pronation, wrist flexion and extension, finger flexion, hip extension and abduction, knee extension and ankle plantar flexion,. Some of these movements are for the left side of the body, some are for the right side and some are for both sides.

In addition to stretching the prime movers you will need to stretch their antagonists and the joint stabiliser and neutraliser muscles.

Batting	Head		Cervical				Thoracic				Lumbar			
	F	E	F	E	S	R	F	E	S	R	F	E	S	R
Direction	O	X	X	X	X	X	X	X	X	X	X	X	X	x
Range	O	X	.	.	X	X	.	.	X	.	.	.	X	X
Contraction	.	X	.	X	X	.	O	X	X	.	.	X	X	X
Stretch	.	X	.	X	X	X	.	X	X	X	.	X	X	X

	Scapula				Shoulder					
	Re	Pr	El	De	F	E	Ab	Ad	Ir	Er
Direction	X	X	X	X	X	O	O	O	X	X
Range	X	X	.	.	X	O	O	O	X	X
Contraction	X	X	.	.	X	.	.	.	X	X
Stretch	X	X	.	.	X	X	.	.	X	X

	Elbow				Wrist				Hand		SI	
	F	E	P	Su	F	E	Ab	Ad	F	E	F	E
Direction	X	O	X	X	X	X	X	X	X	O	O	O
Range	X	O	.	.	.	.	.	.	O	O	O	O
Contraction	X	.	.	.	X	X	.	.	X	.	.	.
Stretch	X	.	X	X	X	X	.	.	X	X	.	.

	Hip						Knee		Foot				Toes	
	F	E	Ab	Ad	Ir	Er	F	E	Pf	Df	In	Ev	F	E
Direction	X	O	X	O	X	X	X	O	X	O	O	O	O	O
Range	.	O	O	O	.	.	.	O	.	O	O	O	O	O
Contraction	.	X	X	.	.	.	O	X	X	O	.	.	O	O
Stretch	.	X	X	.	.	.	.	X	X	.	.	.	O	O

Key: None (O) partial (.) full (X) Range = Range of joint movement, Contraction = Level of muscle contraction, Direction = Direction of movement Direction may be Flexion (F), Extension (E), Sidebending (S), Rotation (R), Retraction (Re), Protraction (Pr), Elevation (El), Depression (De), Abduction (Ab), Adduction (Ad), Internal rotation (Ir), External rotation (Er), Pronation (P), Supination (Su), Plantar flexion (Pf), Dorsi flexion (Df), Inversion, (In), Eversion (Ev)

Weekly stretching program for batting

Day 1	Day 2	Day 3	Day 4	Day 5	Day 6	Day 7
1.4a	1.3a	1.7c	1.3b	1.7f	2.0b	1.8
1.5	1.4c	2.5b	2.9a	2.4a	2.0b	2.3
3.1a	3.0a	2.9b	2.8	2.6b	2.5c	3.0c
3.0e	3.3	3.2a	3.4	3.5	3.1b	4.0a
3.8d	3.8c	4.0b	4.0e	4.0d	4.0c	3.8a
4.0f	4.0g	4.1	4.3	4.4	4.2	5.9
5.2a	4.8	4.9c	5.0a	5.7c	5.8c	6.7a
5.3a	5.5	5.6a	6.5e	5.7d	5.8d	6.0a
6.4d	6.7c	6.6a	6.9a	6.7f	7.1b	7.1f

691

Bodyboarding (boogieboarding)

Bodyboarding, also known as Boogieboarding is a surface water sport in which the surfer rides a bodyboard on the crest, face or curl of a wave towards the shore using swim fins for additional propulsion and control while riding the wave.

The bodyboard is a short, rectangular piece of hydrodynamic foam, sometimes containing a short graphite rod within the core. There are three ways of riding a bodyboard prone, dropknee, or stand-up. Prone riding is riding the wave on your stomach. Dropknee is when one places one fin forward flat on the front of the deck and with the opposing knee on the bottom end of the board with his fin dragging behind in the water. Stand-up consists of standing upright on the board and performing tricks on the face of the wave as well as in the air.

Bodyboarding requires coordination and balance. The prone method is described here under bodyboarding. Stretches for the stand-up method are described under windsurfing and surfing.

Prone bodyboarding involves: head, cervical, thoracic and lumbar extension, thoracolumbar rotation, sacroiliac flexion, scapula retraction, shoulder flexion and extension, elbow flexion and extension, wrist flexion, hip extension, knee flexion and extension, ankle dorsiflexion and plantar flexion.

Bodyboarding	Head		Cervical				Thoracic				Lumbar			
	F	E	F	E	S	R	F	E	S	R	F	E	S	R
Direction	O	X	O	X	X	O	O	X	O	O	O	X	O	X
Range	.	.	O	.	.	O	O	X	O	O	O	.	O	.
Contraction	.	X	.	X	.	.	O	X	.	.	O	.	.	.
Stretch	.	X	.	X	.	.	.	X	.	.	O	X	.	X

	Scapula				Shoulder					
	Re	Pr	El	De	F	E	Ab	Ad	Ir	Er
Direction	X	X	O	O	X	O	O	O	O	O
Range	.	.	O	O	.	O	O	O	O	O
Contraction	X	X	.	.	X	X	.	.	.	.
Stretch	X	X	.	.	X	X	.	.	.	.

	Elbow				Wrist				Hand		SI	
	F	E	P	Su	F	E	Ab	Ad	F	E	F	E
Direction	X	X	X	X	X	X	X	X	X	O	X	O
Range	X	X	.	.	.	.	.	.	.	O	.	O
Contraction	X	X	.	.	X	.	.	.	.	O	.	O
Stretch	X	X	.	.	X	.	.	.	.	O	.	O

	Hip						Knee		Foot				Toes	
	F	E	Ab	Ad	Ir	Er	F	E	Pf	Df	In	Ev	F	E
Direction	O	X	O	O	O	O	X	X	X	X	O	O	O	O
Range	O	.	O	O	O	O	X	X	X	X	O	O	O	O
Contraction	.	X	O	O	.	.	X	X	X	X	.	.	O	O
Stretch	.	X	O	O	.	.	X	X	X	X	.	.	O	O

Key: None (O) partial (.) full (X) Range = Range of joint movement, Contraction = Level of muscle contraction, Direction = Direction of movement Direction may be Flexion (F), Extension (E), Sidebending (S), Rotation (R), Retraction (Re), Protraction (Pr), Elevation (El), Depression (De), Abduction (Ab), Adduction (Ad), Internal rotation (Ir), External rotation (Er), Pronation (P), Supination (Su), Plantar flexion (Pf), Dorsi flexion (Df), Inversion, (In), Eversion (Ev)

Weekly stretching program for prone bodyboarding

Day 1	Day 2	Day 3	Day 4	Day 5	Day 6	Day 7
1.3b	1.4a	1.4b	1.4c	1.7a	1.7b	1.9
2.0b	1.7c	2.4a	2.4b	2.4c	2.5b	2.6c
3.1a	3.1b	3.0a	3.0e	2.6d	3.2b	2.9b
2.9a	4.7	4.8	4.5	4.0h	4.0b	4.0f
5.2a	5.3a	4.9a	4.9c	5.0a	6.0b	5.4
6.1b	6.1c	6.1f	6.2c	6.3d	6.5j	6.6c
6.6d	6.7a	6.7b	6.7f	5.8b	6.9a	7.0a
6.9c	6.0a	6.3c	7.1c	5.9	7.5a	7.1b
7.1f	7.1g	7.4b	7.2b	7.5b	7.4a	7.6

Ten-pin bowling, flat green bowling and crown green bowling - Bowling Underarm

Ten-pin bowling is a sport and popular leisure activity where players compete to knock down as many pins as possible standing at the end of a wooden or synthetic bowling lane with a large ball.

Bowls or lawn bowls is a sport leisure activity where the objective is to roll large balls over grass surfaces so that they stop as close as possible to a smaller ball called a jack. The large ball is weighted on one side or biased so that it rolls in a slight arc.

In flat-green bowls the green is flat and bowling occurs along parallel playing strips called rinks. In crown-green bowls the green is convex or uneven. Both types are normally played outdoors on manicured grass and there are many variations in the shapes and sizes of greens. There are however more indoor clubs starting up which play on synthetic surface.

All the underarm bowling sports require skill and good shoulder flexibility especially full shoulder flexion and scapula protraction and good elbow movement. Stretch the agonists (the muscles that contract) because they will shorten with use and stretch the antagonists to allow movement to occur.

Bowling involves head extension, upper cervical extension and lower cervical flexion, thoracic and lumbar flexion, lumbar sidebending and rotation, sacroiliac flexion and extension, scapula retraction, protraction, elevation and depression, shoulder flexion, extension and abduction, elbow flexion, extension and supination, wrist flexion and extension, finger flexion and extension, hip flexion, extension and abduction, knee flexion and extension, ankle dorsiflexion and plantar flexion and toe flexion and extension.

Bowling underarm	Head		Cervical				Thoracic				Lumbar			
	F	E	F	E	S	R	F	E	S	R	F	E	S	R
Direction	O	X	X	X	X	X	X	O	O	O	X	O	X	X
Range	O	.	.	.	.	.	.	O	O	O	.	O	.	.
Contraction	.	X	.	X	.	.	.	X	.	.	.	X	.	.
Stretch	.	X	.	X	.	.	X	X	.	.	.	X	X	X

	Scapula				Shoulder									
	Re	Pr	El	De	F	E	Ab	Ad	Ir	Er				
Direction	X	X	X	X	X	X	X	O	O	O				
Range	X	.	.	.	X	X	O	O	O	O				
Contraction	X	X	.	.	X	X	.	.	.	.				
Stretch	X	X	.	.	X	X	X	.	.	.				

	Elbow				Wrist				Hand		SI			
	F	E	P	Su	F	E	Ab	Ad	F	E	F	E		
Direction	X	X	O	X	X	X	O	O	X	X	X	X		
Range	X	X	O	.	X	X	O	O	.	.	.	.		
Contraction	X	.	.	.	X	.	O	O	X	.	.	.		
Stretch	X	X	.	.	X	X	O	O	X	X	.	.		

	Hip						Knee		Foot				Toes	
	F	E	Ab	Ad	Ir	Er	F	E	Pf	Df	In	Ev	F	E
Direction	X	X	X	O	O	O	X	X	X	X	O	O	X	X
Range	.	X	O	O	O	O	X	X	X	X	O	O	.	.
Contraction	.	X	X	.	.	.	X	X	X	.	.	.	.	.
Stretch	X	X	X	.	.	.	X	X	X	X	.	.	X	X

Key: None (O) partial (.) full (X) Range = Range of joint movement, Contraction = Level of muscle contraction, Direction = Direction of movement Direction may be Flexion (F), Extension (E), Sidebending (S), Rotation (R), Retraction (Re), Protraction (Pr), Elevation (El), Depression (De), Abduction (Ab), Adduction (Ad), Internal rotation (Ir), External rotation (Er), Pronation (P), Supination (Su), Plantar flexion (Pf), Dorsi flexion (Df), Inversion, (In), Eversion (Ev)

Weekly stretching program for bowling underarm

Day 1	Day 2	Day 3	Day 4	Day 5	Day 6	Day 7
1.3c	1.4a	1.3b	1.4c	1.7a	1.8	1.9
2.1b		2.4a	2.4b	1.7b	2.5c	2.5a
2.5b	1.7c	2.6a	2.6d	2.0a	3.0a	2.9b
4.1	1.7f	4.0a	4.0e	3.3	3.8a	4.0g
4.8	2.9a	4.4	4.3	4.0c	3.8d	4.5
4.9b	2.9a	5.2a	5.3a	4.2	3.8e	4.9e
5.5	5.7b	5.9	6.0a	6.1a	3.9a	5.6b
6.1e	5.8b	6.2a	6.2b	6.4a	6.4d	6.6a
6.7a	6.7f	6.9a	7.1b	7.1e	7.2b	7.3a

Boxing and martial arts punching

Boxing is a combat sport in which two people throw punches at each other with gloved hands. Boxing requires strength, speed, endurance and fast reflexes. Also included here under the heading Boxing are mixed martial arts punching and martial art punching such as in karate. Karate punches are straight thrusts and arguably less powerful than a boxer's follow-through punches. Types of movements in boxing include jabs (punches which retract) and hooks and uppercuts (follow-through punches).

Boxing involves head flexion and extension, cervical flexion, sidebending and rotation, thoracic flexion and extension, lumbar flexion and extension, sidebending and rotation, scapula retraction, protraction, elevation and depression, shoulder flexion and extension, adduction and internal rotation, elbow flexion and extension, supination and pronation, wrist flexion and extension and finger flexion, hip flexion, abduction, adduction, internal rotation and external rotation, knee flexion, ankle plantar flexion and foot inversion and eversion.

It is important to stretch both the agonist muscles and the antagonist muscles. During the punch the agonists must contract to produce joint movement and the antagonists must relax to allow the joint movement and the muscles to lengthen. For example in boxing and punching you should stretch the scapula protractor and retractor muscles and the shoulder flexor and extensor muscles.

Boxing	Head		Cervical				Thoracic				Lumbar			
	F	E	F	E	S	R	F	E	S	R	F	E	S	R
Direction	X	X	X	X	X	X	X	X	O	O	X	X	X	X
Range	.	.	.	.	.	.	X	.	O	O	X	.	.	.
Contraction	.	.	.	.	.	.	.	.	.	.	X	X	X	X
Stretch	X	X	.	.	.	.	X	.	.	.	X	X	X	X

	Scapula				Shoulder					
	Re	Pr	El	De	F	E	Ab	Ad	Ir	Er
Direction	O	X	X	X	X	O	X	X	X	O
Range	O	X	X	X	X	O	.	.	X	O
Contraction	X	X	.	.	X	X	.	X	X	.
Stretch	X	X	X	X	X	X	X	X	X	.

	Elbow				Wrist				Hand		SI	
	F	E	P	Su	F	E	Ab	Ad	F	E	F	E
Direction	X	X	X	X	X	X	O	O	X	O	O	O
Range	X	X	.	.	.	X	O	O	X	O	O	O
Contraction	X	X	.	.	X	.	O	O	X	O	.	.
Stretch	X	X	.	.	X	X	.	.	X	.	.	.

	Hip						Knee		Foot				Toes	
	F	E	Ab	Ad	Ir	Er	F	E	Pf	Df	In	Ev	F	E
Direction	X	O	X	X	X	X	X	O	X	O	X	X	O	O
Range	.	O	.	.	.	.	O	X	O	.	.	.	O	O
Contraction	.	X	X	X	.	.	.	X	X	.	.	.	.	.
Stretch	X	X	X	X	.	.	X	X	X	X	X	X	.	.

Key: None (O) partial (.) full (X) Range = Range of joint movement, Contraction = Level of muscle contraction, Direction = Direction of movement Direction may be Flexion (F), Extension (E), Sidebending (S), Rotation (R), Retraction (Re), Protraction (Pr), Elevation (El), Depression (De), Abduction (Ab), Adduction (Ad), Internal rotation (Ir), External rotation (Er), Pronation (P), Supination (Su), Plantar flexion (Pf), Dorsi flexion (Df), Inversion, (In), Eversion (Ev)

Weekly stretching program for boxing and punching

Day 1	Day 2	Day 3	Day 4	Day 5	Day 6	Day 7
1.3a	2.0a	1.3b	2.4b	1.9	1.4a	1.4b
2.5c	2.5b	2.6b	2.6d	2.5a	1.5	2.7a
2.9a	2.9b	3.0a	4.1	3.2a	1.7c	3.4
2.8	4.0c	3.5	4.3	4.0e	3.1a	4.0g
4.4	4.2	5.0a	4.9c	4.5	4.7	4.8
5.2c	5.1a	5.2a	5.5	5.4	5.3a	5.6a
5.6b	5.7b	5.9	6.0a	6.0c	6.1a	6.1e
6.2a	5.8b	6.4b	6.2b	6.4d	6.5d	6.5m
6.6b	6.7b	6.9a	6.7f	7.1b	7.1e	7.3a

697

Catching a ball (Baseball, Cricket, Rounders, Softball)

Catching a ball requires good hand-eye coordination. Catching a ball involves head extension, cervical flexion and extension, thoracic flexion, lumbar flexion and extension, scapula retraction, protraction, elevation and depression, shoulder flexion, extension, abduction, adduction and internal rotation, elbow flexion, supination and pronation, wrist extension, abduction and adduction, finger flexion and extension, hip flexion, abduction and external rotation, knee flexion, ankle plantar flexion and toe flexion.

Catching a ball	Head		Cervical				Thoracic				Lumbar			
	F	E	F	E	S	R	F	E	S	R	F	E	S	R
Direction	O	X	X	X	O	O	X	O	O	O	X	X	O	O
Range	O	X	.	.	O	O	.	O	O	O	.	.	O	O
Contraction	.	X	.	X	.	.	.	X	.	.	.	X	.	.
Stretch	X	X	X	X	.	.	.	X	.	.	X	X	.	.

	Scapula				Shoulder					
	Re	Pr	El	De	F	E	Ab	Ad	Ir	Er
Direction	X	X	X	X	X	X	X	X	X	O
Range	.	X	.	.	X	.	.	.	.	O
Contraction	.	X	.	.	X	X	.	X	X	.
Stretch	X	X	.	.	X	X	X	.	X	X

	Elbow				Wrist				Hand		SI	
	F	E	P	Su	F	E	Ab	Ad	F	E	F	E
Direction	X	O	X	X	O	X	X	X	X	X	O	O
Range	.	O	.	.	O	.	.	.	X	.	O	O
Contraction	X	X	.	.	.	X	.	.	X	.	.	.
Stretch	X	X	X	X	X	X	.	.	X	X	.	.

	Hip						Knee		Foot				Toes	
	F	E	Ab	Ad	Ir	Er	F	E	Pf	Df	In	Ev	F	E
Direction	X	O	X	O	O	X	X	O	X	O	O	O	X	O
Range	X	O	.	O	O	.	X	O	X	O	O	O	.	O
Contraction	.	X	X	.	.	.	.	X	X	.	.	.	.	.
Stretch	X	X	X	.	X	X	X	X	X	.	.	.	X	.

Key: None (**O**) partial (.) full (**X**) Range = Range of joint movement, Contraction = Level of muscle contraction, Direction = Direction of movement Direction may be Flexion (F), Extension (E), Sidebending (S), Rotation (R), Retraction (Re), Protraction (Pr), Elevation (El), Depression (De), Abduction (Ab), Adduction (Ad), Internal rotation (Ir), External rotation (Er), Pronation (P), Supination (Su), Plantar flexion (Pf), Dorsi flexion (Df), Inversion, (In), Eversion (Ev)

Weekly stretching program for catching a ball

Day 1	Day 2	Day 3	Day 4	Day 5	Day 6	Day 7
1.2	1.3b	1.4a	1.4b	1.7c	1.4c	1.8
1.9	2.0a	1.5	2.4c	1.7f	2.5a	2.5b
2.5c	2.7a	3.6	3.2a	2.9a	3.0a	2.9b
4.0e	4.0c	3.7	4.1	2.8	4.0g	4.0b
4.5	4.2	3.8a	4.9a	5.0a	4.3	4.9e
5.2a	5.1b	3.8c	5.5	5.4	5.3a	5.6a
6.0a	6.1a	3.8d	6.1e	6.2a	5.8e	6.2b
6.4c	6.4h	3.8e	6.5f	6.6a	5.9	6.7b
6.7e	6.7f	6.9a	7.1b	7.1g	7.1e	7.3a

Climbing

Climbing is a physical activity requiring great strength and agility. It involves the use of one's limbs to ascend any steep object, natural or manmade. It may be done competitively, recreationally, professionally or as part of an emergency rescue or military exercise. Types of climbing considered here include indoor climbing such as an artificial wall in a climbing gym, rock climbing or mountaineering, net climbing, industrial climbing and tree climbing.

Climbing mainly involves upper limb muscles such as pectoralis major and latissimus dorsi and lower limb muscles such as gluteus maximus. It requires strength and flexibility throughout the whole body. Specifically climbing involves head extension, cervical extension, thoracic extension, lumbar extension and sidebending, sacroiliac flexion, scapula retraction, protraction, elevation and depression, shoulder flexion, extension, abduction, adduction, internal rotation and external rotation, elbow flexion, extension, supination and pronation, wrist flexion, extension, abduction and adduction, finger flexion, hip flexion, extension, abduction, adduction, internal rotation and external rotation, knee flexion and extension, ankle dorsiflexion and plantar flexion and foot eversion.

Considering the direction and range of movement, the level of muscle contraction and other criteria climbers should stretch muscles responsible for head flexion and extension, cervical flexion and extension, thoracic extension, lumbar extension and sidebending, scapula retraction, protraction, elevation and depression, shoulder flexion, extension, abduction, adduction, internal rotation and external rotation, elbow flexion, extension, supination and pronation, wrist flexion, extension, abduction and adduction, finger flexion, sacroiliac flexion, hip flexion, extension, abduction, adduction, internal rotation and external rotation, knee flexion and extension, ankle dorsiflexion and plantar flexion and foot eversion. Climbing is a whole body activity involving an extensive number of muscles and this is reflected in the large number of muscles listed in the table that need to be stretched.

Climbing	Head		Cervical				Thoracic				Lumbar			
	F	E	F	E	S	R	F	E	S	R	F	E	S	R
Direction	.	X	.	X	.	.	.	X	.	.	.	X	X	.
Range	.	X	.	.	.	.	.	.	.	.	.	.	.	.
Contraction	X	.	X	.	.	.	.	X	.	.	X	X	X	.
Stretch	X	X	X	X	.	.	.	X	.	.	.	X	X	.

	Scapula				Shoulder					
	Re	Pr	El	De	F	E	Ab	Ad	Ir	Er
Direction	X	X	X	X	X	X	X	X	X	X
Range	X	X	X	X	X	.	X	X	.	X
Contraction	X	.	.	X	.	X	.	X	X	.
Stretch	X	X	X	X	X	X	X	X	X	X

	Elbow				Wrist				Hand		SI	
	F	E	P	Su	F	E	Ab	Ad	F	E	F	E
Direction	X	X	X	X	X	X	X	X	X	.	X	.
Range	X	X	X	X	X	X	X	X	X	.	X	.
Contraction	X	.	X	X	X	X	.	.	X	.	X	.
Stretch	X	X	X	X	X	X	X	X	X	.	X	.

	Hip						Knee		Foot				Toes	
	F	E	Ab	Ad	Ir	Er	F	E	Pf	Df	In	Ev	F	E
Direction	X	X	X	X	X	X	X	X	X	X	.	X	.	O
Range	X	X	X	X	X	X	X	X	X	X	.	.	.	O
Contraction	X	X	X	X	X	X	X	X	X	X	.	X	.	O
Stretch	X	X	X	X	X	X	X	X	X	X	.	X	.	O

Key: None (O) partial (.) full (X)
Range = Range of joint movement, Contraction = Level of muscle contraction, Direction = Direction of movement of Body Part Direction may be Flexion (F), Extension (E), Sidebending (S), Rotation (R), Retraction (Re), Protraction (Pr), Elevation (El), Depression (De), Abduction (Ab), Adduction (Ad), Internal rotation (Ir) or External rotation (Er), Pronation (P) or Supination (Su), Plantar flexion (Pf) or Dorsi flexion (Df), Inversion, (In), Eversion (Ev)

Weekly stretching program for climbing

Day 1	Day 2	Day 3	Day 4	Day 5	Day 6	Day 7
1.4a	1.3b	2.9a	1.4b	1.3a	1.4c	2.0a
1.5	1.8	2.8	1.2	2.6b	2.5c	2.5a
1.7c	2.4c	2.4a	4.0f	1.7d	3.0a	4.0g
4.0c	3.4	3.1a	4.9c	4.3	3.8a	4.5
4.8	4.1	4.0e	5.5	5.3a	3.8d	5.2a
5.9	4.0d	4.2	6.0c	5.6b	5.6a	5.7c
6.2c	4.9b	5.0a	6.1e	5.8c	6.0a	5.7d
6.3d	6.2b	3.0e	6.5g	5.8d	6.7f	6.4d
6.6c	6.5h	6.7b	6.9a	7.1b	7.1f	7.3b

Cricket - Bowling Overarm

Overarm bowling commonly used in cricket is the action of propelling a ball toward a wicket defended by a batsman. Overarm bowling is different from throwing in that the bowler's arm must not extend during the bowling action, only the rotation of the shoulder can be used to impart velocity to the ball. Most bowlers hold their elbows fully extended as they bowl. They rotate their arm through an arc and release the ball as it nears the top of the arc above the shoulder joint.

Pace bowlers or fast bowlers emphasise increasing the speed of the ball with a faster run up or a sling action delivery, whereas spin bowlers impart rotation to the ball with the subtle contraction of wrist or finger muscles.

Bowling requires skill and good all round flexibility. It involves a complex system of changing movements. Scapula retraction becomes protraction, shoulder abduction becomes extension, elbow flexion becomes extension and wrist extension becomes flexion. As well as stretching the agonists (the muscles that contract) it is necessary to stretch the antagonist muscles

The movements involved in the run up phase of bowling include: hip flexion, extension, abduction and adduction, knee flexion and extension, ankle dorsiflexion and plantar flexion and toe flexion and extension. The movements involved in the bowling phase include: head extension, upper cervical extension and lower cervical flexion, thoracic flexion, lumbar flexion, sidebending and rotation, scapula retraction, protraction, elevation and depression, shoulder flexion, extension and abduction, elbow flexion and extension, wrist flexion and extension and finger flexion.

The stretches selected in the weekly program cover all the muscles used in bowling but with an upper limb bias. For a more comprehensive list of lower limb stretches see Running.

Cricket bowling	Head		Cervical				Thoracic				Lumbar			
	F	E	F	E	S	R	F	E	S	R	F	E	S	R
Direction	O	X	X	X	X	X	X	O	O	O	X	O	X	X
Range	O	.	.	.	.	.	.	O	O	O	.	O	.	.
Contraction	.	.	X	.	.	.	.	X	.	.	X	X	.	.
Stretch	.	X	X	X	.	.	X	X	.	.	X	X	X	X

	Scapula				Shoulder					
	Re	Pr	El	De	F	E	Ab	Ad	Ir	Er
Direction	X	X	X	X	X	X	X	O	X	X
Range	X	X	.	.	X	X	X	O	X	X
Contraction	X	X	.	.	X	X	X	.	.	.
Stretch	X	X	.	.	X	X	X	X	X	X

	Elbow				Wrist				Hand		SI	
	F	E	P	Su	F	E	Ab	Ad	F	E	F	E
Direction	X	X	X	X	X	X	O	O	X	O	X	X
Range	X	X	.	.	X	.	O	O	.	O	.	.
Contraction	X	.	.	.	X	.	.	.	X	.	.	.
Stretch	X	X	.	.	X	X	X	X	X	X	.	.

	Hip						Knee		Foot				Toes	
	F	E	Ab	Ad	Ir	Er	F	E	Pf	Df	In	Ev	F	E
Direction	X	X	X	O	O	O	X	X	X	X	O	O	X	X
Range	X	X	O	O	O	O	X	X	X	X	O	O	.	.
Contraction	.	X	X	.	.	.	X	X	X	X	.	.	.	.
Stretch	X	X	X	X	.	.	X	X	X	X	.	.	X	X

Key: None (O) partial (.) full (X) Range = Range of joint movement, Contraction = Level of muscle contraction, Direction = Direction of movement Direction may be Flexion (F), Extension (E), Sidebending (S), Rotation (R), Retraction (Re), Protraction (Pr), Elevation (El), Depression (De), Abduction (Ab), Adduction (Ad), Internal rotation (Ir), External rotation (Er), Pronation (P), Supination (Su), Plantar flexion (Pf), Dorsi flexion (Df), Inversion, (In), Eversion (Ev)

Weekly stretching program for cricket - overarm bowling

Day 1	Day 2	Day 3	Day 4	Day 5	Day 6	Day 7
1.2	1.3a	1.4b	1.4a		1.7c	1.9
2.5b	2.4c	2.4b	1.5	2.1a	1.7f	1.8
3.0a	3.0e	3.1a	2.5c	2.5a	2.6b	2.9a
2.9b	3.2b	4.1	3.8a	3.4	4.0c	2.8
4.0b	4.0e	4.7	3.8d	4.2	4.3	4.0g
4.4	4.5	5.5	3.8e	5.4	4.9e	4.9c
5.2a	5.3a	5.9	5.6b	5.8c	5.7c	5.6a
6.0b	6.1e	6.2a	6.2b	5.8d	5.7d	6.4b
6.4d	6.5h	6.6a	6.7b	6.7f	7.1b	7.3c

703

Cue sports

Cue sports is a general term for pool, snooker and billiards - games where the players use a cue stick to strike billiard balls and move them around a cloth-covered table bounded by rubber cushions.

Cue sports involves head extension, cervical extension and sidebending, thoracic flexion, lumbar flexion, sidebending and rotation, scapula retraction, protraction and elevation, shoulder flexion, extension, abduction, adduction, elbow flexion and extension, wrist extension, finger flexion, hip flexion, knee extension, ankle plantar flexion and toe extension.

Cue sports	Head		Cervical				Thoracic				Lumbar			
	F	E	F	E	S	R	F	E	S	R	F	E	S	R
Direction	O	X	O	X	X	O	X	O	O	O	X	O	X	X
Range	O	X	O	X	.	O	.	O	O	O	X	O	.	.
Contraction	.	X	.	X	X	.	.	X	.	.	.	X	.	.
Stretch	X	X	X	X	X	.	X	X	X	.	X	X	X	X

	Scapula				Shoulder					
	Re	Pr	El	De	F	E	Ab	Ad	Ir	Er
Direction	X	X	X	O	X	X	X	X	O	O
Range	X	X	.	O	X	X	.	X	O	O
Contraction	.	.	.	.	X	.	.	.	.	.
Stretch	X	X	X	.	X	X	X	X	.	.

	Elbow				Wrist				Hand		SI	
	F	E	P	Su	F	E	Ab	Ad	F	E	F	E
Direction	X	X	O	O	O	X	O	O	X	X	O	X
Range	X	X	O	O	O	X	O	O	X	X	O	X
Contraction	.	X	.	.	O	.	.	.	X	.	O	.
Stretch	X	X	.	.	.	X	.	.	X	X	.	X

	Hip						Knee		Foot				Toes	
	F	E	Ab	Ad	Ir	Er	F	E	Pf	Df	In	Ev	F	E
Direction	X	O	O	O	O	O	O	X	X	O	O	O	O	X
Range	X	O	O	O	O	O	O	X	.	O	O	O	O	X
Contraction	.	X	.	.	O	O	.	.	X	.	.	.	X	.
Stretch	X	X	.	.	.	.	X	X	X	X	.	.	X	X

Key: None (**O**) partial (**.**) full (**X**) Range = Range of joint movement, Contraction = Level of muscle contraction, Direction = Direction of movement Direction may be Flexion (F), Extension (E), Sidebending (S), Rotation (R), Retraction (Re), Protraction (Pr), Elevation (El), Depression (De), Abduction (Ab), Adduction (Ad), Internal rotation (Ir), External rotation (Er), Pronation (P), Supination (Su), Plantar flexion (Pf), Dorsi flexion (Df), Inversion, (In), Eversion (Ev)

Weekly stretching program for cue sports (pool, snooker and billiards)

Day 1	Day 2	Day 3	Day 4	Day 5	Day 6	Day 7
1.2	1.3b	1.4a	1.3a	1.7a	1.4c	1.7d
2.0a	2.1b	1.5	1. 7i	2.4a	2.4b	2.5a
2.1a	2.5b	3.0e	1.8	2.6b	2.9a	3.0a
3.1a	2.9b	3.3	3.4	3.5	2.8	3.6
4.8	4.0b	4.0c	4.0h	4.5	4.7	3.7
5.5	4.3	4.9a	5.3a	4.9e	5.2a	3.8a
6.0a	5.6b	5.8b	6.1c	5.8e	5.4	3.8e
6.6a	6.4d		6.7b	5.9	6.6d	6.7c
6.7f	6.9a	7.1a	7.1f	7.1b	7.2b	7.3b

Cycling

Cycling takes many forms, racing, mountain biking, utilitarian and recreational. Racing bicycles have dropped handlebars requiring the rider to bend forward which reduces air resistance and use stronger muscles such as the gluteus maximus to generate high speeds. In contrast town bikes and mountain bike have a more upright arrangement and shorter wheelbase for greater manoeuvrability.

Bicycles are a great way to improve cardiovascular fitness and strength, especially in the lower limb. As a non weight bearing system of exercise it is especially useful for anyone who needs to keep fit yet has a lower limb dysfunction such as osteoarthritis and cycling is useful because it can combine the need stay fit with the need to commute.

Cycling has one disadvantage, it is done seated. Sitting does little to promote flexibility, good posture and healthy levels of bone density. Excessive cycling can lead to overuse injuries in the neck, knees, hips, hands and back. Disc disease increases in the lumbar spine with prolonged sitting and when the spine is held in a fixed flexed position characteristic of cycling.

Stretching helps counter some of the negative effects of cycling. Ensure the bicycle is set up correctly for the rider, with a seat that is wide and supports the buttocks and take regular breaks to walk when cycling long distances. Cycling mainly requires the contraction of lower limb muscles such as gluteus maximus and the hamstrings, calf and quadriceps muscles. The static nature of the cycling posture causes muscle shortening in the spine and upper limbs.

Cycling involves head extension, cervical extension, thoracic and lumbar flexion, sacroiliac extension, scapula protraction and elevation, shoulder and elbow flexion, forearm supination (dropped handlebars) or pronation (other bikes), wrist extension, finger flexion, hip flexion, knee flexion and ankle dorsiflexion. These positions tend to be greatest in racing type bikes.

Cycling	Head		Cervical				Thoracic				Lumbar			
	F	E	F	E	S	R	F	E	S	R	F	E	S	R
Direction	O	X	O	X	O	O	X	O	O	O	X	O	O	O
Range	O	X	O	.	O	O	X	O	O	O	X	O	O	O
Contraction	.	X	.	X	.	O	O	X	.	O	.	X	.	.
Stretch	.	X	.	X	.	O	.	X	.	.	X	X	.	.

	Scapula				Shoulder					
	Re	Pr	El	De	F	E	Ab	Ad	Ir	Er
Direction	O	X	X	O	X	O	O	O	O	O
Range	O	X	.	O	.	O	O	O	O	O
Contraction	.	O	.	O	.	O	O	O	O	O
Stretch	.	X	.	.	X	.	.	.	.	.

	Elbow				Wrist				Hand		SI	
	F	E	P	Su	F	E	Ab	Ad	F	E	F	E
Direction	X	O	.	.	O	X	O	O	X	O	O	X
Range	.	O	.	.	O	.	O	O	X	O	O	X
Contraction	.	.	.	.	.	X	O	O	X	.	O	.
Stretch	.	.	.	.	.	X	.	.	X	.	O	X

	Hip						Knee		Foot				Toes	
	F	E	Ab	Ad	Ir	Er	F	E	Pf	Df	In	Ev	F	E
Direction	X	X	O	O	O	O	X	X	X	X	O	O	O	O
Range	.	.	O	O	O	O	.	.	.	X	O	O	O	O
Contraction	.	X	.	.	O	O	.	X	X	O	O	O	O	O
Stretch	X	X	.	.	.	.	X	X	X	X	.	.	.	O

Key: None (O) partial (.) full (X) Range = Range of joint movement, Contraction = Level of muscle contraction, Direction = Direction of movement of Body Part. Direction may be Flexion (F), Extension (E), Sidebending (S), Rotation (R), Retraction (Re), Protraction (Pr), Elevation (El), Depression (De), Abduction (Ab), Adduction (Ad), Internal rotation (Ir) or External rotation (Er), Pronation (P) or Supination (Su), Plantar flexion (Pf) or Dorsi flexion (Df), Inversion, (In) or Eversion (Ev)

Weekly stretching program for cycling

Day 1	Day 2	Day 3	Day 4	Day 5	Day 6	Day 7
1.7c	1.3b	1.3a	1.4a	1.4b	1.2	1.9
1.7f	1.8	2.2b	1.5	2.4c	2.9a	2.6b
2.0a	2.5a	2.7a	1.7a	3.0a	2.8	3.1c
4.0c	3.8a	4.0a	2.5c	3.7	4.0g	4.0d
4.2	3.8d	4.8	4.1	3.8b	4.3	4.5
5.0a	3.8e	5.2a	5.5	3.8c	5.3a	5.6b
6.1e	6.1a	6.4b	6.4c	6.0a	6.4d	6.4g
6.5m	6.6a	6.5c	6.5j	6.5k	6.6d	6.6f
7.2b	6.7f	6.7b	6.9a	7.5a	7.1b	7.1g

Solo Freeform Dancing (i.e. Pop, Disco and Techno)

Dancing requires good spine and limb flexibility. The demand of the dance on the body is determined by the type of dance, the intensity of the dance and the available dance floor space for the dancer. As there are many dance variations involving many different movements a generalised stretching program for freeform dancing is selected here. On a dance floor that is packed full of people there is less space and less scope for adventurous dancing, especially with respect to the lower limb. The stretches list are therefore is based on the joints and muscles are most likely to be moved in this environment.

Freeform Dancing mainly involves the cervical and thoracolumbar spine and the upper limbs. It involves many of the joints in the body including head extension and flexion, cervical, thoracic and lumbar flexion, extension, sidebending and rotation, scapula retraction, protraction, elevation and depression, shoulder flexion, extension, abduction, adduction, internal rotation and external rotation, elbow flexion, extension, supination and pronation, wrist flexion, extension, abduction and adduction, finger flexion and extension, hip flexion, extension, abduction, adduction, internal rotation and external rotation, knee flexion and extension and ankle dorsiflexion and plantar flexion.

Most the joints of the body are used in freeform dancing but the level of muscle contraction is generally low. It varies considerably between upper and lower limbs and is lowest in the spine and lower limbs where it acts to maintain standing posture and produce limited movement. The agonists, antagonists, joint stabiliser and neutraliser muscles are all considered in determining which stretches are selected.

Dancing	Head		Cervical				Thoracic				Lumbar			
	F	E	F	E	S	R	F	E	S	R	F	E	S	R
Direction	X	X	X	X	X	X	X	X	X	X	X	X	X	X
Range	X	X	X	.	X	X	X	.	X	.	X	.	X	X
Contraction	.	X	.	X	.	.	.	X	X	.	.	X	X	X
Stretch	.	X	.	X	X	X	.	X	X	X	.	X	X	X

	Scapula				Shoulder					
	Re	Pr	El	De	F	E	Ab	Ad	Ir	Er
Direction	X	X	X	X	X	X	X	X	X	X
Range	X	X	X	X	X	X	X	X	X	X
Contraction	.	.	.	.	X	.	X	.	X	X
Stretch	X	X	X	X	X	X	X	X	X	X

	Elbow				Wrist				Hand		SI	
	F	E	P	Su	F	E	Ab	Ad	F	E	F	E
Direction	X	X	X	X	X	X	X	X	X	X	X	x
Range	X	X	X	X	X	X	X	X	X	X	.	.
Contraction	.	.	.	.	.	.	.	.	.	.	.	.
Stretch	X	X	X	X	X	X	X	X	X	X	.	.

	Hip						Knee		Foot				Toes	
	F	E	Ab	Ad	Ir	Er	F	E	Pf	Df	In	Ev	F	E
Direction	X	X	X	X	X	X	X	X	X	X	O	O	O	O
Range	.	O	O	O	.	.	.	O	.	O	O	O	O	O
Contraction	.	X	X	.	.	.	O	X	X	O	.	.	O	O
Stretch	.	X	X	.	.	.	.	X	X	.	.	.	O	O

Key: None (O) partial (.) full (**X**) Range = Range of joint movement, Contraction = Level of muscle contraction, Direction = Direction of movement Direction may be Flexion (F), Extension (E), Sidebending (S), Rotation (R), Retraction (Re), Protraction (Pr), Elevation (El), Depression (De), Abduction (Ab), Adduction (Ad), Internal rotation (Ir), External rotation (Er), Pronation (P), Supination (Su), Plantar flexion (Pf), Dorsi flexion (Df), Inversion, (In), Eversion (Ev)

Weekly stretching program for dancing (freeform, pop, disco and techno)

Day 1	Day 2	Day 3	Day 4	Day 5	Day 6	Day 7
1. 3a	1.7b	1.3b	1.7c	1.4b	1.5	1.4c
2.0a	2.4c	2.1b	1.7f	2.2b	1.4a	2.3
2.6a	3.1a	2.6c	2.9b	2.6d	3.4	2.7a
2.9a	3.8a	4.0c	4.0g	3.8d	4.1	3.0a
4.0b	3.8c	4.2	4.3	3.8e	4.5	4.6b
4.8	4.9c	5.0a	4.9d	5.1a	5.2a	4.7
5.3a	5.5	5.6a	5.4	6.0a	6.1a	6.1d
6.2a	6.4b	6.4d	6.5c	6.6a	6.3c	6.6d
6.7f	6.9a	7.1b	7.1c	7.1g	6.7a	7.1f

Partner Dancing (i.e. Waltz, Foxtrot, Quickstep, Tango etc.)

Partner dancing involves the coordinated dancing of two people who maintain some degree of connection with each other. One partner, usually the man, is the leader, and the other, usually the woman, is the follower. Types of partner dancing included in this section include the Waltz, Foxtrot, Quickstep and Tango.

Many joints are used in partner dancing but the direction of joint movement is limited and determined by the fact the two partners move together and mostly face each other. Partner dancing requires good cervical and lumbar extension and good lower limb flexibility generally. It involves head, cervical and lumbar extension, lumbar flexion, sidebending and rotation scapula retraction and protraction, shoulder flexion, extension, abduction, adduction, internal rotation and external rotation, elbow flexion and extension, hip flexion, extension, abduction, adduction, internal rotation and external rotation, knee flexion and extension and ankle dorsiflexion and plantar flexion.

Partner Dancing	Head		Cervical				Thoracic				Lumbar			
	F	E	F	E	S	R	F	E	S	R	F	E	S	R
Direction	X	X	X	X	X	X	X	X	X	X	X	X	X	X
Range	.	X	.	X	.	.	.	.	.	.	.	X	.	X
Contraction	X	X	.	X	.	.	.	.	.	.	X	X	.	X
Stretch	X	X	.	X	.	.	.	.	.	.	.	X	.	X

	Scapula				Shoulder					
	Re	Pr	El	De	F	E	Ab	Ad	Ir	Er
Direction	X	X	X	X	X	X	X	X	X	X
Range	X	X	.	.	X	.	X	.	.	.
Contraction	.	.	.	.	X	X	X	.	.	.
Stretch	X	X	X	X	X	X	X	X	X	X

	Elbow				Wrist				Hand		SI	
	F	E	P	Su	F	E	Ab	Ad	F	E	F	E
Direction	X	X	X	X	X	X	X	X	X	O	X	X
Range	X	X	.	.	.	.	.	.	X	O	.	.
Contraction	X	X	.	.	.	.	.	.	.	.	.	.
Stretch	X	X	.	.	X	X	X	X	X	X	.	.

	Hip						Knee		Foot				Toes	
	F	E	Ab	Ad	Ir	Er	F	E	Pf	Df	In	Ev	F	E
Direction	X	X	X	X	X	X	X	X	X	X	X	X	X	X
Range	X	X	X	X	X	X	X	X	X	X	X	X	X	X
Contraction	X	X	X	X	X	X	X	X	X	X	.	.	.	.
Stretch	X	X	X	X	X	X	X	X	X	X	X	X	.	.

Key: None (O) partial (.) full (X) Range = Range of joint movement, Contraction = Level of muscle contraction, Direction = Direction of movement Direction may be Flexion (F), Extension (E), Sidebending (S), Rotation (R), Retraction (Re), Protraction (Pr), Elevation (El), Depression (De), Abduction (Ab), Adduction (Ad), Internal rotation (Ir), External rotation (Er), Pronation (P), Supination (Su), Plantar flexion (Pf), Dorsi flexion (Df), Inversion, (In), Eversion (Ev)

Weekly stretching program for partner dancing

Day 1	Day 2	Day 3	Day 4	Day 5	Day 6	Day 7
1. 3a	1.7b	1.3b	1.8	1.4b	1.4a	1.2
2.0a	2.4c	2.6b	2.9a	2.5c	1.5	2.3
2.9b	3.1a	3.0e	2.6d	2.7a	3.4	1.7c
3.2b	3.0a	4.0c	4.0g	3.2a	4.1	1.7f
4.0b	4.9c	4.2	4.3	5.1a	4.5	4.7
4.8	5.2a	5.0a	4.9d	6.0a	5.7b	5.8b
5.3a	5.5	5.6a	5.9	6.6c	6.1a	6.5g
6.2a	6.4b	6.4d	6.5c	6.7g	6.3c	6.6d
6.7f	6.9a	7.1b	6.8a	6.7b	7.1f	7.3a

Darts

Darts is a throwing game in which small missiles or darts are thrown at a circular target or dartboard hanging on a wall. Darts is a traditional pub game that has evolved into a professional competitive sport.

Darts involves head extension, cervical extension, thoracic flexion and sidebending, lumbar flexion, sidebending and rotation, scapula protraction and retraction, shoulder flexion and abduction, elbow flexion, extension, supination and pronation, wrist flexion, extension and adduction, finger flexion, hip abduction and ankle dorsiflexion.

Darts	Head		Cervical				Thoracic				Lumbar			
Movement	F	E	F	E	S	R	F	E	S	R	F	E	S	R
Direction	O	X	O	X	O	O	X	O	X	O	X	O	X	X
Range	O	X	O	.	O	O	.	O	.	O	.	O	.	.
Contraction	O	X	.	X	.	.	O	.	.	O	.	.	.	X
Stretch	.	X	.	X	.	O	.	.	.	.	.	X	X	X
Body Part	Scapula				Shoulder									
Movement	Re	Pr	El	De	F	E	Ab	Ad	Ir	Er				
Direction	X	X	O	O	X	O	X	O	O	O				
Range	O	X	.	O	.	O	O	O	O	O				
Contraction	X	X	O	O	.	O	O	O	O	O				
Stretch	X	X	.	.	X	.	.	.	.	.				
Body Part	Elbow				Wrist				Hand		SI			
Movement	F	E	P	Su	F	E	Ab	Ad	F	E	F	E		
Direction	X	X	X	X	X	X	X	X	X	O	O	O		
Range	X	X	.	.	.	.	.	.	X	O	O	O		
Contraction	.	X	.	.	.	X	.	X	X	.	O	O		
Stretch	X	X	X	X	X	X	.	X	X	.	O	O		
Body Part	Hip						Knee		Foot				Toes	
Movement	F	E	Ab	Ad	Ir	Er	F	E	Pf	Df	In	Ev	F	E
Direction	.	O	X	O	O	O	O	O	O	X	O	O	O	O
Range	.	.	.	O	O	O	O	O	O	.	O	O	O	O
Contraction	O	.	X	O	O	O	O	.	X	O	O	O	O	O
Stretch	.	.	X	O	O	O	.	.	X	.	O	O	.	.

Key: None (O) partial (.) full (X) Range = Range of joint movement, Contraction = Level of muscle contraction, Direction = Direction of movement of Body Part. Direction may be Flexion (F), Extension (E), Sidebending (S), Rotation (R), Retraction (Re), Protraction (Pr), Elevation (El), Depression (De), Abduction (Ab), Adduction (Ad), Internal rotation (Ir) or External rotation (Er), Pronation (P) or Supination (Su), Plantar flexion (Pf) or Dorsi flexion (Df), Inversion, (In) or Eversion (Ev)

Weekly stretching program for darts

Day 1	Day 2	Day 3	Day 4	Day 5	Day 6	Day 7
1.3b	1.4b	1.2	1.4a	1.3a	1.9	1.4c
2.0a	2.1b	2.3	1.5	1. 7i	1.7d	1.7a
3.1a	2.5b	3.0a	2.4c	2.4d	2.7a	1.7h
4.0a	2.9a	3.1b	3.9a	3.2a	3.5	3.4
4.4	4.0e	4.3	4.7	4.0b	4.8	4.0h
4.9e	5.4	5.0a	5.2c	4.9a	5.3a	4.9c
5.6b	5.7a	5.7c	5.5	5.6a	5.8c	5.8e
6.0a	6.1c	6.2b	6.4b	6.4g	6.4d	5.9
6.5g	6.6a	6.7a	7.1a	6.9a	7.1e	7.3b

Stretches for domestic work

These stretches are for domestic work such as washing dishes, vacuuming, cleaning and general home duties. Domestic work is most demanding on the muscles of the shoulders, upper thoracic and lower lumbar spine. It places some demand on the hips, arms, forearms, hands and feet.

Domestic work involves head, cervical, thoracic and lumbar flexion and extension, sacroiliac flexion and extension, scapula retraction and protraction, shoulder flexion and extension, elbow flexion, extension, supination and pronation, wrist flexion and extension, finger flexion and extension, hip flexion and extension and knee flexion and extension.

Domestic work	Head		Cervical				Thoracic				Lumbar			
	F	E	F	E	S	R	F	E	S	R	F	E	S	R
Stretch	X	X	X	X	.	O	X	X	.	.	X	X	.	.

	Scapula				Shoulder									
	Re	Pr	El	De	F	E	Ab	Ad	Ir	Er				
Stretch	X	X	.	.	X	X	.	.	O	O				

	Elbow				Wrist				Hand		SI			
	F	E	P	Su	F	E	Ab	Ad	F	E	F	E		
Stretch	X	X	X	X	X	X	O	O	X	X	X	X		

	Hip						Knee		Foot				Toes	
	F	E	Ab	Ad	Ir	Er	F	E	Pf	Df	In	Ev	F	E
Stretch	X	X	.	O	O	O	X	X	.	.	O	O	O	O

Key: None (**O**) partial (**.**) full (**X**) Range = Range of joint movement, Contraction = Level of muscle contraction, Direction = Direction of movement of Body Part. Direction may be Flexion (F), Extension (E), Sidebending (S), Rotation (R), Retraction (Re), Protraction (Pr), Elevation (El), Depression (De), Abduction (Ab), Adduction (Ad), Internal rotation (Ir) or External rotation (Er), Pronation (P) or Supination (Su), Plantar flexion (Pf) or Dorsi flexion (Df), Inversion, (In) or Eversion (Ev)

Weekly stretching program for domestic work

Day 1	Day 2	Day 3	Day 4	Day 5	Day 6	Day 7
1.1a	1.3b	1.4a	1.1c	1.3c	1.8	2.0a
2.4a	2.4c	1.5	1.2	1.4b	2.5b	2.5a
2.6a	3.0e	1.7c	2.9a	1.7i	2.9b	3.0a
4.0a	4.0d	1.7f	4.0g	3.6	3.2a	4.8
4.9c	5.2c	3.1b	5.2a	3.7	5.3a	4.9b
5.5	5.6b	5.4	4.4	3.8d	4.5	5.6a
6.0a	6.1e	6.1c	6.2b	3.8c	6.1a	6.4d
6.7a	6.6a	6.7c	6.7b	3.8d	6.7f	7.0a
7.1a	6.9a	7.1b	7.1g	3.8e	7.5b	7.6

Stretches for driving a car or truck

These stretches are for driving a vehicle and especially for prolonged periods of time. Driving a car is a form of sitting that also involves the coordination of the arms to steer and legs to accelerate or brake.

Both arms and leg muscles are used in driving. In the upper limb they include triceps brachii, pectoralis major, anterior and posterior deltoid, infraspinatus, biceps brachii and teres major. Some are prime movers and others are stabilizers. Which upper limb muscles are used depend on whether steering is clockwise or anticlockwise and on the technique of the driver. In the lower limb they are the gastrocnemius, soleus and tibialis anterior.

A common problem when driving is contracting muscles that are not needed for turning the wheel. Driving can be stressful and upper trapezius and levator scapulae may be inappropriately contracted at times, resulting in muscle shortening and fibrous changes within these shoulder muscles.

Driving a car mainly involves the contraction of the muscles responsible for head, cervical, upper thoracic and lumbar extension, scapula retraction, shoulder flexion, shoulder extension, elbow flexion, elbow extension, wrist extension, finger flexion and ankle plantar flexion.

Prolonged periods of driving causes postural fatigue, and cause muscles to shorten, atrophy and change structurally for example with fibrous infiltration. These changes affect other muscles and joints during standing, walking, sports and other physical activities, sometime with adverse consequences.

Muscles that are held in a prolonged shortened state during driving include the muscle responsible for head extension, upper cervical extension and lower cervical flexion, thoracic and lumbar flexion, scapular protraction and elevation, shoulder adduction and internal rotation, elbow flexion, wrist extension, finger flexion, sacral extension, hip flexion, knee flexion and ankle dorsiflexion.

Other muscle involved in driving include brachialis, brachioradialis, supinator, pronator teres, pronator quadratus, extensor carpi radialis longus and brevis, extensor carpi ulnaris, flexor digitorum superficialis and profundus and 7licis longus.

Muscles that may shorten as a result of poor posture include sternocleidomastoid, anterior scalene pectoralis major and minor and the posterior suboccipital muscles. Postural fatigue affects the posterior cervical muscles, thoracic erector spinae, middle trapezius, rhomboid major and rhomboid minor. Muscle atrophy and weakness occurs as a result of the inactivity during driving. Most significant are the abdominal muscles, important for maintaining trunk postural alignment and supraspinatus, important for maintaining shoulder joint integrity. Lower limb muscles that shorten as a result of being held in a prolonged shortened state include iliopsoas, the hamstrings and the hip abductors, adductors and rotators.

For optimal health take a break from driving at least every hour and walk for 1 minute. Allow your arms to swing freely like a pendulum alternating with your legs. Walking is important for relaxing muscles used in driving, stimulating circulating blood and lymph and mobilising the sacrum, ilium, lumbar and thoracolumbar spine. Also use the stretches listed.

Use a dedicated lumbar support or place a small pillow behind you lumbar spine if your car seat does not provide adequate support. Hold the steering wheel firmly but comfortably with both hand and control the wheel. Adjust your steering wheel to the optimal position to see all the dials and readouts on the dashboard and adjust your side and rear view mirrors so you have a full view behind and so they keep your head in a position that maintains good posture.

The weekly stretching program for driving is similar to the program for sitting in a chair except with the addition or emphasis of stretches for the upper and lower limb. When taking a break from driving it is not always practical to lie on the ground by the side of the road. Standing or sitting stretches have therefore been favoured over stretches lying on the floor.

Weekly stretching program for driving a car or truck (see criteria table on following page)

Day 1	Day 2	Day 3	Day 4	Day 5	Day 6	Day 7
1.2	1.8	1.4a	1.3b	1.7f	1.9	1.4c
2.1c	2.4c	1.5	2.1b	3.1a	2.4b	2.0a
2.9b	1.7d	1.7b	2.5a	2.5b	3.2a	2.0b
3.2b	4.0b	4.0e	4.2	4.1	4.0g	3.3
4.5	4.8	4.6a	4.7	4.9a	4.9e	4.3
5.3a	5.0a	4.9d	5.5	5.1a	5.6b	5.2a
5.8e	3.8b	3.8c	6.0a	5.6a	5.7a	5.7b
5.9	6.4a	6.6a	6.4a	6.4b	6.5h	5.7c
6.7a	6.7f	7.2b	6.7b	6.9a	7.1b	5.7d

717

Car driving	Head		Cervical				Thoracic				Lumbar			
	F	E	F	E	S	R	F	E	S	R	F	E	S	R
Direction	O	X	O	X	O	O	X	O	O	O	X	O	O	O
Range	O	.	O	.	O	O	.	O	O	O	.	O	O	O
Contraction	O	X	O	X	O	O	O	X	O	O	O	X	O	O
Stretch	O	X	.	X	.	.	X	X	.	.	X	X	.	.

	Scapula				Shoulder					
	Re	Pr	El	De	F	E	Ab	Ad	Ir	Er
Direction	O	X	X	O	X	X	O	X	O	O
Range	O	.	.	O	.	.	O	.	O	O
Contraction	X	O	.	O	.	.	O	O	O	O
Stretch	X	X	X	.	.	.	.	X	X	.

	Elbow				Wrist				Hand		SI	
	F	E	P	Su	F	E	Ab	Ad	F	E	F	E
Direction	X	X	X	X	O	X	X	X	X	O	O	X
Range	X	.	.	.	O	.	.	.	.	O	O	X
Contraction	.	.	.	.	O	X	O	O	.	.	X	.
Stretch	X	X	.	.	.	X	X	X	X	.	X	X

	Hip						Knee		Foot				Toes	
	F	E	Ab	Ad	Ir	Er	F	E	Pf	Df	In	Ev	F	E
Direction	X	O	O	O	O	O	X	O	O	X	O	O	O	O
Range	X	O	O	O	O	O	.	O	O	.	O	O	O	O
Contraction	.	O	O	O	O	O	O	O	X	X	O	O	O	O
Stretch	X	X	.	.	.	.	X	X	X	X	O	O	O	O

Easy stretches for a light morning workout

Easy stretches are undemanding, gentle on the body and most suited for warming up before work or other activities. The focus is general - a light stretch for the whole body. Easy stretches are for the maintenance of flexibility and to stimulate capillary circulation and venous and lymphatic drainage. Sometime the body needs a light workout that does not place large demands on the body. A person with low vitality or who is recovering from illness for example may need easy stretches.

Easy stretches involves head flexion and extension, cervical flexion, extension, sidebending and rotation, thoracic and lumbar flexion, extension, sidebending and rotation, sacroiliac flexion and extension, scapula retraction, protraction, elevation and depression, shoulder flexion, extension, abduction, adduction, internal rotation and external rotation, elbow flexion, extension, supination and pronation, wrist flexion, extension, abduction and adduction, finger flexion and extension, hip flexion, extension, abduction, adduction, internal rotation and external rotation, knee flexion and extension, ankle dorsiflexion and plantar flexion, foot inversion and eversion and toe flexion and extension.

Easy stretches	Head		Cervical				Thoracic				Lumbar			
	F	E	F	E	S	R	F	E	S	R	F	E	S	R
Stretch	X	X	X	X	X	X	X	X	X	X	X	X	X	X

	Scapula				Shoulder					
	Re	Pr	El	De	F	E	Ab	Ad	Ir	Er
Stretch	X	X	X	X	X	X	X	X	X	X

	Elbow				Wrist				Hand		SI	
	F	E	P	Su	F	E	Ab	Ad	F	E	F	E
Stretch	X	X	X	X	X	X	X	X	X	X	X	X

	Hip						Knee		Foot				Toes	
	F	E	Ab	Ad	Ir	Er	F	E	Pf	Df	In	Ev	F	E
Stretch	X	X	X	X	X	X	X	X	X	X	X	X	X	X

Weekly easy stretching program

Day 1	Day 2	Day 3	Day 4	Day 5	Day 6	Day 7
1.1a	1.3b	1.4a	1.3c	1.2	1.7c	1.4b
2.2b	1.8	1.5	2.1c	2.1b	1.7f	2.4b
2.5a	2.3	1.6	2.5b	3.2b	2.0a	2.9a
2.6a	4.0b	1.7a	3.0a	3.6	2.0b	2.8
3.4	4.3	3.3	3.0e	3.7	3.1a	3.7
4.0a	4.4	5.0b	4.9b	3.8a	4.0g	3.8b
5.6b	5.4	5.1b	5.5	3.8c	5.2c	3.8d
6.0a	6.2b	6.1g	6.3a	3.8d	6.5a	3.9a
6.6b	6.7a	7.1a	7.1f	3.8e	7.4b	7.3b&c

Fencing

Fencing is a sport where two combatants fight with swords in an attempt to land a touch or make blade contact with a valid target area on the opponent's body. There are two types of fencing classical fencing, which is a type of martial art and competitive fencing, also known as Olympic fencing. Both types have three weapon categories: foil, sabre and épée.

A foil is a light thrusting weapon with a small circular hand guard that protects the hand. An épée is also a thrusting weapon but much heavier than the foil. With foil and épée points are scored only when the tip hits the target. Hits with the side of the blade do not count. A sabre is a light cutting and thrusting weapon that targets the entire body above the waist (and not the hands) and points can be gained by hitting the target with the tip or with the side of the blade.

Techniques used in fencing are offensive, defensive or combinations of both. Offensive techniques have the goal of landing a hit on the opponent while defensive protect against a hit or gain priority or right of way. Offensive techniques include the attack or thrust, feint, lunge, disengage, remise and flick. Defensive techniques include the parry, riposte and point in line.

The stretches selected are for offensive lunging and thrusting. In this regard fencing mainly involves head extension, cervical extension and sidebending, thoracic flexion and sidebending, lumbar flexion or extension, sidebending and rotation, sacroiliac flexion, scapula protraction, retraction, scapula elevation and depression, shoulder abduction, elbow flexion or extension, forearm supination or pronation, wrist extension, finger flexion, hip flexion, extension, abduction and external rotation, knee flexion and extension, ankle plantar flexion.

Scapula protraction and retraction and hip flexion and extension and knee flexion and extension occur on opposite sides of the body. The thoracic and lumbar spine can be in flexion or extension during the fencing thrust and so equal weight is given to both. Similarly with forearm supination and pronation, wrist flexion, extension, abduction and adduction and shoulder internal and external rotation.

Fencing	Head		Cervical				Thoracic				Lumbar			
Movement	F	E	F	E	S	R	F	E	S	R	F	E	S	R
Direction	O	X	O	X	X	O	X	X	X	O	X	X	X	X
Range	O	X	O	.	.	O	X	.	X	O	X	.	X	.
Contraction	.	.	.	.	.	O	.	.	.	O	.	.	.	.
Stretch	.	X	.	X	.	O	X	X	X	.	X	X	X	X

Body Part	Scapula				Shoulder					
Movement	Re	Pr	El	De	F	E	Ab	Ad	Ir	Er
Direction	X	X	X	X	O	O	X	O	X	X
Range	X	X	.	.	O	O	X	O	.	.
Contraction	X	X	.	.	.	.	X	.	.	.
Stretch	X	X	X	X	.	.	X	.	X	X

Body Part	Elbow				Wrist				Hand		SI	
Movement	F	E	P	Su	F	E	Ab	Ad	F	E	F	E
Direction	O	X	X	X	X	X	X	X	X	O	X	O
Range	O	X	.	.	.	.	.	.	X	O	X	O
Contraction	.	X	.	.	X	X	X	X	X	.	.	.
Stretch	X	X	X	X	X	X	X	X	X	.	X	.

Body Part	Hip						Knee		Foot				Toes	
Movement	F	E	Ab	Ad	Ir	Er	F	E	Pf	Df	In	Ev	F	E
Direction	X	X	X	O	O	X	X	X	X	X	X	X	X	O
Range	X	X	.	O	.	.	X	X	.	X	.	.	O	O
Contraction	X	X	.	.	.	X	.	X	X	.	.	.	.	O
Stretch	X	X	X	.	.	.	X	X	X	.	.	.	.	O

Weekly stretching program for fencing (thrusting and lunging)

Day 1	Day 2	Day 3	Day 4	Day 5	Day 6	Day 7
1.1a	1.2	1.3a	1.4a	1.3c	1.7a	2.0a
2.3	2.4a	2.4c	1.7c	2.5a	2.5b	2.0b
2.6a	2.9a	2.7a	1.7f	3.0a	6.1a	2.5c
4.0d	2.8	3.2b	3.1a	4.0g	4.1	4.0c
4.4	4.5	4.3	4.2	5.0a	4.9a	4.8
5.2a	5.3a	4.9e	5.8b	5.6b	5.5	6.0b
5.7b	5.7c	6.0a	6.5m	5.9	5.8c	6.3c
6.4d	5.7d	6.2b	6.6b	6.4c	5.8d	6.6f
6.7f	7.1d	6.7b	7.1g	6.9a	7.1b	7.3a

Golf

Golf is a sport in which competing players use different types of clubs to hit a ball into a series of holes on a course using the fewest number of strokes. Each golf course is unique and consists of a series of nine or eighteen holes. Each hole on includes a tee box to start from, a putting green containing the actual hole and a variety of hazards which each player must avoid such as rough grass and sandy bunkers.

Golf involves thoracic rotation, lumbar extension, sidebending and rotation, sacroiliac flexion, scapula retraction and protraction, shoulder flexion, abduction, adduction, internal rotation and external rotation, elbow flexion and extension, wrist flexion, extension, abduction and adduction, finger flexion, hip extension, abduction and adduction, knee extension, ankle plantar flexion, foot inversion and eversion.

Shoulder abduction and adduction, internal rotation and external rotation, elbow flexion and extension, wrist flexion, extension, abduction and adduction, hip abduction and adduction and foot inversion and eversion occur in limbs on opposite sides of the body.

Golf mainly involves the hamstrings and quadriceps, shoulder, arm and forearm muscles such as triceps and wrist muscle, as well as core muscles such as erector spinae, latissimus dorsi and the abdominal muscles.

Golf	Head		Cervical				Thoracic				Lumbar			
	F	E	F	E	S	R	F	E	S	R	F	E	S	R
Direction	O	O	O	O	O	O	O	O	O	X	O	X	X	X
Range	O	O	O	O	O	O	O	O	O	.	O	X	X	X
Contraction	.	.	.	.	.	.	O	.	.	X	.	X	X	X
Stretch	.	.	.	.	X	X	.	.	.	X	.	X	X	X

	Scapula				Shoulder					
	Re	Pr	El	De	F	E	Ab	Ad	Ir	Er
Direction	X	X	O	O	X	X	X	X	X	X
Range	X	X	O	O	X	X	X	X	.	.
Contraction	X	X	.	.	X	X	X	X	.	.
Stretch	X	X	.	.	X	X	X	X	X	X

	Elbow				Wrist				Hand		SI	
	F	E	P	Su	F	E	Ab	Ad	F	E	F	E
Direction	X	X	O	O	X	X	X	X	X	O	X	O
Range	X	X	O	O	.	.	.	.	X	O	.	O
Contraction	.	.	.	.	X	X	.	.	.	O	X	O
Stretch	X	X	.	.	X	X	X	X	X	.	X	O

	Hip						Knee		Foot				Toes	
	F	E	Ab	Ad	Ir	Er	F	E	Pf	Df	In	Ev	F	E
Direction	O	X	X	X	O	O	O	X	X	O	X	X	O	O
Range	O	X	.	.	O	O	O	.	.	O	.	.	O	O
Contraction	.	X	X	.	.	.	.	X	.	.	.	.	.	.
Stretch	.	X	X	.	.	.	.	X	X	.	.	.	.	.

Key: None (O) partial (.) full (X) Range = Range of joint movement, Contraction = Level of muscle contraction, Direction = Direction of movement Direction may be Flexion (F), Extension (E), Sidebending (S), Rotation (R), Retraction (Re), Protraction (Pr), Elevation (El), Depression (De), Abduction (Ab), Adduction (Ad), Internal rotation (Ir), External rotation (Er), Pronation (P), Supination (Su), Plantar flexion (Pf), Dorsi flexion (Df), Inversion, (In), Eversion (Ev)

Weekly stretching program for golf

Day 1	Day 2	Day 3	Day 4	Day 5	Day 6	Day 7
2.9a	1.2	1.7c	1.3b	2.4a	2.6b	3.0a
2.8	2.6d	1.7f	3.1a	3.1b	2.9b	3.2b
3.3	3.7	2.0b	4.0c	4.0g	3.2a	4.5
4.4	3.8a	2.5c	4.8	4.9a	4.7	5.2a
5.0a	3.8c	3.4	5.3a	5.4	5.5	5.6a
5.7a	6.0a	6.1c	5.8c	6.2a	5.8e	6.4c
6.4d	6.4g	6.5d	5.8d	6.5h	5.9	6.6a
6.6d	6.7b	6.7c	6.7f	6.9a	7.0a	7.1b
7.1g	7.2b	7.3b	7.5a	7.4b	6.9c	7.6

Harder stretches for an end of day workout

Harder stretches are more demanding on the body and appropriate for developing greater flexibility. After an adequate warm up period these stretches can be done at any time or they can be done at the end of the day. The focus is on stretching muscles that are frequently short because they are used a lot. These are developmental stretches for increasing flexibility and strength.

Harder stretches mainly involves head flexion, cervical, thoracic and lumbar flexion, extension, sidebending and rotation, sacroiliac extension, scapula retraction, protraction and depression, shoulder flexion, extension, abduction, adduction, internal rotation and external rotation, elbow flexion and extension, wrist flexion and extension, finger flexion and extension, hip flexion, extension, abduction, adduction, internal rotation and external rotation, knee flexion and extension, ankle dorsiflexion and plantar flexion and toe flexion and extension.

Hard stretches	Head		Cervical				Thoracic				Lumbar			
	F	E	F	E	S	R	F	E	S	R	F	E	S	R
Stretch	X	.	X	X	X	X	X	X	X	X	X	X	X	X

	Scapula				Shoulder					
	Re	Pr	El	De	F	E	Ab	Ad	Ir	Er
Stretch	X	X	.	X	X	X	X	X	X	X

	Elbow				Wrist				Hand		SI	
	F	E	P	Su	F	E	Ab	Ad	F	E	F	E
Stretch	X	X	.	.	X	X	.	.	X	X	.	X

	Hip						Knee		Foot				Toes	
	F	E	Ab	Ad	Ir	Er	F	E	Pf	Df	In	Ev	F	E
Stretch	X	X	X	X	X	X	X	X	X	X	.	.	X	X

Key: None (**O**) partial (**.**) full (**X**) Range = Range of joint movement, Contraction = Level of muscle contraction, Direction = Direction of movement Direction may be Flexion (F), Extension (E), Sidebending (S), Rotation (R), Retraction (Re), Protraction (Pr), Elevation (El), Depression (De), Abduction (Ab), Adduction (Ad), Internal rotation (Ir), External rotation (Er), Pronation (P), Supination (Su), Plantar flexion (Pf), Dorsi flexion (Df), Inversion, (In), Eversion (Ev)

Weekly harder stretching program

Day 1	Day 2	Day 3	Day 4	Day 5	Day 6	Day 7
1.3a	1.4a	1.4b	1.4c	1.8	1.9	2.0b
2.4a	1.5	2.4b	2.4d	2.7a	2.5b	2.5c
2.6b	1.7c	3.5	2.7c	3.0c	2.9b	3.3
3.1c	1.7f	3.7	4.5	4.8	4.0d	4.0c
5.2b	3.1b	3.8a	4.9b	5.9	5.4	6.0b
6.0a	6.1b	3.8d	6.1e	6.2a	6.2b	6.3d
6.4a	6.5d	6.5f	6.5l	6.5h	6.5m	6.4d
6.6a	6.6d	6.7b	6.7d	6.9b	6.7f	7.0c
7.1b	7.1c	7.1f	7.1g	7.2b	7.3a	7.5a

Stretches for heavy manual labour

These stretches are for heavy work such as digging, lifting, wheel barrowing and general labouring. They can be done before and after heavy work. Heavy manual labour is most demanding on the muscles of the middle and lower back, shoulders and hips, and to a lesser extent, on the muscles of the arms, forearms and knees and legs.

Heavy manual labour involves head, cervical and thoracic flexion and extension, lumbar flexion, extension, sidebending and rotation, sacroiliac flexion and extension, scapula retraction and protraction, shoulder flexion and extension, elbow flexion, extension, supination and pronation, wrist flexion and extension, finger flexion, hip flexion, extension, abduction, adduction and knee flexion and extension.

Heavy manual labour	Head		Cervical				Thoracic				Lumbar			
	F	E	F	E	S	R	F	E	S	R	F	E	S	R
Stretch	X	X	X	X	.	.	X	X	.	.	X	X	X	X

	Scapula				Shoulder									
	Re	Pr	El	De	F	E	Ab	Ad	Ir	Er				
Stretch	X	X	.	.	X	X	.	.	.	.				

	Elbow				Wrist				Hand		SI			
	F	E	P	Su	F	E	Ab	Ad	F	E	F	E		
Stretch	X	X	X	X	X	X	O	O	X	.	X	X		

	Hip						Knee		Foot				Toes	
	F	E	Ab	Ad	Ir	Er	F	E	Pf	Df	In	Ev	F	E
Stretch	X	X	X	X	.	.	X	X	.	.	O	O	O	O

Key: None (O) partial (.) full (X) Range = Range of joint movement, Contraction = Level of muscle contraction, Direction = Direction of movement Direction may be Flexion (F), Extension (E), Sidebending (S), Rotation (R), Retraction (Re), Protraction (Pr), Elevation (El), Depression (De), Abduction (Ab), Adduction (Ad), Internal rotation (Ir), External rotation (Er), Pronation (P), Supination (Su), Plantar flexion (Pf), Dorsi flexion (Df), Inversion, (In), Eversion (Ev)

Weekly stretching program for heavy manual labour

Day 1	Day 2	Day 3	Day 4	Day 5	Day 6	Day 7
1.4b	1.4a	2.1a	1.7d		2.0a	1.9
1. 7i	1.7c	2.4c	2.9a	2.5b	2.0b	2.3
2.4b	1.7f	2.4d	2.8	2.6d	2.5c	2.5a
2.6a	2.6b	2.9b	2.6c	3.0a	3.0c	3.0e
3.1a	3.1c	3.2b	3.4	3.2a	3.3	3.5
3.1b	4.9b	3.6	4.8	4.0f	4.0c	4.0a
4.9a	5.2a	3.7	6.0a	4.9e	6.1a	6.1e
6.2b	6.4d	3.8a	6.5e	6.6a	6.6f	6.7b
6.7a	7.6	6.7f	6.9a	6.9c	7.1b	7.4b

High jump

The high jump is a track and field event where each competitor jumps over a horizontal bar placed at a defined height and without the aid of a prop.

A jumper must take off on one foot and pass over the bar without dislodging it. If the bar is dislodged or there is a jumping error on three consecutive jumps the jumper is eliminated from competition and victory goes to the jumper who clears the greatest height.

The high jump involves head extension, thoracic extension, sacroiliac flexion and extension, scapula retraction, protraction and elevation, shoulder flexion and abduction, elbow extension, supination and pronation, hip flexion, extension, knee flexion and extension, ankle plantar flexion and toe flexion.

For stretches for the first phase of the high jump the run up see Running Sprinting.

High jump	Head		Cervical				Thoracic				Lumbar			
	F	E	F	E	S	R	F	E	S	R	F	E	S	R
Direction	O	X	O	O	O	O	O	X	X	O	O	X	X	X
Range	O	.	O	O	O	O	O	.	.	O	O	X	.	.
Contraction	.	O	X	.	.	.	O	X	.	.	.	X	.	.
Stretch	.	.	.	.	.	.	.	X	.	.	X	X	.	.

	Scapula				Shoulder					
	Re	Pr	El	De	F	E	Ab	Ad	Ir	Er
Direction	X	X	X	O	X	O	X	O	O	O
Range	.	.	.	O	X	O	.	O	O	O
Contraction	.	.	.	O	.	.	.	.	.	.
Stretch	X	X	X	.	X	X	X	X	X	X

	Elbow				Wrist				Hand		SI	
	F	E	P	Su	F	E	Ab	Ad	F	E	F	E
Direction	O	X	X	X	O	O	O	O	O	O	X	X
Range	O	X	.	.	O	O	O	O	O	O	X	.
Contraction	.	X	.	.	O	O	O	O	O	O	X	X
Stretch	X	X	.	.	.	.	O	O	.	.	X	X

	Hip						Knee		Foot				Toes	
	F	E	Ab	Ad	Ir	Er	F	E	Pf	Df	In	Ev	F	E
Direction	X	X	O	O	O	O	X	X	X	O	O	O	X	O
Range	.	X	O	O	O	O	.	X	X	O	O	O	X	O
Contraction	.	X	X	.	.	.	.	X	X	.	.	.	X	.
Stretch	X	X	X	.	.	.	X	X	X	.	.	.	X	X

Key: None (O) partial (.) full (X) Range = Range of joint movement, Contraction = Level of muscle contraction, Direction = Direction of movement Direction may be Flexion (F), Extension (E), Sidebending (S), Rotation (R), Retraction (Re), Protraction (Pr), Elevation (El), Depression (De), Abduction (Ab), Adduction (Ad), Internal rotation (Ir), External rotation (Er), Pronation (P), Supination (Su), Plantar flexion (Pf), Dorsi flexion (Df), Inversion, (In), Eversion (Ev)

Weekly stretching program for high jump

Day 1	Day 2	Day 3	Day 4	Day 5	Day 6	Day 7
1.3b	1.4a	1.4c	1.8	1.7e	2.4b	2.5a
2.6b	1.5	2.5b	3.0a	2.0a	2.9a	3.0d
3.4	1.7a	4.0c	3.7	3.1a	2.8	4.0g
4.8	4.4	4.2	3.9a	4.9c	5.0a	5.2a
5.7b	6.0a	6.1a	6.0b	6.1c	6.0c	6.1f
5.8b	6.2a	6.4a	6.2b	6.4b	6.4c	6.4h
6.5c	6.6a	6.5f	6.6c	6.5k	6.6d	6.5m
6.7a	6.7f	6.7b	6.7g	6.7c	6.8a	6.7e
6.9a	7.1a	7.1d	7.1b	7.1f	7.1g	7.3b

729

Hockey

Hockey, also known as field hockey is a sport where two teams attempt to manoeuvre a ball into the opponent's goal using a hockey stick. Each team contains eleven players including the goalie. Goal keepers are the only players allowed to touch the ball with any part of their body. The field players must use the flat side of their wood or fibre glass hockey sticks to hit the hard rubber ball.

Hockey involves head extension, upper cervical extension and lower cervical flexion, thoracic and lumbar flexion, sidebending and rotation, sacroiliac extension, scapula retraction, protraction, elevation and depression, shoulder flexion, extension, abduction, adduction, internal rotation and external rotation, elbow flexion, extension, supination and pronation, wrist flexion, extension, abduction and adduction, finger flexion, hip flexion, extension, abduction, adduction, internal rotation and external rotation, knee flexion and extension, ankle dorsiflexion and plantar flexion, foot inversion and eversion and toe flexion and extension.

Hockey is a complex series of movements requiring stretching exercises for the whole body and the actions listed in the table below reflects this. The stretches selected in the weekly stretching program for hockey however have an upper limb bias. For a more comprehensive list of lower limb stretches see Running.

Hockey	Head		Cervical				Thoracic				Lumbar			
	F	E	F	E	S	R	F	E	S	R	F	E	S	R
Direction	O	X	X	X	O	O	X	O	X	X	X	O	X	X
Range	O	X	X	X	O	O	X	O	.	.	X	O	X	X
Contraction	.	X	.	X	.	.	.	X	.	.	.	X	X	X
Stretch	.	X	X	X	X	.	X	X	.	.	X	X	X	X

	Scapula				Shoulder					
	Re	Pr	El	De	F	E	Ab	Ad	Ir	Er
Direction	X	X	X	X	X	X	X	X	X	X
Range	.	X	.	.	.	.	X	X	.	.
Contraction	X	X	.	.	X	X	X	X	X	X
Stretch	X	X	.	.	X	X	X	X	X	X

	Elbow				Wrist				Hand		SI	
	F	E	P	Su	F	E	Ab	Ad	F	E	F	E
Direction	X	X	X	X	X	X	X	X	X	O	O	X
Range	.	.	.	.	.	.	.	.	X	O	O	.
Contraction	X	X	X	X	X	X	.	.	.	.	.	X
Stretch	X	X	X	X	X	X	X	X	X	.	X	X

	Hip						Knee		Foot				Toes	
	F	E	Ab	Ad	Ir	Er	F	E	Pf	Df	In	Ev	F	E
Direction	X	X	X	X	X	X	X	X	X	X	X	X	X	X
Range	.	.	.	.	,	,	.	.	.	X	.	.	.	.
Contraction	.	X	X	X	.	.	.	X	X	.	.	.	.	.
Stretch	X	X	X	X	.	.	X	X	X	X	X	X	.	.

Key: None (O) partial (.) full (X) Range = Range of joint movement, Contraction = Level of muscle contraction, Direction = Direction of movement Direction may be Flexion (F), Extension (E), Sidebending (S), Rotation (R), Retraction (Re), Protraction (Pr), Elevation (El), Depression (De), Abduction (Ab), Adduction (Ad), Internal rotation (Ir), External rotation (Er), Pronation (P), Supination (Su), Plantar flexion (Pf), Dorsi flexion (Df), Inversion, (In), Eversion (Ev)

Weekly stretching program for hockey

Day 1	Day 2	Day 3	Day 4	Day 5	Day 6	Day 7
1.3b	1.7b	1.3a	1.8	1.4a	2.0a	1.4b
2.4a	2.4b	2.5a	2.5b	1.5	2.5c	2.6b
2.6c	2.6d	3.0d	2.9b	1.7f	2.9a	3.0a
3.1a	3.8a	4.0a	3.2a	3.1b	3.4	3.5
4.0c	3.8c	4.0g	4.3	4.5	4.8	4.9a
4.2	5.0a	5.2a	5.3a	5.4	5.5	5.6a
5.6b	5.7b	5.8c	5.8d	5.9	6.0a	6.1c
6.2a	6.4d	6.4b	6.5d	6.5m	6.6a	6.7b
6.7f	6.9a	7.1b	7.3a	7.1f	7.4a	7.5a

Horse riding

Horse riding, also known as equestrianism or horseback riding may be done for practical reasons such as working or transportation, as a cultural exercise, or for recreation or competitive sport. Competitive equestrianism includes horse racing, dressage, jumping and eventing, also known as horse trials.

During riding the rider has to react to the horse's movement and stay balanced in the saddle. This involves relaxing and contracting many different muscles. Stretching is particularly important in horse riding because there is contraction but very little range of movement. The rider must remain in the saddle and most of the muscle contraction is isometric.

The psoas, iliacus and rectus abdominis contract to pull the torso forwards into a vertical position and as close as possible to its centre of gravity. Other muscles assisting with maintaining balance and posture include gluteus maximus, quadriceps and erector spinae and muscles of the shoulders. The calf and hip muscles are used for holding onto the horse and for delivering cues to the horse. For example closing the knees by contracting the adductor muscles slow a horse down and opening the knees by contracting the abductor muscles speed a horse up.

Horse riding requires flexibility, strength, coordination and balance. It involves head extension, cervical extension, thoracic flexion, lumbar extension, sacroiliac extension, scapula retraction, shoulder extension, abduction, internal rotation and external rotation, elbow flexion, wrist flexion, extension, finger flexion, hip flexion, abduction and internal rotation, knee flexion and ankle dorsiflexion.

Horse Riding	Head		Cervical				Thoracic				Lumbar			
	F	E	F	E	S	R	F	E	S	R	F	E	S	R
Direction	O	X	O	X	O	O	X	O	O	O	O	X	O	O
Range	O	.	O	.	O	O	.	O	O	O	O	X	O	O
Contraction	.	X	.	X	.	.	.	X	.	O	X	X	.	.
Stretch	.	X	.	X	.	.	.	X	.	.	X	X	.	.

	Scapula				Shoulder					
	Re	Pr	El	De	F	E	Ab	Ad	Ir	Er
Direction	X	O	O	O	O	X	X	O	X	X
Range	X	O	O	O	O	.	.	O	.	.
Contraction	X	O	O	O	.	X	.	O	.	.
Stretch	X	.	.	O	X	X	.	.	.	.

	Elbow				Wrist				Hand		SI	
	F	E	P	Su	F	E	Ab	Ad	F	E	F	E
Direction	X	O	O	O	X	X	O	O	X	O	O	X
Range	X	O	O	O	.	.	O	O	X	O	O	.
Contraction	X	O	O	O	X	.	.	.	X	O	O	.
Stretch	X	.	O	O	X	X	.	.	X	.	.	X

	Hip						Knee		Foot				Toes	
	F	E	Ab	Ad	Ir	Er	F	E	Pf	Df	In	Ev	F	E
Direction	X	O	X	O	X	O	X	O	X	X	O	O	O	O
Range	.	O	X	O	.	O	.	O	.	X	O	O	O	O
Contraction	X	.	.	X	.	.	.	X	X	.	O	O	O	O
Stretch	X	X	X	X	.	.	X	X	X	.	O	O	O	O

Key: None (O) partial (.) full (X) Range = Range of joint movement, Contraction = Level of muscle contraction, Direction = Direction of movement Direction may be Flexion (F), Extension (E), Sidebending (S), Rotation (R), Retraction (Re), Protraction (Pr), Elevation (El), Depression (De), Abduction (Ab), Adduction (Ad), Internal rotation (Ir), External rotation (Er), Pronation (P), Supination (Su), Plantar flexion (Pf), Dorsi flexion (Df), Inversion, (In), Eversion (Ev)

Weekly stretching program for horse riding

Day 1	Day 2	Day 3	Day 4	Day 5	Day 6	Day 7
1.3b	1.7c	1.3c	1.7d	1.4a	2.0a	1.4b
2.4a	2.5a	2.5b	2.5c	1.5	2.6b	2.4c
3.0a	2.9a	4.0b	4.0c	3.1a	2.9b	3.2b
1.2	4.3	4.8	4.9d	4.9c	5.2a	5.7b
5.8b	5.8c	5.9	6.0a	6.0c	6.1a	6.1c
6.2b	5.8d	6.2c	6.3c	6.4b	6.4d	6.5a
6.5c	6.5j	6.5i	6.5d	6.5l	6.5f	6.6a
6.6d	6.7a	6.7f	6.7b	6.9a	7.5b	7.0a
7.1a	7.1d	7.1e	7.1g	7.2b	7.6	7.1h

Ice Skating

Ice skating is moving on ice with ice skates for exercise, leisure, travelling and as part of various sports including figure skating, speed skating and ice hockey. Ice skating may be done indoor, outdoor or on naturally occurring bodies of frozen water, such as lakes and rivers.

Figure Skating involves a series of complex dance movements such as circles, jumps, steps, spirals, and figure eights on ice and usually set to music. It may be done as an individual, coordinated pair or group. Speed skating is ice skating in which the competitors race each other over short or long distances. Ice hockey is a team sport played on ice in which skaters use sticks to shoot a hard rubber hockey puck into their opponent's net to score points. All of these different forms of ice skating requires coordination and balance, especially with respect to the spine and lateral hip and ankle muscles.

Ice skating involves head extension, cervical flexion, extension, sidebending and rotation, thoracic and lumbar flexion, extension, sidebending and rotation, scapula retraction and protraction, shoulder flexion, extension and abduction, hip flexion, extension, abduction, adduction, internal rotation and external rotation, knee flexion and extension, ankle dorsiflexion and plantar flexion, and foot inversion and eversion.

For Figure Skating combine Ice Skating with Gymnastics stretches and for Ice Hockey combine Ice Skating with Hockey stretches.

Ice Skating	Head		Cervical				Thoracic				Lumbar			
	F	E	F	E	S	R	F	E	S	R	F	E	S	R
Direction	O	X	X	X	X	O	X	O	X	O	X	O	X	X
Range	O	.	.	.	.	O	.	O	.	O	X	O	.	.
Contraction	.	X	.	X	X	.	.	X	.	.	X	X	X	.
Stretch	.	X	.	X	X	.	.	X	X	.	X	X	X	.

	Scapula				Shoulder					
	Re	Pr	El	De	F	E	Ab	Ad	Ir	Er
Direction	X	X	O	O	X	X	O	O	O	O
Range	.	.	O	O	.	.	O	O	O	O
Contraction	.	.	O	O	.	.	.	O	O	O
Stretch	.	.	O	O	.	X	.	O	O	O

	Elbow				Wrist				Hand		SI	
	F	E	P	Su	F	E	Ab	Ad	F	E	F	E
Direction	X	X	O	O	O	O	O	O	O	O	X	X
Range	.	.	O	O	O	O	O	O	O	O	.	.
Contraction	.	.	O	O	O	O	O	O	O	O	.	.
Stretch	.	.	O	O	O	O	O	O	O	O	.	.

	Hip						Knee		Foot				Toes	
	F	E	Ab	Ad	Ir	Er	F	E	Pf	Df	In	Ev	F	E
Direction	X	X	X	O	O	O	X	X	X	X	X	X	O	O
Range	.	.	O	O	O	O	.	.	X	.	O	O	O	O
Contraction	.	X	X	X	.	.	.	.	X	.	X	X	O	O
Stretch	X	X	X	X	.	.	X	X	X	.	X	X	O	O

Key: None (O) partial (.) full (X) Range = Range of joint movement, Contraction = Level of muscle contraction, Direction = Direction of movement Direction may be Flexion (F), Extension (E), Sidebending (S), Rotation (R), Retraction (Re), Protraction (Pr), Elevation (El), Depression (De), Abduction (Ab), Adduction (Ad), Internal rotation (Ir), External rotation (Er), Pronation (P), Supination (Su), Plantar flexion (Pf), Dorsi flexion (Df), Inversion, (In), Eversion (Ev)

Weekly stretching program for ice skating

Day 1	Day 2	Day 3	Day 4	Day 5	Day 6	Day 7
1.8	1.3a	1.4a	1.4c	1.7f	1.7e	2.1b
2.4a	2.1a	1.7a	2.5a		2.2a	2.5b
2.6b	2.7a	3.0a	3.0c	2.0b	2.8	3.0e
4.8	4.5	4.0g	3.1c	4.0c	2.9a	3.7
5.2a	4.9c	6.0a	6.1a	6.1e	6.0c	3.9a
6.2a	6.2b	6.3a	6.4a	6.4b	6.4c	6.4d
6.4g	6.4h	6.5a	6.5f	6.5m	6.6a	6.6d
6.7a	6.7b	6.7f	6.7g	6.8a	6.9a	6.9c
7.1a	7.1f	7.1b	7.2b	7.1d	7.5a	7.6

Juggling

Juggling is the skill of using one or both hands to toss and catch one or several objects, while keeping them in constant motion. Juggling is a form of art, recreation, entertainment or sport and features in fairs, festivals, theatres, circuses and as part of street performance.

The most common objects juggled are balls, clubs and rings but sometimes jugglers use more dramatic objects such as knives or fire torches.

Juggling requires good coordination especially with regards to eye-hand-object movement. It involves head and cervical extension, shoulder flexion, extension, internal rotation and external rotation, elbow flexion, extension, supination and pronation, wrist flexion and extension and finger flexion and extension and hip abduction and ankle inversion and eversion for lower limb stabilisation.

Juggling	Head		Cervical				Thoracic				Lumbar			
	F	E	F	E	S	R	F	E	S	R	F	E	S	R
Direction	O	X	O	X	O	O	O	O	O	O	O	O	O	O
Range	O	X	O	X	O	O	O	O	O	O	O	O	O	O
Contraction	.	.	.	.	.	O	O	.	.	O	O	.	.	O
Stretch	X	X	.	X	.	O	O	.	.	O	O	.	.	O

	Scapula				Shoulder					
	Re	Pr	El	De	F	E	Ab	Ad	Ir	Er
Direction	O	O	X	O	X	X	O	O	X	X
Range	O	O	.	O	.	.	O	O	.	.
Contraction	.	.	.	.	.	.	.	O	.	.
Stretch	.	.	.	.	X	X	.	.	X	X

	Elbow				Wrist				Hand		SI	
	F	E	P	Su	F	E	Ab	Ad	F	E	F	E
Direction	X	X	X	X	X	X	O	O	X	X	O	O
Range	X	X	.	.	.	.	O	O	.	.	O	O
Contraction	.	.	.	.	.	.	.	.	.	.	O	O
Stretch	X	X	X	X	X	X	.	.	X	X	O	O

	Hip						Knee		Foot				Toes	
	F	E	Ab	Ad	Ir	Er	F	E	Pf	Df	In	Ev	F	E
Direction	O	O	X	O	O	O	O	O	O	O	X	X	O	O
Range	O	O	O	O	O	O	O	O	O	O	O	O	O	O
Contraction	O	.	X	.	O	O	O	X	X	X	X	X	X	X
Stretch	.	X	X	.	.	.	.	X	.	.	.	.	O	O

Key: None (O) partial (.) full (X) Range = Range of joint movement, Contraction = Level of muscle contraction, Direction = Direction of movement Direction may be Flexion (F), Extension (E), Sidebending (S), Rotation (R), Retraction (Re), Protraction (Pr), Elevation (El), Depression (De), Abduction (Ab), Adduction (Ad), Internal rotation (Ir), External rotation (Er), Pronation (P), Supination (Su), Plantar flexion (Pf), Dorsi flexion (Df), Inversion, (In), Eversion (Ev)

Weekly stretching program for juggling

Day 1	Day 2	Day 3	Day 4	Day 5	Day 6	Day 7
1.3b	1.4a	1.2	1.4c	1.7b	1.8	1.7c
2.5c	2.0a	2.9b	2.5b	2.4b	2.9a	1.7f
3.0a	2.0b	3.8b	3.2a	3.0e	3.6	4.0c
4.0a	4.0e	3.8a	4.0g	4.0d	3.7	4.1
4.7	4.2	3.8c	4.3	4.5	3.8a	4.6b
5.3b	5.0a	3.8d	4.8	5.1a	3.9a	4.9b
5.6b	5.4	3.8e	5.5	5.6a	5.2c	5.2a
5.8c	6.0a	6.7f	6.1e	5.7c	7.1e	6.4b
5.8d	6.4d	6.4h	6.6a	5.7d	6.7b	7.1b

Soccer and Football – Kicking a ball

Soccer also known as football or association football is a sport played between two teams of eleven players on a rectangular field with a goal at each end. The object of the game is to put a spherical ball into the opposing goal using any part of the body except the arms and hands. Only the goalkeeper is allowed to touch the ball with their hands. These are stretches for kicking a stationary ball such as taking a penalty or free kick. They are applicable to soccer, rugby, American gridiron, Australian rules football and other types of football.

Soccer requires lower limb flexibility, power and strength and whole body balance and coordination. Kicking a ball primarily involves rectus femoris and the other quadriceps muscles, iliacus, psoas, gluteus maximus, sartorius, tensor fascia latae, the hip adductors, especially adductor magnus, the hamstrings and the calf muscles. The abdominal muscles help maintain balance and work with erector spinae and psoas to stabilise the trunk. Shoulders muscles including anterior, posterior and middle deltoid, supraspinatus, infraspinatus, teres minor, pectoralis major and latissimus dorsi align the upper body square with the ball and maintain balance.

Kicking a ball can be broken down into the preparation stage which involves the run up and approach to the ball and then planting one foot on the ground adjacent to the ball. The kick involves swinging the other leg backwards and then forwards until there is foot contact with the ball. After striking the ball the final stage is the follow through where the kicking leg is decelerated. For the run up stage please see the stretches for walking, running and sprinting.

In the first part of the kick the hamstrings and gluteus maximus extend the hip and the hamstrings also flex the knee. This is the backward swing of the leg. During this phase the head and spine are partially flexed so the eyes can focus on the ball. The arm on the opposite side to the kicking leg is flexed to counter the rotation of body. By the end of the backward swing there is a build-up of elastic energy in front of the hip and thigh which assists in the next phase of kicking the ball.

In the second part of the kick iliopsoas initiates hip flexion, then quadriceps flexes the hip and then quadriceps extends the knee. The forward swing phase involves combined movements of the thigh and leg. The thigh moves forward and downward, then slows and transfers momentum to the leg which accelerates taking the leg and foot forward.

Quadriceps contraction is combined with the release of stored elastic energy in the muscle from the backward swing. Hip rotator muscles including gluteus maximus and adductor muscles, especially adductor magnus, control the hip joint for accurate contact with the ball.

Gastrocnemius, soleus, tibialis anterior and other leg muscles control the foot between dorsiflexion and plantarflexion during different phases of the kick. At ball strike gastrocnemius and soleus contract to plantar flex the foot while the abdominal muscle and lower back muscles stabilize the trunk.

Kicking is a ballistic movement with agonists and antagonist working together using a combination of concentric and eccentric muscle contraction. For example the quadriceps contract eccentrically to decelerate the leg at the end of the backward swing and the hamstrings contract eccentrically to decelerate the leg at the end of the forward swing. Controlled hamstring deceleration is particularly important in preventing the hamstrings from being over stretched and injured at the end of the kick.

In the following description of kicking a ball the weight bearing leg is the left leg and the kicking leg is the right leg. During the approach and backward swing stages of kicking a ball the abdominals, psoas and erector spinae stabilise the trunk. Gluteus maximus and the hamstrings extend the right hip.

Gluteus medius maintains body weight over the left hip. The hamstrings and popliteus flex the right knee. The quadriceps extends the left knee. The right plantar flexors concentrically plantar flex the right ankle and the left plantar flexors eccentrically plantar flex the left ankle.

738

Middle deltoid and supraspinatus abduct both shoulders. The left anterior deltoid and pectoralis major flex or horizontally flex the left shoulder and the right posterior deltoid and triceps extend or horizontally extend the right shoulder.

During the forward swing and follow through stages of kicking a ball iliopsoas, rectus femoris and sartorius work concentrically and the hamstrings and gluteus maximus work eccentrically to flex the right hip. Gluteus medius maintains body weight over the left hip. Piriformis and external rotators abduct and externally rotate the right hip. The quadriceps extends the right knee. Gastrocnemius and soleus plantar flex the right ankle. Middle deltoid and supraspinatus maintain abduction. The right anterior deltoid and pectoralis major flex or horizontally flex the right shoulder and the left posterior deltoid and triceps extend or horizontally extend the left shoulder.

Kicking a ball involves head flexion, cervical flexion, thoracic and lumbar flexion and sidebending, sacroiliac flexion on one side and extension on the other, scapula retraction then protraction, shoulder abduction and horizontal adduction, hip extension then flexion of the kicking leg, hip abduction of the weigh bearing leg, hip adduction, internal rotation and external rotation for fine control, knee flexion and the extension of the kicking leg, ankle dorsiflexion and plantar flexion.

Kicking	Head		Cervical				Thoracic				Lumbar			
	F	E	F	E	S	R	F	E	S	R	F	E	S	R
Direction	X	O	X	O	O	O	X	O	X	X	X	O	X	X
Range	.	O	.	O	O	O	.	O	.	.	.	O	.	.
Contraction	O	X	.	X	.	.	.	.	.	.	.	X	.	X
Stretch	.	X	.	X	.	.	.	X	.	.	X	X	X	X

	Scapula				Shoulder					
	Re	Pr	El	De	F	E	Ab	Ad	Ir	Er
Direction	X	X	O	O	X	X	X	O	O	O
Range	X	X	O	O	X	X	X	O	O	O
Contraction	X	X	.	.	.	.	.	.	.	.
Stretch	X	X	.	.	X	X	X	.	.	.

	Elbow				Wrist				Hand		SI	
	F	E	P	Su	F	E	Ab	Ad	F	E	F	E
Direction	X	O	O	O	O	O	O	O	O	O	X	X
Range	.	O	O	O	O	O	O	O	O	O	.	.
Contraction	.	O	O	O	O	O	O	O	O	O	.	.
Stretch	.	.	O	O	O	O	O	O	O	O	X	X

	Hip						Knee		Foot				Toes	
	F	E	Ab	Ad	Ir	Er	F	E	Pf	Df	In	Ev	F	E
Direction	X	X	X	X	X	X	X	X	X	X	X	X	X	X
Range	X	X	.	.	.	.	X	X	X	X	.	.	.	.
Contraction	X	X	.	X	.	.	X	X	X	X	.	.	.	.
Stretch	X	X	X	X	X	X	X	X	X	X	.	.	X	X

Key: None (O) partial (.) full (X) Range = Range of joint movement, Contraction = Level of muscle contraction, Direction = Direction of movement Direction may be Flexion (F), Extension (E), Sidebending (S), Rotation (R), Retraction (Re), Protraction (Pr), Elevation (El), Depression (De), Abduction (Ab), Adduction (Ad), Internal rotation (Ir), External rotation (Er), Pronation (P), Supination (Su), Plantar flexion (Pf), Dorsi flexion (Df), Inversion, (In), Eversion (Ev)

Weekly stretching program for kicking a ball

Day 1	Day 2	Day 3	Day 4	Day 5	Day 6	Day 7
1.3b	1.4a	1.4b	1.8	1.9	2.0a	2.1b
2.4a	1.5	2.5a	2.5b	2.5c	2.6a	2.6b
2.7a	1.6	3.0e	3.1a	2.8	3.1b	3.0a
	1.7b	4.0b	4.0d	4.0e	4.0f	4.0g
4.5	1.7f	4.8	6.1c	4.9c	5.1a	5.2a
6.0a	6.0c	6.1a	6.4d	6.1e	6.2a	6.2b
6.5a	6.4b	6.4a	6.5m	6.4g	6.5g	6.5h
6.6a	6.7f	6.5c	6.8a	6.6e	7.2b	6.9a
6.7a	7.1b	6.7b	7.1g	6.7c	7.1e	7.6

740

Long jump

The long jump is a track and field event where each competitor has to run down a runway and jump as far as possible across a pit filled with finely ground sand.

The long jump consists of the run-up, the last two strides, take-off, movement adjustments in the air, and landing. A foul line is marked on a wooden board at the start of the jump point and the long jumper cannot jump from any point past this line or the jump is declared a foul. Each competitor has a set number of attempts.

Successful long jumping depends on the high speed of the run-up, the correct angle of take-off, effective body streamlining during the jump and effective landing. The main muscles used in the long jump are Gluteus Maximus, Quadriceps, Hamstrings and Calf Muscles.

The long jump involves head flexion, thoracic and lumbar flexion, sacroiliac flexion and extension, scapula protraction, shoulder flexion and extension, elbow extension, hip flexion, extension, abduction, adduction, internal rotation and external rotation, knee flexion and extension, ankle dorsiflexion and plantar flexion, and toe flexion and extension.

For stretches for the first phase of the long jump the run up see Running Sprinting.

Long jump	Head		Cervical				Thoracic				Lumbar			
	F	E	F	E	S	R	F	E	S	R	F	E	S	R
Direction	X	O	O	O	O	O	X	O	O	O	X	O	O	O
Range	.	O	O	O	O	O	.	O	O	O	.	O	O	O
Contraction	.	.	.	.	O	O	.	.	O	O	.	.	.	O
Stretch	.	.	.	.	.	.	.	.	.	.	X	X	.	.

	Scapula				Shoulder					
	Re	Pr	El	De	F	E	Ab	Ad	Ir	Er
Direction	O	X	O	O	X	X	O	O	O	O
Range	O	.	O	O	X	X	O	O	O	O
Contraction	.	.	.	O	X	X	.	.	.	.
Stretch	X	X	.	.	X	X	X	.	.	.

	Elbow				Wrist				Hand		SI	
	F	E	P	Su	F	E	Ab	Ad	F	E	F	E
Direction	X	X	O	O	O	O	O	O	O	O	X	X
Range	X	X	O	O	O	O	O	O	O	O	X	X
Contraction	X	X	.	.	O	O	O	O	O	O	X	X
Stretch	X	X	.	.	.	.	O	O	.	.	X	X

	Hip						Knee		Foot				Toes	
	F	E	Ab	Ad	Ir	Er	F	E	Pf	Df	In	Ev	F	E
Direction	X	X	X	X	X	X	X	X	X	X	X	X	X	X
Range	X	X	X	.	.	.	X	X	X	X	.	.	X	X
Contraction	X	X	X	.	.	.	X	X	X	X	.	.	X	X
Stretch	X	X	X	X	X	X	X	X	X	X	X	X	X	X

Key: None (**O**) partial (**.**) full (**X**) Range = Range of joint movement, Contraction = Level of muscle contraction, Direction = Direction of movement Direction may be Flexion (F), Extension (E), Sidebending (S), Rotation (R), Retraction (Re), Protraction (Pr), Elevation (El), Depression (De), Abduction (Ab), Adduction (Ad), Internal rotation (Ir), External rotation (Er), Pronation (P), Supination (Su), Plantar flexion (Pf), Dorsi flexion (Df), Inversion, (In), Eversion (Ev)

Weekly stretching program for long jump

Day 1	Day 2	Day 3	Day 4	Day 5	Day 6	Day 7
1.3c	2.0a	1.7a	2.4b	1.4a	2.5a	1.7d
2.5c	2.8	1.7f	3.0a	1.5	2.9b	1.8
3.4	2.9a	4.0c	4.0e	4.5	5.0a	4.9d
5.2a	5.4	6.0a	6.0b	5.1b	6.0c	4.8
6.1a	6.2a	6.1c	6.2b	6.1e	6.3a	6.1f
6.4a	6.3d	6.4b	6.4d	6.4g	6.5b	6.5d
6.5f	6.5g	6.5i	6.5k	6.5m	6.6a	6.6d
6.7b	6.6a	6.7c	6.7e	6.7f	6.9a	6.9c
7.1a	7.1f	7.1b	7.1g	7.1c	7.3b	7.4b

Stretches for riding a motorcycle

Riding a motorcycle involves sitting with the hips abducted, thighs and knees apart and with both feet on foot rests, using the arms to steer, fingers of the left hand to operate the clutch, fingers of the right hand to operate the front brake, left foot to change gear, right foot to operate the rear brake and right hand to turn the throttle on the right handlebar.

Motorcycles come in many forms - sports, off-road, scooters, cruisers are a few examples. But the stretches listed here are for the standard general purpose street motorcycle. These motorcycles mainly involves the contraction of the muscles responsible for head, cervical, upper thoracic and lumbar extension, scapula retraction, shoulder flexion and extension, elbow flexion and extension, wrist flexion and extension, finger flexion and extension, hip adduction and ankle plantar flexion and dorsiflexion.

The major muscles used when riding a motorcycle are the posterior cervical muscles, shoulder retractor muscles (rhomboids and middle trapezius) erector spinae, abdominals, anterior and posterior deltoids, biceps brachii, triceps brachii, pectoralis major, wrist flexors (flexor carpi radialis and ulnaris) and wrist extensors (extensor carpi radialis longus and brevis and extensor carpi ulnaris), finger flexors (flexor digitorum superficialis and profundus and flexor pollicis longus), hip adductors (gracilis, pectineus, adductors longus, brevis and magnus), calf muscles (gastrocnemius and soleus) and ankle dorsiflexor (tibialis anterior).

Prolonged periods of motorcycle riding can cause postural fatigue and pain. Helmets can be heavy and contribute toward neck pain. Hand and forearm muscles can tire from long period of twisting a throttle, operating a clutch or repeated braking. Leg and foot pain can result from frequent gear changing and hip pain from griping the seat, especially if you ride over rough roads. Like riding a horse the adductors muscles get tired. Long periods hunched over a motorcycle can cause postural fatigue and pain in middle trapezius and rhomboid major and minor and in lumbar and thoracic spinal muscles. Riding into a wind can be beneficial by neutralising a forward slouching posture or it can be problematic by forcing the rider backwards.

Muscles held in a prolonged shortened state will remain short unless stretched. Muscles that may become short include the muscle responsible for head extension (posterior suboccipital muscles), upper cervical extension (posterior cervical muscles) and lower cervical flexion (sternocleidomastoid and anterior scalene), thoracic and lumbar flexion, scapular protraction (pectoralis minor) and elevation (upper trapezius and levator scapulae), shoulder adduction and internal rotation (such as pectoralis major), elbow flexion, wrist extension, finger flexion, sacral extension, hip flexion, knee flexion and ankle plantar flexion. In the lower limb these are iliopsoas, hamstrings and the hip abductors.

For optimal health take a break from riding a motorcycle every hour and take a short walk and allow your arms to swing freely like a pendulum alternating with your legs. Also use the stretches listed. Adjust your motorcycle to the optimal position to operate controls, see the instruments and mirrors and maintain a good posture.

Motorcycling	Head		Cervical				Thoracic				Lumbar			
	F	E	F	E	S	R	F	E	S	R	F	E	S	R
Direction	O	X	X	O	O	O	X	O	O	O	X	O	O	O
Range	O	.	.	O	O	O	.	O	O	O	X	O	O	O
Contraction	.	X	X	X	.	.	.	X	.	.	.	X	.	O
Stretch	.	X	X	X	.	.	X	X	.	.	X	X	.	.

	Scapula				Shoulder					
	Re	Pr	El	De	F	E	Ab	Ad	Ir	Er
Direction	O	X	O	O	X	O	X	O	X	O
Range	O	X	O	O	.	O	.	O	X	O
Contraction	X	.	.	.	X	X	.	.	.	O
Stretch	.	X	X	.	X	X	X	X	X	.

	Elbow				Wrist				Hand		SI	
	F	E	P	Su	F	E	Ab	Ad	F	E	F	E
Direction	X	O	O	O	X	X	O	O	X	X	O	X
Range	.	O	O	O	X	X	O	O	X	X	O	.
Contraction	.	.	.	.	X	X	.	.	X	X	X	.
Stretch	X	X	.	.	X	X	.	.	X	X	X	X

	Hip						Knee		Foot				Toes	
	F	E	Ab	Ad	Ir	Er	F	E	Pf	Df	In	Ev	F	E
Direction	X	O	X	O	O	X	X	O	X	X	O	O	X	X
Range	X	O	X	O	O	.	.	O	X	X	O	O	.	.
Contraction	.	.	.	X	.	.	.	.	X	X	.	.	X	X
Stretch	X	X	X	X	.	X	X	X	X	X	.	.	X	X

Key: None (O) partial (.) full (X) Range = Range of joint movement, Contraction = Level of muscle contraction, Direction = Direction of movement Direction may be Flexion (F), Extension (E), Sidebending (S), Rotation (R), Retraction (Re), Protraction (Pr), Elevation (El), Depression (De), Abduction (Ab), Adduction (Ad), Internal rotation (Ir), External rotation (Er), Pronation (P), Supination (Su), Plantar flexion (Pf), Dorsi flexion (Df), Inversion, (In), Eversion (Ev)

Weekly stretching program for riding a motorcycle

Day 1	Day 2	Day 3	Day 4	Day 5	Day 6	Day 7
1.2	1.3b	1.4a	1.8	1.7d	1.9	2.0a
3.2b	4.3	1.6	3.2a	2.4b	2.1b	2.5b
3.8b	2.1a	1.7a	4.0e	4.0f	4.0g	3.3
3.8c	4.0b	1.7f	4.5	4.1	4.8	4.0c
3.8d	4.9e	5.0a	5.1a	5.2a	5.8e	4.9d
3.8e	5.4	5.7a	5.7b	6.0a	5.9	6.0c
6.1e	6.2a	5.8a	6.2b	6.2c	6.4a	6.4b
6.4c	6.5i	6.6a	6.5h	6.5m	6.6c	6.7b
6.7a	7.1e	6.7f	7.2b	6.9a	7.1b	7.3a

Polo

Polo is a team sport played on horseback on a large grass field. Each team consists of four riders and their horses. Players score goals by hitting a small white wooden or plastic ball into the opposing team's goal using a long-handled mallet.

Polo has all the challenges of regular horse riding but the rider has to control the horse with one hand and hit the ball with the mallet held in the other hand. So in addition to the stretches for normal horse riding there need to stretches for the upper limb which controls the horse and stretches for the upper limb which is used to hit the ball.

As with horse riding the iliopsoas and rectus abdominis keep the riders torso in a vertical position and the hip and calf muscles keep the rider on the horse, help maintain balance and control the horse. But in polo, in order to strike the ball the rider has to rotate the spine, abduct and extend the shoulder and then flex the shoulder.

Like horse riding, polo requires flexibility, strength, coordination and balance. It involves head extension, cervical extension, thoracic flexion, lumbar flexion, sidebending and rotation, sacroiliac extension, scapula retraction, shoulder flexion, extension, abduction, adduction, elbow flexion, extension, supination and pronation, wrist flexion and extension, finger flexion, hip flexion, abduction, internal rotation and external rotation, knee flexion and ankle dorsiflexion.

Polo	Head		Cervical				Thoracic				Lumbar			
	F	E	F	E	S	R	F	E	S	R	F	E	S	R
Direction	O	X	O	X	O	O	X	O	O	O	X	O	X	X
Range	O	.	O	.	O	O	X	O	O	O	.	O	.	.
Contraction	.	X	.	X	.	.	.	X	.	.	X	X	.	.
Stretch	.	X	.	X	.	.	.	X	.	.	X	X	.	.

	Scapula				Shoulder							
	Re	Pr	El	De	F	E	Ab	Ad	Ir	Er		
Direction	X	O	O	O	X	X	X	O	O	O		
Range	X	O	O	O	X	X	X	O	O	O		
Contraction	X	X	.	.	X	X	X	.	.	.		
Stretch	X	.	.	O	X	X	.	.	.	.		

	Elbow				Wrist				Hand		SI	
	F	E	P	Su	F	E	Ab	Ad	F	E	F	E
Direction	X	O	X	X	X	X	O	O	X	O	O	X
Range	X	O	.	.	.	.	O	O	X	O	O	.
Contraction	X	X	.	.	X	.	.	.	X	O	.	.
Stretch	X	X	.	.	X	X	.	.	X	.	.	X

	Hip						Knee		Foot				Toes	
	F	E	Ab	Ad	Ir	Er	F	E	Pf	Df	In	Ev	F	E
Direction	X	O	X	O	X	O	X	O	X	X	O	O	O	O
Range	.	O	X	O	.	O	.	O	.	X	O	O	O	O
Contraction	X	.	.	X	.	.	.	X	X	.	O	O	O	O
Stretch	X	X	X	X	.	.	X	X	X	.	O	O	O	O

Key: None (O) partial (.) full (X) Range = Range of joint movement, Contraction = Level of muscle contraction, Direction = Direction of movement Direction may be Flexion (F), Extension (E), Sidebending (S), Rotation (R), Retraction (Re), Protraction (Pr), Elevation (El), Depression (De), Abduction (Ab), Adduction (Ad), Internal rotation (Ir), External rotation (Er), Pronation (P), Supination (Su), Plantar flexion (Pf), Dorsi flexion (Df), Inversion, (In), Eversion (Ev)

Weekly stretching program for polo

Day 1	Day 2	Day 3	Day 4	Day 5	Day 6	Day 7
1.4b	1.7c	1.8	1.3b	1.4a	2.3	2.4d
2.6b	2.0a	2.9a	3.0c	1.5	2.5a	2.5c
4.3	4.0b	2.8	4.0g	4.1	3.4	4.5
4.9a	4.9e	5.2c	5.3a	5.0b	5.5	5.4
5.6b	5.8b	5.8c	5.7b	5.9	6.0a	6.0c
6.1a	6.2a	5.8d	6.3b	6.4a	6.4c	6.4g
6.5a	6.5c	6.6a	6.5e	6.6e	6.5h	6.5m
6.7a	6.9a	6.7b	7.0a	6.7c	7.1a	6.7f
7.1b	7.2a	7.1d	7.1e	7.1g	7.5a	7.1h

Rowing, canoeing and kayaking

In rowing a boat is propelled by the force of an oar blade, as it is pushed against the water. Rowing may be competitive or recreational. It may be done as an individual activity or as a team sport which can vary from two to eight persons. Propulsion may be as a result of a single oar or two oars. In rowing the oar is held in place at a pivot point that is in a fixed position relative to the boat, whereas in other types of rowing such as canoeing or kayaking the oar is not fixed. In racing rowing boats the seats slide to allow the use of the legs to apply power to the oar and the thoracic and lumbar spinal muscles contract to produce extension. In contrast in canoeing and kayaking there is more upper body power and more spinal rotation.

Rowing involves head and cervical extension, thoracic and lumbar flexion, lumbar rotation, scapula retraction and protraction, shoulder flexion, extension and adduction, elbow flexion and extension, wrist flexion and extension, finger flexion, hip flexion and extension and knee flexion and extension. The thoracic and lumbar spine tend to be fixed in a flexed position.

Rowing is cyclic activity divided into the catch, the drive, the finish and the recovery. In the catch the elbows are extended by the triceps and the hip and knees flexed by the iliacus and hamstrings in preparation for the drive. In the drive and finish erector spinea produces back extension, the hips are extended by the gluteus maximus and hamstrings, the knees are extended by the quadriceps and the feet are plantar flexed by the gastrocnemius and soleus. The elbows are flexed by biceps, brachialis and brachioradialis and the scapula is stabilised by serratus anterior and trapezius. The shoulders are extended and internally rotated by latissimus dorsi, teres major and pectoralis major. Other muscles assist as shoulder stabilisers and wrist adductors and stabilisers. In the recovery phase the elbows are returned to full extension by triceps, the arm is flexed by anterior deltoid and biceps, and the torso is flexed by abdominal contraction.

Rowing	Head F	Head E	Cervical F	Cervical E	Cervical S	Cervical R	Thoracic F	Thoracic E	Thoracic S	Thoracic R	Lumbar F	Lumbar E	Lumbar S	Lumbar R
Direction	O	X	O	X	O	O	X	O	O	O	X	O	O	X
Range	O	X	O	.	O	O	X	O	O	O	X	O	O	.
Contraction	O	X	.	X	.	O	.	X	O	O	.	X	.	.
Stretch	.	X	.	X	.	.	.	X	.	.	.	X	.	X

	Scapula Re	Pr	El	De	Shoulder F	E	Ab	Ad	Ir	Er
Direction	X	X	O	O	X	X	O	X	X	O
Range	X	X	O	O	.	X	O	.	.	O
Contraction	X	X	.	.	X	X	.	X	.	.
Stretch	X	X	.	.	X	X	X	X	.	.

	Elbow F	E	P	Su	Wrist F	E	Ab	Ad	Hand F	E	SI F	E
Direction	X	X	O	O	O	X	O	X	X	O	O	X
Range	X	X	O	O	O	.	O	.	X	O	O	.
Contraction	X	X	.	.	.	X	O	.	X	.	O	.
Stretch	X	X	.	.	.	X	O	.	X	.	.	X

	Hip F	E	Ab	Ad	Ir	Er	Knee F	E	Foot Pf	Df	In	Ev	Toes F	E
Direction	X	X	O	O	O	O	X	X	X	X	O	O	O	O
Range	X	X	O	O	O	O	X	X	X	.	O	O	O	O
Contraction	.	X	O	O	O	O	X	X	.	.	O	O	O	O
Stretch	X	X	.	.	O	O	X	X	X	.	O	O	O	O

Key: None (O) partial (.) full (X) Range = Range of joint movement, Contraction = Level of muscle contraction, Direction = Direction of movement Direction may be Flexion (F), Extension (E), Sidebending (S), Rotation (R), Retraction (Re), Protraction (Pr), Elevation (El), Depression (De), Abduction (Ab), Adduction (Ad), Internal rotation (Ir), External rotation (Er), Pronation (P), Supination (Su), Plantar flexion (Pf), Dorsi flexion (Df), Inversion, (In), Eversion (Ev)

Weekly stretching program for rowing

Day 1	Day 2	Day 3	Day 4	Day 5	Day 6	Day 7
1.2	1.3b	1.4a	1.3a	1.4b	1.7b	1.8
1.9	2.9a	1.5	2.3	2.1b	2.0a	2.4b
2.5b	3.0e	1.6	2.6a	2.6d	2.8	2.7a
4.0a	3.1a	1.7a	3.0a	3.8b	3.2a	3.1b
4.4	3.5	2.9b	4.0d	3.8c	4.1	4.0c
4.8	4.0g	4.5	4.9c	5.1a	4.9a	5.2a
5.3a	5.6b	5.8b	5.7b	6.0a	5.5	5.4
6.1e	6.4b	6.5h	6.5m	6.7a	6.6a	6.0c
6.7f	6.9a	6.7e	6.9c	7.1b	6.7b	7.1e

Stretches for sedentary work sitting at a desk in a chair

These stretches are for sedentary activities involving prolonged periods of sitting in an office chair using a computer at home or in an office environment.

Sitting at a desk and typing on a keyboard mainly involves the contraction of the muscles responsible for head, cervical, upper thoracic and lumbar extension, scapula retraction, wrist extension and finger flexion and extension. Long periods of sitting may result in postural fatigue, muscle strain, atrophy and shortness and over time prolonged sitting may also result in structural changes such as an increase in fibrous tissue within muscles.

The postural muscles most affected by sitting include the posterior cervical muscles, the extensor muscles of the spine (erector spinae) and the shoulder retractor muscles (rhomboids and middle trapezius).

Muscle atrophy is a result of the prolonged disuse of muscles during sitting. Most significant is the atrophy and weakness of abdominal muscles, which are important for maintaining trunk postural alignment. Also of significance is the atrophy and weakness of the supraspinatus muscles. Combined with shortness in the pectoralis muscle this can predispose towards a rotator cuff tendon injury.

Shortness occurs in muscles that are held in a prolonged shortened state during sitting. These include the muscle responsible for head extension, upper cervical extension and lower cervical flexion, thoracic and lumbar flexion, scapular protraction and elevation, shoulder adduction and internal rotation, elbow flexion, wrist extension, finger flexion, sacral extension, hip flexion, knee flexion, ankle dorsiflexion and ankle plantar flexion.

Shortness in the iliopsoas, hip external rotators, hamstrings and calves has significant effect on other muscles and joints of body during standing, walking, sports and other physical activities. The chin out posture combined with weak deep neck flexors and overactive upper trapezius, levator scapula and rhomboid muscles can result in postural fatigue and shoulder pain. Poor sitting posture can result in acute lumbosacral or mid thoracic pain and predispose towards early joint degeneration. This is the characteristic slouching posture with the thoracic and lumbar spine in flexion, the sacrum in extension and the top of the pelvis tilting backwards.

In addition to contributing to changes in muscles and joints prolonged sitting can result in obesity, diabetes, heart disease, deep vein thrombosis, depression, low sex drive and other physical and emotional problems.

Good sitting involves sitting on your two buttock bones (ischial tuberosities) with your pelvis erect and supported against the back of the chair. An erect pelvis provides the platform for an erect spine and a well-balanced shoulder posture with both scapulae in a horizontally neutral position relative to the rib cage, not protracted or retracted. Your chair should have a straight back that maintains a neutral body position and keeps your vertebrae aligned. Your knees should be level with or a little bit lower than your hips. The soles of both feet should be planted on the floor.

Adjust the height of the table so that the middle of your forearms rest on the edge of the table and your fingertips resting comfortably on the keyboard. The table edge is a fulcrum around which the forearms pivot. An optimum table height positions the shoulders with both scapulae in a vertically neutral position relative to the rib cage, not elevated or depressed.

If your chair does not have a good ergonomic design or is not adjustable then you may need to place a dedicated lumbar support or a small pillow behind your lumbar spine. Do not cross your legs. Get up and walk every half hour.

Sitting	Head		Cervical				Thoracic				Lumbar			
	F	E	F	E	S	R	F	E	S	R	F	E	S	R
Direction	O	X	O	X	O	O	X	O	O	O	X	O	O	O
Range	O	.	O	.	O	O	X	O	O	O	X	O	O	O
Contraction	O	X	O	X	.	O	O	X	O	O	O	X	O	O
Stretch	O	X	.	X	.	.	X	X	.	.	X	X	.	.

	Scapula				Shoulder					
	Re	Pr	El	De	F	E	Ab	Ad	Ir	Er
Direction	O	X	X	O	O	O	O	X	X	O
Range	O	.	.	O	O	O	O	.	.	O
Contraction	X	O	O	O	.	.	O	.	.	O
Stretch	.	X	.	.	.	.	.	X	X	.

	Elbow				Wrist				Hand		SI	
	F	E	P	Su	F	E	Ab	Ad	F	E	F	E
Direction	X	O	O	O	O	X	O	O	X	O	O	X
Range	X	O	O	O	O	.	O	O	.	O	O	X
Contraction	O	.	.	O	O	X	O	O	.	.	X	.
Stretch	X	.	.	.	.	X	.	.	X	.	X	X

	Hip						Knee		Foot				Toes	
	F	E	Ab	Ad	Ir	Er	F	E	Pf	Df	In	Ev	F	E
Direction	X	O	O	O	O	X	X	O	O	X	O	O	O	O
Range	X	O	O	O	O	.	X	O	O	.	O	O	O	O
Contraction	.	O	O	O	O	O	O	X	O	O	O	O	O	O
Stretch	X	X	.	.	.	X	X	X	X	X	.	.	.	.

Key: None (O) partial (.) full (X) Range = Range of joint movement, Contraction = Level of muscle contraction, Direction = Direction of movement Direction may be Flexion (F), Extension (E), Sidebending (S), Rotation (R), Retraction (Re), Protraction (Pr), Elevation (El), Depression (De), Abduction (Ab), Adduction (Ad), Internal rotation (Ir), External rotation (Er), Pronation (P), Supination (Su), Plantar flexion (Pf), Dorsi flexion (Df), Inversion, (In), Eversion (Ev)

751

Weekly stretching program for sedentary work sitting in a chair

Day 1	Day 2	Day 3	Day 4	Day 5	Day 6	Day 7
1.2	1.3c	1.4a	1.3b	1.3a	1.4b	1.4c
1.8	1. 7i	1.7b	2.1b	1.7d	2.4b	2.0a
1.9	2.4c	1.7f	2.5a	2.5b	2.7a	2.0b
2.5c	2.6a	2.6d	3.0a	3.0e	3.0c	2.8
3.2a	3.2b	3.6	3.4	4.0a	3.9a	3.3
4.0d	4.0e	3.7	4.0f	4.0g	4.1	4.0h
4.5	4.8	3.8a	6.0a	5.3a	4.9b	5.2a
6.0c	6.2a	3.8b	6.2b	6.4b	6.5h	6.6a
6.7a	6.7f	3.8c	6.7b	6.9a	7.1b	7.6

Supreme stretches suggested by the author

This is a general group of the best all round stretches as determined by the author Rowland Benjamin. They can be done any time of the day and cover the whole body.

Day 1	Day 2	Day 3	Day 4	Day 5	Day 6	Day 7
1.1a	1.2	1.3a	1.4a	1.4b	2.0a	2.4b
2.5a	2.9a	2.6a	1.5	2.7a	2.0b	2.5b
3.0a	2.8	3.0e	1.6	3.6	3.1a	4.8
4.5	3.4	4.0g	1.7a	3.7	3.1b	4.9b
5.3a	5.4	5.0a	1.7b	3.8a	4.0c	5.2a
6.0a	5.8d	6.2a	1.7f	3.8b	5.1a	5.5
6.2b	5.8c	6.5a	6.4d	3.8c	6.1a	5.6a
6.5h	6.6a	6.7b	6.7f	3.8d	6.5m	6.9a
7.1b	7.1f	7.1g	7.2b	3.8e	7.3a	7.6

Skateboarding

Skateboarding is an activity which involves riding and performing tricks on a skateboard. It requires balance, coordination, flexibility, strength and power. It puts demand on ligaments and muscles but from only one direction. Skateboarding can be ambidextrous. But commonly skateboarders stand on their skateboard facing one direction and so favour one side of the body. One sided skateboarding causes an increase in the development of muscles down one side of the body. When muscles on one side get bigger and stronger they can pull the body to one side and it movement may be reduced in the other direction. Stretches for skateboarding should be on both sides of the body, left and right, but if the skateboarder favours one side then they should do more stretches and stretch harder on the side that is stiffest.

Skateboarding places great demand on the whole body but it places the greatest demand on the calf muscles which keep the body balanced on the skateboard and the quadriceps muscles which produce explosive knee extension. Gluteus maximus, medius and minimus, tensor fascia latae, the hamstrings and the hip adductors and external rotators are responsible for balance, performing tricks, and various skateboarding skills. Tensor fascia latae and gluteus maximus work hard together to stabilize the hip joint. The abdominal muscles, iliopsoas, erector spinae, latissimus dorsi and lower trapezius stabilize the upper body and also maintain balance.

Skateboarding may use any combination of posture but commonly involves head extension, cervical flexion, sidebending and rotation, thoracic and lumbar flexion, sidebending and rotation, sacroiliac extension, scapula retraction or protraction, elevation, shoulder abduction, elbow flexion, wrist extension, hip flexion and abduction, knee flexion and extension, ankle plantar flexion, foot inversion or eversion and toe flexion.

Skateboarding	Head		Cervical				Thoracic				Lumbar			
	F	E	F	E	S	R	F	E	S	R	F	E	S	R
Direction	O	X	X	O	X	X	X	O	X	X	X	O	X	X
Range	O	.	.	O	.	.	.	O	.	.	X	.	.	.
Contraction	.	X	.	X	.	.	.	X	.	.	.	X	.	.
Stretch	.	X	.	X	.	.	.	X	.	.	.	X	.	.

	Scapula				Shoulder					
	Re	Pr	El	De	F	E	Ab	Ad	Ir	Er
Direction	X	X	O	O	O	O	X	O	O	O
Range	.	.	O	O	O	O	X	O	O	O
Contraction	X	X	.	.	.	.	X	.	.	.
Stretch	X	X	.	.	.	.	X	.	.	.

	Elbow				Wrist				Hand		SI	
	F	E	P	Su	F	E	Ab	Ad	F	E	F	E
Direction	X	O	O	O	O	X	O	O	O	O	O	X
Range	.	O	O	O	O	.	O	O	O	O	O	O
Contraction	.	.	.	.	.	.	.	.	.	.	X	X
Stretch	.	.	.	.	.	.	.	.	.	.	X	X

	Hip						Knee		Foot				Toes	
	F	E	Ab	Ad	Ir	Er	F	E	Pf	Df	In	Ev	F	E
Direction	X	O	X	O	O	O	X	X	X	X	X	X	X	O
Range	X	O	X	O	O	O	X	X	X	X	.	.	.	O
Contraction	.	X	X	X	.	.	.	X	X	.	X	X	X	.
Stretch	X	X	X	X	.	.	X	X	X	X	X	X	X	X

Key: None (O) partial (.) full (X) Range = Range of joint movement, Contraction = Level of muscle contraction, Direction = Direction of movement Direction may be Flexion (F), Extension (E), Sidebending (S), Rotation (R), Retraction (Re), Protraction (Pr), Elevation (El), Depression (De), Abduction (Ab), Adduction (Ad), Internal rotation (Ir), External rotation (Er), Pronation (P), Supination (Su), Plantar flexion (Pf), Dorsi flexion (Df), Inversion, (In), Eversion (Ev)

Weekly stretching program for skateboarding

Day 1	Day 2	Day 3	Day 4	Day 5	Day 6	Day 7
1.3b	1.4b	1.4a	1.7d	1.8	1.9	2.0b
2.4a	2.5a	1.7c	2.5b	2.4b	2.5c	2.0b
2.8	2.9b	1.7f	3.0a	3.0e	3.1c	3.2a
2.9a	3.9a	4.0g	4.0b	4.1	4.4	4.5
4.8	4.9b	5.0a	5.1b	5.2a	5.1a	6.0c
6.0a	6.1e	6.1c	6.2b	6.2a	6.4a	6.4b
6.4d	6.4g	6.5a	6.5c	6.5e	6.5f	6.5h
6.5m	6.6a	6.6d	6.6f	6.7a	6.7e	6.7f
6.9a	6.9c	7.1b	7.1c	7.1d	7.1e	7.1g

Skydiving

Skydiving or parachuting is the sport of jumping out of an aircraft, free-falling for a period of time and then using a parachute to slow down and return to Earth. During the free-fall phase the body accelerates to terminal velocity. When the parachute is deployed the body decelerates until it is moving at a speed appropriate for a ground landing.

Skydiving is a recreational and military activity and a competitive sport. It requires coordination and a moderate degree of flexibility, particularly with regard to extension of the spine, hips and shoulders.

Skydiving involves head extension, cervical extension, thoracic and lumbar extension, sacroiliac flexion, scapula retraction, shoulder extension, abduction and external rotation, elbow flexion, wrist flexion, finger flexion, hip extension and abduction and knee flexion.

Skydiving	Head		Cervical				Thoracic				Lumbar			
	F	E	F	E	S	R	F	E	S	R	F	E	S	R
Direction	O	X	O	X	O	O	O	X	O	O	O	X	O	O
Range	O	X	O	.	O	O	O	X	O	O	O	X	O	O
Contraction	.	X	.	X	.	O	.	.	O	O	.	X	.	o
Stretch	.	X	X	X	.	.	X	X	.	.	X	X	.	.

	Scapula				Shoulder					
	Re	Pr	El	De	F	E	Ab	Ad	Ir	Er
Direction	X	O	O	O	O	X	X	O	O	X
Range	X	O	O	O	O	X	X	O	O	X
Contraction	.	X	.	.	X	.	.	.	X	.
Stretch	X	X	.	.	X	X	X	.	X	X

	Elbow				Wrist				Hand		SI	
	F	E	P	Su	F	E	Ab	Ad	F	E	F	E
Direction	X	O	O	O	X	O	O	O	X	O	X	O
Range	.	O	O	O	.	O	O	O	.	O	.	O
Contraction	.	.	O	O	X	.	O	O	.	.	X	.
Stretch	X	.	O	O	.	.	O	O	.	.	X	X

	Hip						Knee		Foot				Toes	
	F	E	Ab	Ad	Ir	Er	F	E	Pf	Df	In	Ev	F	E
Direction	O	X	X	O	O	O	X	O	O	O	O	O	O	O
Range	O	X	X	O	O	O	.	O	O	O	O	O	O	O
Contraction	X	.	X	.	O	O	.	.	O	O	O	O	O	O
Stretch	X	X	X	X	.	.	.	.	.	O	O	O	O	O

Key: None (O) partial (.) full (X) Range = Range of joint movement, Contraction = Level of muscle contraction, Direction = Direction of movement Direction may be Flexion (F), Extension (E), Sidebending (S), Rotation (R), Retraction (Re), Protraction (Pr), Elevation (El), Depression (De), Abduction (Ab), Adduction (Ad), Internal rotation (Ir), External rotation (Er), Pronation (P), Supination (Su), Plantar flexion (Pf), Dorsi flexion (Df), Inversion, (In), Eversion (Ev)

Weekly stretching program for skydiving

Day 1	Day 2	Day 3	Day 4	Day 5	Day 6	Day 7
1.3a	1.4a	1.9	1.7c	1.4b	1.3b	2.0a
2.4a	1.5	2.5a	2.5c	2.4d	2.5b	2.6b
2.7a	2.7b	2.9a	2.7c	3.5	2.9b	3.1a
3.0a	3.0c	3.4	3.0e	4.0d	3.6	4.0c
4.0e	4.0f	4.0g	4.0h	4.1	3.7	4.2
4.4	4.5	4.7	4.8	4.9a	3.8a	4.3
5.2a	4.9e	5.4	5.3a	5.1b	3.8d	5.0a
6.0a	6.0c	6.1c	6.2a	6.4b	6.5h	6.4d
6.5g	6.6a	6.7b	6.7f	7.0a	7.1b	6.9a

Tennis

Tennis is a racquet sport between two or four people. The racquet is strung with cord to hit a ball over a net and into the opponent's court and land in such a way that the opponent is unable to play a good return ball. Tennis balls are made of hollow rubber with a felt coating.

Tennis is a skill that requires good upper limb flexibility, good hand-eye-ball coordination and a muscular system trained for strength, power, endurance and speed. Tennis involves powerful explosive movements and frequent bursts of short-distance running, decelerating and stopping and split second changes of direction. This is particularly good for strengthening ligaments and fast-twitch muscle fibres.

The tennis serve involves scapula retraction then protraction, shoulder flexion, abduction and external rotation then extension, adduction and internal rotation, elbow flexion then extension, wrist extension and then flexion and increasing finger flexion. Tennis also involves head extension then flexion, cervical extension then flexion, lumbar and thoracolumbar extension then flexion, sacral flexion then extension and thoracolumbar rotation with sidebending.

These are stretches for tennis and especially the tennis serve. The tennis stretches are similar to the stretches for throwing except in tennis there is greater stretching of the calf, forearm muscles and muscles that extend the spine.

The main muscles used in tennis are gastrocnemius, soleus, hamstrings, quadriceps, gluteus maximus and medius, rectus abdominis and abdominal obliques, latissimus dorsi and erector spinae, pectorals, deltoids, supraspinatus, infraspinatus, teres minor and subscapularis, rhomboid, trapezius, biceps, triceps and wrist flexors and extensors. During a tennis serve some muscles contract to stabilises the lower limb. The iliopsoas, gluteus maximus, hamstrings, hip abductors and adductors hold the lower limb in position during the serve.

Tennis	Head		Cervical				Thoracic				Lumbar			
	F	E	F	E	S	R	F	E	S	R	F	E	S	R
Direction	X	X	X	X	O	O	X	X	X	O	X	X	X	X
Range	.	X	.	.	O	O	.	.	.	O	.	.	.	.
Contraction	X	.	X	.	.	.	.	.	.	.	X	X	.	.
Stretch	X	X	X	X	.	.	X	X	.	.	X	X	X	X

	Scapula				Shoulder					
	Re	Pr	El	De	F	E	Ab	Ad	Ir	Er
Direction	X	X	X	O	X	X	X	X	X	X
Range	X	X	.	O	X	X	X	X	X	X
Contraction	X	X	.	.	X	X	X	X	X	.
Stretch	X	X	.	.	X	X	X	X	X	X

	Elbow				Wrist				Hand		SI	
	F	E	P	Su	F	E	Ab	Ad	F	E	F	E
Direction	X	X	X	X	X	X	X	X	X	O	X	X
Range	X	X	.	.	X	X	.	.	.	O	.	.
Contraction	X	X	.	.	X	X	.	.	X	.	.	.
Stretch	X	X	.	.	X	X	X	X	X	X	X	X

	Hip						Knee		Foot				Toes	
	F	E	Ab	Ad	Ir	Er	F	E	Pf	Df	In	Ev	F	E
Direction	O	O	O	O	O	O	X	X	X	X	O	O	X	X
Range	O	O	O	O	O	O	O	O	.	.	O	O	.	.
Contraction	X	X	X	X	.	.	.	.	X	.	.	.	.	.
Stretch	X	X	X	.	.	.	X	X	X	X	.	.	X	X

Key: None (O) partial (.) full (X) Range = Range of joint movement, Contraction = Level of muscle contraction, Direction = Direction of movement Direction may be Flexion (F), Extension (E), Sidebending (S), Rotation (R), Retraction (Re), Protraction (Pr), Elevation (El), Depression (De), Abduction (Ab), Adduction (Ad), Internal rotation (Ir), External rotation (Er), Pronation (P), Supination (Su), Plantar flexion (Pf), Dorsi flexion (Df), Inversion, (In), Eversion (Ev)

Weekly stretching program for tennis

Day 1	Day 2	Day 3	Day 4	Day 5	Day 6	Day 7
1.3b	1.3a	1.4b	1.4a	2.0a	1.7c	1.9
2.5b	2.4a	2.4b	1.5	2.1b	1.7f	1.8
3.0a	2.7a	3.1a	2.5c	2.5a	2.6b	2.9a
2.7c	4.0e	4.1	3.8a	3.4	4.0c	2.8
4.4	4.3	3.5	3.8d	5.1a	4.8	4.0g
5.2a	4.5	5.5	3.8e	5.4	5.3a	5.6a
5.9	5.3a	5.8e	4.9c	5.8c	5.7b	5.8b
6.1a	6.5m	6.6a	6.2b	5.8d	6.1e	6.4b
6.7b	7.1g	6.7f	6.0a	7.2b	7.1b	7.1f

Throwing a ball

Throwing is used in many sports to propel an object over distance. The object is usually a ball but may be a knife, axe, or javelin. The type of object, its shape and size will influence how the object is thrown. These are the stretches for throwing a small ball with one hand from a stationary position.

Overarm throwing involves the scapula, arm, forearm and hand to impart velocity to the ball. Whereas in bowling (cricket) the elbow is extended in throwing the elbow is allowed to flex. Throwing is a more natural action than bowling.

Throwing requires skill and good upper limb flexibility. The throw involves scapula retraction then protraction, shoulder flexion, abduction and external rotation then extension, adduction and internal rotation, elbow flexion then extension and wrist extension and then flexion and some finger flexion. Throwing also involves head extension then flexion, cervical extension then flexion, lumbar and thoracolumbar extension then flexion, sacral flexion then extension and thoracolumbar rotation with sidebending. Stretch the muscles that contract (agonists) to produce movement and the muscles that need to be flexible to allow movement to occur (antagonists).

There is little or no movement in the lower limb during a throw from a stationary position but there is muscle contraction. The iliopsoas, gluteus maximus, hamstrings, hip abductors and adductors act as stabilises holding the lower limb in position during the throw.

Throwing	Head		Cervical				Thoracic				Lumbar			
	F	E	F	E	S	R	F	E	S	R	F	E	S	R
Direction	X	X	X	X	O	O	X	O	O	O	X	X	X	X
Range	.	.	.	.	O	O	.	O	O	O	.	.	.	.
Contraction	.	.	.	.	.	.	.	.	.	.	X	X	.	.
Stretch	X	X	X	X	.	.	.	.	.	.	X	X	X	X

	Scapula				Shoulder					
	Re	Pr	El	De	F	E	Ab	Ad	Ir	Er
Direction	X	X	O	O	X	X	X	X	X	X
Range	X	X	O	O	X	X	X	X	X	X
Contraction	X	X	.	.	X	X	X	X	X	X
Stretch	X	X	.	.	X	X	X	X	X	X

	Elbow				Wrist				Hand		SI	
	F	E	P	Su	F	E	Ab	Ad	F	E	F	E
Direction	X	X	O	O	X	X	O	O	X	O	X	X
Range	X	X	O	O	X	X	O	O	.	O	.	.
Contraction	X	X	.	.	X	X	.	.	X	.	.	.
Stretch	X	X	.	.	X	X	.	.	X	X	.	.

	Hip						Knee		Foot				Toes	
	F	E	Ab	Ad	Ir	Er	F	E	Pf	Df	In	Ev	F	E
Direction	O	O	O	O	O	O	O	O	O	O	O	O	O	O
Range	O	O	O	O	O	O	O	O	O	O	O	O	O	O
Contraction	X	X	X	.	.	.	.	.	X	.	.	.	.	.
Stretch	.	.	.	.	.	.	.	.	.	.	.	.	.	.

Key: None (O) partial (.) full (X) Range = Range of joint movement, Contraction = Level of muscle contraction, Direction = Direction of movement Direction may be Flexion (F), Extension (E), Sidebending (S), Rotation (R), Retraction (Re), Protraction (Pr), Elevation (El), Depression (De), Abduction (Ab), Adduction (Ad), Internal rotation (Ir), External rotation (Er), Pronation (P), Supination (Su), Plantar flexion (Pf), Dorsi flexion (Df), Inversion, (In), Eversion (Ev)

Weekly stretching program for throwing

Day 1	Day 2	Day 3	Day 4	Day 5	Day 6	Day 7
1.7d	1.3a	1.4b	1.4a	2.0a	1.7c	1.9
2.5b	2.4a	2.4b	1.5	2.1b	1.7f	1.8
3.0a	2.7a	3.1a	2.5c	2.5a	2.6a	2.9a
2.9b	3.2b	4.1	3.8a	3.4	4.0c	2.8
4.0b	4.0e	3.5	3.8d	4.2	4.8	4.0g
4.4	4.5	5.5	3.8e	5.4	4.9e	4.9c
5.2a	5.3a	5.8e	5.6b	5.8c	5.7b	5.6a
5.8a	5.7a	5.9	6.2b	5.8d	6.1e	5.8b
6.1a	6.5m	6.6a	6.0a	6.7f	7.1b	6.4b

Volleyball and beach volleyball

Volleyball is a team sport involving two teams of six players separated by a net. It is played inside or outside on a rectangular court that is wood, grass or on sand as beach volleyball. Each team attempts to score points by grounding a ball on the other team's court. Rules allow the ball to be touch up to 3 times but individual players may not touch the ball twice consecutively.

Volleyball requires flexibility, agility and good eye ball coordination. It involves head flexion and extension, cervical flexion, extension, sidebending and rotation, thoracic and lumbar flexion and extension and sidebending, sacroiliac flexion and extension, scapula retraction, protraction and elevation, shoulder flexion, extension, abduction, adduction, internal rotation and external rotation, elbow flexion, extension, supination and pronation, wrist flexion, extension, abduction and adduction, finger flexion and extension, hip extension, abduction and adduction, knee flexion and extension, ankle dorsiflexion and plantar flexion, foot inversion and eversion and toe flexion and extension. In beach volleyball there is greater foot plantar flexion, inversion and eversion and toe flexion because of the greater demand on the lower limb to push against sand.

Volleyball	Head		Cervical				Thoracic				Lumbar			
	F	E	F	E	S	R	F	E	S	R	F	E	S	R
Direction	X	X	X	X	X	X	X	X	X	O	X	X	X	O
Range	.	X	.	X	X	.	X	X	X	O	X	X	X	O
Contraction	X	.	X	.	.	.	X	X	X	X	X	X	X	X
Stretch	X	X	X	X	X	.	X	X	X	.	X	X	X	.

	Scapula				Shoulder					
	Re	Pr	El	De	F	E	Ab	Ad	Ir	Er
Direction	X	X	X	O	X	X	X	X	X	X
Range	X	X	.	O	X	.	X	.	.	X
Contraction	X	X	X	X	X	X	X	X	X	X
Stretch	X	X	X	X	X	X	X	X	X	X

	Elbow				Wrist				Hand		SI	
	F	E	P	Su	F	E	Ab	Ad	F	E	F	E
Direction	X	X	X	X	X	X	X	X	X	X	X	X
Range	.	X	.	.	.	X	.	.	.	X	X	.
Contraction	X	X	.	.	X	X	.	.	X	.	.	X
Stretch	X	X	X	X	X	X	X	X	X	X	X	X

	Hip						Knee		Foot				Toes	
	F	E	Ab	Ad	Ir	Er	F	E	Pf	Df	In	Ev	F	E
Direction	X	X	X	X	O	O	X	X	X	X	X	X	X	X
Range	.	X	.	X	O	O	.	X	X	X	.	.	.	X
Contraction	.	X	X	X	.	.	.	X	X	.	.	.	X	.
Stretch	X	X	X	X	.	.	X	X	X	X	X	X	X	X

Key: None (O) partial (.) full (X) Range = Range of joint movement, Contraction = Level of muscle contraction, Direction = Direction of movement Direction may be Flexion (F), Extension (E), Sidebending (S), Rotation (R), Retraction (Re), Protraction (Pr), Elevation (El), Depression (De), Abduction (Ab), Adduction (Ad), Internal rotation (Ir), External rotation (Er), Pronation (P), Supination (Su), Plantar flexion (Pf), Dorsi flexion (Df), Inversion, (In), Eversion (Ev)

Weekly stretching program for volleyball

Day 1	Day 2	Day 3	Day 4	Day 5	Day 6	Day 7
1.9	1.3a	1.4a	1.4b	1.4c	1.7a	1.7d
1.2	2.0a	1.5	2.1a	1.8	1.7f	2.1b
2.5c	2.5a	1.7b	2.5b	2.4a	2.4d	2.6c
2.6a	2.9b	2.6b	3.0a	2.7a	3.0e	3.4
3.2a	4.0c	3.9a	3.8d	4.1	3.8b	4.0g
4.0b	4.2	4.5	3.8e	5.4	3.8c	4.8
4.9b	5.0a	5.2a	6.6a	6.4h	6.0a	5.8c
6.1c	6.2b	6.4a	6.7f	6.5f	6.1e	5.8d
7.1b	6.5h	7.2b	7.1f	6.7b	7.3a	6.9a

Walking, running and sprinting

Walking, running and sprinting are the actions of moving the body forward. Similar muscles are used in all these actions. But the mechanics and the level of muscle contraction and aerobic respiration are different. Muscles are mainly used for support and forward propulsion. They work harder during running and sprinting and some muscles and tendons function differently, soleus and the Achilles tendon for example.

Running and sprinting differs from walking in several ways: the time spent in the stance phase, whether the knees are flexed of locked in extension and the level of involvement of the Achilles tendon in recovering energy from ground contact for propulsion. Aerobic respiration in running is greater than in walking.

Running is over longer distances for endurance and sprinting is over shorter distances and for speed. Running includes jogging, road racing, cross country running, fell running, trail running and marathons. Other forms of running include running and jumping over hurdles and running and weaving such as in rugby and some types of football. Weaving will increase contraction and tighten the lateral muscles of the body, for example tensor fasciae latae, gluteus maximus and medius and cause shortening of the iliotibial band.

During walking one foot is always on the ground and at regular points during the walking cycle both feet are on the ground at the same time and the stance phase is more than half of the gait cycle. During running there is no period when both feet are in contact with the ground and at regular points in the running cycle both feet are off the ground. As the body moves faster less time is spent in stance and sprinters spend the least time in the stance phase, about a quarter of the gait cycle.

During walking the knees are locked and a straight leg moves like an inverted pendulum pivoting around the foot. In contrast the knees are unlocked during running and the legs move more like a wheel. Also during running the Achilles tendon and other tendons play a greater role in recycling impact energy into propulsion. The elasticity of the tendon is used to spring the body forward. About half of the propulsion comes from the Achilles tendon and the other half comes from muscle contraction.

With greater knee flexion during running the quadriceps are able to contract more strongly and this increases the force exerted on the ground. Greater force is exerted by soleus, gastrocnemius, gluteus maximus and the hamstrings during running. Soleus has a more significant role in forward propulsion during walking and a more stabilising role during running. Upper limb muscle contraction also increases during running and this also helps stabilize the body.

Running involves the coordinated alternating movement of the left and right sides of the body: scapula retraction and protraction, shoulder extension and flexion, elbow flexion and extension, hip flexion and extension, knee flexion and extension, ankle plantar flexion and dorsiflexion and foot and toe flexion and extension. Other movements include head extension, upper cervical extension and lower cervical flexion, thoracic flexion, rib inhalation and exhalation, lumbar flexion, sidebending and rotation, shoulder abduction, finger flexion, hip abduction and foot inversion and eversion.

Walking, running and sprinting requires muscle strength, good joint integrity, cardiovascular and respiratory fitness and all round flexibility. Stretching helps by lengthening muscles and fascia and this facilitates joint movement.

When deciding which stretches to use for the weekly program all of these different muscle groups are considered: the prime movers which move the body, the antagonists which allow movement, the stabilisers which stabilise joints and the neutralisers which cancel out unwanted actions by other muscles.

Walking, running and sprinting	Head		Cervical				Thoracic				Lumbar			
	F	E	F	E	S	R	F	E	S	R	F	E	S	R
Direction	O	X	X	X	X	X	X	O	O	O	X	O	X	X
Range	O	.	.	.	.	.	.	O	O	O	.	O	.	.
Contraction	.	.	.	.	.	.	.	X	.	.	X	X	.	.
Stretch	.	X	X	X	.	.	X	X	.	.	X	X	X	X

	Scapula				Shoulder					
	Re	Pr	El	De	F	E	Ab	Ad	Ir	Er
Direction	X	X	O	O	X	X	X	O	O	O
Range	X	X	O	O	X	X	.	O	O	O
Contraction	X	X	.	.	X	X	.	.	.	.
Stretch	X	X	.	.	X	X	X	.	.	.

	Elbow				Wrist				Hand		SI	
	F	E	P	Su	F	E	Ab	Ad	F	E	F	E
Direction	X	X	O	O	O	O	O	O	X	O	X	X
Range	X	X	O	O	O	O	O	O	X	O	.	.
Contraction	X	X	.	.	.	.	.	.	X	.	.	.
Stretch	X	X	.	.	.	.	.	.	X	.	X	X

	Hip						Knee		Foot				Toes	
	F	E	Ab	Ad	Ir	Er	F	E	Pf	Df	In	Ev	F	E
Direction	X	X	X	O	O	O	X	X	X	X	X	X	X	X
Range	X	X	.	O	O	O	X	X	X	X	X	X	.	.
Contraction	X	X	.	.	.	.	X	X	X	X	.	.	.	.
Stretch	X	X	X	X	.	.	X	X	X	X	X	X	X	X

Key: None (O) partial (.) full (X) Range = Range of joint movement, Contraction = Level of muscle contraction, Direction = Direction of movement Direction may be Flexion (F), Extension (E), Sidebending (S), Rotation (R), Retraction (Re), Protraction (Pr), Elevation (El), Depression (De), Abduction (Ab), Adduction (Ad), Internal rotation (Ir), External rotation (Er), Pronation (P), Supination (Su), Plantar flexion (Pf), Dorsi flexion (Df), Inversion, (In), Eversion (Ev)

Weekly stretching program for walking, running and sprinting

Day 1	Day 2	Day 3	Day 4	Day 5	Day 6	Day 7
1.3a	1.4a	1.4b	1.3b	1.7d	1.8	1.9
2.1b	1.5	2.5a	2.5b	2.0a	2.1a	2.4a
2.6a	1.6	3.0a	3.0e	2.0b	2.6b	2.8
3.6	1.7a	3.5	3.2a	3.1a	3.1b	2.9a
3.7	1.7f	4.5	4.0b	4.0e	4.0g	4.1
3.8a	4.8	5.1a	5.2a	5.9	5.3a	4.9a
6.0a	6.1a	6.0c	6.4a	6.1e	6.4d	6.5c
6.5h	6.6a	6.5l	6.7a	6.7b	6.7f	6.9a
7.1a	7.1d	7.1b	7.1f	7.1c	7.2b	7.3b

Windsurfing and surfing

Windsurfing combines aspects of surfing and sailing. A windsurfer is like a surfboard fitted with a movable mast and sail and powered by the wind. A windsurfer rides it by standing upright on the board and manoeuvres the sail so as to catch the wind. Windsurfing requires coordination, balance, strength, flexibility, and physical fitness. Wind and wave forces can be strong and place great demand on muscles, ligaments and tendons, especially in rotator cuff tendons, wrist extensor tendons and ligaments and in the lumbar spine.

Day 1	Day 2	Day 3	Day 4	Day 5	Day 6	Day 7
1.1a	1.3b	1.4b	1.4a	1.7d	1.9	1.7c
2.0b	2.1b	1.8	1.5	2.4a	2.4d	1.7f
2.5c	2.5b	2.9a	1.6	3.0a	3.0e	3.1a
3.2b	4.0b	2.8	1.7a	3.7	4.0c	4.0g
4.4	4.5	3.5	4.8	3.8a	4.9b	5.0a
5.1a	5.2a	5.3a	5.5	3.8c	5.6b	5.7b
5.4	6.0b	6.1c	5.8b	3.9a	6.2c	6.3d
6.4b	6.4d	6.5a	6.5f	6.5h	6.5m	6.6a
6.7f	6.7b	6.9a	7.1d	7.1f	7.2b	7.6

Weekly stretching program for whole body flexibility involving all the joints in the body, suitable for ballet, gymnastics and wrestling.

Day 1	Day 2	Day 3	Day 4	Day 5	Day 6	Day 7
1.1c	1.3c	1.4c	1.4a	1.7c	2.2b	2.4a
2.0a	2.1c	1.7i	1.5	1.7f	2.5b	2.6b
2.6d	2.7c	2.9a	1.6	3.0c	3.1a	3.3
3.4	4.0d	2.8	1.7a	3.8a	4.0e	4.0h
4.2	4.5	4.6b	5.4	3.8c	4.9c	5.0a
5.1b	5.2c	5.5	5.6a	3.8e	5.7c	5.7d
5.9	6.0c	6.1e	6.2a	3.9b	6.3a	6.3b
6.4c	6.4g	6.5c	6.5g	6.5j	6.5m	6.6f
6.7b	6.7g	7.0a	7.1a	7.1e	7.3a	7.3d

Appendix

Joint ranges of movement

<u>Temporomandibular joint (TMJ)</u>
Opening 35 – 55 mm measured from the upper incisal edge to the lower.
Side to side or lateral movement 7 – 12 mm measured from the mid-line to one side.
Protrusion retraction total is 6 – 10 mm Protrusion = 4 – 7 mm Retraction = 2 – 3 mm
Protrusion is taking the chin forwards and retraction is taking the chin and backwards.

<u>Atlanto-occipital joint</u>
Occiput and atlas (C1) is mostly concerned with flexion and extension or nodding of the head. Total flexion extension is quite variable, even between left and right sides, and is between 8 and 20 degrees. Sidebending is less than 5 degrees on each side. Rotation is less than 5 degrees on each side.

<u>Atlanto-axial joint</u>
Atlas (C1) and axis (C2) is mostly concerned with rotation of the head and accounts for about half of the total head rotation.
Rotation is 45 degrees but varies between people and can be as low as 35 degrees on each side. Flexion is about 5 degrees. Extension is about 10 degrees. Sidebending is between 1 and 3 degrees on each side.

<u>Lower cervical spine</u> (C2 to C7)
Rotation in the lower cervical spine is about 45 degrees, and the amount of rotation diminishes progressively as you decend the lower cervical spine. Other movements increase as you decend so that most flexion, extension and sidebending occurs between C5 and C6. This is because at this level the facet joint are 45 degrees which is the optimum angle for movement. Also there is greater range of movement in women than men.

Range of movement decreases in the lower cervical spine with age, mainly due to loss of disc height and the presence of pathology. The greatest level of pathology limiting range of movement is between C5 and C6, folowed by C6 and C7, and then C4 and C5.

<u>Total cervical and suboccipital spine</u>
Flexion 40 to 50 degrees. Extension 80 to 90 degrees.
Sidebending (lateral flexion) is 35 to 45 degrees and most occurs between C2 and C7
Rotation is 80 to 90 degrees in each direction – most occuring at the atalantoaxial joint.

<u>Thoracic movement</u>
Flexion 40 to 50 degrees
Extension 20 to 30 degrees
Sidebending 20 degrees
Rotation 25 to 35 degrees (add 15 degrees for passive rotation).

<u>Lumbar movement</u>
Flexion 40 to 60 degrees
Extension 20 to 40 degrees
Sidebending 20 degrees
Rotation 5 degrees

Zygapophyseal facet joint orientation is extremely variable throughout the lumbar spine but in general favors flexion and extension and limits sidebending and rotation.

<u>Total thoracic and lumbar movement</u>
Flexion 90 to 110 degrees.
Extension 40 to 60 degrees
Sidebending 30 to 40 degrees
Rotation 30 to 40 degrees (add 15 degrees for passive rotation)

The mid to lower thoracic spine is most mobile in rotation and is about 8 degrees per segment. In general in the thoracic and lumbar spine the areas of least flexibility are C7 to T3 and L1 to L4, and the areas of greatest flexibility are T11 to L1 and T6 to T8.

Thoracic and lumbar movement at each vertebral level

Lumbar rotation is only about 1 degree per vertebra throughout the lumbar spine. But flexion, extension and sidebending are greater. In general the range of flexion and extension increases as you decend the spine from L1/2 to L4/5 but then decreases slightly between L5/S1. Flexion-extension at L1/2 is 8 degrees, L2/3 is 9 degrees, L3/4 is 12 degrees, L4/5 is 12 degrees, and L5/S1 is 10 degrees but extremely variable.

In general the range of sidebending and rotation decreases as you decend the spine from L1/2 to L5/S1. It is usually least at L5/S1 because of the common 45 deg orientation of the facets to the sagital plane, but the L5/S1 facet orientation show conciderable variation and the range varies accordingly.

The total range of sacroiliac nutation and counter-nutation is between one and three degrees. The sacroiliac joints show considerable variation in shape and surface features. Surface irregularities increase with age and its range of movement decreases with age.

Shoulder

Movement at the shoulder is a combination of scapulothoracic, acromioclavicular, sternoclavicular and glenohumeral joint movement. Shoulder flexion is a combination of glenohumeral flexion, scapular protraction, backward tilt and upward rotation. Shoulder extension is a combination of glenohumeral extension, scapular retraction, forward tilt and downward rotation.

Total shoulder flexion or abduction is between 170 and 180 degrees (add 10 to 15 degrees for passive movement). This is a combination of glenohumeral joint and scapulothoracic joint movement. As an average over the whole range of movement, for every 2 degrees of glenohumeral abduction there will usually be about 1 degree of scapular rotation. So there is 120 degrees glenohumeral joint and 60 degrees scapulothoracic joint movement.

When the arm is slightly abducted total scapulothoracic and glenohumeral internal rotation is between 90 and 110 degrees (add 10 degrees for passive movement) and external rotation is 50 to 80 degrees (add 15 degrees for passive movement).

The scapula rests 5 cm from the midline between ribs 2 and 7. It sits 30 to 40 degrees to the frontal plane and 10 to 20 degrees from vertical.

Scapulothoracic movement

Medial to lateral movement of the scapula along the rib cage is about 14 cm, a combination of 10 cm protraction and 4 cm retraction. There is a total of 60 degrees of upward-downward rotation of the scapular during abduction-adduction of the shoulder. There is a total of 20 to 30 degrees of forward-backward tilting of the scapular during flexion-extension of the shoulder. Total scapular elevation-depression is between 10 and 12 cm, of which elevation is about 10 cm and depression is between 1 and 2 cm.

Glenohumeral movement

Abduction and Flexion. There is between 90 and 120 degrees of pure glenohumeral movement (flexion and abduction) and the remainder is a combination of acromioclavicular, sternoclavicular and scapulothoracic movement, with additional movement in the lumbar spine during unilateral action. Total abduction is about 180 degrees.

Due to the greater tubercle contacting the coracoacromial arch, only 60 degrees abduction is possible at the glenohumeral joint when the arm is internally rotated and only 90 degrees abduction is possible when the arm is in neutral. But when the arm is externally rotated greater glenohumeral abduction is possible. Between 90 and 120 degrees of active abduction may be possible at the glenohumeral joint when the arm is externally rotated.

Extension is between 50 and 60 degrees (Add 30 degrees for passive movement).

Rotation
With the arm adducted close to the side of the body, total medial-lateral rotation at the glenohumeral joint is only about 50 or 60 degrees. Medial rotation is limited by the lesser tubercle making contact with the anterior glenoid fossa, and lateral rotation is limited by the greater tubercle making contact with the acromion. Most of the rotation is therefore coming from the scapula moving on the rib cage.

Rotation at the glenohumeral joint increases when the arm is abducted because the tubercles are able to clear the joint. When the forearm hits the front of the body at about 70 degrees internal rotation, any further internal rotation can only be obtained by abducting the arm and passing the forearm behind the back.

With the arm abducted to 90 degrees this allows a much greater amount of rotation because movement is only limited by the tension of the capsule and muscles. Approximately 120 degrees of active rotation is possible when the glenohumeral joint is at 90 degrees abduction, consisting of about 70 degrees external rotation and 50 degrees internal rotation.

Horizontal abduction or horizontal extension 30 to 40 degrees
Horizontal adduction or horizontal flexion 140 degrees
Adduction in extension 5 to 10 degrees. Adduction in flexion 30 to 45 degrees.

Sternoclavicular joint (SC)
Shoulder elevation results in about 10 cm superior movement at the distal end of the clavicle, and about 30 degrees upward movement of the clavicle at the SC joint.
Shoulder depression results in about 3 cm inferior movement at the distal end of the clavicle and about 5 degrees downward movement of the clavicle at the SC joint.
Shoulder protraction results in about 10 cm anterior movement at the distal end of the clavicle and about 15 degrees forward movement of the clavicle at the SC joint.
Shoulder retraction results in about 3 cm posterior movement at the distal end of the clavicle.
Shoulder flexion-extension results in between 30 and 50 degrees rotation of the clavicle and about 15 degrees backward movement of the clavicle at the SC joint.

Clavicular elevation is 45 degrees and depression is 15 degrees.
Clavicular rotation 30 to 50 degrees.
Posterior clavicular rotation occurs with additional scapular backward tilt and anterior clavicular rotation occurs with additional scapular forward tilt.

Elbow
Supination (rotation outward) 90 degrees.
Pronation (rotation inward) 90 degrees.
Flexion Active is 135 to 150 degrees and passive is 150 to 160 degrees.
In most men there is no extension at the elbow due to the bony anatomy of the joint.
In women and hypermobile people there may be 15 degrees hyperextension at the elbow.
The carrying angle at the elbow is about 5 degrees in men and 15 degrees in women and anything greater is regarded as abnormal and is called a cubitus valgus.

Wrist
Flexion 80 to 90 degrees (add 10 degrees for passive flexion)
Extension 75 to 85 degrees (add 10 degrees for passive extension)
Although some flexion and extension occur at both the radiocarpal joints and midcarpal joints most wrist flexion occurs at the radiocarpal joint and most wrist extension occurs at the midcarpal joint.
Wrist abduction (radial deviation) is 15 to 20 degrees
Wrist adduction (ulnar deviation) 40 to 45 degrees
Most adduction occurs at the radiocarpal joint but abduction is equally split between radiocarpal and midcarpal joints.

Hand
Metacarpophalangeal joint (MCP) abduction 20 to 25 degrees.
MCP adduction 20 degrees.
MCP flexion 90 degrees at index finger progressing to 110 degrees at the little finger.
MCP extension 10 degrees (add 20 degrees for passive extension) is consistent between fingers but varies widely between individuals. Passive MCP extension is a measure of the generalized mobility of an individual.
The range of proximal interphalangeal joint (PIP) flexion increases from about 100 degrees at the index finger to 135 degrees at the little finger.
The range of distal interphalangeal joint (DIP) flexion increases from about 80 degrees at the index finger to 90 degrees at the little finger.
Metacarpophalangeal joint of thumb abduction 0-50 degrees.
MCP of thumb adduction 40 degrees.
MCP of thumb flexion 70 to 80 degrees.
MCP of thumb extension is negligible but there may be 15 degrees passive extension.
Interphalangeal joint of thumb flexion 90 degrees.

Motion of the thumb between the trapezium and the first metacarpal bone is 50 to 55 degrees flexion/extension and 40 to 45 degrees abduction/adduction and 15 to 20 degrees rotation. Flexion/extension of the thumb occurs around an oblique anteroposterior axis so motion occurs nearly parallel to the palm. Abduction/adduction of the thumb occurs around an oblique coronal axis so motion is nearly perpendicular to the palm.

Hip
Flexion 120 to 130 degrees when knee is flexed but 90 degrees when knee is extended due to hamstring tension.
Extension 10 to 20 (30) degrees (add 10 degrees for passive extension) but is limited to between 5 and 10 degrees when the knee is flexed due to rectus femoris tension.
Abduction 45 degrees (Passive abduction may be 90 degrees).
Adduction 20 to 35 degrees (Passive adduction may be 45 degrees).
Internal rotation (with the hip in neutral or flexion) 35 to 45 degrees.
(Add 10 to 20 degrees for passive internal rotation).
External rotation (with the hip in neutral or flexion) 40 to 50 degrees.
(Add 10 to 20 degrees for passive external rotation).

Knee
Flexion is 130 to 140 degrees. Add 20 degrees for passive flexion, so for example when squatting there is usually at least 160 degrees flexion at the knee.
Extension is usually zero, but between 5 and 10 degrees hyperextension is considered normal. In hypermobile people there may be 10 to 15 degrees hyperextension.
At 90 degrees knee flexion, between 60 and 70 degrees active or passive tibial rotation is possible. The knee joint capsule and ligaments are at their most lax state and the knee in it most loose packed position at 90 degrees flexion. The range of rotation decreases progressively as the knee moves toward greater flexion or extension.
Tibial internal/inwards/medial rotation (with the knee flexed) is 30 degrees.
Tibial external/outwards/lateral rotation (with the knee flexed) is 40 degrees.

Ankle (talocrural joint)
Plantarflexion and dorsiflexion are the primary movements occurring at the ankle. But between 20% and 50% of movement may occur in the intertarsal joints.
Plantarflexion (downward movement of the foot) is 30 to 50 degrees and dorsiflexion (movement upward) is 20 to 30 degrees. Dorsiflexion is greater by about 10 degrees when the knee is flexed due to the release of tension on gastrocnemius.
Plantarflexion and dorsiflexion occur on an oblique axis. So during plantarflexion, in addition to the downward movement, the foot also moves medial to the leg (toe-in) and longitudinally to the midline (supination or inversion), and during dorsiflexion, in addition to the upward movement, the foot also moves lateral to the leg (toe-out) and longitudinally away from the midline (pronation or eversion).
There is between 5 and 10 degrees rotation and tilt of the talus within the mortise of the ankle joint - adduction/abduction and inversion/eversion.

Foot

There may be a considerable individual differences in the range of movement in the foot, and a considerable difference between active and passive ranges of movement.

The primary movement at the subtalar joint is supination and pronation which is a composite of inversion and eversion, and adduction and abduction and a small amount of plantarflexion and dorsiflexion. In the non-weight bearing foot inversion (longitudinal axis), adduction (vertical axis) and plantarflexion (coronal axis) occur together, and eversion, abduction and dorsiflexion occur together.

Inversion/ varus (turned inward) is 20 to 30 degrees.

Eversion/ valgus (turned outwards) is 5 to 15 degrees.

Flexion of metatarsophalangeal joints 30 degrees.

Extension of metatarsophalangeal joints 80 degrees.

Abduction/adduction are secondary movements of the metatarsophalangeal joints.

Flexion of interphalangeal joints of toe 60 degrees (add 10 degrees for passive flexion)

Extension of interphalangeal joints of toes 50 degrees (add 30 degrees for passive extension)

Limiting factors in the spine

Flexion

Tectorial membrane, posterior atlantoaxial ligament and osseous contact at the atlanto-occipital joint - above C2.

Ligamentum nuchae - between the occiput and C7.

Posterior longitudinal ligament - from C2 to sacrum (especially in the cervical and thoracic).

Supraspinous and interspinous ligament (especially in the thoracic spine).

Rib cage.

Zygapophyseal joint capsule (especially in upper thoracic and thoracolumbar spine).

Ligamentum flavum and interspinous ligament (especially in the lumbar spine).

Compression of the annulus fibrosis of the intervertebral disc.

Extension

Anterior atlantoaxial ligament - between C1 and C2.

Anterior longitudinal ligament - from C2 to sacrum (especially in the cervical, lumbar and lower thoracic spine).

Contact between spines and laminae of vertebrae (especially in the cervical and thoracic).

Contact between zygapophyseal facet joints (especially in the thoracic spine).

Tension of abdominal muscles and other anterior muscles.

Tension of zygapophyseal joint capsule.

Sidebending

Uncinate processes of cervical vertebrae (also posterior translation).

Zygapophyseal facet joint closure.

Tension of the rib cage.

Compression of the annulus fibrosis of the intervertebral disc.

Intertransverse ligaments (especially in the lumbar).

Iliolumbar ligaments (lumbar spine).

Zygapophyseal joint capsule.

Lateral muscles of the trunk.

Rotation

Annulus fibrosis of the intervertebral disc - true for rotation of vertebrae of the spine in general (also distraction and translation of vertebral bodies).

Zygapophyseal joint capsules (especially in upper thoracic and thoracolumbar spine).

Rib cage

Aging and degeneration (especially in the thoracic, lower cervical and lower lumbar spine)

Zygapophyseal facet joint orientation - lumbar rotation is extremely limited.

Rotation and sidebending

Alar ligament - between C1 and C2.

Flexion, extension, sidebending, rotation and anterior sliding of L5 on the sacrum.

Iliolumbar ligaments

Table of anatomical movements

Joints / body parts and directions of movement			
Cervical spine			
Flexion	Extension	Sidebending	Rotation
Thoracic spine (& Lumbar)			
Flexion	Extension	Sidebending	Rotation
Scapulothoracic joint (scapular)			
Elevation	Depression	Protraction	Retraction
Downward rotation	Upward rotation	Backward tilt	Forward tilt
Glenohumeral (shoulder) joint			
Flexion	Extension	Abduction	Adduction
Horizontal abduction	Horizontal adduction	External rotation	Internal rotation
Elbow & forearm			
Flexion	Extension	Supination	Pronation

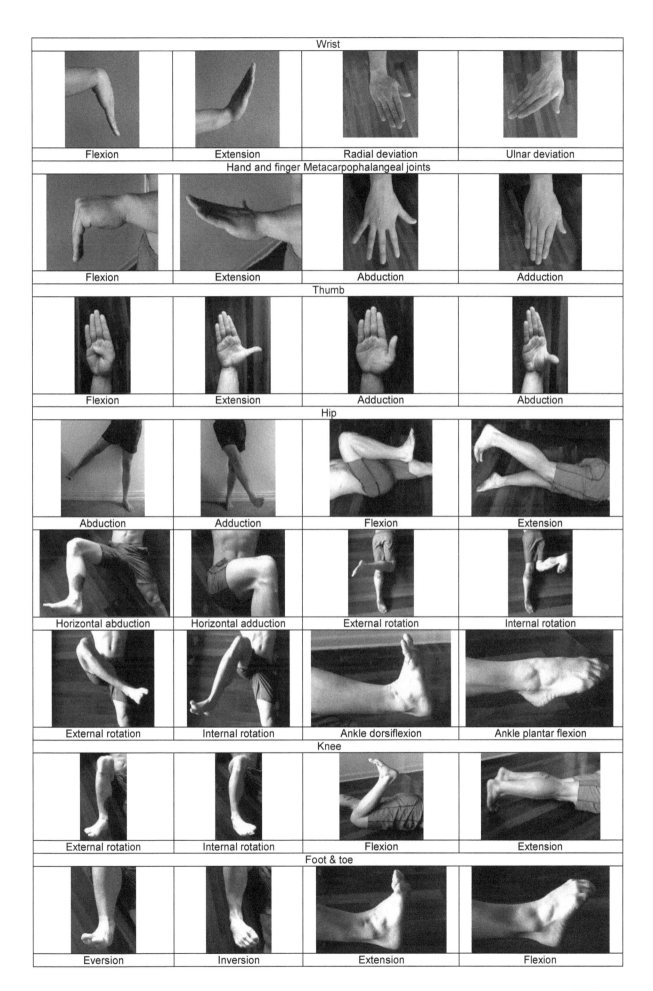

Tables of muscle actions

Shoulder joint / Arm

Muscle contracted / Movement	Flex	Ext	Hyp Ext	Abd	Add	Out Rot	In Rot	Horiz Flex	Horiz Ext	Out rot @ 90	Int rot @ 90
Middle deltoid				X							
Supraspinatus				X							
Latissimus dorsi		X	X		X		X		X		X
Teres major		X	X		X		X		X		X
Anterior deltoid	X				x lo		X	X			x
Pectoralis major clavicular fibres	X		X				X	X			
Pectoralis major sternal fibres		X			X		X	x			X
Coracobrachialis	x				x		x	x			
Subscapularis					x 90+		X	X			
Posterior deltoid		X			x lo	X			X		
Infraspinatus				x up	x lo	X			x		
Teres minor					X	X			X		
Biceps brachii	x				x			x			
Triceps brachii long head		x	x		x	x					

Muscle stretched / Movement /	Flex 90+	Hyp Ext	Abd 90+	Add ant	Add post	Out Rot	In Rot	Horiz Flex	Horiz Ext	Out rot @ 90	Int rot @ 90
Middle deltoid				X	X						
Supraspinatus				X	X						
Latissimus dorsi	X		X			x		x		x	
Teres major	X		X			x		x		x	
Anterior deltoid		X				X			X	x	
Pectoralis major clavicular fibres		x				X			X		
Pectoralis major sternal fibres	X		X						X	X	
Coracobrachialis		X							X		
Subscapularis						X					
Posterior deltoid	x						X	X			
Infraspinatus							X	x			x
Teres minor	x						X	x			
Biceps brachii		x							x		
Triceps brachii long head	x		x								

X = prime mover or primary muscle stretched
x = secondary mover or secondary muscle stretched
up = upper fibres
lo = lower fibres
an = anterior fibres
90+ = above 90 degrees
@ 90 = arm is at 90 degrees abduction

Shoulder girdle / Scapula

Muscle contracted / Movement	Elevation	Depression	Abd'n / Protraction (+ lat tilt + up rotn)	Add'n / Retraction (+ med tilt + down rotn)	Upward rot'n	Downward rot'n	Upward tit	Downward tilt
Subclavius		X clav						
Pectoralis minor		X	X			X	X	
Latissimus dorsi		X		X		x	X	
Serratus anterior upper			X		x			
Serratus ant lower fibres	X		x		X			x
Pectoralis major clavicular fibres	X		X					
Pectoralis major sternal fibres		X	X				x	
Levator scapulae	X					X	x	
Trapezius 1	X							
2	X			x	X			
3				X				
4		X		x	X			
Rhomboid min	X			X		x		x
Rhomboid maj	x			X		X		x

Muscle stretched / Movement	Elevation	Depression	Abd'n / Protraction (+ lat tilt + up rotn)	Add'n / Retraction (+ med tilt + down rotn)	Upward rot'n	Downward rot'n	Upward tit	Downward tilt
Subclavius	X clav							
Pectoralis minor	X			X	X			X
Latissimus dorsi	x		x		x			x
Serratus ant upper fibres		X		X				
Serratus ant lower fibres						X	x	
Pectoralis major clavicular fibres		x		x				
Pectoralis major sternal fibres	x			x	x			x
Levator scapulae		X					x	x
Trapezius 1		X						
2		X	x			X		
3		x	X					
4	X		x			X		
Rhomboid min		X	X					
Rhomboid maj		X	X		X		x	

Elbow & Radioulnar joint / Forearm

Muscle contracted / Movement	Flexion	Extension	Pronation	Supination
Biceps brachii	X			X
Brachialis	X			
Brachioradialis	X			
Pronator teres	x		X	
Pronator quadratus			X	
Triceps brachii		X		
Aconeus		X		
Supinator				X
Ext carpi ulnaris	x			
Ext carpi rad longus	x			
Ext carpi rad brevis	x			

Muscle stretched / Movement	Flexion	Extension	Pronation	Supination
Biceps brachii		X	X	
Brachialis		X		
Brachioradialis		X	x	x
Pronator teres		x		X
Pronator quadratus				X
Triceps brachii	X			
Aconeus	X			
Supinator			X	
Ext carpi ulnaris		x		
Ext carpi rad longus		x		
Ext carpi rad brevis		x		

Wrist and hand

Muscle contracted / Movement	Wrist				Finger	
	Flexion	Extension	Radial dev'n / Abduction	Ulnar dev'n / Adduction	Flexion	Extension
Ext carpi ulnaris		X		X		
Ext carpi radialis longus		X	X			
Ext carpi radialis brevis		X	X			
Flex carpi ulnaris	X			X		
Flex carpi radialis	X		x			
Palmaris longus	X					
Ext digit communis		x				X
Ext digiti minimi		x				X
Ext indicis		x				X
Flex digit profundus	x				X	
Flex digit superficialis	x				X	
Flex pollicis longus	X				X	
Abd pollicis longus	x		X		x	

Muscle stretched / Movement	Wrist				Finger	
	Flexion	Extension	Radial dev'n / Abduction	Ulnar dev'n / Adduction	Flexion	Extension
Ext carpi ulnaris	X		X			
Ext carpi radialis longus	X			X		
Ext carpi radialis brevis	X			X		
Flex carpi ulnaris		X	X			
Flex carpi radialis		X		x		
Palmaris longus		X				X
Ext digit communis	x				X	
Ext digiti minimi					X	
Ext indicis	x				X	
Flex digit profundus		x				X
Flex digit superficialis		x				X
Flex pollicis longus		X				X
Abd pollicis longus		x		X		x

Hip joint / Thigh

Muscle contracted / Movement	Flex	Ext	Add	Abd	Out Rot	In Rot	Add @ 90	Abd @ 90 deg	Out rot @ 90	Int rot @ 90
Psoas major	X				x					
Iliacus	X				x					
Sartoroius	X			x	x					
Pectineus	X		x							
Tensor fasiae latae	X			x		x				
Rectus femoris	X									
Gluteus maximus		X	x lo	x up	X			X lo	x	
Biceps femoris		X			x					
Semitendinosus		X				x				
Semimembranosus		X								
Gluteus medius				X		X an		X		
Gluteus minimus				X		X		x		X
Gracilis	x		X							
Adductor longus	x		X							
Adductor brevis	x		X							
Adductor magnus		X	X			x lo	x		x	
Piriformis				x	x			X		
Obturator internus					X			x		
Obturator externus					X					
Gamelus superior					X			x		
Gamelus inferior					X			x		
Quadratus femoris					X					

Muscle stretched / Movement	Flex	Ext	Add	Abd	Out Rot	In Rot	Add @ 90	Abd @ 90 deg	Out rot @ 90	Int rot @ 90
Psoas major		X				x				
Iliacus		X				x				
Sartorius		X	x			x				
Pectineus		X		x						
Tensor fasciae latae		X	x							
Rectus femoris		X								
Gluteus maximus	X		X up	X lo		X	X lo			x
Biceps femoris	X					x				
Semitendinosus	X				x					
Semimembranosus	X									
Gluteus medius		X			X an		X			
Gluteus minimus		X			X		x		X	
Gracilis		x		X						
Adductor longus		x		X						
Adductor brevis		x		X						
Adductor magnus	X			X	X lo			x		X up
Piriformis			x			x	X			
Obturator internus						X	x			
Obturator externus						X				
Gamelus superior						X	x			
Gamelus inferior						X	x			
Quadratus femoris						X				

@ 90 = hip at 90 degrees flexion
an = anterior fibres
up = upper fibres
lo = lower fibres

Knee joint / Leg

Muscle contracted / Movement	Flex	Ext	Out Rot	In Rot
Rectus femoris		X		
Vastus intermedius		X		
Vastus lateralis		X		
Vastus medialis		X		
Biceps femoris	X		X	
Semitendinosus	X			X
Semimembranosus	X			X
Sartoroius	X			x
Gracilis	X			x
Popliteus	x			X
Tensor fasciae latae		x		
Gastrocnemius	x			

Muscle stretched / Movement	Flex	Ext	Out Rot	In Rot
Rectus femoris	X			
Vastus intermedius	X			
Vastus lateralis	X			
Vastus medialis	X			
Biceps femoris		X		X
Semitendinosus		X	X	
Semimembranosus		X	X	
Sartorius		X	x	
Gracilis		X	x	
Popliteus		x	X	
Tensor fasiae latae	x			
Gastrocnemius		x		

780

Ankle, Foot and toes

Muscle contracted / Movement	Ankle		Foot				Toes	
	Dorsi flexion	Plantar flexion	Dorsi flexion	Plantar flexion	Supination inversion adduction	Pronation eversion abduction	Flex	Ext
Tibials ant	X		X		X			
Ext dig long	X		X			x		X
Ext hal long			X					X
Peroneus tertius	X		X			X		
Gastrocnem		X						
Soleus		X						
Tibialis post		x		X	X			
Flex dig lon		x		X	x		X	
Flex hal lon		x		X	x		X	
Peroneus l		X		X		X		
Peroneus b		x		X		X		

Muscle stretched / Movement	Ankle		Foot				Toes	
	Dorsi flexion	Plantar flexion	Dorsi flexion	Plantar flexion	Supination inversion adduction	Pronation eversion abduction	Flex	Ext
Tibials ant		X		X		X		
Ext dig long		X		X	x		X	
Ext hal long				X			X	
Peroneus tertius		X		X	X			
Gastrocnem	X							
Soleus	X							
Tibialis post	x		X			X		
Flex dig lon	x		X			x		X
Flex hal lon	x		X			x		X
Peroneus l	X		X		X			
Peroneus b	x		X		X			

Head and Neck

Muscle contracted / Movement	Flexion	Extension	Sidebending	Rotation same side	Rotation opp side
Prevertebral muscles	X		X		
Hyoid muscles	x				
Scalenus anterior	X		X		x
Scalenus medius			X		
Scalenus posterior			X		
Sternocleidomastoid	X		X		X
Levator scapulae		x	X	x	
Suboccipitals**		X head	X head	X head	x sup oblique
Splenius capitis and cervicis		X	X	X	
Erector spinae* Capitis and cervicis		X	X	X	
Semispinalis capitis and cervicis		X	X		X
Trapezius		X	X		X

Muscle stretched / Movement	Flexion	Extension	Sidebending opp side	Rotation same side	Rotation opp side
Prevertebral muscles		X	X		
Hyoid muscles		x			
Scalenus anterior		X posterior translation	X	x	
Scalenus medius			X		
Scalenus posterior			X		
Sternocleidomastoid		X	X	x	
Levator scapulae	x		X		x
Suboccipitals**	x head		X head	x sup oblique	X head
Splenius capitis and cervicis	X		X		X
Erector spinae* capitis and cervicis	X		X		X
Semispinalis capitis and cervicis	X		X	X	
Trapezius	X		X	X	

* Longissimus, spinalis and iliocostalis   *** Multifidus and rotatores

** Rectus capitus posterior major and minor, obliqus capitus superior and inferior

Thoracic and Lumbar joints / Trunk

Muscle contracted / Movement	Flexion	Extension	Sidebending	Rotation same side	Rotation opposite side
Rectus abdominis	X		X		
External oblique	X		X		X
Internal oblique	X		X	X	
Quadratus lumborum			X		
Psoas	X		X		x
Erector spinae					
Longissimus		X	X	x	
Spinalis		X	x	x	
Iliocostalis		X	X	x	
Semispinalis thoracis		X	X		X
Deep popsterior muscles		X	x		X

Muscle stretched / Movement	Flexion	Extension	Sidebending	Rotation same side	Rotation opposite side
Rectus abdominis		X	X		
External oblique		X	X	X	
Internal oblique		X	X		X
Quadratus lumborum			X		
Psoas		X	X	x	
Erector spinae					
Longissimus	X		X		x
Spinalis	X		x		x
Iliocostalis	X		X		x
Semispinalis thoracis	X		X	X	
Deep popsterior muscles***	X		x	X	

782

Glossary

Abduction - taking the arm or leg sideways, up and away from the midline of the body or away from the midline of a limb. For the fingers and toes, it is moving the digits apart, away from the centerline of the hand or foot. Abduction of the wrist is also called radial deviation.

Abnormal barrier - a pathological barrier occurring within the limits of motion at a joint, caused by structural changes in muscle, fasciae, ligament, bone, skin or by oedema.

Acetabulum - a cup-shaped joint cavity on the lateral surface of the pelvis in which the head of the femur articulates.

Actin - a protein found in a wide variety of animal and plant cells, which forms, but is not limited to, the structure of muscles, and is responsible for the contraction and relaxation of muscle fibres.

Active motion - the voluntarily movement of a joint by the muscles to the physiological barrier.

Active stretching - exercise technique done using voluntary muscle contraction to overcome the resistance offered by another muscle or muscles or soft tissue on the opposite side of the limb, spine or body; one group of muscles (agonists) acting directly against opposing muscles (antagonists), while reciprocal inhibition facilitates the stretch.

Active tension - the tension generated within a muscle as a result of the sliding of actin and myosin filaments in the contracting muscle.

Acute - a disease or illness with a rapid onset and short duration, for example a cold or sprain. Acute symptoms may range from mild to intense.

Adduction - taking the arm or leg down and towards the midline of body or towards the midline of a limb. For the fingers and toes, it is bringing the digits together, towards the centerline of the hand or foot. Adduction of the wrist is also called ulnar deviation..

Adhesion - a band of scar tissue that joins two internal body surfaces that are not usually connected; they may be caused by surgery, infection or injury.

Aerobic - the use of oxygen by the body to meet energy demands during exercise and includes walking, swimming, cycling and running.

Ageing - the process of becoming older occurs on a cellular level and a whole body level and is influenced by a complex mixture of environmental and genetic factors.

Agonist - a muscle that produces the primary contraction and motion at a joint; also known as a prime mover.

Ambidextrous - a person with both left and right handedness.

Anatomical barrier - the total range of movement that can be produced in a joint.

Anatomy - a branch of biology dealing with the study of the structure of organisms, including human anatomy.

Ankle joint - this can refer specifically to the talocrural joint between the talus in the foot, and the tibia and fibula in the leg, or generally to the region where the foot meets the leg; including the talocrural joint, the subtalar joint and the inferior tibiofibular joint.

Ankylosing spondylitis - a type of arthritis that primarily affects the joints of the spine, causing inflammation, new bone formation and fusion in a fixed forward-bent posture or kyphosis.

Ankylosis - stiffness and rigidity or complete fusion of a joint due to adhesions or inflammation as a result of injury or disease.

Annulus fibrosus - the outer part of the intervertebral disc, which with the inner part, the nucleus pulposus, provides shock absorption for the spine.

Antagonist - in a general sense it is something that opposes; in anatomy is it usually referring to a muscle that opposes the contraction of an agonist muscle, for example, biceps opposing the triceps muscle.

Anterior - the front or towards the front of the body.

Anterior head posture - the forward movement of the occiput on the atlas, and the forward movement of the head relative to the body but without any flexion occurring.

Anterior translation - the forward shifting or sliding movement of one bone or area of the body on another, for example the forward movement of the head relative to the rest of the body (not flexion) or the forward sliding of the tibia on the femur after an anterior cruciate ligament tear.

Anxiety - an unpleasant state of inner turmoil characterised by persistent feelings of nervousness, worry or dread of imminent death or future threats, real or perceived, plus physical symptoms including muscular tension, panic attacks, restlessness, fatigue and poor concentration, which don't subside when the original stressor is removed. Types of anxiety includes generalised anxiety disorder, social phobia, obsessive compulsive disorder, post-traumatic stress disorder, and panic disorders.

Aponeuroses - sheets of dense white compact collagen fibres, penetrating and surrounding muscles, and serving to more evenly distribute the forces generated by muscle contraction.

Arterial - relating to the system of arteries taking blood to the body.

Artery - a blood vessel taking oxygen-rich blood from the heart to the tissues of the body.

Asana - a type of yoga stretching exercise and part of a system of mind-body awareness.

Atlanto-axial joints - a complex grouping of three synovial joints between the first cervical vertebra (atlas or C1) and the second cervical vertebra (axis or C2). The middle or median joint between the anterior surface of the odontoid process and the posterior surface of the anterior arch of atlas, and the anterior surface of the transverse ligament and the posterior surface of the odontoid process form a pivot joint. The two lateral atlanto-axial joints between the articular processes of the two bones are plane, arthrodial or gliding joints.

Atlanto-occipital joints - the uppermost joints of the spine are bilateral, symmetrical, ellipsoidal synovial joints between the superior articular facets of the first cervical vertebra (atlas or C1) and the condyles of the occipital bone (C0).

Atrophy - decrease in size or wasting of an organ or tissue, such as a muscle.

Autogenic - produced from within; self-generating or self-regulating, usually with regard to circulation, breathing and heart rate.

Ballistic movements - an extremely rapid movement of the limbs which, once initiated, cannot be modified. For example hitting a nail with a hammer or throwing a ball.

Ballistic stretching - a type of exercise which uses the momentum of a moving limb and bouncing into the stretch position to force a muscle to lengthen beyond its range of motion.

Barrier - an obstruction that restricts free movement in a joint in the body and can be a normal or abnormal.

Biomechanics - the study of the structure and function of biological systems. When applied to human movement is termed sports biomechanics, although it may be applied to any action.

Bipedalism / Bipedal / Biped - a form of terrestrial locomotion where the organism moves by means of its two rear limbs, for example walking, running and hopping.

Body types - a system for classifying the general structure and shape of the human body, especially the musculoskeletal structure and assessing its influence on function; dividing people into three types: ectomorph, endomorph and mesomorph.

Bones - a dynamically active tissue that forms the skeleton. Bones have a complex structure, come in a range of shapes and sizes, and have many functions: they enable mobility, provide support, protect organs, produces blood cells and store minerals.

Brain - a complex organ containing billions of neurons, which is at the centre of the nervous system in nearly all animals. The largest part of the human brain is the cerebrum, and with the cerebellum, midbrain, brain stem and spinal cord has motor and autonomic control over muscles and organs and receives sensory information from all over the body.

Brain plasticity - see **Neuroplasticity**.

Breathing - the movement of the ribs and diaphragm produces inhalation and exhalation which moves air in and out of the lungs; part of the respiration process required to sustain life.

Bunions - swelling, tenderness and thickening of the soft tissues, bursa and bone on the medial side of the first metatarsophalangeal joint and base of the big toe, caused by genetic factors and from pressure from tight-fitting shoes forcing the big toe inwards towards, and sometimes under or over, the other toes, while the head of the metatarsal bone tilts sideways and stick out; also known as a hallux valgus.

Bursitis - painful swelling of bursae that cushion the movement of tendons passing over joints. Bursae commonly become inflamed near joints that perform frequent repetitive movement such as the shoulder and hip or where there is a lot of pressure on a joint such as the elbow knee, heel and the base of the big toe.

Capillary - the smallest of a body's blood vessels, capillaries are only one cell layer thick. They connect arterioles and venules, and enable the exchange of oxygen, carbon dioxide, water, nutrients and waste substances between the blood and the surrounding tissues.

Carpal tunnel syndrome - a medical condition where the median nerve is compressed as it passes through the carpal tunnel at the wrist, causing pain, numbness and tingling in the part of the hand supplied by the median nerve. Predisposing factors include diabetes, obesity, pregnancy, hypothyroidism and a genetically determined narrower carpal tunnel.

Cartilage - a flexible connective tissue found in the joints, rib cage, nose, ear, bronchial tubes and the intervertebral discs. It is classified as fibrocartilage, elastic and hyaline cartilage.

Central canal stenosis - a narrowing of the central canal within the spinal column as a result of degenerative changes in the joints, discs and bones from osteoarthritis or other arthritides, impacting on the spinal cord.

Centre of gravity (COG) - an imaginary point in a body of matter where the weight of the body is concentrated. In the human body the centre of gravity depends on the shape of the body and its position. In the anatomical position it lies just in front of the second sacral vertebra.

Cerebral palsy - a movement disorder arising in early childhood with symptoms ranging from stiffness, weakness, tremors, seizures, poor coordination, changes in sensation, vision, and hearing and difficulty swallowing, speaking and reasoning. It is caused by abnormal development in areas of the brain that control movement, balance and posture, either during pregnancy, childbirth or shortly after birth.

Cervical spine - the upper seven vertebrae of the spine, usually forming a posteriorly concave lordotic curve and enabling the movement of the head.

Chronic - a health condition or disease that persists for a long duration or at least three months, for example osteoarthritis, asthma, cancer and diabetes.

Circulation - usually referring to blood circulation, but may apply to lymph, cerebrospinal fluid or any other fluids moving through a closed system. The movement of blood through the body by the action of the heart, takes oxygen, nutrients and other materials to the tissues and removes wastes from them.

Circumduction - conical movement combining flexion, extension, adduction and abduction; occuring in ball and socket joints, such as the hip and shoulder, as well as in the fingers, hands, feet, spine and head.

Close-packed position - a joint that is locked, least free to move and in its most stable state because its surfaces have maximum congruence and most surface contact; its joint capsule it tight, and its overlying soft tissues are at high levels of tension. Joint play cannot be done.

Collagen - different types of proteins that give ligaments, tendons, menisci, joint capsules, intervertebral discs and other tissues their strength.

Collateral ligaments - ligaments running down the inside (medial collateral) or outside (lateral collateral) of the knee, elbow, wrist, finger and toe joints.

Concentric - towards the centre.

Concentric isotonic contraction - the joint angle changes, the contracting muscle shortens and movement takes place because the tension generated by the contracting muscle is greater than the load on the muscle; for example when you contract your triceps muscle and raise your body off the floor during a push-up.

Congenital - a condition that is present at birth regardless of the cause, characterised by structural deformities or birth defects, congenital heart disease is the most common type of congenital disorder.

Congruence - joints fitting together with maximum surface contact.

Connective tissue (CT) - is found everywhere in the body and includes: loose CT in the dermis layer of the skin; dense CT in tendons and ligaments; adipose tissue, lining organs and body cavities; cartilage; bone; blood; and lymph. Apart from blood and lymph it consists of fibres, ground substance and cells. It binds, supports, connects, holds in place or separates different types of tissues and organs in the body.

Contraction - see **Isometric contraction**, **Isotonic** or **Muscle contraction**.

Contracture - abnormal shortness, thickening and inextensibility, especially in the hands, fingers or toes, caused by fibrosis in a muscles, tendons, fasciae and ligaments. It develops in muscles or tendons that have remained short for too long, thus becoming even shorter. Examples include Dupuytren's contracture, Volkmann's contracture and ischemic contracture.

Coronal - a plane or line running in a left right direction and dividing the body into front and back halves; relating to the coronal suture separating the frontal and parietal bones.

Counter-nutation - backward bending or extension of the sacrum on the ilium

Coccyx - the tail bones at the bottom of the spinal column, comprising of three to five separate or fused coccygeal vertebrae.

Creep is a time-dependent elongation or deformation that occurs in connective tissues and other viscoelastic materials when prolonged forces are applied.

Crimp phase - the unwinding and straighten out of crimps in the collagen fibres of ligaments and joint capsules during the initial phase of stretching requires little energy because no major chemical bonds need to be broken.

Crimping / Crimps - the buckled or wavy orientation of collagen fibre which determines the elongation or deformation direction of different tissues.

Cross-bridges - the bonds formed and broken between actin and myosin during muscle contraction.

Deep Fasciae - a tensional network of dense fibrous connective tissue, which penetrates and surrounds muscles, divides groups of muscles into fascial compartments and surrounds bones, cartilage, blood vessels and nerves. It includes aponeuroses, ligaments, tendons, retinacula, joint capsules and septa. Also known as investing fascia.

Depression - a state of low mood, sadness, emptiness, low energy, hopeless, poor concentration, helpless, low sense of well-being, loss of interest in activities that were once pleasurable. Types of depressive disorders include clinical depression, bipolar disorder, cyclothymic disorder and seasonal affective disorder.

Depression - movement in an inferior or downwards direction.

Developmental stretch - a stretch requiring strong force a longer than average hold to increase muscle length and flexibility.

Diaphragm - this can refer to the urogenital diaphragm or pelvic diaphragm, but the diaphragm usually refers to the thoracic diaphragm, a dome-shaped sheet of skeletal muscle and fibrous tissue that extends across the bottom of the thoracic cavity separating it from the abdominal cavity. The diaphragm is mainly involved with breathing but assists with some non-respiratory functions such as aiding digestion and by increasing intra-abdominal pressure it enables vomiting and defication.

Distal - a relative term comparing the position of two points further from the midline of the body to each other, for example, the wrist is distal to the elbow.

Dopamine - a neurotransmitter released by nerve cells to send signals to other nerve cells. In the brain it plays a major role in reward-motivated behaviour, while in the rest of the body it has many functions including noradrenaline inhibitor, vasodilator and a local chemical messenger controlling insulin production and digestive motility.

Dorsiflexion - movement of the foot where the toes are brought closer to the shin, decreasing the angle between the dorsum (top) of the foot and the leg, for example, the foot is dorsiflexed when walking on the heels.

Dowager hump - an abnormal forward curvature or kyphosis in the upper thoracic spine due to poor posture, genetic susceptibility or disease such as osteoporosis.

Dynamic stretching - a controlled muscle contraction to generate continuous swinging or to-and-fro quick movements, to take a muscle through its stiffness barrier, and sometimes involving a bouncing action at the end of the movement.

Dystrophin - a protein that connects the muscle cell membrane to the surrounding extracellular matrix, thereby strengthening muscles and protect them from injury.

Eccentric isotonic contraction - the joint angle changes, the contracting muscle lengthens and movement take place because the tension generated by the contracting muscle is less than the load on the muscle, for example when you contract your triceps muscle and lower your body to the floor during a push-up.

Ectomorph - a tall thin person with a light frame and small bone, muscle and ligament mass, enabling greater flexibility but without the benefit of stability.

Ehlers-Danlos syndrome - an connective tissue disorder caused by genetic mutations which result in problems with the production of collagen. The condition has great variability and is often misdiagnosed. Symptom include depression, fatigue, pain, joint hypermobility, early onset osteoarthritis, increased curvatures of the spine and skin problems.

Elastic barrier - the limit to the passive range of movement. When a muscle approaches the elastic limit, tension within the muscle increases dramatically and stretching the muscle beyond this limit results in tissue damage.

Elastic phase - the phase of extensibility or deformation of any elastic material including ligaments and muscles; when a load is applied to an elastic material it will change shape and when that load is removed it returns to its original shape.

Elasticity - a change in shape of a material at low stress that is recoverable after the stress is removed.

Elastin - a yellow coloured protein which gives ligaments and other tissues their elasticity.

Electromyography (EMG) - a technique for evaluating and recording the electrical activity of skeletal muscles; an electromyograph detects the electrical potential of muscle cells, to work out the activation level or recruitment order of muscles and if there are any medical problems.

Elevation - movement in a superior or upwards direction, for example, shrugging the shoulders is elevation of the scapula.

Elongation - a type of deformation; the act of lengthening an elastic material such as a muscle by applying an external load, such as the force of gravity or an upper limb of the body, or an internal force, such as muscle contraction.

End-feel - sensation perceived by an examiner when the end of a joints range of motion is reached, and which varies according to the limiting structure or tissue; capsular, muscular or bone-on-bone, or the presence of pathology.

Endomorph - a short stocky person with large bone mass, muscle bulk, ligament thickness and joint size, ensuring high resistance to stretching and giving the body great stability.

Endorphins - a group of peptides produced in the pituitary gland and other parts of the brain, in the spinal cord and throughout the nervous system. They resemble opiates and react with the brain's opiate receptors to raise the pain threshold, and like opiates they can produce feelings of euphoria, for example during exercise. They are also neurotransmitters, enabling or inhibiting signals from one neuron to the next, and there main function is to inhibit the transmission of pain signals.

Eversion - tilting the sole of the foot away from the median plane so the outside is raised.

Extension - a straightening movement, increasing the joint angle in saggital plane, for example straightening the knee; but in joints that can move forward and backwards such as the spine and wrist, extension is backward bending or movement in a posterior direction.

External rotation - turning a limb or body part away from the midline of the body, also known as lateral rotation.

Facet joints / Zygapophysial joints - small, plane, gliding, synovial joints located posteriorly between the articular processes of adjacent vertebrae at every spinal level except the top where they are modified. Facet orientation enables forward, backward and sidebending movements but limited rotation. As well as a guiding function they have a stabilising function.

Fasciae / Fascia - fibrous connective tissue, primarily collagen, that form sheets or bands beneath the skin (superficial fascia), around and between muscles (deep fascia) and around organs (visceral fascia).

Fast-twitch fibres - muscle fibres that are fast to contract but fatigue quickly.

Fatigue - feeling of tiredness which may be physical, mental, normal or abnormal. Physical fatigue is the inability of a muscle to maintain tone and postural support; mental fatigue is a temporary decrease in performance resulting from prolonged periods of cognitive activity; normal fatigue can usually be alleviated by periods of rest and may be the result of prolonged working or other activity, mental stress, jet lag, boredom and lack of sleep; abnormal fatigue may be due to disease, minor illness, mineral or vitamin deficiency, blood loss and anaemia.

Fatty infiltration - the pathological accumulation fat deposits in and between cells of tissues.

Fibres - have different meanings in the body depending on their location. In fasciae, tendons and ligaments fibres are proteins such as collagen and elastin, in muscles they cells, while in nerves they are the axons that conducts electrical impulses away from the cell body.

Fibrocartilage - fibrous tissue with variable amounts of cartilage and other materials depending on it location and function; is present in menisci, articular discs, the annulus fibrosus of intervertebral discs, the glenoid and acetabular labra, discs of the symphysis pubis and temporomandibular joints, and at the tendon bone interface as dense white fibrocartilage, and in the external ears and larynx as yellow elastic fibrocartilage.

Fibronectin - a fibrous protein that binds collagens and other proteins to cell membranes. It also plays a crucial role in wound healing, cell growth, migration and differentiation.

Fibrosis - the deposition of excess fibrous connective tissue in a gland, organ or tissue, as a result of injury, burns, disease or anything that has caused long periods of inflammation. It can occur in the liver, heart and lung but of relevance to stretching is muscular fibrosis.

Fibrous muscle - similar to scarring in that the muscle is less elastic and there is a firm hard end feel when stretching the muscle. There may be weakness, fatigue and other dysfunction. Structural changes may be the result of prolonged use or postural fatigue.

Flexibility - an attribute of any viscoelastic tissue to lengthen or be compressed, but in the context of this book it the active or passive extensibility of a muscle.

Flexion - narrowing of a joint angle in a saggital plane, for example bending the knee; but in joints that can move forwards and backwards such as in the spine and wrist, flexion is forward bending or movement in a anterior direction.

Force - energy exerted to changes a body from a state of rest to one of motion or changes its rate of motion, including muscle contraction and gravity.

Frontal - a plane or line dividing the body into front and back halves, as well as parallel planes; also known as the coronal plane.

Gait - walking or locomotion of the human body through the movement of limbs; the cyclic loss and recovery of balance with the least expenditure of energy; two phases of gait - stance and swing are further divided into smaller components, including heel strike and toe off.

Gender - the range of characteristics belonging to, and differentiating men and women.

Generalised - a general truth or statement about something based on limited or incomplete evidence or broader understanding.

Genes - the molecular units of heredity; blueprints containing the codes for the production of proteins, and which determine the shape, structure and function of all living things.

Genetics - the study of genes, heredity, and genetic variation in living organisms.

Genu recurvatum - excessive extension, backward bending or hyperextension of the knee joint; more common in women; and is associated with congenital hypermobility.

Genu varum - an outward bowing of the lower limbs or bow-leggedness, which starts in childhood and may be caused by rickets or anything preventing ossification of the bones.

Genu valgum - a childhood deformity, where the knees are together but the ankles are far apart or knock-knees; due to a growth irregularity in the long bones of the lower limbs.

Gibbus deformity - an increased thoracic or thoracolumbar kyphosis, where one or more adjacent vertebrae become wedged, and the spine becomes sharply angulated and hunched.

Gland - an organ or cluster of cells that secrete a substance for release into the bloodstream (endocrine gland) or into cavities inside the body or its outer surface (exocrine gland).

Gluteal fold - a prominent horizontal skin furrow formed by the lower margin of gluteus maximus and overlying fat, that defines the border of the posterior upper thigh and the lower buttock, also known as the gluteal sulcus or gluteal crease.

Glycoproteins - a carbohydrate attached to a protein; they have many functions but have a structural role in connective tissues, binding together cells, fibres and ground substance.

Golgi tendon organs - sensory receptors located at the junction between skeletal muscles and tendons that are sensitive to tension either from active muscle contraction or stretching.

Gravity - a natural phenomenon by which all things attract one another; a constant external force acting on any object and giving weight to physical objects including the human body.

Ground substance - an amorphous material, composed of proteins, metabolites, water and other substances, depending on the tissue, in which the cells and fibres of connective tissue are embedded, also known as extrafibrillar matrix.

Habituation - the decrease or cessation in response to a repeated stimulus; a tolerance to the effects of a stimulus acquired through continued use; a learned adaptation where it takes greater effort to move from one fixed state to another.

Hallux valgus - the medial deviation of the first metatarsal and lateral deviation of the big toe.

Hip joint - a ball and socket joint between the femur and acetabulum of the pelvis whose primary function is to support the weight of the body in standing, walking or running and for retaining balance.

Homeostasis - a system of feedback control; the process of maintaining equilibrium and stability of the human body's internal environment, in response to changes in external conditions, for example the regulation of pH and temperature.

Hormones - a group of molecules produced by glands and transported by the circulatory system to target distant organs to regulate physiology and behaviour, including growth, mood, metabolism and reproduction.

Hydration - having adequate fluid in the body tissues; the act or process of taking water or fluids into the body for a variety of functions, including maintaining metabolism, removing waste and reducing the concentration of toxic substances in the tissues, and controlling temperature, heart rate and blood pressure.

Hyperextension - movement of a joint beyond its normal limit or range of movement.

Hypermobile joints - joints that move beyond their normal range because the ligaments around them are too loose and the muscles are too weak, also called ligament laxity, joint laxity, and double-jointedness or hypermobility syndrome.

Hypermobility - increase in mobility in one joint usually due to injury or multiple joints, due to a connective tissue disease or genetic susceptibility.

Hypertonic - excessive tone or tension in a muscle resulting in shortness and increased resistance to stretching.

Hypertrophy - increase in size, bulk and volume of an organ or tissue due to the enlargement of its component cells; often associated with muscle enlargement due to increased demand.

Hypomobility - stiffness; decrease in mobility in a joint due to injury, disease or other factors.

Idiopathic - a disease of unknown cause, origin or pathogenesis, or of spontaneous origin.

Iliac crests - the curved upper ridge of the wing the pelvic or hip bone.

Immune system - formed by many cells and structures in the body and protects against disease, especially infection from bacteria, viruses and other foreign bodies.

Incisal - the cutting edge or surface of an incisor tooth.

Inhibition - see **Reciprocal inhibition**

Internal rotation - turning a limb towards the midline of the body, also called medial rotation.

Intervertebral disc - a fibrocartilagenous disc acting as a shock absorber between vertebrae, helping hold the vertebral bodies together, and faciltating movement of the spinal column.

Intervertebral foramina - a natural opening or passage between two adjacent vertebrae through which spinal nerves from the spinal cord pass; also called neural foramina or IVF.

Inversion - tilting the sole of the foot towards the midline of the body so the inside of the foot is raised.

Ischial tuberosities - two bony swellings at the base of the pelvis that bear the weight of the body during sitting; also called sit bones, sitting bones or buttock bones.

Isometric - relating to a muscle, which during contraction keeps the same length.

Isometric contraction - increased tension in a muscle but the joint angle and muscle length does not change and no movement takes place; occurs when the load on the muscle equals the tension generated by the contracting muscle, for example when you attempt to push or pull an immovable object during an isometric exercise.

Isotonic - relating to a muscle, where during contraction, the muscle maintains the same tension or tone but allows a change in length.

Joint capsule - an envelope surrounding a synovial joint, made up of an outer fibrous layer and an inner synovial layer or membrane.

Joint degeneration - joint disease that results from the breakdown of joint cartilage; also known as osteoarthritis; symptoms include joint pain and stiffness and muscle pain.

Joint instability - is a lack of ligament support in a joint, which may result in dislocation, injury and eventually to osteoarthritis; it may be genetic or due to injury, or in the spine it may be due to a break and separation in a vertebra, called a spondylolisthesis or pars defect.

Joint movement - the degree of movement varies according to the type of joint so most fibrous joints such as in the skull permit little or no mobility, cartilaginous joints such as in the intervertebral discs permits slight mobility, and synovial joints are freely movable.

Joint stiffness - inability or difficulty moving a joint or the partial or complete loss of range of motion; may be associated with pain, swelling and other symptoms; may be caused by injury or disease in the joint, such as osteoarthritis, or injury or inflammation in an adjacent area, such as a bursae; when a joint does not move at all it is said to be ankylosed.

Joint - a location two bones connect to allow movement and provide mechanical support.

Joint fusion - where no mobility occurs due to disease or surgery, also called ankylosis.

Knee hyperextension - see **Genu recurvatum**

Knee joint - joint between the thigh and the leg and consists of two articulations: one between the femur and tibia, and one between the femur and patella.

Knock knees - see **Genu valgum**

Kyphosis - a normal outward convex curvature of the thoracic spine; when exaggerated it is called a hyperkyphosis, increased kyphosis or more commonly as a hunchback.

Laminin - proteins, binding cell membranes and tissues and forming sheets of scaffolding.

Lateral - the outer side of the body, or a body part that is farther from the middle of the body.

Lateral flexion - to move the spine or head sideways, also known as sidebending.

Lateral translation - sideshifting movement to the right or left but without any sidebending.

Lever - a beam or rigid rod (bone) pivoted at a fixed hinge or fulcrum (joint), to amplify an input force (muscle contraction), provide a greater output force (movement) and confer a mechanical advantage (leverage).

Lifestyle - the way a person lives plays a role in shaping their lifestyle: their behavior, interests and activities, including their politics, religion, health, levels of intimacy and more.

Ligaments - fibrous connective tissue that connects bones to other bones, controlling movement and providing stability.

Ligament laxity is the loss of structural integrity in a ligament because of overstretching, injury or for genetic reasons resulting in the loss of support and stability in joints.

Ligament sprain - a joint that is forced beyond its normal range of motion causing overstretched or torn ligaments; symptoms usually include swelling and pain, and, depending on the severity of the sprain, joint hypermobility and instability, for example rolling your ankle.

Ligamentous creep - time dependent elongation of a ligament when subjected to a constant stress. Most elongation first occurs quickly, over minutes, and then the rate slows but still continues even when the load is constant; the deformation over time is non-linear.

Linear - where the output is directly proportional to the input.

Load - a force which is applied to a structure; a weight or mass that is supported or carried.

Localisation - something confined to a small area of the body, for example a sign such as redness, swelling or a soft tissue mass or a symptom, such as pain or numbness.

Loeys-Dietz syndrome - a genetic disorder that affects the connective tissues of the body, with a wide range of symptoms including, kyphosis, scoliosis and joint hypermobility.

Longitudinal - running in the direction of the long axis of the body or body part.

Longitudinal stretches - stretching along the long axis of the body, creating less angulation and sidebending.

Loose fatty tissue - also known as adipose tissue, is loose connective tissue composed of fat cells; primarily located under the skin, it is also found providing padding around internal organs, and functions to store energy and nutrients, and cushion and insulate the body.

Loose packed position - a joint that is unlocked and free to move because its joint capsule is lax, overlying soft tissues are relaxed, joint surfaces have limited contact and are not congruent. High levels of joint play are also possible.

Lordosis - a normal inward, concave curvature of the lumbar or cervical spine; when exaggerated is called a hyperlordosis, increased lordosis, or commonly called a sway back.

Lumbar spine - the lower five vertebrae of the spine, usually forming a posteriorly concave lordotic curve and enabling the movement of the trunk and upper body.

Lymphatic system - part of the circulatory system and made up of a network of lymphatic vessels that carry a clear fluid or lymph towards the heart; as well as functioning to return interstitial fluid to the blood, it has an important role in defense as part of the immune system.

Macrofailure - a major tear in a tissue, for example a rupture in the middle of a tendon or ligament or an avulsion at the junction of a tendon and a bone.

Maintenance stretch – a mild to moderate force to maintain flexibility.

Malleoli - the two bony protuberances on either side of the ankle, formed by the lower ends of the tibia and fibula.

Manual therapy - hands-on physical therapy to correct abnormal structural changes in tissues, restore normal function in joints and reduce symptoms such as pain, by mobilising restricted joints, relaxing tense muscles, increasing circulation and breaking up scar tissue.

Marfan syndrome - a genetic disorder that affects the body's connective tissue; caused by a mutation in the gene that tells the body how to make a critical protein

Membrane - the outer layer of a cell that allows the passage of some components into and out of the cell but not others, and retains other constituents found in the cell.

Mesomorph - broad shouldered person with moderate structural characteristics, enabling average flexibility and stability.

Metacarpophalangeal joint - articulation between the distal end of a metacarpal bone and the proximal end of a phalanx or finger bone of the hand.

Microfailure - the failure, at the microscopic level, of any material when is subjected to an excessive load, but in this book the word relates primarily to ligament tissue and to a lesser extent to muscle and tendon.

Micro-tearing - the breaking of actin-myosin bonds where the muscle filaments are forced apart; a natural process, usually resulting in muscle pain after vigorous exercise.

Microtrauma - small microscopic injuries to soft tissues such as muscles and their sheaths, plus tendons, fasciae and ligaments. Repetitive overuse and ballistic activities that are not allowed time to recover may cause low levels of inflammation resulting in more serious problems later.

Midfoot - the part of the foot between the hindfoot and forefoot and comprised of the navicular, cuboid and the three cuneiform bones.

Mind-body - the idea that the physical body and the mind should be thought of as a single integrated unit, in contrast to the dualist conception of a separate body and mind; the interrelationship between the body and the mind, and between physical and mental health.

Mobility - the ability to move a joint, actively or passively, through a range of motion; may also be called motion or movement.

Motor fatigue - the ability to detect a stimulus but inability to respond to it efficiently.

Multitasking - an attempt to do many tasks or activities at once; a limited and rapidly switching focus may result in more errors and reduced performance, depending on the task.

Muscle contraction - the activation of actin-myosin to generate tension within a muscle; skeletal muscle requires synaptic input from a motor neuron whereas smooth and cardiac muscle contraction is modulated by the autonomic nervous system.

Muscle energy technique (MET) - a group of manual techniques, which enable a therapist to lengthen shortened muscles and increase movement at joints.

Muscle fibres - a term used when describing muscle cells.

Muscle power - the ability of muscles to produce force in or at a given time.

Muscle spasm - a sudden, involuntary contraction of a muscle or group of muscles, usually accompanied by pain, also known as a muscle cramp.

Muscle spindle - a sensory receptor within a muscle that detects changes in the muscles length for the regulation of muscle contraction and stretching.

Muscle strain - an injury to a muscle where the muscle fibres are torn as a result of overstretching, commonly known as a pulled muscle.

Muscle tension - the continuous and passive contraction of a muscle, and which affects the muscle's resistance to passive stretching, also known as muscle tone. Normal muscle tension helps maintain posture but increased or decrease tension can cause problems.

Muscle tone - see **Muscle tension**.

Muscles - a soft tissue responsible for maintaining posture, locomotion and movement of joints, and present in some organs, such as the heart and gut. Muscle cells contain the proteins actin and myosin that slide over one another producing muscle contraction and generating force and motion.

Myofascial manipulation - a form of massage for muscle and fasciae.

Myofibril - composed of proteins such as actin, myosin and titin, they are the basic unit of a muscle; each muscle cell or fibre contains many chains of myofibrils.

Myosin - a protein responsible for motility in a wide variety of cells, including muscles, where it is responsible for the contraction and relaxation of muscle fibres.

Myotatic reflex - see **Stretch reflex**.

Nervous system - consists of the central nervous system containing the brain and spinal cord and the peripheral nervous system consisting of nerves; uses electrical and chemical mechanisms to send and receive signals from different parts of the body, enables the parts to communicate with each other, and reacts to changes both outside and inside the body.

Neural adaptation - see **Sensory adaptation**.

Neutraliser muscles - simultaneous contraction of two muscles which cancel out or neutralise an undesired motion to ensure that movement occurs in a desired plane.

Neuromuscular coordination - the ability of the nervous system to efficiently recruit a muscle or group of muscles in order to perform a specific task.

Neuromuscular inhibition - see **Reciprocal inhibition**

Neuroplasticity - the brain's ability to reorganize itself by forming new neural connections. Healthy neurons in the brain can grow new nerve ending, connect with other neurons and form new neural pathways to increase function in response to changes in their environment or compensate for loss if part of the brain is damaged by injury or disease.

Neurotransmitter - chemical messengers that transmit signals across a synapse from one neuron (nerve cell) to another; they are released on one side of the synapse and they are received by receptors on other synapses.

Non-contractile components of muscle - part of a muscle not directly involved with active contraction; epimysium, perimysium and endomysium layers of connective tissue surround the muscle fibre, and connect to a network extending throughout the muscular system.

Normal barrier - a naturally occurring restriction within a joints range of movement; examples of normal barrier include the physiological, elastic and anatomical barriers.

Nutation - the forward bending or flexion of the sacrum on the ilium

Occupational overuse syndrome - see **Repetitive strain injury**.

Odontoid process - a bony projection arising on the axis (C2 vertebra), passing superiorly behind the anterior arch of the atlas (C1) and articulating with it and the transverse ligament, also called the odontoid peg or dens.

Oedema - the build-up of fluid or swelling; it can be localised such as in an ankle after a ligament strain or more general such as after heart or kidney failure. It may occur anywhere in the body but it is most common in the feet and ankles, as peripheral oedema.

Organ - an organised collection of tissues joined in a structural unit to serve a common function. For example, the heart which pumps blood around the body is primarily made of myocardium which is combined with connective tissues plus nerves and blood vessels.

Osteoarthritis - a form of joint disease or degeneration where the protective cartilage that cushions the ends of bones wears down, causing swelling, pain, the development of osteophytes, or bony spurs and eventual loss of movement. It can occur as a result of major or minor trauma, infection, genetic factors, compensation and natural ageing processes.

Osteophytes - bony growth or spur associated with osteoarthritis.

Osteoporosis - loss of calcium in bones more quickly than the body can replace it, causing a loss of bone density or mass which can lead to fractures. There may be no symptoms until a broken bone occurs. The most common sites are the hip, spine, forearm and wrist.

Overstretching - stretching ligaments beyond their elastic limits of can result in permanent lgament deformation and laxity and joint hypermobility.

Overuse - see **Repetitive strain injury**

Pars defect - see **Spondylolisthesis**

Passive range of motion - the range a joint can be moved either by one's self or by another person with the body part relaxed. The limit of passive range of motion, the elastic barrier, is the point at which there is resistance to movement and any further movement will cause tissue damage.

Passive motion or movement - involuntary movement; movement induced in a joint by another person or gravity or an external prop or by one's self using another body part, usually an upper limb, while the muscles around the joint being moved are relaxed.

Passive stretching - movement done by the person doing the stretch using one limb, the weight of the body (gravity) or a prop to stretch another limb or body part; or when another person holding the limb or body part, moves it while the person relaxes.

Passive tension - the result of the viscoelastic properties of a ligament, fasciae or the non-contractile part of a muscle.

Patella - the knee cap is a thick, rounded, triangular sesamoid bone overlying and protecting the anterior surface of the knee joint and articulating with the femur.

Pes cavus - a high-arched and supinated foot.

Pes planus - a low-arched and pronated foot or flat foot.

Phasic muscles - muscles that provide movement; their fibres are at rest a lot of the time but are frequently called on for brief bouts of intense dynamic activity; they can contract quickly but are fast to fatigue and slow to recover.

Physiological barrier - the range that active movement can produce.

Plantar flexion - movement where the foot is taken away from the shin, thereby increasing the angle between the foot and the front of the leg, for example, the foot is plantar flexed like when walking on tiptoes.

Plastic phase - the final phase of deformation before complete tissue failure of a viscoelastic material such as a ligaments. This is a non-linear phase and follows the linear elastic phase, where the material it returns to its original shape when the load is removed.

Poor posture - an extreme posture requiring high energy input to maintain; typically a forward slouching posture where posterior positioned spinal muscles have to work harder against the continuous pull of gravity.

Posterior - the back or towards the back of the body.

Posterior head posture - the backward movement of the occiput (head) on the atlas but without flexion or extension occurring.

Posterior translation - the backward shifting or sliding movement of one bone or area of the body on another, for example the backward movement of the head on the upper cervical spine or the backward sliding of the tibia on the femur after a posterior cruciate ligament tear.

Post-isometric stretching - a type of static stretching that combines an initial low intensity isometric muscle contraction with passive or active stretching. After the contraction there is a refractory period where the muscle automatically relaxes and when it can be lengthening.

Post-synaptic - the wave of electrical excitation situated behind or occurring after a synapse of two connecting neurones.

Posture - the position of a person's body when standing or sitting; good posture depends on bony alignment, structural integrity of ligaments and muscle, and muscle tone and power supporting the joints of the body.

Postural fatigue - the exhaustion of a muscle after prolonged contraction, especially after attempting to maintain a poor posture.

Proprioceptive neuromuscular facilitation stretching (PNF) - a group of techniques used by manual therapists to increase range of movement and optimise performance.

Primary scoliosis - the main curvature in a group of lateral curvatures in the spine.

Prone - lying on the floor or on a table flat on your front, face downwards.

Pronation - the inward rotation of the forearm when the elbow is at 90 degrees flexion; also, the outward movement of the foot as it rolls to distribute the force of impact of the ground during walking or running, so that more weight is borne on the medial side of the foot.

Proprioception - a perception governed by proprioceptors which provide the brain with important feedback about the position of the body in space and the direction of movement.

Proprioceptors - sensory receptors found in muscles and joints, for example muscle spindles and Golgi tendon organs.

Proteins - large molecules made up of long chains of amino acids, which perform an extensive range of functions in living organisms.

Protraction - lateral movement of the scapula along the rib cage and away from the spine.

Proximal - a relative term comparing the position of two points nearer to the midline of the body to each other. For example, the elbow is proximal to the wrist.

Psoriatic arthritis - a type of arthritis associated with the skin condition psoriasis and characterised by pain, swelling and joint stiffness.

Psychoemotional - a psychological condition involving interaction with the emotions.

Quadrupedalism - terrestrial locomotion in animals using four limbs or legs. Most quadrupeds are vertebrates, including mammals such as sheep, cats and dogs.

Race - a group of people sharing similar and distinct physical characteristics.

Range of movement (ROM) - distance a joint can move between two opposite positions, for example full flexion and extension.

Reciprocal inhibition - an automatic process controlled by the nervous system whereby muscles on one side of a joint are made to relax to allow contraction of muscles on the other side of that joint. For example, for forearm flexion to occur freely, forearm extensor muscle contraction must be inhibited by the nervous system.

Refractory period - a short period of a time after a muscle has contracted before it can contract again, when the muscle is in a relaxed state and conditions are optimal for stretching.

Repetitive strain injury (RSI) - symptoms such as pain, swelling, numbness and stiffness caused by repetitive movements, patterns of overuse or maintaining an awkward or bad posture for a long time. Problems commonly occur in the fingers, hands, wrists and elbows.

Retraction - the medial movement of the scapula along the rib cage and towards the spine.

Reversed kyphosis - reversal of the normal outward convex curvature of the thoracic spine, so the thoracic spine is straight or is extended inwards, sometimes called a poker back.

Reversed lordosis - reversal of the normal inward, concave curvature of the lumbar or cervical spine so these parts of the spine are flexed.

Rheumatoid arthritis - a systemic inflammatory disease causing the joints of the wrist and hands to become warm, swollen, painful and stiff. The disease may also affect other parts of the body including the lungs and heart.

Rotation - a twisting or turning motion in the spine, head and limbs.

Rotator cuff tendon tears - a tear of one or more of the tendons of the four rotator cuff muscles of the shoulder, usually the supraspinatus, as it passes below the acromion.

Rounded shoulders - a faulty posture characterized by an increase thoracic kyphosis, two protracted scapula and short pectoralis muscles.

Sacral torsion - abnormal positioning and movement of the sacrum between the two hip or ilium bones with the sacrum twisted on a diagonal axis.

Sacroiliac joints - two joints between the sacrum and the right and left ilium of the pelvis are supported by strong ligaments and formed by irregular interlocking elevations and depressions; they are highly variable from person to person.

Safe stretching - a stretching system that takes into consideration the age of the person stretching, the presence of disease and genetic differences in people, especially with regard to joint mobility and muscle flexibility, so as to produce an optimal outcome and reduce the probability of injury.

Sagittal - a plane or line dividing the body into left and right halves, as well as parallel planes; relating to the sagittal suture on top of the skull separating the parietal bones and running in a front to back direction.

Scarring - the deposition of fibrous connective tissue mainly collagen, as a result of injury, burns, disease, surgery or anything that has caused tissue damage.

Scoliosis - a lateral curvature of the spine, which may involve the cervical, thoracic, thoracolumbar, lumbar or sacroiliac spine and single, double or multiple curves; usually combined with rotation.

Secondary scoliosis - one or more lateral curvatures of the spine, sometimes compensating for a primary scoliosis.

Sensory adaptation - diminished sensitivity to a stimulus by the sensory system (receptors, neurons, spine cerebral cortex) as a consequence of constant exposure to that stimulus. When sensory neurons are stimulated there is an initial response but then they respond less until there may be no response at all; for example getting use to a low level noise.

Sensory receptor - a sensory nerve ending that responds to a stimulus in the internal or external environment of an organism, for example mechanoreceptors, photoreceptors and taste, touch and smell receptors.

Sidebending - to move the spine or head sideways, also known as lateral flexion

Sidelying - lying on your right or left side, also known as lateral recumbent position.

Skin - the outer layer of the human body is made up of epidermis, dermis and hypodermis. It contains fat, connective tissue, hair follicles, sweat glands, receptors and sensory nerve endings and which provide information on pain, touch, heat, and cold. Also it regulates body temperature and protects us from the outside environment.

Sliding filament theory - explains how the actin and myosin filaments in muscles, slide past one another to produce tension and force and shorten the muscle.

Slow-twitch fibres - muscle fibres that are slow to contract but can go for a long time before they fatigue.

Soft tissue - tissues that connect, support or surround other structures; all tissues except bone, teeth, nails, hair, and cartilage.

Somafeedback - a technique for assessing the ability to relax muscles and correcting the problems identified.

Spasm - a sudden involuntary muscle contraction or cramp often accompanied by pain.

Spasmodic or spastic torticollis - painful involuntarily neurological disorder causing the neck to bend to one side; may be congenital, chronic, acquired and acute. (a wry neck).

Spine - made up of 24 bones called vertebrae, divided into three groups: cervical, thoracic and lumbar, plus five fused bones forming the sacrum. In between each vertebrae is an intervertebral disc that acts as a cushion.

Spinal motion - the product of the combined interaction of multiple vertebrae; starting from the neutral position the four movements are flexion, extension, sidebending and rotation.

Spondylolisthesis - the forward displacement of a vertebra, usually the fifth lumbar vertebra, after a break or fracture; also known as a pars defect.

Sprain - see **Ligament sprain**.

Stability - is concerned with the proper alignment of joints so that the bones are taking most of the stress, not the overlying tissues. Joint stability depends on the resistance offered by various tissues that surround a joint.

Stabiliser muscles - to stabilise a body part, holding a bone in place while joint movement occurs elsewhere, also called fixator muscles.

Stamina - strength of constitution; endurance, vitality, power to resist disease and fatigue.

Static stretching - slow progressive small ratchet-like movements, often with breathing.

Stimulus - anything that arouses activity, energy, thought in someone causing a physiological or psychological response.

Stretch reflex - a muscle contraction in response to stretching, which provides automatic regulation to maintain skeletal muscle at a constant length; when a muscle lengthens, the muscle spindle, a sensory receptor within the muscle, is stretched, which increases nerve activity, causing the muscle fibre to contract, and thus resist the stretching.

Stretching - a type of physical exercise that increases or maintains muscle flexibility and joint mobility; an instinctive activity performed by humans and many animals.

Subacromial bursitis - painful swelling of the bursae situated within the subacromial space of the shoulder, usually after irritation by the supraspinatus tendons passing over it.

Subcutaneous layer - the deepest layer of the skin, containing superficial fascia, collagen, fat, blood and lymphatic vessels, sweat glands; nerves, hair follicle roots; used mainly for fat storage; also known as the hypodermis.

Superficial fascia - loose areolar, and fatty adipose connective tissue forming much of the deepest layer of the skin, where it defines the shape of the body, and surrounding organs, glands and neurovascular bundles, and as a fill for otherwise unoccupied space.

Supine - in a position lying on the floor or on a table flat on your back, face up.

Supination - rotating the forearm outwards

Synergist muscles - the simultaneous contraction of agonist and antagonist muscles producing a secondary joint movement, for example when wrist flexors combine with wrist extensors to produce radial or ulna deviation.

Synovial fluid - viscous fluid found in the cavities of synovial joints and functioning to reduce friction between the articular cartilage of joints during movement.

Synovial membrane - inner membrane of synovial joints which secretes synovial fluid into the joint cavity.

Talin - a protein that helps stabilise the cytoskeleton by binding integrin to actin.

Tarsals - the seven irregularly shaped bones of the foot: talus, calcaneus, navicular, cuboid and three cuneiform bones.

Temporomandibular joint (TMJ) - hinge synovial joint between the mandible (jawbone) and the temporal bones of the skull.

Tendinitis - acute tendon injury or irritation accompanied by inflammation, examples include Achilles tendinitis, patellar tendinitis and tennis elbow.

Tendons - tough fibrous connective tissue, mainly of collagen, that connect muscle to bone.

Tennis elbow strain - overuse or repetitive use of the extensor muscles of the forearm resulting in inflammation and pain of the tendon or tendonitis on the outside of the elbow; it is usually caused by work related activity rather than tennis; also known as lateral epicondylitis.

Tension - may be related to increased psychoemotional stress or muscle tension.

Thoracic spine - the middle twelve vertebrae of the spine, usually forming a posteriorly convex kyphotic curve and enabling the movement of the trunk, ribs and upper body.

Tonic Fibres - relating to slow-twitch postural muscles that contract slowly, but can go for a long time before they fatigue; they are slow to fatigue and quick to recover.

Translation - gliding of the head or a vertebra in the spine forwards, backwards or sideways but without nodding or sidebending the head or tilting the vertebra by sidebending, flexing or extending. Sideways or lateral translation is the same as sideshifting.

Transverse - situated or extending across something.

Transverse plane - an imaginary plane that divides the body into upper and lower parts; also called the horizontal plane. This plane is perpendicular to the coronal and sagittal planes and longitudinal axis of the body.

Varicose veins - superficial veins, most commonly in the legs, that have become enlarged, distended and twisted; caused by faulty valves within veins that allow the blood to flow backwards and to pool, causing even more enlargement of the veins.

Veins - blood vessels that return blood from the general circulation back to the heart.

Venous system - a network of veins that return blood from the circulation back to the heart.

Vertebra - one of a series of small bones forming the spinal column, made up of a body at the front and projections for articulation and muscle attachments at the back, with a hole through the middle where the spinal cord passes.

Vinculin - a protein that helps stabilise the cytoskeleton by binding integrin to actin.

Visceral fascia - a thin, fibrous membrane that envelops, suspends, binds and partitions organs and glands; it forms two layers, the visceral layer and the parietal layer, separated by a thin serous membrane.

Viscosity - a measure of a fluids resistance to deformation, which can vary from low in a freely flowing fluid such as water, to medium in a thick and sticky fluid such as honey, to high in the case of pitch, where the substance has a solid appearance.

Vitality - a state of being healthy, lively and energetic.

Wellbeing - having high levels of physical and mental health, emotional happiness.

Yoga - a system of physical, mental, and spiritual practice or discipline which originated in India; there are a range of schools but Hatha yoga, a system for controlling the body and the mind is the most popular.

Bibliography and References

1. Influence of posture on the range of axial rotation and coupled lateral flexion of the thoracic spine. J Manipulative Physiol Ther. 2007 Mar-Apr; 30(3):193-9.
http://www.ncbi.nlm.nih.gov/pubmed/17416273

2. Gray's Anatomy 36th edition Williams and Warwick

3. Aging Does Not Cause Stiffness: Stiffness Causes Aging
Jon Burras http://www.jonburras.com/pdfs/Aging-Does-Not-Cause-Stiffness.pdf

4. Why Stretching is Great For Older Adults
Margaret Richard http://seniorliving.about.com/od/exercisefitnes1/a/stretching.htm

5. Does stretching induce lasting increases in joint ROM? A systematic review.
Harvey L1, Herbert R, Crosbie J., School of Physiotherapy, University of Sydney, Australia.
Physiotherapy Research International. 2002 7(1):1-13. harveyl@doh.health.nsw.gov.au

6. Does stretching increase ankle dorsiflexion range of motion? A systematic review.
Radford JA1, Burns J, Buchbinder R, Landorf KB, Cook C. British Journal of Sports Medicine.
2006 Oct; 40(10):870-5.

School of Biomedical and Health Sciences, University of Western Sydney, Campbelltown,
Australia. j.radford@uws.edu.au

7. To stretch or not to stretch: the role of stretching in injury prevention and performance.
McHugh MP1, Cosgrave CH., Nicholas Institute of Sports Medicine and Athletic Trauma,
Lenox Hill Hospital, New York, USA. mchugh@nismat.org Scand J Med Sci Sports. 2010 Apr;
20(2):169-81. doi: 10.1111/j.1600-0838.2009.01058.x. Epub 2009 Dec 18.

8. Stretching and Flexibility - Everything you never wanted to know
Brad Appleton http://web.mit.edu/tkd/stretch/stretching_1.html

9. What Multitasking Does to Our Brains
Leo Widrich 26 June 2012
http://blog.bufferapp.com/what-multitasking-does-to-our-brains

10. Think You're Multitasking? Think Again
Jon Hamilton 2 October 2008
http://www.npr.org/templates/story/story.php?storyId=95256794

11. The Science Behind How We Learn New Skills
Thorin Klosowski
http://lifehacker.com/the-science-behind-how-we-learn-new-skills-908488422

12. Effect of Acute Dynamic and Static Stretching on Maximal Muscular Power in a Sample of
College Age Recreational Athletes
Murphy, Jeffrey Christopher (2008). Doctoral Dissertation, University of Pittsburgh. J Athl
Train. 2005 Apr-Jun; 40(2): 94–103. PMCID: PMC1150232

13. Acute Effects of Static and Proprioceptive Neuromuscular Facilitation Stretching on
Muscle Strength and Power Output

Sarah M Marek, Joel T Cramer, A. Louise Fincher, Laurie L Massey, Suzanne M
Dangelmaier, Sushmita Purkayastha, Kristi A Fitz, and Julie Y Culbertson

14. Does Static Stretching Reduce Maximal Muscle Performance?
Ian Shrier, MD, PhD, Malachy McHugh, PhD
Clinical Journal of Sport Medicine 2012; 22(5):450-451.
http://www.medscape.com/viewarticle/777155

15. Does Acute Static Stretching Reduce Muscle Power?
Journal of Physiotherapy & Sports Medicine Dec 2012 Volume 1, Issue 2

16. Acute Effects of Static, Dynamic, and Proprioceptive Neuromuscular Facilitation
Stretching on Muscle Power in Women
Manoel, Mateus; Harris-Love, Michael; Danoff, Jerome; Miller, Todd.
Journal of Strength & Conditioning Research:
September 2008 - Volume 22 - Issue 5 - pp 1528-1534

17. Duration Of Static Stretching Influences Muscle Force Production In Hamstring Muscles.
Ogura, Yuji; Miyahara, Yutetsu; Naito, Hisashi; Katamoto, Shizuo; Aoki, Junichiro
Journal of Strength & Conditioning Research August 2007

18. Does pre-exercise static stretching inhibit maximal muscular performance? A meta-
analytical review.
Simic L1, Sarabon N, Markovic G., Scand J Med Sci Sports. 2013 March

19. Application of Passive Stretch and Its Implications for Muscle Fibers
Patrick G De Deyne, PT, PhD, Assistant Professor, Departments of Orthopaedic Surgery,
Physiology, and Physical Therapy, University of Maryland School of Medicine, Baltimore, Md.

20. The influence of immobilization and stretch in protein turnover of rat skeletal muscle.
Goldspink G., J Physiol Jan 1977; 264: 267–282.

21. Changes in muscle mass and phenotype and the expression of autocrine and systemic
growth factors by muscle in response to stretch and overload.
Goldspink G., J Anat 1999; 194: 323–334.

22. Physiological and structural changes in the cat's soleus muscle due to immobilization at
different lengths by plaster casts.
J. C. Tabary, C. Tabary, C. Tardieu, G. Tardieu, and G. Goldspink.
J Physiol. Jul 1972; 224(1): 231–244.

23. The morphological basis of increased stiffness of rabbit tibialis anterior muscles during
surgical limb-lengthening.
Pamela Williams, Peter Kyberd, Hamish Simpson, John Kenwright, Geoffrey Goldspink
J Anat. Jul 1998; 193(Pt 1): 131–138.

24. Muscle Testing and Function.
Baltimore: Williams & Wilkins, 1993.
Kendall FP, McCreary EK, Provance PG:

25. Therapeutic Exercise for Body Alignment and Function.
Lucille Daniels MA and Catherine Worthingham Ph.D. Sep 1972
W.B. Saunders Company

26. Normative data for strength and flexibility of women throughout life.
Brown DA, Miller WC:. Eur J Appl Physiol 1998; 78: 77–82.

27. Exercising and elderly person
Brown M., Phys Ther Pract 1992; 1: 34–42.

28. Biomechanical role of lumbar spine ligaments in flexion and extension: determination
using a parallel linkage robot and a porcine model.
Gillespie KA1, Dickey JP.
Spine (Phila Pa 1976). 2004 Jun 1. http://www.ncbi.nlm.nih.gov/pubmed/15167660

29. US AMA Guides to the Evaluation of Permanent Impairment, 3rd edition (revised), copyright 1990 and adopted by the US Department of Consumer & Business Services. http://www.cbs.state.or.us/wcd/policy/bulletins/docconv_9557/2278.pdf

30. Physical Therapy. Merck Manual Professional. November 2005. http://www.merck.com/mmpe/sec22/ch336/ch336b.html

31. The Study of Joint Hypermobility and Q Angle in Female Football Players
H. Daneshmandi and F. Saki
Faculty of Physical Education and Sport Sciences, Guilan University. World Journal of Sport Sciences 3 (4): 243-247, 2010 ISSN 2078-4724 IDOSI Publications, 2010

32. Patterns of glenohumeral joint laxity and stiffness in healthy men and women
P. A Borsa., E. L. Sauers, and D. E. Herling.
Med. Sci. Sports Exerc., Vol. 32, No. 10, pp. 1685–1690, 2000.

33. Normal range of motion of joints in male subjects.
Boone DC, Azen SP.,
J Bone Joint Surg [Am]. 1979; 61:756-759.

34. Joint Structure and Function (3rd edition)
Pamela K. Levangie and Cynthia C. Norkin
(MacLennan & Petty)

35. Proprioceptive neuromuscular facilitation stretching: mechanisms and clinical implications.
Sharman MJ1, Cresswell AG, Riek S.
Sports Med. 2006;36(11):929-39.
Abstract: http://www.ncbi.nlm.nih.gov/pubmed/17052131

36. The effect of muscle energy technique on hamstring extensibility: the mechanism of altered flexibility.
Ballantyne. F., Fryer. G., McLaughlin. P. (2003).
Journal of Osteopathic Medicine. 6(2):59-63.

37. Principles of physiology (5th ed.).
Berne, R.M. & Levy, M.N. (1996).
Pub. Mosby.

38. Muscle Energy Techniques (2nd ed.).
Chaitow,L (2001).
Churchill: Livingston.

39. Greenman's principles of manual medicine (4th ed.).
DeStefano, L.A. (2011). Philadelphia:
Lippincott Williams & Wilkins.

40. Footwear Science, vol 1.
Taylor & Francis
Official Journal of the Footwear Biomechanics Group

42. Barefoot Lies - Funny Feet
Laura Spinney
New Scientist 24th January 2015

43. Strength Training by Children and Adolescents
AMERICAN ACADEMY OF PEDIATRICS, Committee on Sports Medicine and Fitness
http://pediatrics.aappublications.org/content/107/6/1470.full.pdf

44. Myofaction - Myofascial Manipulation
Rowland Benjamin D.O.

45. The Anatomy of the Achilles Tendon
Michael Benjamin, P. Theobald, D. Suzuki, and H. Toumi

46. Functional anatomy of the Achilles tendon
Mahmut Nedim Doral, Mahbub Alam, Murat Bozkurt, Egemen Turhan, Ozgu¨r Ahmet Atay,
Gu¨rhan Do¨nmez, Nicola Maffulli
Knee Surg Sports Traumatol Arthrosc (2010) 18:638–643. DOI 10.1007/s00167-010-1083-7

47. Stretch and Reach: The Unexaggerated Truth About Stretching
Kelle Walsh, Experience Life Magazine June 2008
https://experiencelife.com/article/stretch-and-reach-the-unexaggerated-truth-about-stretching/

48. Active fascial contractility: Fascia may be able to contract in a smooth muscle-like manner
and thereby influence musculoskeletal dynamics.
Schleip R, Klingler W, Lehmann-Horn F.
Med Hypotheses. 2005; 65 (2): 273-7. Department of Applied Physiology, Ulm University,
Albert-Einstein-Allee 11, 89069 Ulm, Germany.

49. Clinical Anatomy of the Lumbar Spine and Sacrum
Nikolai Bogduk, Elsevier Health Sciences, 2005

50. Changes in muscle fibre type, muscle mass and IGF-I gene expression in rabbit skeletal
muscle subjected to stretch.
Shiyu Yang, Majed Alnaqeeb, Hamish Simpson, and Geoffrey Goldspink
J Anat. Jun 1997; 190(Pt 4): 613–622.

51. Kinesiology - The Scientific Basis of Human Motion
Katharine F. Wells, PhD
Pubished by W.B. Saunders Company

52. Review of Gross Anatomy
Ben Pansky Ph.D.,M.D.
Macmillan Publishing Co., Inc.

53. The Physiology of the Joints
I.A. Kapandji
Churchill Livingstone Volume 1 - 3

Index

Cervical prevertebral muscles 259, 268-270, 292, 297, 337, 340, 524, 544-547, 781, 782.
Cervical spine 6, 8, 10, 11, 14, 16, 17, 22, 25, 31, 37, 38, 42, 45, 49, 53-71, 87-90, 94-96, 102-111, 128,129, 244-246, 249-253, 258-298, 336-341, 348-354, 355-376, 535, 543-555, 633-635, 653, 654, 668, 671, 672, 674, 675, 682, 686, 690, 694-720, 726, 730-736, 739, 743, 746-764, 769, 773, 774, 784, 785, 790, 792, 793.
Chronic 5, 19, 31, 33, 508, 536, 548, 668, 785, 794.
Circulation 2, 9, 10, 15, 34, 38 548, 718, 784, 785, 790, 795.
Circumduction 265, 266, 270, 785.
Close-packed position 23, 38, 497, 601, 785.
Coccyx 99, 196, 316, 566, 601, 605, 785.
Collagen 5, 12, 526-532, 535, 621, 784-787, 794, 795.
Collateral ligaments 7, 346, 452, 465, 474, 531, 590, 593, 595, 597, 617, 619-621, 625, 785.
Common peroneal nerve 247, 619.
Concentric contraction 27, 269, 293, 532, 534-536, 555, 671, 672, 681, 738, 739, 785.
Congenital 5, 15, 25, 28, 37, 252, 271, 294, 334, 338, 346, 353, 361, 407, 422, 425, 435, 474, 486, 489, 497, 551, 593, 785, 788.
Congruence 23, 38, 507, 584, 785.
Connective tissue 8, 10, 18, 39, 526-532, 534, 535, 537, 785-795.
Contraction 2, 10, 18, 20, 22-24, 30-32, 37-39, 45, 528, 530, 532, 533-537, 547, 555, 558, 560, 622, 776-782, 783-789, 791-795 plus multiple listings in parts A, B & C.
Contracture 26, 34, 785.
Coracobrachialis 143-147, 333, 382, 383, 399, 406, 407, 417-423, 434, 520, 521, 581, 586, 671, 672, 776.
Coronal 279, 299, 303, 315, 353, 452, 538, 568, 772, 773, 785, 788, 795.
Creep 26, 527, 536, 785, 790.
Crimp phase/ Crimping 9, 526, 527, 529, 530, 535, 786.
Cross-bridges 32, 45, 526, 532, 786.
Deep Fasciae 527, 529, 532, 540, 547, 551, 560, 563, 579, 582, 583, 586, 587, 591, 603, 605, 611, 615, 622-629, 786, 787.
Deltoid 144, 574, 575, 578, 581, 582-586, 641-643, 670-672, 716, 738, 739, 743, 748, 758, 776.
Deltoid ligament 625.
Deep peroneal nerve 247, 626, 627, 628.
Depression (psychoemotional) 7, 36, 786.
Depression (anatomical) 556, 568, 580, 619, 680, 770, 771, 786.
Developmental stretch 19, 29, 30, 32, 39, 724, 786.
Dopamine 7, 786.
Dorsal scapular nerve 552, 572, 573.
Dorsal tunnels of wrist 598.
Dowager hump 7, 13, 283, 284-286, 298, 322, 338, 358, 786.
Dynamic stretching 15, 23, 24, 32, 34, 35, 41, 44, 45, 531, 786.
Dystrophin 532, 786.
Eccentric contraction 27, 256, 268, 270, 292, 343, 532, 534-536, 555, 671, 672, 681, 738, 739, 786.
Ectomorph 3, 4, 784, 786.
Ehlers-Danlos syndrome 5, 786,
Elastic barrier 6, 18, 32, 33, 37, 48, 680, 786, 787, 791, 792.
Elastic phase 526, 527, 529, 786, 792.
Elastic / Elasticity 3-10, 15, 18, 23, 24, 32, 33-41, 45, 48, 526, 528, 530-537, 568, 570, 623, 786, 787.
Elastin 5, 12, 526-529, 532, 786.
Elbow 585-593, 597, 643, 644, 662, 663, 671-675, 684-764, 771, 774, 778, 784, 795.
Elbow collateral ligaments 7, 590, 593.
Electromyography (EMG) 787.
End-feel 20, 787.
Endomorph 3, 4, 784, 787.
Endorphins 2, 7, 787.
Erector spinae 10, 37, 41, 72-80, 249-253, 258-261, 262-267, 275-291, 299-354, 373-376, 535, 550, 551, 556-562, 601, 635-639, 670, 671, 716, 722, 732, 738, 743, 748, 750, 754, 758, 781, 782.
Extensor carpi radialis brevis (wrist) 115, 154, 155, 157, 367-372, 436-439, 597, 673, 716, 743, 778, 779.
Extensor carpi radialis longus (wrist) 115, 154, 155, 157, 367-372, 436-439, 596, 597, 673, 716, 743, 778, 779.
Extensor carpi ulnaris (wrist) 115, 154, 155, 156, 367-372, 436-439, 594, 596, 673, 716, 743, 778, 779.
Extensor digitorum brevis (toes) 509-515, 628, 673, 778, 779.
Extensor digitorum communis (fingers) 116, 370, 438, 597, 673, 778, 779.
Extensor digitorum longus (toes) 233, 234, 238, 363, 364, 479, 507, 509-515, 626, 627, 781.
Extensor hallucis brevis (big toe) 233, 234, 238, 509-515.
Extensor hallucis longus (big toe) 233, 234, 238, 363, 364, 479, 507, 509-515, 626, 627, 781.

Hip 4, 8, 9, 12, 14, 15, 21, 25, 29-31, 38, 164-224, 239-242, 535, 601, 600-613, 619, 638, 645-650, 664-666, 670, 671, 682, 700, 738, 743, 772, 775, 779, 780, 788.

Homeostasis 8, 788.

Hormones 2, 6, 529, 788.

Hydration 23, 529, 530, 788.

Hyoid muscles 542, 546, 547, 675, 781.

Hyperextension 6, 12, 554, 771, 772, 788, 789.

Hypermobile 5, 6, 8, 16, 19, 20, 21, 25, 28, 33-35, 38-40, 44, 46, 48, 568, 593, 771, 772, 788.

Hypermobility 3, 5, 6, 9, 12, 18, 20, 21, 25, 27, 35, 37, 40-42, 48, 88, 568, 668, 786, 788-790, 792.

Hypertonic 34, 535, 580, 605, 609, 626, 628, 789.

Hypertrophy 11, 789.

Hypomobility 9, 18-21, 25, 27, 39, 42, 48, 568, 789.

Hypothenar eminence 149, 246, 598, 599.

Ilium / Iliac 14, 16, 134, 221-224, 550, 555, 558, 562, 563, 566-568, 600-604, 606, 608, 613-616, 793.

Iliacus 164, 165, 248, 221-224, 248, 600, 601, 607, 645, 670, 732, 738, 732, 748, 779, 780.

Iliocostalis cervicis 65, 550, 556, 557.

Iliocostalis thoracis and lumborum 556, 557, 782.

Intercostal nerves 562, 563, 565.

Iliotibial tract 531, 601, 602, 605, 614, 764.

Immune system 2, 789, 790.

Inferior gluteal nerve 602.

Inferior hyoid muscles 546, 547, 675, 781, 782.

Infraspinatus 36, 574, 575, 642, 671, 672, 716, 738, 758, 776.

Inguinal ligament 248, 562-565, 605.

Internal abdominal oblique muscles 535, 564, 565, 652, 670-672, 675, 716, 722, 738, 743, 748, 750, 754, 758, 773, 786.

Internal intercostal muscles 562, 563, 579, 580, 635, 636, 675.

Interspinous ligament 551, 565, 570, 773.

Intervertebral disc 9, 11, 12, 15, 23, 26, 34, 526, 554, 555, 568, 569, 570, 600, 668, 773, 783, 785, 787, 789, 794.

Intervertebral foramina 13, 789.

Ischial tuberosity 15, 29, 60, 213, 221-224, 247, 566, 607, 608, 610, 611, 616, 618, 750, 789.

Isometric contraction 14, 19, 20, 27, 37, 45, 532, 535-537, 789, 792 plus multiple listings in parts A - C.

Isotonic contraction 27, 532, 536, 671, 680, 681, 785, 786, 789.

Joint capsule 12, 13, 26, 32, 34, 526, 528, 577, 586, 603, 613, 614, 620, 622,

Joint degeneration/disease 2, 8, 10, 15, 21, 22, 25-28, 33, 34, 39, 569, 668, 706, 750, 751, 789, 792.

Joint fusion 39, 40, 568, 569, 783, 789.

Joint stability / instability 3-5, 12, 17, 18, 22, 38, 39, 48, 528, 533, 567, 568, 584, 614, 615, 622, 668, 786-790, 794.

Joint movement / mobility 2-6, 9, 11, 12, 15, 17-23, 25, 26, 28, 29, 32-35, 38-40, 43-46, 48, 87, 88, 526, 527, 530-533, 535-537, 542, 552, 554, 555, 560, 566-570, 584, 593, 594, 599, 613, 621, 654-667, 680, 681, 774, 775, 776-782, 789.

Joint stiffness 7, 8, 9, 19, 20, 23, 32, 33, 34, 39, 41, 48, 668, 783, 785, 786, 789, 793.

Joints 4-26, 30-48, 570 also see individual joints by name in parts A and B.

Knee collateral ligaments 7, 12, 19, 38, 617, 785.

Knee hyperextension (Genu recurvatum) 5, 12, 772, 788, 789.

Knee joint 5, 666, 667, 670, 671, 682-768, 772, 775, 780, 789, 792.

Knock knees (Genu valgum) 12,

Kyphosis 6, 7, 9, 11-17, 41, 42, 47, 568, 569, 783, 786, 788, 789, 790, 793.

Laminin 532, 789.

Lateral flexion 554, 789.

Latissimus dorsi 37, 80, 86, 126, 185, 535, 561, 563, 575-577, 586, 636, 640, 671, 672, 700, 722, 738, 754, 758, 777.

Levator scapulae 7, 10, 31, 41, 56, 64, 66, 68, 69, 535, 548, 551, 552, 571, 572, 634, 635, 716, 743, 777, 781, 782.

Lever / Leverage 13, 20, 23, 34, 35, 37, 39, 45, 48, 102-105, 222, 229, 234, 235, 534, 535, 789.

Lifestyle 2-4, 7-12, 15, 16, 18, 26, 40, 46, 48, 568, 569, 789.

Ligament laxity 6, 7, 10, 18, 20, 27, 34, 37, 48, 568, 790, 792.

Ligament sprain 3, 5, 7, 12, 568, 628, 783, 790.

Ligaments 2-14, 18-23, 26-28, 31, 34, 35, 37-41, 44, 48, 526-531, 539, 550, 551, 553, 554, 556, 559, 560-568, 570-572, 578, 590, 592-595, 597-601, 603, 605, 609, 613, 615, 617-621, 624, 625, 627, 628, 630, 651, 668, 669, 680, 681, 754, 758, 767, 772, 773, 783, 784-790, 792-794.

Linear 526, 527, 790, 792.

Load / Loading 9, 13, 25, 26, 31, 43, 45, 526, 527, 529-531, 535, 536, 552, 569, 572, 668, 785-792.

Loeys-Dietz syndrome 5, 790.

Long thoracic nerve 581.

Longissimus capitis 543, 557, 782.

Patella 614, 615, 620, 792.

Pectineus 609, 610, 612, 743, 779, 780.

Pectoral nerve 579, 580.

Pectoralis major 10, 31, 41, 110, 119-126, 535, 578, 579, 580, 586, 639, 640, 661, 662, 670, 671, 672, 675, 700, 716, 738, 739, 743, 748, 776, 777.

Pectoralis minor 10, 41, 110, 119-126, 134, 579, 580, 639, 640, 641, 659, 671, 743, 777.

Peroneus brevis and longus 230, 535, 627, 628, 630, 651, 667, 781.

Peroneus tendons 627-630.

Pes cavus 12, 792.

Pes planus 5, 12, 631, 792.

Phasic muscles 533, 535, 792.

Physiological barrier 32, 33, 783, 792, 794.

Piriformis 167, 175, 239, 247, 535, 603, 606, 607, 609, 645, 646, 652, 739, 779, 780.

Plantar aponeurosis 626, 629-631, 669.

Plantar flexion 12, 204, 223, 233, 237, 622, 624-627, 649, 651, 652, 667, 781, 792.

Plastic phase 527, 530, 536, 792.

Poor posture 7, 12, 13, 16, 41, 536, 668, 716, 786, 792, 793.

Popliteus 216, 217, 226, 617, 619, 620, 650, 738, 780.

Posterior cervical muscles 13, 41, 56, 57, 543, 549, 551, 555, 633, 654, 716, 743, 750.

Posterior compartment 622, 623, 625.

Posterior sacroiliac ligament 550, 556, 559, 566-568, 600, 793.

Posterior head posture or posterior translation 61, 62, 71, 87, 142, 258-261, 275-290, 773, 782, 792.

Post-isometric stretching 3, 19, 24, 28, 31, 37, 45 537, 792 plus multiple listings in parts A and B.

Post-synaptic 537, 793.

Postural fatigue 2, 5, 16, 29, 33, 573, 668, 669, 716, 743, 750, 793.

Posture 2, 7, 9, 10-18, 20, 22, 24, 26, 27, 36, 40-42, 45-48, 54, 64, 99, 140, 530, 535, 536, 562, 580, 605, 612, 613, 668, 675, 706, 708, 716, 732, 743, 750, 754, 783, 785, 786, 791-793, 796.

Prevertebral muscles (cervical) 544-546, 781, 782.

Primary scoliosis 10, 14, 36, 793, 794.

Pronator teres 152, 153, 244, 588, 590, 595, 596, 643, 663, 716, 778.

Proprioception 530, 793.

Proprioceptive neuromuscular facilitation (PNF) stretching 24, 793.

Protein 5, 526, 528, 529, 531, 532, 536, 783, 786, 787, 790, 791, 795.

Psoas major 31, 41, 164-166, 248, 535, 600, 601, 645, 664, 670-672, 716, 732, 738, 743, 746, 750, 754, 758, 760, 779, 780, 782.

Psoriatic arthritis 25, 793.

Psychoemotional 15, 27, 48, 668, 793, 795.

Quadratus femoris 606, 608, 609, 779, 780.

Quadratus lumborum 37, 80, 185, 186, 535, 560, 561, 635, 636, 647, 672, 782.

Quadriceps 31, 203-208, 602, 605, 614, 615, 620, 648, 649, 670, 671, 706, 722, 738-741, 748, 754, 758, 764, 780.

Quadriceps tendon 615, 620.

Quadrupedalism 27, 793.

Race 4, 793.

Radial nerve 245, 586, 589, 590, 596, 597.

Range of movement (ROM) 2-6, 9-11, 15-20, 22-27, 29, 32-34, 38, 40, 41, 45, 48, 537, 552, 554, 569, 584, 680, 681, 769, 773 793.

Reciprocal inhibition 19, 35, 37, 536, 783, 789, 793.

Rectus abdominis 243, 535, 562-564, 672, 732, 746, 758, 782.

Rectus capitis anterior and lateralis 65, 546, 633-635, 654.

Rectus capitis posterior major and minor 65, 543, 633-635, 654.

Rectus femoris 37, 535, 614, 615, 672, 738, 739, 772, 779, 780.

Refractory period 37, 537, 792, 793.

Repetitive strain injury (RSI) 45, 791-793.

Reversed kyphosis 41, 568, 793.

Reversed lordosis 13, 41, 568, 793.

Rheumatoid arthritis 18, 25, 27, 568, 793.

Rhomboid major and minor 10, 41, 535, 550, 562, 571, 573, 671, 672, 716, 743, 750, 777.

Rotation stretches for spine 45, 60, 65, 67-70, 90, 102-109, 555, 558, 560, 569, 634, 638, 639, 654, 656.

Rotator cuff tendon tears 31, 38, 583, 669, 750, 767, 793.

Rounded shoulders 7, 793.

Sacral torsion 555, 793.

Sacroiliac joints 4, 10, 12, 15, 30, 38, 40, 555, 566, 567, 568, 570, 600, 606, 609, 770, 793.

Sacrospinous and sacrotuberous ligaments 556, 565, 566, 601, 605, 617, 618.

Safe stretching 3, 6, 30, 36, 37, 535, 569, 793.

Sartorius 226, 248, 605, 611, 614-616, 618, 672, 738-740, 780.

Scalene / Scalenus 10, 41, 61, 62, 64, 65, 548, 572, 675, 716, 743, 781, 782.
Scarring 9, 18, 23, 33, 34, 787, 794.
Sciatic nerve 247, 609, 611, 619.
Scoliosis 10-17, 36, 42, 47, 118, 555, 568, 790, 793, 794.
Secondary scoliosis 794.
Semimembranosus and semitendinosus 165, 209-214, 218, 224, 226, 239, 481-487, 490-498, 516-518, 615-620, 649-651, 664, 779, 780.
Semispinalis capitis and cervicis 65, 543, 550, 558, 781, 782.
Semispinalis thoracis 550, 557, 558, 782.
Sensory receptor 24, 536, 537, 788, 791, 793, 794.
Sensory (neural) adaption 47.
Serratus anterior 563, 571, 579-581, 671, 672, 748, 777.
Sidebending stretches 26, 37, 42, 61-70, 72-80, 83, 89, 117, 118, 558, 560-562, 569, 634-636, 769.
Skin 9, 10, 23, 528, 529, 599, 611, 631, 655, 656, 783, 785, 787, 788, 790, 793, 794, 795.
Sliding filament theory 32, 532, 533, 553, 621, 794.
Slow-twitch fibres 533, 535, 794, 795.
Soft tissue 29, 32, 783, 790, 791, 794.
Soleus 225, 229-232, 533, 535, 622, 624, 651, 670, 682, 716, 738, 739, 743, 748, 758, 764, 781.
Somafeedback 45, 794.
Spasm 15, 34, 631, 668, 791, 794.
Spasmodic / Spastic torticollis 537, 794.
Spasticity 18, 34.
Spinal motion 794.
Spinalis capitis, cervicis and thoracis 65, 556-558, 782.
Splenius capitis and cervicis 65, 549, 550, 557, 782, 781.
Spondylolisthesis 25, 26, 38, 789, 792, 794.
Sprain 3, 5, 7, 8, 12, 22, 28, 30, 35, 38, 40, 568, 628, 783, 790, 794.
Stabiliser or fixator muscles 555, 573, 574, 582, 681, 684, 686, 688, 690, 708, 748, 764, 794.
Stability 3-5, 7, 12, 17-19, 22, 23, 32, 38, 40, 44, 46, 48, 528, 533, 584, 614, 615, 622, 786-790, 794.
Stamina 2, 43, 44, 794.
Static stretching 31, 32, 44, 45, 531, 535, 792, 794, 794.
Sternocleidomastoid 62, 70, 535, 543, 547, 548, 550, 557, 571, 635, 675, 716, 743, 781, 782.
Stretch reflex / Myotatic reflex 23, 24, 31, 35, 45, 536, 537, 794.
Subacromial bursitis 38, 573, 795.
Subcutaneous layer 529, 626, 631, 795.
Suboccipital muscles 37, 38, 41, 543-546, 555, 569, 633-635, 716, 743, 769, 781, 782.
Subscapular nerve 576, 577.
Subscapularis 535, 577, 578, 641, 671, 658, 776.
Superficial fascia 529, 547, 562, 563, 579, 583, 625, 795.
Superficial peroneal nerve 247, 627.
Superior gluteal nerve 603, 604, 605.
Superior hyoid muscles 546, 675, 781, 782.
Supinator 151, 245, 716, 778.
Suprascapular nerve 573, 574.
Supraspinatus 573, 574, 669, 670, 716, 738, 739, 750, 758, 776, 793, 795.
Supraspinous ligament 773.
Synergist muscles 551, 556, 560-562, 565, 570-572, 670, 795.
Synovial fluid 7, 9, 23, 25, 26, 38, 570, 789, 795.
Synovial membrane 9, 18, 567, 586, 595, 596, 598, 620, 624, 627, 628, 789, 795.
Talin 532, 795.
Temporalis 540, 633, 769.
Temporomandibular joint 14, 540-542, 769, 787, 795.
Tendinitis 5, 795.
Tendons 2, 18, 23, 26, 44, 526-530, 532, 534-537, 764, 767, 784, 785-788, 790, 793, 795.
Tennis elbow strain 31, 795.
Tension 2, 7, 15, 18, 19, 22-24, 26, 29, 30, 32, 36-38, 40, 41, 45, 529, 532, 535-537, 668, 675, 771, 772, 783, 785, 786, 788, 789, 791, 792, 794, 795.
Tensor fasciae latae 181, 183, 185-187, 226, 604, 605, 646, 647, 672, 764, 780.
Teres major 36, 575-577, 670, 672, 716, 748, 776.
Teres minor 36, 574, 575, 671, 672, 738, 758, 776.
Thenar eminence 244, 594, 598.
Theoretical considerations 2.
Thoracolumbar 10, 13, 16, 17, 21, 38, 42, 73, 80, 83, 95, 551, 557, 558, 560, 561, 564, 565, 569, 576, 635, 636, 638, 655, 656, 658, 666, 674, 692, 708, 716, 758, 760, 773, 788, 794.
Tibial nerve 247, 619, 620, 622, 624, 625.
Tibialis anterior 203, 226, 233, 535, 626, 627, 648, 649, 651, 652, 671, 716, 738, 743, 781.
Tibialis posterior 230, 623-625, 630, 650, 651, 670, 781.